Angiography/ Scintigraphy

Symposium of the European Association of Radiology
Mainz 1—3 October, 1970

Edited by

L. Diethelm

With 262 Figures

Springer-Verlag Berlin · Heidelberg · New York 1972

EUROPEAN ASSOCIATION OF RADIOLOGY

Honorary President: Prof. B. RAJEWSKY, Frankfurt
President: Prof. J. C. VON RONNEN, Leiden
Secretary General: Prof. CH. GROS, Strasbourg

German Organizing Comittee

Joint Presidents:

Prof. H. POPPE
Chairman of the Deutsche Röntgengesellschaft

Prof. H. HUNDESHAGEN
Chairman of the Gesellschaft für Nuclearmedizin

Executive Committee

Chairman: Prof. W. FROMMHOLD

Secretary General: Prof. L. DIETHELM

Treasurer: Dr. med. habil. WEISSWANGE

Secretary: Prof. J. P. HAAS

Prof. A. DÜX
Prof. U. FEINE
Prof. H. HUNDESHAGEN
Med.-Dir. Dr. A. JAKOB
Prof. H. OESER
Prof. H. W. PABST
Prof. H. POPPE
Prof. W. RÜBE
Prof. E. SCHERER
Prof. H.-ST. STENDER
Prof. F. E. STIEVE
Prof. P. THURN
Prof. K. H. VAN DE WEYER
Frau WEISSWANGE
Prof. K. ZUM WINKEL
Prof. R. WOLF

Programme Committee

Prof. L. DIETHELM

Scientific Exhibition

Prof. K. H. VAN DE WEYER

Social Programme

Frau WEISSWANGE

ISBN 3-540- 05804-4 Springer-Verlag Berlin Heidelberg NewYork
ISBN 0-387- 05804-4 Springer-Verlag NewYork Heidelberg Berlin

Foreword

The symposium on Angiography/Scintigraphy brought to Mainz in the fall of 1970 not only many European colleagues with an interest in these techniques, but also a number of visitors from overseas. These busy, work-filled days are beginning to fade in the memory of those who were there. Nevertheless, the scientific results reported on that occasion still supply the guidelines for what is currently being done in radiology and nuclear medicine.

Anyone who has kept abreast of the literature over the past few years will have noted with some surprise how comparisons of the results obtained with these two important diagnostic aids continue to provoke controversy. One thing is certain: the emblem chosen for the Mainz symposium could hardly have been more appropriate. Like two cogwheels meshing in some complex piece of machinery, these radiological procedures demand the highest level of skill and precision before they will function properly on engaging so as to produce optimal results. Their findings complement each other in almost ideal fashion.

Even though development in these two diagnostic disciplines has not exactly stood still since 1970, the papers given at this symposium established the fundamentals from which have stemmed many an intelligent adaptation of a method, many a cunning modification of an instrument and, not least, many a new research lead. This is why we applaud the initiative of Professor Diethelm of Mainz, whose brainchild this symposium was, in making the proceedings available to a wider audience.

On 16th December, 1972, the European Association of Radiology celebrates its tenth anniversary. When, following the proposal of Professor Boris Rajewsky, President of the Ninth International Congress of Radiology held in Munich in 1959, the national societies amalgamated in order to lend more weight to European radiology, it was hardly predictable that the AER symposia would rival the European Congresses in importance. After Montreux and Strasbourg, the Ossium Symposium in London in 1968 was enthusiastically received, above all by clinicians whose concern is with diagnosis and therapy, while the 1969 Brussels meeting impressed the experts with its debate on the use of computers in radiology. Professor Diethelm, with the keen eye of the radiologist experienced in both research and teaching, recognized the topicality and future importance of achieving close correlation between angiographic procedures and the methods of localization afforded by nuclear medicine. Thus, the Mainz symposium was yet another peak in what may already be termed the tradition of AER working meetings. May the reports presented in this book speed the dynamic progress of the radiologic specialty!

Moreover, may the symbolism of the frictionless meshing of the cogwheels remind us that what is needed is nothing less than full and frank cooperation, based on mutual respect and recognition, between the various disciplines of medicine.

Tübingen, August 1972 W. Frommhold

Contents

Space-Occupying Intracranial Lesions

HÜNIG, R. WELLAUER, J.: Angiography and Scintigraphy in the Preoperative Diagnosis of Intracranial Tumors . . . 1
KLAUS, E., KUBA, J., SEVČÍK, M.: Gegenüberstellung der Angiographie und Hirnszintigraphie in der Diagnostik von intrakraniellen raumfordernden Prozessen 15
VAN ECK, J. H. M., PENNING, L.: Isotope Encephalography and Cerebral Angiography in the Diagnosis of Brain Lesions . . . 18
AKERMAN, M., HERTZOG, E., ZILBERBERG, CH., KOUTOULIDIS, C.: L'imprégnation des tumeurs cérébrales. Etude artériographique, scintigraphique et angioscintigraphique au pertechnétate de ^{99m}Technétium de 100 tumeurs opérées . . . 23
GALLI, G., SIMONE, F., TRONCONE, L., DE ROSSI, G.: La détection des metastases intracraniennes par scintigraphie et gammacisternographie . . . 31
SCHMIDT-WITTKAMP, E., PIEPGRAS, U., OHLMANN, F.: The Value of Diagnostic Procedures in Brain Tumor Identification . . . 41
ZEIDLER, U., KOTTKE, S., SEEBERG, A., HUNDESHAGEN, H.: Vergleichende Untersuchungen zur Aussagekraft verschiedener szintigraphischer Untersuchungsverfahren und der Angiographie in der Hirntumorlokalisationsdiagnostik . . . 43
WALDBAUR, H., WALTER, W., KRÖNERT, E., WOLF, F.: The Value of Brain Scintigraphy (Technetium-99m) in the Topographic Diagnosis of Space-Occupying Intracranial Lesions . . . 45
NORDMAN, E., REKONEN, A.: ^{75}Se-Scintigraphy in Differential Diagnosis of Benign and Malign Cerebral Processes . . . 49
SANGUINETI, M., SCOPINARO, G., GOTTLIEB, A., DAMIANI, S. GROSSI, G.: Differential Scintigraphic Diagnosis of Focal Brain Lesions . . . 51
ASKIENAZY, S., DI PAOLA, R., CONSTANT, J. P., CHOTKIEWICZ, J. P., SCHLIENGER, M.: Apport d'une technique de double marquage dans le diagnostic differentiel des lésions cérébrales . . . 60
LAUSBERG, G., SCHEPELMANN, F., GELETNEKY, C. L.: Die Bedeutung des Abklingfaktors bei Untersuchung mit ^{203}Hg (Chlormerodrin) . . . 62
HEILMANN, H. P., FEINE, U., FISCHBACH, U.: Differenzierung hirnszintigraphischer Befunde durch RIHSA-Szintigramm . . . 63
BÖCK, F., BRENNER, H., BERGMANN, H., HÖFER, R.: Nuklearmedizinische Differentialdiagnostik der Hirntumoren. Angioszintigraphie und a.v.-Shuntbestimmung . . 66
HINCK, V. C., JUDKINS, M. P.: Femorocerebral Angiography: A New Technic Using Preformed Ducor Catheters . . . 70

Cerebral Vascular Lesions

GÖKAY, H.: Optic Atrophy Due to Intracranial Aneurysms . . . 73
LOKEN, M. K., GOLD, L.: Radioisotopic Evaluation of Cerebral Vascular Lesions 77
BÜCHELER, E., KÄUFER, C.: The Determination of Cerebral Death by Cerebral Angiography . . . 84
DEISENHAMMER, E., HAMMER, B.: Correlation of Angiography and Angioscintigraphy in Diffuse Cerebral Vascular Lesions . . . 87

ARNAIZ BUENO, F., CARRILLO YAGÜE, R., CHAMORRO ROMERO, J. L., ORTIZ BERROCAL, J.: Application of the Anger Camera in the Evaluation of the Permeability of Pudenz Valves. Evaluation of a New Method 89
KLAUSBERGER, E. M.: The Use of Angiokinematography in Diseases and Closures of Cerebral Vessels 96
WALDBAUR, H., WALTER, W., WOLF, F., SCHIEFER, W.: The Value of Brain Scintigraphy (Technetium-99m) in the Differential and Follow-Up of Cases of Cerebro-Vascular Disease 97
HACKER, H.: Zur Differentialdiagnose früh abführender Venen im Carotisangiogramm 99
SALOMON, G., GIUTICELLI, G., CASTAN, P., MITARD, D.: Opacification des veines de l'orbite au cours de l'angiographie carotidienne externe 100

Pathological Processes of the Spinal Canal

DJINDJIAN, R.: L'artériographie médullaire étude clinique 101
HERSCHAFT, H., GLEIM, F.: The Significance of the Magnetic-Tape Recording of Myelographies with Duroliopaque for the Diagnosis of Small Space-Narrowing Processes in the Cervico-Thoracic Region of the Spinal Canal 104
VOGELSANG, H.: Space Occupying Processes of the Spinal Canal and Their Diagnosis through Intraosseous Spinal Venography 115
PIEPGRAS, U., VOETS, P.: Diagnosis by Scanning in Pathological Processes of the Spinal Canal (Intravenous Myelo-Scanning) 117
ZEITLER, E.: Möglichkeiten und Grenzen der Rückenmarkszintigraphie 121
OTTO, H., SAUER, J., FIEBACH, O., BETTAG, W.: A Comparison of Myeloscintography, Myelography and Discography in Detection of Spinal Block Lesions 127

Thyroid Lesions

WELLMANN, H. N., MACK, J. F., SAENGER, E. L., GOLDSMITH, R. E., SODD, V. J.: A Study of the Parameters Influecing the Clinical Use of Iodine-123 129
FEINE, U., SCHMIDT, H., HOFFMANN, K.: Die kombinierte Angio- und Szintigraphie in der Schilddrüsendiagnostik 138
ROSSI, P.: Thyroid Angiography 141

Pulmonary Vascular Lesions

RANNIGER, K.: Comparison of Pulmonary Arteriography with Lung Scintigraphy in the Diagnosis of Pulmonary Emboli 144
WELLMAN, H. N., MACK, J. F., ROMHILT, D. W., HOLMES, J. C., GANDEL, P., SPI Z, H. B., FENTON, J. C.: Scintigraphy in Screening Pulmonary Emboli-Prospective Comparison with Angiography 146
NÄGELE, E., LASCH, H. G., WICK, E., GREBE, S., NOLTE, D., SCHOEN, U.: Radiographic Angiographic and Scintigraphic Findings after Relapsing Pulmonary Embolism 154
BORY, M., DUMON, J. F., DJIANE, P., SERRADIMIGNI, A.: Indications respectives de la scintigraphie et de l'angiographie dans l'embolie pulmonaire 156
SCHRÖDER, H., PLECHL, S. CH.: Über den quantitativen Nachweis von Durchblutungsstörungen der Lungen, über deren Ursache und Ausmaß bei Patienten mit einer cavernösen Siliko-Tuberkulose 162
FELIX, R., VAN DE WEYER, H. J., ASSHEUER, J., BÜCHELER, E., H., WINKLER, C.: Analysis of the Function of the Pulmonary Vascular System 163
FERNHOLZ, H.-J., DIHLMANN, W.: Semiquantitative and Planimetric Investigations of Pulmonary Scintiscans for the Estimation of Functional Disturbances of Lungs after Lymphography 170
KOPPENHAGEN, K., ERNST, H., MEINHOLD, H., PAEPRER, H., LIEBENSCHÜTZ, H. W.: Perfusionslungenszintigraphie bei primär vasculärer pulmonaler Hypertonie . . . 172

Novak, D., Frenzel, H., Wieners, H.: Angiography and Scintiscanning in Preoperative Assessment of Congenital and Acquired Lung Diseases 174
Pauwels, R., Schelstraete, K., Verhaeghe, L., Tasson, J., Kunnen, M., van Vaerenbergh, M., Barbier, F.: Comperative Study of the Pulmonary Perfusion as Determined by Different Scintigraphic Techniques and by Angiography . . 181
Greco, S., Beritelli, F., Loreto, C., Cotroneo, G. B., Tafuri, G.: Selective catheterization of the Bronchial Arteries and Their Diagnostic and Therapeutic Use 183
Loken, M. K.: Evaluation of Pulmonary Function and Blood Flow Using 133-Xenon and a Scintillation (Anger) Camera 187

Diseases Pulmonary and Mediastinum

Ježek, V., Vančura, J., Teichmann, Vl., Kolář, J., Ort, J.: Angiographic and Scintigraphic Evaluation of the Circulation in Patients with Bronchial Cancer 194
Bollaert, A., Schockert, J., Yernault, J. C., Payfa, M., de Costre, Ph., Ermans, A. M., de Coster, A.: Comparasion de l'angiographie et de la scintigraphie en pathologie pulmonaire 196
Kaneko, M.: A Radio-Isotope Approach in the Diagnosis of Lung Cancer 204
Staib, I., Maroske, D., Würdinger, H.: Lungenszintigraphische Funktionskontrolle im Vergleich zu Röntgenuntersuchungen nach Thoraxtraumen 207
Reschke, H.: Selective Arteriography of Tumours and First Experiences with Angioscintigraphy of the Mediastinum 209

Diseases of the Liver

Winkler, C., Düx, A., Bücheler, E.: Vergleichende vasographische und szintigraphische Untersuchungen zum Nachweis von Lebertumoren 213
Raschke, E.: A Comparison of Angiographic and Scintigraphic Examinations of the Liver and the Results of Histology 226
Bischof-Delaloye, A., Delaloye, B.: Diagnose primärer und sekundärer Lebertumoren 227
Rahmouni, Dj.: Scintigraphie et angiographie dans le diagnostic du kyste hydatique du foie 231
Rossi, P., Gould, H. R.: Comparative Study of Angiography and Scanning in Deseases of the Liver 232
Höfer, R.: Angiographische und szintigraphische Untersuchungen der Abdominalorgane 233
Freemann, L. M.: Combined Angiographic and Scintigraphic Investigations of the Liver 236
Claus, H. G., Haas, J. P.: Zur Angiographie-Szintigtaphie im Abdominalraum . . 237
Imhof, H., Jantsch, Ch., Kratochwill, A., Pokieser, H., Umek, H.: Comperative Studies on the Informational Value of Angiography, Scintigraphy and Ultrasonic Scanning in Hepatic Disorders 241
Kaneko, M.: Pharmacoangiography by Intra-arterial Injection of Nor-adrenalin . . 244
Sasaki, T.: Comparative Study of Angiography and Scintigraphy in the Diagnosis of Liver Disease 249
Steckenmesser, R., Bayindir, S., Heger, N., Grebe, S. F.: Angiography and Comparative Scintigraphic Findings in Space-occupying Lesions of the Liver 251
Wood, E. J., Tavill, A. S., Kreel, L.: Hepatic Scintigraphy and Venography in the Budd-Chiari-Syndrome 253
Beduhn, D., Kampmann, H.: Vergleichende angio- und szintigraphische Untersuchungen beim experimentellen Verschlußikterus 258
Alfidi, R. J.: A Comparison of Isotope Scanning and Angiography in the Diagnosis of Liver Disease 263
Hupe, K., Maroske, D., Dombrowski, H., Joseph, K.: Hepatic Scan and Arteriogram in the Preoperative Diagnosis of Circumscribed Liver Diseases 265
Wenz, W., Wawersik, J.: Diagnostische Wertigkeit der abdominalen Arteriographie 267

Diseases of the Spleen

HENNIG, K., FRANKE, W.-G., PLATZBECKER, H.: Szintigraphische und angiographische Milzdiagnostik. Ein Vergleich bei Hämoblastosen 269
FISCHER, J.: Möglichkeiten und Grenzen der Milzszintigraphie 280
GOULD, H. R., ROSSI, P.: Comparative Study of Angiography and Scanning in Diseases of the Spleen 283
BURAGGI, G. L., RINGHINI, R., RODARI, A.: Anwendungsmöglichkeiten von Radioisotopen mit kurzer Halbwertszeit in der Milzszintigraphie 286

Diseases of the Pancreas

CEN, M., FERNHOLZ, H.-J.: Combined Angiographic and Scintigraphic Examination of the Pancreas 287
HUNDESHAGEN, H., CREUTZIG, H., DOPSLAFF, H.: Doppelradionuklid Pankreas-Funktionsszintigraphie mit einem Prozeßrechner 289
RODRIGUEZ-ANTUNEZ, A., ALFIDI, R. J.: Pancreatic Scanning in Clinical Practice and its Comparison with Splanching Angiography 299
GROS, CH., WARTER, P., VERGNES, R., TRUCHOT, M., TONGIO, J., HAEHNEL, P.: Resultats comparés de la scintigraphie et de l'artériographie pancréatique 302
BESSLER, W., JUCKER, A.: Angioscintigraphy of the Pancreas 304
VAN DE WEYER, K. H., CLAUSEN, C., HECKRODT, J.: Perfusionsangioszintigraphie in der Diagnostik von Erkrankungen der Bauchspeicheldrüse 308
PREVOT JR., H.: Kombination von Szintigraphie und Angiographie in der radiologischen Pankreasdiagnostik 312
SCHERER, H., MUTZENBACH, P., MAURER, P., SCHOLZE, H.: The Endocrine Disorder of the Pancreas and Its Comparative Investigations Between Clinical, Angiographical and Operative Findings 320
RIUS CHORNET, J. M.: El tronco celiaco y la mesenerica superior en las pancreatitis cronica 324
MADSEN, B.: Angiographic Localisation of Insulomas 325
DEINIGER, H. K., HEUCK, F.: The Scintigraphy of the Panceras 326

Tumours of Stomach and Colon

WÓJTOWICZ, J.: Angiographic Diagnosis and Evaluation of the Extent of Tumours of the Stomach and Colon 329

Adrenal-Lesions

RESCHKE, H.: Adrenal Angiography 332
VAN DE WEYER, K. H.: Angioszintigraphie der Nebennieren 336

Retroperitoneal-Tumours

BÜCHELER, E.: Angiographical Examination of the Retroperitoneal Space 341
HEGER, N., BAYINDIR, S., STECKENMESSER, R., GREBE, S. F.: Die angiographische Darstellung primärer Retroperitonealtumoren 348
DIETHELM, L.: Angioszintigraphie der retroperitonealen Tumoren 352

Disease of the Kidney

RODRIGUEZ-ANTUNEZ, A.: Assessment of Function in the Transplanted Kidney with ^{133}I Hippuran 356
VARGHA, G., KELEMEN, J., MILTÉNYI, L., SZÜCS, L.: Vx2-Carcinoma as a Tumor Model Induced in the Stomach and Kidney of Rabbits. Pharmacoangiographical Examinations 358
KELEMEN, J., KELENTEY, B., KÉKI, M., VARGHA, G.: Investigations in Connection with the Effect of the Alpha and Beta Stimuli and Blocking Agents of the Sympathetic Nervous System on the Evolution of Renal Angiograms 370

Frik, W., Cen, M.: Intraarterial Pressure During Pharmacoangiography 380
Kaneko, M.: Renal Glomerulography in the Diagnosis of Renal Tumor 383
Schmidt, H.: Außergewöhnliche radiologische Befunde bei Nierentumoren 385
Shida, H., Ohara, I.: Evaluation of Peripheral Circulation by Angioscintigraphy 386
zum Winkel, K., Sonderkamp, H.-M., Jost, H., Marx, F., Hermann, H.-J.: Angiography and Scintigraphy of the Kidney 387
Freeman, L. A.: Rapid Sequential Renal Blood Flow Scintigraphy 392
Hör, G., Buttermann, G., Heinze, H. G., Klein, U., Langhammer, H., Müller-Fassbender, H., Pabst, H. W.: Selective Angioszintigraphy and Angiography in Kidney Diseases 393
Haas, J. P., Claus, H. G.: Ergebnisse der renalen Angio-Szintigraphie 397
Vogler, E.: Ergebnisse der Radiologischen Untersuchungen bei vaskulären Nierenerkrankungen 402
Ludin, H.: Die klinische Bedeutung der Weite und Konfiguration der Nierenarterien 406
Stephan, G., Zimmer, R.: Comparison of Angiographic and Scintigraphic Findings in Localized and Generalized Alterations of the Renal Arteries 408
Laubenberger, Th., Oberhausen, G.: Angiography and Scintigraphy of Inflammatory Renal 411
Wieners, H., Novak, D.: Comparison of Angiographic and Scintigraphic Findings in Unilateral Renal Lesions Accompanied by Hypertension 413
Habighorst, L. V., Schmidt, K. J.: Comparative Angiographic and Scintigraphic Studies in Chronic Renal Disease 417
Nuic, M., Wagner, H. H.: Comparing Scintigraphic and Angiographic Tests with Peripheral Renal Processes 420
Fuchs, F. S., Ogris, E., Olbert, F.: Comparative Angiographic and Isotope Studies of the Kidneys 426
Kempe, H., Pfannenstiel, P., Hoffmann, G., Weissleder, H.: Vergleichende szintigraphische und angiographische Untersuchungen der Nieren 434
Pfeifer, K. J., Frey, K. W., Heinze, H. G., Klein, U., Müller-Fassbender, H., Langhammer, H.: Comparison of the Diagnostic Value of Renal Scan and Angiography (Together with I. V. P. and Isotope Nephron) 436
Anatkov, J., Kumanov, Chr.: Selective Nephrophlebography 438
Catalano, D.: The Role of Angiography in the Detection of Polycystic Renal Disease and Associated Aneurysm of the Splenic Artery 444

List of Contributors

Akerman, M., Dr., Unité de Neurophysiologie Chirurgicale – I. N. S. E. R. M. Laboratoire des Radio-Isotopes, Hopital Foch, F-92 Suresnes

Alfidi, R. J., M. D., Director, Hospital Radiology Department, The Cleveland Clinic, Cleveland, Ohio 44106/USA

Anatkov, J., Dr., Oberass. am Lehrstuhl für Röntgenologie und Radiologie der Medizinischen Fakultät, Bd. Georgi Sofijski 1, Sofia 31/Bulgarien

Arnaiz Bueno, F., Dr., Centro nacional de Investigationes medico-quirurgicas de la seguridad social. Clinica Puerta de Hierro, Nuklearmedizinische Abteilung, San Martin de Porres 4, Madrid 20/Spanien

Askienazy, S., Dr., Laboratoire des isotopes du centre neurochirurgical, Hôpital Sainte-Anne, 1 Rue Cabanis, Paris XIV/France

Assheuer, J., Dr., Nuklearmedizinische Abteilung der Universität D-5300 Bonn-Venusberg

Barbier, F., Prof. Dr., Dienst voor Inwendige Ziekten, Akademisch Ziekenhuis, University of Ghent, B-9000 Gent, De Pintelaan 135

Bayindir, S., Prof. Dr., Leiter der Röntgenabteilung der Chirurg. Universitätsklinik und Poliklinik, D-6300 Gießen, Klinikstr. 37

Beduhn, D., Priv.-Doz. Dr., Chirurg. Universitätsklinik, Röntgenabteilung, D-6900 Heidelberg, Kirschnerstr. 1

Bergmann, H., Dr., II. Medizinische Klinik der Universität Wien, A-1000 Wien, Garnisonsgasse 13

Beritelli, F., Dr., Università di Catania, Instituto di Radiologica Medica, Ospedale Garibaldi, I-95123 Catania

Bessler, W., Dr., Chefarzt des Röntgeninstituts des Kantonspitals Winterthur, CH-8400 Winterthur

Bettag, W., Prof. Dr. med., Neurochirurg. Klinik des Klinikum Essen, D-4300 Essen, Hufelandstr. 55

Bischof-Delaloye, A., Dr., Département de Médecine Nucléaire, CHUV, CH-1011 Lausanne

Böck, F., Dr., Neurochirurgische Klinik der Universität Wien, A-1000 Wien, Garnisonsgasse 13

Bollaert, A., Dr., Chef de service de radiodiagnostic de l'Hôpital Universitaire Saint Pierre, Université Libre de Bruxelles, B-1000 Bruxelles, Rue Haute 322

Bory, M., Dr., Clinique medicale, Hôpital de la Timone, Boulevard d'Ales, F-13 Marseille

Brenner, H., Doz. Dr., Neurochirurgische Klinik der Universität Wien, A-1000 Wien, Garnisonsgasse 13

Bücheler, E., Prof. Dr., Radiologische Klinik der Universität Bonn, D-5300 Bonn-Venusberg

Burragi, G. L., Prof. Dr., Direttore, Laboratorio Radioisotopi dell'Instituto Nazionale Tumori, V. Venezian 1, I-20133 Milano

Buttermann, G., Dr., Nuklearmedizinische Klinik und Poliklinik rechts der Isar der TU München, D-8000 München 80, Ismaningerstr. 22

Carrillo, Yagüe, R., Dr., Centro nacional de investigationes medico-quirurgicas de la seguridad social. Clinica Puerta de Hierro, Nuklearmedizinische Abteilung, Madrid/Spanien

Castan, P., Dr., Hôpital de la Timone, F-13 Marseille 5e

Catalano, D., Prof. Dott., Radiological Department, Ospedale S. Gennaro, Via Constantinopoli 84, I-80138 Napoli

Cen, M., Prof. Dr., Abteilung Radiologie der Med. Fakultät an der Rhein.-Westf. TH Aachen, D-5100 Aachen, Goethestr. 27–29

Chamorro Romero, J., Dr., Centro nacional de investigationes medico-quirurgicas de la seguridad social. Clinica Puerta de Hierro, Nuklearmedizinische Abteilung, Madrid/Spanien

Chodkiewicz, J. P., Dr., Laboratoire des isotopes de centre neurochirurgical, Hôpital Sainte-Anne, 1 Rue Cabanis, Paris XIV/France

Claus, H. G., Professor Dr., Chefarzt der Röntgenabteilung der Städt. Krankenhausanstalten, D-5630 Remscheid

Clausen, C., Dr., Institut für klinische Strahlenkunde der Universität D-6500 Mainz, Langenbeckstr. 1

Constant, J. P., Dr., Laboratoire des isotopes du centre neurochirurgal, Hôpital Sainte-Anne, 1 Rue Cabanis, Paris XIV/France

Coster, A. De, Dr., Department des Voies Respiratoires de l'Hôpital Universitaire Saint Pierre, Université Libre de Bruxelles, B-1000 Bruxelles, Rue Haute 322

Costre, Ph. De, Dr., Service de radiodiagnostic de l'Hôpital Universitaire Saint Pierre, Université Libre de Bruxelles, B-1000 Bruxelles, Rue Haute 322

Cotroneo, G. B., Dr., Università di Catania, Instituto di Radiologica, Medica, Ospedale Garibaldi, I-95123 Catania

Creutzig, H., Dr., Institut für Nuklearmedizin, Department Radiologie der Medizinischen Hochschule Hannover, D-3000 Hannover, Roderbruchstr. 101

Damiani, S., Dr., Ospedali Galliera di Genova, Servizio di Radiodiagnostica, Via A. Volta 8, I-16128 Genova

Deininger, H. K., Dr. Oberarzt, Zentral-Röntgeninstitut im Katharinenhospital der Stadt D-7000 Stuttgart 1, Kriegsbergstr. 60

Deisenhammer, E., Dr., Wagner-Jauregg-Krankenhaus des Landes Oberösterreich, A-4024 Linz, Wagner-Jauregg-Weg 15

Delaloye, B., Dr., Département de Médecine Nucléaire, CHUV CH-1011 Lausanne

Diethelm, L., Prof. Dr., Direktor des Instituts für Klinische Strahlenkunde der Universitäts-Kliniken Mainz, D-6500 Mainz, Langenbeckstr. 1

Dihlmann, W., Prof. Dr., Abteilung Radiologie der Medizinischen Fakultät an der Rhein.-Westf. TH Aachen, D-5100 Aachen, Goethestr. 27–28

Djiane, P., Dr., Clinique medicale, Hôpital de la Timone, Boulevard d'Ales, F-13 Marseille

Djindjian, R., Dr. Prof., agrégé, Rue de l'Université 16, Paris 7ième, France

Dombrowski, H., Priv.-Doz. Dr., Universitätsklinik, D-3550 Marburg/Lahn

Dopslaff, H., Institut für Nuklearmedizin, Department Radiologie der Medizinischen Hochschule Hannover, D-3000 Hannover, Roderbruchstr. 101

Düx A., Prof. Dr., Röntgeninstitut des Krankenhauses Maria Hilf, D-4050 Mönchen-Gladbach

Dumon, J. F., Clinique medicale, Hôpital de la Timone, Boulevard d'Ales, F-13 Marseille

Eck, J. H. M. van, M. D., University Hospital of Groningen, Department of Neuroradiology, Groningen/The Netherlands

Ermans, A., Dr., Service des Radioisotopes de l'Hôpital Universitaire Saint Pierre, Université Libre de Bruxelles, B-1000 Bruxelles, Rue Haute 322

Ernst, H., Prof. Dr., Strahlenklinik und -institut der FU Berlin im Klinikum Steglitz, D-1000 Berlin 45, Hindenburgdamm 30

Feine, U., Dr. med., Prof., Oberarzt des Medizinischen Strahleninstituts, Nuklearmedizinische Abteilung der Universität, D-7400 Tübingen, Röntgenweg 11

Felix, R., Priv.-Doz. Dr., Radiologische Klinik der Universität D-5300 Bonn-Venusberg

Fenton, J. C., M. D., Cardise Research Laboratories Department of Medicine, Cincinnati General Hospital, Cincinnati, Ohio 45229/USA

Fernholz, H.-J., Priv.-Doz. Dr., Abteilung Radiologie der Medizinischen Fakultät an der Rhein.-Westf. TH Aachen, D-5100 Aachen, Goethestr. 27–28

Fiebach, O., Dr., Röntgeninstitut und Strahlenklinik des Klinikum Essen, D-4300 Essen, Hufelandstr. 55

Fischbach, U., Dr., Medizinisches Strahleninstitut, Universität Tübingen, D-7400 Tübingen, Röntgenweg 11

Fischer, J., Prof. Dr., I. Medizinische Klinik der Universität, D-6500 Mainz, Langenbeckstraße 1

Franke, W.-G., Dr., Oberarzt der Nuklearmedizinischen Abteilung der Medizinischen Akademie „Carl Gustav Carus“, DDR-8019 Dresden, Fetscher Str. 74

Freeman, L. A., M. D., Department of Radiology, Albert Einstein College of Medicine, Bronx, New York, N.Y. 10461/USA

Frenzel, H., Prof. Dr., I. med. Universitätsklinik, D-2000 Hamburg 20, Martinistr. 52

Frey, K. W., Prof. Dr., Klinik und Poliklinik für Radiologie der Universität München, D-8000 München 2, Ziemsenstr. 1

Frik, W., Prof. Dr., Vorstand der Abteilung Radiologie der Med. Fakultät an der Rhein.-Westf. TH Aachen. D-5100 Aachen, Goethestr. 27–29

Fuchs, F. S., Dr., Urologische Abteilung des Krankenhauses der Stadt Wien-Lainz, A-1130 Wien, Wolkersbergenstr. 1

Galli, G., Prof. Dr., Università Cattolica S. Cuore, Istituto di Radiologia, I-Roma

Gandel, P., M. D., Cardise Research Laboratories Department of Medicine, Cincinnati General Hospital, Cincinnati, Ohio 45229/USA

Geletneky, C. L., Dr., Neurochirurg. Universitätsklinik, D-6300 Gießen, Klinikstr. 37

Gleim, F., Dr., Neurologische Klinik, Krankenhaus Nordwest, D-6000 Frankfurt/Main 90, Steinbacher Hohl 2–26

Gökay, H., M. D., Prof. of Neurosurgery, Istanbul University, Fakulty of Medicine, Çopa, Istanbul/Turkey

Gold, L., M. D., Assist. Prof., Department of Radiology University of Minnesota-Hospital, MN 55455/USA

Goldsmith, R. E., M. D., Radioisotope Laboratory, Cincinnati General Hospital of the University of Cincinnati, Cincinnati, Ohio 45229/USA

Gottlieb, A., Dr., Ospedali Galliera di Genova, Divisione Neurochirurgica, Via A. Volta 8, I-16128 Genova

Gould, H. R., M. D., St. Vincent's Hospital and Medical Center of New York, Depart. of Radiology, 153 West 11th Street, New York, N.Y. 10011/USA

Grebe, S. F., Prof. Dr., Leiter der Nuklearmedizinischen Abteilung der Medizinischen Kliniken und Polikliniken, D-6300 Gießen, Klinikstr. 37

Greco, S., Prof., Università di Catania, Instituto di Radiologica Medica, Ospedale Garibaldi, I-95123 Catania

Gros, Ch., Prof. Dr., Directeur de Service Central de Radiologie, Hôpital Civil, F-67 Strasbourg

Grossi, G., Dr., Ospedali Galliera di Genova, Divisione Neurochirurgica, Via A. Volta 8, I-16128 Genova

Guidicelli, G., Dr., Hôpital de la Timone, F-13 Marseille 5e

Haas, J. P., Prof. Dr., Institut für Klinische Strahlenkunde der Universitätsklinik, D-6500 Mainz, Langenbeckstr. 1

Habighorst, L. V., Prof. Dr., Institut für Klinische Strahlenkunde der Johannes Gutenberg-Universität, D-6500 Mainz, Langenbeckstr. 1

Hacker, H., Dr., Neurochirurg. Universitätsklinik, D-6000 Frankfurt-Niederrad, Schleusenweg 2–16

Haehnel, P., Dr., Service Central de Radiologie, Hôpital Civil, F-67 Strasbourg

Hammer, B., Dr., Wagner-Jauregg-Krankenhaus des Landes Oberösterreich, A-4024 Linz, Wagner-Jauregg-Weg 15

Heckrodt, J., Dr., Institut für Klinische Strahlenkunde der Universität, D-6500 Mainz, Langenbeckstr. 1

Heger, N., Dr. med., Röntgenabteilung der Chirurg. Universitätsklinik und Poliklinik D-6300 Gießen, Klinikstr. 37

Heilmann, H. P., Dr. med., Medizinisches Strahleninstitut Universität Tübingen, D-7400 Tübingen, Röntgenweg 11

Heinze, H. G., Priv.-Doz. Dr., Klinik und Poliklinik für Radiologie der Universität München, D-8000 München 2, Ziemssenstr. 1

Hennig, K., Prof. Dr. sc. med., Leiter der Nuklearmedizinischen Abteilung der Medizinischen Akademie „Carl Gustav Carus", DDR-8019 Dresden, Fetscher Str. 74

Hermann, H.-J., Dr., Universitäts-Strahleninstitut des Klinikums Westend, D-1000 Berlin 19, Spandauer Damm 130

Herrschaft, H., Dr., Neurologische Klinik, Krankenhaus Nordwest, D-6000 Frankfurt/Main 90, Steinbacher Hohl 2–26

Hertzog, E., Dr., Département de Neuro-Radiologie Hôpital Foch, F-92 Suresnes

Heuck, F., Prof. Dr., Direktor des Zentral-Röntgeninstituts im Katharinenhospital der Stadt, D-7000 Stuttgart 1, Kriegsbergstr. 60

Hinck, V. C., M. D., Prof. and Head, Division of diagnostic radiology, University of Wisconsin, Medical Center, 1300 University Avenue, Madison, Wisconsin 53706/USA

Höfer, R., Prof. Dr., II. Medizinische Klinik der Universität Wien, 1000-Wien, Garnisongasse 13

Hör, G., P. D., Dr., Nuklearmedizinische Klinik und Poliklinik rechts der Isar der TU München, D-8000 München 80, Ismaningerstr. 22

Hoffmann, G., Prof. Dr., Leiter der Abteilung für klinische Nuklearmedizin der Medizinischen Universitätsklinik, D-7800 Freiburg/Br.

Hoffmann, K., Dr., Nuklearmedizinische Abteilung des Medizinischen Strahleninstituts der Universität Tübingen, D-7400 Tübingen, Röntgenweg 11

Holmes, J. C., M. D., Cardise Research Laboratories, Department of Medicine, Cincinnati General Hospital, Cincinnati, Ohio 45229/USA

Hünig, R., M. D., Department of Radiology of the University of Basel, Bürgerspital, CH-4000 Basel

Hundeshagen, H., Prof. Dr., Institut für Nuklearmedizin und spezielle Biophysik, Department Radiologie, Medizinische Hochschule Hannover, 3 Hannover, Roderbruchstr. 101

Hupe, K., Prof. Dr., Chirurg. Universitätsklinik, D-3550 Marburg/Lahn

Imhof, H., Dr., I. Medizinische Universitätsklinik, A-1090 Wien, Spitalgasse 23

Jantsch, Ch., Dr., I. Medizinische Universitätsklinik, A-1090 Wien, Spitalgasse 23

Ježek, V., Dr., Radiologische Klinik FVL UK, Faculty of General Medecine, Charles University, Unemocnice 2, Praha 2/ČSSR

Joseph, K., Priv.-Doz. Dr., Chirurg. Universitätsklinik, D-3550 Marburg/Lahn

Jost, H., Dr. (Frau), Universitäts-Strahleninstitut des Klinikums Westend, D-1000 Berlin 19, Spandauer Damm 130

Jucker, A., Dr., Röntgeninstitut des Kantonspitals Winterthur, CH-8400 Winterthur

Judkins, M. P., M. D., Loma Linda University School of Medecine, Loma Linda, Calif./USA

Käufer, C., Doz. Dr., Radiologische Klinik der Universität Bonn, D-5300 Bonn-Venusberg

KAMPMANN, H., Dr., Chirurg. Universitätsklinik, Röntgenabteilung, D-6900 Heidelberg, Kirschnerstr. 1

KANEKO, M., M. D., Department of Radiology, Nagoya University Branch Hospital, Higashi-ku, Nagoya/Japan

KÉKI, M., M. D., Department of Radiology, University of Medicine, Debrecen, Hungary

KELEMEN, J., M. D., Department of Radiology, University of Medicine Debrecen, Hungary

KELENTEY, B., M. D., Institute of Pharmacology, University of Medicine Debrecen, Hungary

KEMPE, H., Dr., Abteilung für klinische Nuklearmedizin der Medizinischen Universitätsklinik, D-7800 Freiburg/Br.

KLAUS, E., Priv.-Doz. Dr., Neurologische Klinik der Palacký-Universität, Olmouc, ČSSR

KLAUSBERGER, E. M., Univ.-Doz., Dr., Leiter der Neuroradiologischen Abteilung der Psychiatrisch-Neurologischen Universitätsklinik Wien, A-1000 Wien

KLEIN, U., Dr., Klinik und Poliklinik für Radiologie der Universität München, D-8000 München 2, Ziemssenstr. 1

KOLÁR, J., Dr., Radiologische Klinik FVL UK, Faculty of General Medicine, Charles University, Unemocnice 2, Praha 2/ČSSR

KOPPENHAGEN, K., Dr., Strahlenklinik und -institut der FU Berlin im Klinikum Steglitz, D-1000 Berlin 45, Hindenburgdamm 30

KOTTKE, S., Dr., Neurologische Klinik, Department Psychologische und Neurologische Medizin, Medizinische Hochschule Hannover, D-3000 Hannover, Haltenhofsstraße 48

KOUTOULIDIS, C., Dr., Laboratoire des Radio-Isotopes, Hôpital Foch, F-92, Suresnes

KRATOCHWIL. A., Dr., II. Univ.-Frauenklinik, A-1090 Wien, Spitalgasse 23

KREEL, L., M. Z., M. R. C. P., F. F. R., Clinical Research Centre, Northwich Park Hospital, Harrow, Middlesex U.K.

KRÖNERT, E., Dr., Medizinische Klinik der Universität Erlangen-Nürnberg, D-8520 Erlangen, Krankenhausstr. 12

KUBA, J., Dr., Abteilung für Nuklearmedizin des Fakultätskrankenhauses, Olmouc, ČSSR

KUMANOV, CHR., Dr., Abteilung für Röntgenologie und Radiologie der Medizinischen Fakultät, Bd. Georgi, Sofijski 1, Sofia 31/Bulgarien

KUNNEN, M., Dr., Dienst voor Radiologie, Akademisch Ziekenhuis, University of Ghent, B-9000 Gent, De Pintelaan 135

LANGHAMMER, H., Dr., Nuklearmedizinische Klinik und Poliklinik rechts der Isar der TU München, D-8000 München 80, Ismaningerstr. 22

LASCH, H. G., Prof. Dr., Direktor in den Medizinischen Kliniken und Polikliniken der Universität Gießen, D-6300 Gießen, Klinikstr. 32

LAUBENBERGER, T., Prof. Dr., Chef des Strahleninstitutes des Stadtkrankenhauses, D-6450 Hanau

LAUSBERG, G., Prof. Dr., Neurochirurg. Universitätsklinik D-6300 Gießen, Klinikstr. 37

LIEBENSCHÜTZ, H. W., Klinikum Westend der FU Berlin, D-1000 Berlin 19, Spandauer Damm 130

LOKEN, M. K., M. D., Ph. D. Direktor, Division of Nuclear Medicine Department of Radiology, University of Minnesota Hospitals, Minneapolis Minnesota 55455/USA

LORETO, C., Dr., Università di Catania, Instituto di Radiologica Medica, Ospedale Garibaldi, I-95123 Catania

LUDIN, H., Prof. Dr., c/o Verwaltung, Kantonsspital Bruderholz, CH-4101 Bruderholz BL

MACK, J. F., M. D., Bureau of Radiological Health, Nuclear Medicine Laboratory, Cincinnati General Hospital of the University of Cincinnati, Cincinnati, Ohio 45229/USA

MADSEN, B., M. D., Dept. of Radiology, Komunchospitalet, DK-8000 Århus c.

MAROSKE, D., Dr., Chirurg. Universitätsklinik, D-3550 Marburg/L.

MARX, F., Prof. Dr., Universitäts-Strahleninstitut des Klinikums Westend, D-1000 Berlin 19, Spandauer Damm 130

MAURER, P., Dr., Chirurg. Klinik des Klinikums rechts der Isar der TU München, D-8000 München 80, Ismaningerstr. 22

MEINHOLD, H., Dr., Nuklearmed. Abt. im Klinikum Steglitz der FU, D-1000 Berlin 45, Hindenburgdamm 30

MILTÉNYI, L., M. D., Department of Radiology, University of Medicine Debrecen, Hungary

MITARD, D., Dr., Hôpital de la Timone, F-13, Marseille 5^{e}

MÜLLER-FASSBENDER, H., Dr., Klinik und Poliklinik für Radiologie der Universität, D-8000 München 2, Ziemssenstr. 1

MUTZENBACH, P., Dr., Institut für Röntgendiagmostik des Klinikums rechts der Isar der TU München, D-8000 München 80, Ismaningerstr. 22

NÄGELE, E., Prof. Dr., Radiologische Abteilung des Krankenhauses D-7630 Lahr, Klosterstraße 19

NOLTE, D. Dr., Medizinische Kliniken und Polikliniken der Universität Gießen, D-6300 Gießen, Klinikstr. 32

NORDMAN, E., Dr., Department of Radiotherapy, Central Hospital, Jyväskylä/Finnland

NOVAK, D., Doz. Dr., Radiologische Universitätsklinik und Strahleninstitut, D-2000 Hamburg 20, Martinistr. 52

NUIC, M., Dr., Institut für Nuklearmedizin und spez. Biophysik des Radiologischen Zentrums der Medizinischen Hochschule Hannover, D-3000 Hannover, Roderbruchstr. 101

OBERHAUSEN, G., Prof. Dr., Biophysikalisches Institut der Universität des Saarlandes, D-6650 Homburg/Saar

OGRIS, E., Dr., Isotopenlabor d. Sonderabt. für Strahlentherapie des Krankenhauses der Stadt Wien-Lainz, A-1130 Wien, Wolkersbergenstr. 1

OHARA, I., M. D., Department of Second Surgery Tohoku University School of Medicine, Sendai/Japan

OHLMANN, F., M. D., Department of Neuroradiology of the Clinic for Nervous and Mental Diseases of the University of the Saarland, D-6650 Homburg/Saar, Germany

OLBERT, F., Dr., Angiologisches Institut d. I. Chirurg. Abt. des Krankenhauses der Stadt Wien-Lainz, A-1130 Wien, Wolkersbergenstr. 1

ORT, J., Dr., Radiologische Klinik FVL UK, Faculty of General Medicine, Charles University, Unemocnice 2, Praha 2/ČSSR

ORTIZ BERROCAL, J., Dr., Direktor der Nuklearmedizinischen Abteilung, Centro nacional de investigaciones medico-quirurgicas de la seguridad social. Clinica Puerta de Hierro, Madrid/Spanien

OTTO, H., Dr., Neurochirurgische Klinik des Klinikum Essen, D-4300 Esssen, Hufelandstraße 55

PABST, H. W. Prof. Dr., Nuklearmedizinische Klinik und Poliklinik rechts der Isaar der TU München, D-8000 München 80, Ismaningerstr. 22

PAEPRER, H., Prof. Dr., Klinikum Westend der FU Berlin, D-1000 Berlin 19, Spandauer Damm 130

PAOLA, R., Di Dr., Laboratoire des isotopes du centre neurochirurgical, Hôpital Saint-Anne, 1 Rue Cabanis, Paris XIV/France

PAUWELS, R., Dr., Dienst voor Inwendige Ziekten, Akademisch Ziekenhuis, University of Ghent, B-9000 Gent, De Pintelaan 135

PAYFA, M., Dr., Service de radiodiagnostic de l'Hôpital Universitaire Saint Pierre, Université Libre de Bruxelles, B-1000 Bruxelles, Rue Haute 322

PENNING, L., M. D., University Hospital of Groningen, Department of Neuroradiology, Groningen/The Netherlands

PFANNENSTIEL, P., Dr., Abteilung für klinische Nuklearmedizin der Medizinischen Universitätsklinik, D-7800 Freiburg/Br.

Pfeiffer, K. J., Dr. med., Klinik und Poliklinik für Radiologie der Universität München, D-8000 München 2, Ziemssenstr. 1

Piepgras, U., Prof. Dr., Abteilung für Neuroradiologie an der Universitäts-Nervenklinik, D-6650 Homburg/Saar

Platzbecker, H., Dr., Oberarzt der Radiologischen Klinik der Medizinischen Akademie „Carl Gustav Carus", DDR-8019 Dresden, Fetscher Str. 74

Plechl, S. Ch., Dr., Krankenanstalten „Bergmannsheil", D-4630 Bochum

Pokieser, H., Dr., I. Medizinische Universitätsklinik, A-1090 Wien, Spitalgasse 23

Prévôt, H., Priv.-Doz. Dr., Kurfürstenklinik, Bremen, D-2800 Bremen, Sonnebergerstr. 3

Rahmouni, Dj., Dr., Hospital Ait-Idir, Université d'Alger, Alger (Algerien)

Raschke, E., Prof., Chirurg. Universitätsklinik und Poliklinik, D-5300 Bonn-Venusberg

Ranniger, K., Prof. Dr., Department of Radiology, The University of Chicago, 950 East 59th Street Chicago, Illinois 60637 USA

Rekonen, A., M. Sc., Department of Radiotherapy, Central Hospital, Jyväskylä/Finnland

Reschke, H., Prof. Dr., Städt. Krankenhaus, Strahleninstitut, D-8070 Ingolstadt

Ringhini, R., Per. Radiochimico, Laboratorio Radioisotopi dell'Instituto Nazionale Tumori, V. Venezian 1, I-20133 Milano

Rius Chornet, J. M., Dr., Residencia General de la Ciudad Sanitaria de la Seguridad Social, Sectión de Angioradiologica, Barcelona/Spanien

Rodari, A., Dr., Assistente, Laboratorio Radioisotopi dell'Instituto Nazionale Tumori, V. Venezian 1, I-20133 Milano

Rodriguez-Antunes, A., M. D., Director of the Department of Radiation Therapy and Nuclear Medicine, The Cleveland Clinic Foundation, 2020 East 93rd Street, Cleveland, Ohio 44106/USA

Romhilt, D., W., M. D., Cardise Research Laboratories, Department of Medicine, Cincinnati General Hospital, Cincinnati, Ohio 45229/USA

Rossi, G., de, Dr., Università Cattolica S. Cuore, Instituto di Radiologia, I-Roma

Rossi, P., M. D., Chief, Cardiovascular Roentgenology, St. Vincents's Hospital and Medical Center of New York, Depart. of Radiology, 153 West 11th Street, New York, N.Y. 10011/USA

Saenger, E. L., M. D., Radioisotope Laboratory, Cincinnati General Hospital of the University of Cincinnati, Cincinnati, Ohio 45229/USA

Salomon, , G., Prof., Hôpital de la Timone, F-13 Marseille 5e

Sanguineti, M., Prof., Ospedali Galliera di Genova, Servizio di Medicina Nucleare, Via A. Volta 8, I-16128 Genova

Sasaki, T., M. D., Ass. Prof. of Radiology, Nagoya University School of Medicine, 65 Tsurumai-cho, Showa-ku, Nagoya 466/Japan

Sauer, J., Dr., Röntgeninstitut und Strahlenklinik des Klinikum Essen, D-4300 Essen, Hufelandstr. 55

Schelstraete, K., Dr., Dienst voor Nucleaire Geneeskunde, Akademisch Ziekenhuis, University of Ghent, B-9000 Gent, De Pintelaan 135

Schepelmann, F., Dr., Neurochirurg. Universitätsklinik, D-6300 Gießen, Klinikstr. 37

Scherer, H., Priv.-Doz. Dr., Oberarzt Chirurgische Klinik des Klinikums rechts der Isar der TU München, D-8000 München80, Ismaningerstr. 22

Schiefer, W., Prof. Dr., Neurochirurg. Klinik der Universität Erlangen-Nürnberg, D-8520 Erlangen, Krankenhausstr. 12

Schlienger, M., Dr., Laboratoire des isotopes du centre neurochirurgicale, Hôpital Sainte-Anne, 1 Rue Cabanis, Paris XIV/France

Schmidt, H., Prof. Dr. med., Chefarzt der Röntgendiagnostischen Abteilung des Allgemeinen Krankenhauses Altona, D-2000 Hamburg-Altona

SCHMIDT, H., Dr. med., Chefarzt des Radiologischen Instituts des Städt. Krankenhauses, D-7530 Pforzheim

SCHMIDT, K. J., Dr., Kreiskrankenhaus, Radiolog. Abteilung, D-7988 Wangen/Allgäu

SCHMIDT-WITTKAMP, E., M. D., Department of Radiology of the Clinic St. Elisabeth, D-6630, Saarlouis

SCHOCKERT, J., Dr., Service de radiodiagnostic de l'Hôpital Universitaire Saint Pierre, Université Libre de Bruxelles, B-1000 Bruxelles, Rue Haute 322

SCHOEN, U., Dr., Patholog. Inst. I der Universität Gießen, D-6300 Gießen, Klinikstr. 32g

SCHOLZE, H., Dr., Chirurg. Klinik des Klinikums rechts der Isar der TU München, D-8000 München 80, Ismaningerstr. 22

SCHRÖDER, H., Dr. med., Stadtkrankenhaus, D-8940 Memmingen

SCOPINARO, G., Dr., Ospdeali Galliera di Genova, Servizio di Medicina Nucleare, Via A. Volta 8, I-16128 Genova

SEEBERG, A., Dr., Neurologische Klinik, Department Psychologische und Neurologische Medizin, Medizinische Hochschule Hannover, D-3000 Hannover, Haltenhoffstr. 48

SERRADIMIGNI, A., Dr., Clinique medicale, Hôpital de la Timone, Boulevard d'Ales, F-13 Marseille

ŠEVČIK, M., Dr., Neurologische Klinik der Palacký-Universität, Olmouc/ČSSR

SHIDA, H., M. D., Dept. of Radiology, The Mito National Hospital, Mito-Ibaragiken/Japan

SIMONE, F., Dr., Università Cattolica S. Cuore, Istituto di Clinica delle Malattie Nervose e Mentali, Roma/Italia

SODD, V. J., Ph. D., Bureau of Radiological Health, Nuclear Medicine Laboratory, Cincinnati General Hospital of the University of Cincinnati, Cincinnati, Ohio 45229/USA

SONDERKAMP, H.-M., Dr., Universitäts-Strahleninstitut des Klinikums Westend, D-1000 Berlin 19, Spandauer Damm 130

SPITZ, H. B., M. D., Cardise Research Laboratories, Department of Medicine, Cincinnati General Hospital, Cincinnati, Ohio 45299/USA

STAIB, I., Prof. Dr., Chirurg. Universitätsklinik, D-7800 Freiburg/Br.

STECKENMESSER, R., Dr., Röntgenabteilung der Chirurg. Universitätsklinik und Poliklinik, D-6300 Gießen, Klinikstr. 37

STEPHAN, G., Priv.-Doz., Dr., Radiologische Universitätsklinik und Strahleninstitut, D-2000 Hamburg-Eppendorf, Martinistr. 52

SZÜCS, L., M. D., Institute of Pathology University of Medicine Debrecen, Hungary

TAFURI, G., Dr., Università di Catania, Instituto di Radiologica Medica, Ospedale Garibaldi, I-95123 Catania

TASSON, J., Dr., Dienst voor Inwendige Ziekten, Akademisch Ziekenhuis, University of Ghent, B-9000 Gent, De Pintelaan 135

TAVILL, A. S., M. D., M. R. C. P., Dept. of Medicine, The Royal Free Hospital, Gray's Inn Road, London, W.C. 1

TEICHMANN, Vl., Dr., Radiologische Klinik, FVL UK, Faculty of General Medicine, Charles University, Unemocnice 2, Praha 2/ČSSR

TONGIO, J., Dr. (Pavillon Chir. A), Hôpital Civil, F-67 Strasbourg

TRONCONE, L., Dr., Università Cattolica S. Cuore, Istituto di Radiologia Roma/Italia

TRUCHOT, M., Dr., Service Central de Radiologie, Hôpital Civil, F-67 Strasbourg

UMEK, H., Dr., I. Medizinische Universitätsklinik, A-1090 Wien, Spitalgasse 23

VAN VAERENBERCH, M., Prof. Dr., Dienst voor nucleaire Geneeskunde, Akademisch Ziekenhuis, University of Ghent, B-9000 Gent, De Pintelaan 135

VANČURA, J., Dr., Radiologische Klinik FVL UK, Faculty of General Medicine, Charles University, Unemocnice 2, Praha 2/ČSSR

VARGHA, GY., M. D., Prof., Department of Radiology, University of Medicine, Debrecen, Hungary

Vergnes, R., Dr., Service Central de Radiologie, Hôpital Civil, F-67 Strasbourg
Verhaege, L., Dr., Dienst voor Inwendige Ziekten, Akademisch Ziekenhuis, University of Ghent, B-9000 Gent, De Pintelaan 135
Voets, P., Dr., D-6650 Homburg/Saar, Alte Reichsstr. 6
Vogelsang, H., Prof. Dr., Abteilung für Neuroradiologie, Department Radiologie Medizinische Hochschule, D-3000 Hannover-Kleefeld, Roderbruchstr. 101
Vogler, E., Prof. Dr., Vorstand der radiologischen Universitätsklinik, A-8036 Graz
Wagner, H. H., Dr., Institut für Nuklearmedizin und spezielle Biophysik des Radiologischen Zentrums der Medizinischen Hochschule Hannover, D-3000 Hannover, Roderbruchstr. 101
Waldbaur, H., Dr., Neurochirurg. Klinik der Universität Erlangen-Nürnberg, D-8520 Erlangen, Krankenhausstr. 12
Walter, W., Prof. Dr., Neurochirur. Klinik der Universität Erlangen-Nürnberg, D-8520 Erlangen, Krankenhausstr. 12
Warter, P., Prof. Dr., Pavillon Chir. A., Hôpital Civil, F-67 Strasbourg
Wawersik, J., Prof. Dr., Chirurg. Universitätsklinik, Anaesthesieabteilung, D-6900 Heidelberg, Kirschnerstr. 1
Weissleder, H., Dr., Abteilung für klinische Nuklearmedizin der Medizinischen Universitätsklinik, D-7800 Freiburg/Br.
Wellauer, J., Prof. Dr., Department of Diagnostic Radiology of the University of Zurich, Kantonsspital, CH-8000 Zurich
Wellman, H. N., M. D., Chief, NML, DMRE, BRH, Bureau of Radiological Health, Nuclear Medicine Laboratory, Cincinnati General Hospital of the University of Cincinnati, Ohio 45229/USA
Wenz, W., Prof. Dr., Leiter der Röntgenabteilung der Chirurg. Klinik der Universität, D-6900 Heidelberg, Kirschnerstr. 1
Weyer, K. H. van de, Prof. Dr., Chefarzt der Radiologischen Abteilung und Strahlenklinik des Mutterhauses der Borromäerinnen, D-5500 Trier, Auf der Hill
Weyer, H. J. van de, Dr., Medizinische Klinik der Universität, D-5300 Bonn-Venusberg
Wick, E., Dr., Kardiol. Abt. der Medizinischen Kliniken und Polikliniken der Universität Gießen, D-6300 Gießen, Friedrichstr. 27
Wieners, H., Doz. Dr., Radiologische Universitätsklinik und Strahleninstitut, D-2000 Hamburg 20, Martinistr. 52
Winkel, K. Zum, Prof. Dr., Direktor des Universitäts-Strahleninstituts, Klinikum Westend, D-1000 Berlin 19, Spandauer Damm 130
Winkler, C., Prof., Nuklearmedizinische Abteilung der Universität, D-5300 Bonn-Venusberg
Wójtowicz, J., Doz. Dr., Zakíad Radiologii A. M., Poznan, ul. Szkolna 8/12/Poland
Wolf, F., Prof. Dr., Medizinische Klinik der Universität Erlangen-Nürnberg, D-8520 Erlangen, Krankenhausstr. 12
Wood, E. J., MSc, A. Inst. D., Physics. Dept. The Royal Free Hospital, Gray's Inn Road, London, W.C. 1
Würdinger, H., Dr., Röntgen- und Strahlenabteilung der Städt. Krankenanstalten, D-7300 Eßlingen/Neckar
Yernault, J. C., Dr., Service de radiodiagnostic de l'Hôpital Universitaire Saint Pierre, Université Libre de Bruxelles, B-1000 Bruxelles, Rue Haute 322
Zeidler, U., Dr. Priv.-Doz., Institut für Nuklearmedizin und spezielle Biophysik, Department Radiologie, Medizinische Hochschule Hannover, D-3000 Hannover, Roderbruchstr. 101
Zeitler, E., Prof. Dr. med., Leiter der Radiologischen Abteilung der Aggertalklinik, D-5250 Engelskirchen
Zilberberg, Ch., Dr., Laboratoire des Radio-Isotopes, Hopital Foch, F-92 Suresnes
Zimmer, R., Dr., Radiologische Universitätsklinik und Strahleninstitut, D-2000 Hamburg-Eppendorf, Martinistr. 52

Space-Occupying Intracranial Lesions

Angiography and Scintigraphy in the Preoperative Diagnosis of Intracranial Tumors

R. Hünig and J. Wellauer

In order to decide whether an operation is indicated and, if so, what the operative procedure will be, the neurosurgeon needs not only a diagnosis of tumor, but also the most exact information possible as to the location and size of the tumor. In addition to angiography, scintigraphy is also a particularly valuable method for the diagnosis of intracranial neoplasms. Until now there have been no extensive comparisons of the neurosurgical importance of these two procedures. Having a large number of cases available for study, we have undertaken the evaluation of the efficiency of both angiography and scintigraphy in this regard.

Material

This analysis is based on the retrospective evaluation of 953 patients, seen in the Cantonal Hospital of Zurich between January 1, 1964, and spring 1970, with a presumed diagnosis of intracranial tumor. The majority underwent surgery, the remainder a thorough clinical evaluation. The preoperative clinical diagnostic procedures took place partly in the Department of Neurosurgery (Director Prof. H. Krayenbühl), and partly in the Department of Neurology (Director Prof. G. Baumgartner). There were 809 primary tumors, 102 solitary or multiple metastatic lesions and 128 first, second or third recurrences. Included among the recurrences were also the initially non-radically operated tumors. The tumor diagnosis was confirmed in all cases either at surgery or by autopsy. In addition, there were 93 histologically verified acoustic neurinomas, which are not included in this report.

Examination technique

The carotid angiographies[1] were done either under local or general anesthesia by direct puncture of the common carotid artery. In each case, radiographs in the anterior/posterior and lateral projections were made, the latter always using stereoscopic technique. A clear visualization of the arterial, capillary and venous phases was considered manditory to enable accurate diagnosis of the vascular system.

The vertebral arteriograms were always done under general anesthesia by puncture of the left axillary artery with an approximately 15 cm long needle and injection

1 „Urografin 60 %" (Schering Ltd.) was used for all the cerebral angiographies.

of the contrast media into the subclavian artery. The same radiographic technique as for the carotid angiography was used.

With a few exceptions, all angiographic examinations took place in the Department of Diagnostic Radiology of the University of Zurich (Director Prof. J. WELLAUER).

The brain scans were almost exclusively done in the Department of Radiotherapy and Nuclear Medicine of the University Hospital (Director Prof. W. HORST). Initially a scanner with a 3-inch detector was used. After autumn, 1965, a 5-inch detector became available. Of the isotopes or labeled compounds utilized, ^{99m}Tc-Pertechnetate was the most frequent (used in 214 scans), followed by ^{203}Hg Chlormerodrin (in 46 scans) and ^{75}Se-Selenit (in 11 scans). ^{197}Hg-Chlormerodrin, ^{113m}In- and ^{131}I-serum albumin were used once each. In 23 scans the isotope used was not recorded. As a rule, the scintigrams were done in at least two projections (anterior or posterior and lateral) although most patients were examined in three or even four projections (anterior, posterior and both laterals).

The histological preparations were examined, with few exceptions, in the Institute of Pathology of the University of Zurich (Director Prof. E. UEHLINGER). The minute histological differentiations, for example in glioblastomas, astrocytomas and metastases, were not taken into consideration in this report.

In addition to the patients' age and sex, among others the following facts were recorded on IBM punch cards:

1. classification of the tumor (primary, recurrent or metastatic)
2. location, size and number of tumors
3. histology of the tumor
4. neuroradiologic examinations and their results including the criteria used in the evaluation of the skull and angiographic films
5. electroencephalographic and echoencephalographic results
6. The value of each preoperative examination in respect to the surgical procedure was given prospectively by the surgeon himself in a questionaire and recorded in addition with some special positions.
7. date and radicality of the operation
8. date of death
9. autopsy findings

The interpretations of the various examinations used in this study were those of the official reports of the respective diagnostic departments. A re-evaluation of the data in light of the operative or autopsy findings was not done.

Results

A summary of the type and number of primary tumors, metastases and recurrences with regard to their localization is given in table 1. The topographical scheme described by KRAYENBÜHL and YASARGIL was used for localization of the tumors. The recurrent tumors are shown in parentheses. With the exclusion of the 93 acoustic neurinomas but inclusive all recurrences, 232 glioblastomas (22.3%), 187 meningiomas (18%), 147 astrocytomas (14.1%) and 102 metastases (9.8%) formed the main part of the material studied. In addition, there were 86 tumors of the hypophysis cerebri (8.3%), 50 ependymomas (4.8%), 47 oligodendrogliomas (4.5%),

Table 1. *Summary of the type and number of primary tumors, metastases and recurrences with regard to their location*

	Sella region	Frontomedial-parasagittal	Temporal Lobe post. $^{2}/_{3}$	Parietal	Subfrontal medial	Cerebellar Hemispheres	Frontolateral	Parietooccipital	Temporal Lobe ant. $^{1}/_{3}$	Temporo-occipital	Others	Total number
Number of tumors	112 (7)	101 (19)	85 (17)	69 (14)	61 (8)	60 (6)	42 (16)	50 (3)	43 (6)	38 (4)	250 (28)	911 (128)
Glioblastoma multiforma		20 (1)	39 (4)	13 (7)	5 (2)		14 (3)	27	18 (2)	19 (1)	54 (3)	209 (23)
Meningioma		34 (5)	5 (2)	24 (3)	50 (6)		6 (4)	2	1	2	41 (2)	165 (22)
Astrocytoma		18 (8)	15 (3)	6 (2)		8 (3)	12 (4)	5	15 (4)	3 (1)	31 (9)	113 (34)
Metastases	1	12	9	18	2	16	2	7	3	7	25	102
Hypophysis (Adenoma)	84 (2)											84 (2)
Ependymoma		3 (1)	4 (2)	2 (2)		2 (1)	(3)	3 (1)		1 (1)	19 (5)	34 (16)
Oligodendroglioma		11 (4)	2 (2)			3	5 (1)	1	1	2	12 (3)	37 (10)
Spongioblystoma		1	4 (2)	1	1	10		1 (1)		1	16 (2)	35 (5)
Craniopharyngioma	21 (4)										1 (1)	22 (5)
Medulloblastoma						9					17	26
Sarcoma	1		3 (2)	1	1		1	1 (1)	1	1 (1)	6	16 (4)
Others	5 (1)	2	4	4	2	12 (2)	2 (1)	3	4	2	28 (3)	68 (7)

Recurrences in ( )

40 spongioblastomas (3.8%), 27 craniopharyngiomas (2.6%), 26 medulloblastomas (2.5%), and 20 sarcomas (1.9%). The remaining 75 tumors (7.2%) were divided into 14 different groups.

Of the 1039 intracranial tumors which constitute the base of our study, angiography was done in 838 cases (80.6%) and scintigraphy in 298 cases (28.7%). Table 2 shows the frequency of angiography and scintigraphy according to the various tumor types and the results obtained[2]. The percentage of those tumors studied angiographically included: glioblastomas 99.7% (231/232), meningiomas 95.2% (178/187), astrocytomas 90.5% (133/147) and metastases 87.2% (89/102). In marked contrast are those studied scintigraphically: glioblastomas 29.3% (68/232), meningiomas 29.9% (56/187), astrocytomas 29.2% (43/147) and metastases 54.9% (56/102). Among the smaller tumor groups, the medulloblastoma is conspicuous in that the number studied by scanning (8/26 or 30.8%) is larger than that studied by angiography (5/26 or 19.2).

The angiographic results are classified as

1. obviously negative
2. false negative
3. questionable space occupying lesion (those with deviation of the midline structures and/or questionable vascular displacement)
4. definite space occupying lesion (those with definite vascular delineation of the tumor)
5. questionable tumor (those with questionable pathologic vessels), and
6. definite tumor (those with definite pathologic vessels).

In the scintigraphic examinations, two prependicular projections were evaluted separately and classified as negative, questionably positive or positive.

Of the 821 tumors examined angiographically in the correct region, in 52% (424) the diagnosis was "definite tumor", in 8% (64) "questionable tumor", and in 32% (264) a definite space occupying lesion could be confirmed. In that the diagnosis "definite space occupying lesion" includes the diagnosis "definite tumor" and "questionable tumor", the space occupying lesion could definitely be confirmed in 92% (752) of all tumors examined by angiography. In 17 cases the angiography was done in the wrong area and the results were therefore "obviously negative".

Of the 298 scintigraphically examined tumors, the results were definitely positive in two planes in 45% (133) of the cases, in 8% (24) definitely positive in one plane and questionable positive in the other and in 11% (33) positive in one plane and negative in the other. Thus, a clearly pathological concentration in at least one place could be established in 64% (190) of the cases.

The efficiency of angiography and scintigraphy in regard to the tumor location is shown in table 3.

In order to determine if, and to what extent, tumors which cannot be detected by one of the two methods used can be detected by the other, a number of tumors were examined angiographically as well as scintigraphically. The results of these double examinations are summarized in table 4. The angiographic results are shown

2 In tables, 2, 3, 6 and 7 the tumors examined by angiography and scintigraphy were not always the same lesions.

Table 2. *Frequency of angiography and scintigraphy according to tumor type and results obtained*

Histology	Primary tumors, metastases, recurrences Total	Number of Tumors	Results of Angiography: Obviously Negative	False Negative	Questionable SOL	SOL	Questionable Tumor	Tumor	Hydrocephalus*	Number of Tumors	Results of Scintigraphy: ØØ	Ø(+)	Ø+	+(+)	(+)(+)	++
Glioblastoma multiforma	209 (23)	209 (22)		9	4	44 (4)	18 (2)	134 (16)	2 (1)	63 (5)	7	2	10 (1)	3	4 (1)	38 (3)
Meningioma	165 (22)	159 (19)	1	4	5 (2)	27 (5)	11 (1)	111 (11)	2	48 (8)	5	1 (1)	7	3	3	29 (7)
Astrocytoma	113 (34)	105 (28)	1	2	10 (2)	61 (14)	7 (2)	24 (10)	4 (1)	37 (6)	20	4 (1)	4	2 (1)	1 (1)	6 (3)
Metastases	102	89	5	7	5	21	6	45	3	56	11	4	4	10	2	25
Oligodendroglioma	37 (10)	36 (9)	1	1 (1)	4	14 (3)	3	13 (5)	2	15 (2)	8					7 (2)
Ependymoma	34 (16)	23 (10)	1 (1)	1	2	14 (7)	2 (1)	3 (1)	1	5 (4)	(2)	2	2 (1)	(1)		1
Spongioblastoma	35 (5)	19 (4)	2	1		10 (1)	3 (1)	2 (2)	3 (2)	8 (2)	4 (1)					3 (1)
Hypophysis (Adenoma)	84 (2)	20				1		2		2	1					1
Sarcoma	16 (4)	15 (3)			2	3		10 (3)		6 (2)	2		1	1	(1)	2 (1)
Epidermoid Tumors	12 (1)	10		2		5	2	1	1	4	4					
v. Hippel-Lindau's disease	14 (3)	9 (3)	1			2 (1)		7 (2)	1	2 (2)	1 (2)		1			1
Others	90 (8)	45 (1)	4	4	1	29	5 (2)	21 (1)	4	19 (2)	9	2	2	2 (1)	1 (1)	2 (1)
Total number	911 (128)	739 (99)	16 (1)	31 (1)	33 (4)	229 (35)	57 (7)	373 (51)	23 (4)	265 (33)	72 (5)	15 (2)	31 (2)	21 (3)	11 (3)	115 (18)

Recurrences in ( )
* given as a solitary as well as an additional sign

Table 3. *Efficiency of angiography and scintigraphy in regard to tumor location*

Location	primary tumors, metastases, recurrences Total	Number of Tumors	Results of Angiography: Obviously Negative	False Negative	Questionable SOL	SOL	Questionable Tumor	Tumor	Hydrocephalus*	Number of Tumors	Results of Scintigraphy: ØØ	Ø(+)	Ø+	+(+)	(+)(+)	++
Frontomedial-parasagittal	101 (19)	100 (15)		3	4	28 (5)	9 (2)	56 (8)		38 (3)	9	3	1	3 (1)	3	19 (2)
Temporal Lobe post. 2/3	85 (17)	84 (15)			1	34 (5)	8 (1)	41 (9)	1 (1)	19 (5)	5 (1)		3	1		10 (4)
Parietal	69 (14)	68 (13)		1	5 (2)	13 (4)	3 (2)	46 (5)	1	26 (3)	1	2 (1)	4	2	(1)	17 (1)
Subfrontal medial	61 (8)	59 (7)		3	3 (1)	13 (1)	4 (1)	36 (4)	1	19 (4)	1	1 (1)	3	2		12 (3)
Temporal Lobe ant. 1/3	43 (6)	43 (6)			3 (1)	19 (1)	2	19 (4)		15 (1)	7		5			3 (1)
Frontolateral	42 (16)	42 (14)	(1)	1 (1)		12 (4)	5	24 (8)		17 (4)	4 (1)	2	4		2	5 (3)
Temporooccipital	38 (4)	37 (3)				11 (2)	2	24 (1)		9 (2)			2	(1)	1 (1)	6
Cerebellar Hemispheres	60 (6)	29 (4)	6	3	3	7 (1)		9 (3)	9	20 (1)	8	1	2	2 (1)	2	5
Sella region	112 (7)	29	3	3	1	17		5	1	5	4					1
Frontal central	28 (4)	28 (4)	1	2	2	11 (3)	1	11 (1)	3	12	4	1				7
Others	272 (27)	220 (18)	6	16	11	64 (9)	23 (1)	102 (8)	7 (3)	85 (10)	29 (3)	5	7 (2)	11	3 (1)	30 (4)
Total number	911 (128)	739 (99)	16 (1)	31 (1)	33 (4)	229 (35)	57 (7)	373 (51)	23 (4)	265 (33)	72 (5)	15 (2)	31 (2)	21 (3)	11 (3)	115 (18)

Recurrences in ( )

* given as a solitary as well as an additional sign

Table 4. *Correlation of the angiographic and scintigraphic findings in 256 patients with various brain tumors examined by both methods*

		Angiography				
		False Negative	Questionable SOL	Definite SOL	Questionable Tumor	Definite Tumor
Scintigraphy	False Negative	4	7	20	9	15
	Questionable Positive	5	3	7	5	8
	Positive	7	10	37	12	107

Only Angiographically Positive	64 (25 %)
Only Scintigraphically Positive	17 (7 %)
Angiographically and Scintigraphically Positive	156 (61 %)
Total Number Angiographically Positive	220 (86%)
Total Number scintigraphically Positive	173 (68%)
No Diagnosis	19 (7 %)

67	Glioblastomas	4	Metastases (Melanoma)
52	Meningiomas	3	Angioreticulomas
39	Astrocytomas	2	Angiomas
38	Metastases (Carcinoma)	2	Metastases (Hypernephroma)
14	Oligodendrogliomas	1	Metastasis (Sarcoma)
6	Ependymomas	1	Glomustumor
6	Sarcomas	1	Metastasis (Hodgkin)
4	Epidermoid Tumors	1	Adenoma of the Hypophysis (Chromophobic)
4	Malignant Tumors, unclassifiable	1	Medulloblastoma
4	Glial tumors, unclassifiable	1	Radionecrosis
4	Spongioblastomas	1	Metastasis (Thyroid Carcinoma, Langhans)

on the x-axis, the scintigraphic findings on the y-axis. This reveals the number of tumor which could be diagnosed by only one of the examination methods, as well as those demonstrable with both techniques. This group consisted of 256 tumors with differing histology. A space-occupying lesion or tumor was proven angiographically as well as scintigraphically in 61% (156). In 25% (64) of the total number, a space occupying lesion or tumor was detected only with angiography and in 7% (17) only by scintigraphy. The remaining 7% (19) include the false negative results, the angiographic diagnosis „questionable space-occupying lesion" and the scintigraphic diagnosis "questionable positive". It is striking to note that out of 256 tumors, 86% (220) were proven angiographically whereas only 68% (173) were proven scintigraphically. From this table it can also be seen that of the 83 scintigraphically negative tumors, 77% (64) were detected by angiography. Of the 36 angiographically negative tumors, only 47% (17) were scintigraphically positive. We feel that this demonstrates the extent of the complementary nature of the two examination methods.

The correlation between angiographic and scintigraphic findings in the 4 most frequent tumor types are shown in table 5. In brief, 12 out of 14 scintigraphically negative glioblastomas were diagnosed by angiography, as well as 7 out of 9 meningiomas, 8 out of 12 metastases and 20 out of 25 astrocytomas. In contrast, 7 out of 9 angiographically negative glioblastomas were positive by scintigraphy, likewise with 3 out of 5 meningiomas, 4 out of 8 metastases and 1 out of 6 astrocytomas.

Table 5. *Correlation of angiographic and scintigraphic findings in patients examined by both methods. The results are grouped according to type of the four most frequently occurring tumors*

		Glio blastoma	Menin-gioma	Meta-stases	Astro-cytoma
Total		67	52	47	39
Only Angiographically	Positive	12 (18%)	7 (13%)	8 (17%)	20 (51%)
Total Angiographically	Positive	58 (87%)	47 (90%)	39 (83%)	33 (85%)
Only Scintigraphically	Positive	7 (10%)	3 (6%)	4 (9%)	1 (3%)
Total Scintigraphically	Positive	53 (79%)	43 (83%)	35 (74%)	14 (36%)
Angiographically and Scintigraphically	Positive	46 (69%)	40 (77%)	31 (66%)	13 (33%)
No Diagnosis		2 (3%)	2 (4%)	4 (9%)	5 (13%)

The results mentioned thus far give only information regarding the frequency of positive results in angiography and scintigraphy. They provide, however, no definite conclusion as to their usefulness to the clinician in establishing the diagnosis of intracranial tumor.

To answer this question of clinical usefulness, the following points were evaluated:

1. For all cases the significant data, including history, physical findings and radiological, as well as other laboratory studies, was taken from the patients' charts and recorded according to a special protocol. In this way we tried to maintain a maxi-

mum of objectivity in evaluating the relative importance of the various diagnostic procedures.

2. Our neurosurgeons usually made use of a positive scintigram only when it either established the diagnosis, or at least added information supplementing the angiographic or other preoperative studies. Scintigrams which only confirmed the angiographic diagnosis were not considered.

3. To diminish the resulting subjective character of this analysis, we included the positive scans in those cases where angiography showed only a space occupying lesion.

Table 6 and 7 lists the examination results leading up to the diagnosis. The tumors are classified according to histology and location and are divided into two main groups:

1. primary tumors and metastases and
2. recurrences

In those instances where the total number of patients shown in these tables does not correspond to the number of tumors diagnosed angiographically and/or scintigraphically, the difference represents those patients who were diagnosed by other methods.

Angiography was only done when strictly indicated. Scintigraphy, however, was often done for scientific reasons and was sometimes ordered even after the positive angiographic result was known. Therefore, the ratio of the number of examinations performed to the number of those contributing essential results allows no conclusion as to the significance of each of these two procedures.

The ratio of significant angiography to significant scintigraphy gives a more meaningful comparison. These two values and the resulting quotient show the real efficiency of the two methods of examination. This quotient is given in the last line of both tables 6 and 7. For the primary tumors and metastases, the over-all ratio is 672:79 (8.5), with 151:11 (13.7) for meningiomas, 196:15 (13.1) for glioblastomas, and 94:8 (11.7) for astrocytomas, as evident in table 6. The value of angiography was therefore clearly superior to that of scintigraphy for primary tumors of these types. The highest percentage of scintigraphically positive results was found among the larger tumor groups: metastases 75:28 (2.7), spongioblastomas 17:4 (4.2) and ependymomas 20:3 (6.6).

In the diagnosis of recurrent tumors, the angiography was again proven to be more efficient among the more frequently encountered tumor types. This is especially true for the glioblastomas with 22:2, the astrocytomas with 26:4 and the meningiomas with 18:3. This gives an average value of 94:15 (6.3). However, scintigraphy is a particularly valuable method for the diagnosis of recurrent sarcomas (3:1), oligodendrogliomas (8:2) and ependymomas (9:2). In comparing the diagnostic results in patients with recurrent tumors and in those with primary tumors, we have to take into account that the first group includes some patients which were originally considered to be inoperable. Angiography was, therefore, not always indicated or done. Out of 128 diagnosed recurrences, only 76 were operated.

Table 7 shows the preoperative studies listed according to the tumor localization. The over-all result remains the same; in the case of primary tumors and metastases, however, angiography is especially important for the diagnosis of tumors in the frontolateral region (with a ratio of 39:2), as well as those located in the anterior

Table 6. *Relative importance of preoperative studies according to tumor histology*

	Glioblastoma multiforma	Meningioma	Astrocytoma	Metastases	Adenoma of the Hypophysis	Ependymoma	Oligodendro-glioma	Spongio-blastoma	Cranio-pharyngioma	Medullo-blastoma	Sarcoma	Others	Total number
Total number of tumors	209 (23)	165 (22)	113 (34)	102	84 (2)	34 (16)	37 (10)	35 (5)	22 (5)	26	16 (4)	68 (7)	911 (128)
Number of angiographies performed	209 (22)	159 (19)	105 (28)	89	20	23 (10)	36 (9)	19 (4)	5	5	15 (3)	54 (4)	739 (99)
Those contributing to the diagnosis	196 (22)	151 (18)	94 (26)	75	14	20 (9)	32 (8)	17 (4)	3	3	15 (3)	52 (4)	672 (94)
Number of scintigrams performed	63 (5)	48 (8)	37 (6)	56	2	5 (4)	15 (2)	8 (2)	1	8	6 (2)	16 (4)	265 (33)
Those contributing to the diagnosis	15 (2)	11 (3)	8 (4)	28	1	3 (2)	3 (2)	4		2	2 (1)	2 (1)	79 (15)
Meaningful Angiography/Meaningful Scintigraphy Primary Tumor and Mestastases	13,1	13,7	11,7	2,7	14	6,6	10,6	4,2	3:0	1,5	7,5	26	8,5

Recurrences in ( )

Table 7. *Relative importance of preoperative studies according to tumor location*

	Sella Region	Frontomedial-parasagittal	Temporal Lobe post. $^{2}/_{3}$	Parietal	Subfrontal medial	Cerebellar Hemispheres	Frontolateral	Parietooccipital	Temporal Lobe ant. $^{1}/_{3}$	Temporo-occipital	Others	Total number
Total number of tumors	112 (7)	103 (19)	84 (17)	67 (14)	62 (8)	60 (6)	42 (16)	49 (3)	43 (6)	38 (4)	251 (28)	911 (128)
Number of angiographies performed	29	105 (15)	84 (15)	65 (13)	60 (7)	29 (4)	42 (14)	48 (3)	43 (6)	37 (3)	197 (19)	739 (99)
Those contributing to the diagnosis	20	97 (15)	83 (15)	59 (12)	56 (6)	21 (4)	39 (12)	43 (3)	40 (5)	36 (3)	178 (19)	672 (94)
Number of scintigrams performed	5	38 (3)	19 (5)	26 (3)	19 (4)	20 (1)	17 (4)	13 (1)	16 (1)	9 (2)	83 (24)	265 (33)
Those contributing to the diagnosis	1	14 (1)	7 (1)	8 (1)	6 (1)	9	2 (2)	8 (1)	3 (1)	3 (2)	18 (5)	79 (15)
Meaningful Angiography / Meaningful Scintigraphy Primary Tumors and Metastases	20	6,9	11,8	7,4	9,3	2,3	19,5	5,4	13,3	12	9,9	8,5

Recurrences in ( )

third of the temporal lobe (with 40:3), in the temporo-occipital area (with 36:3) and the posterior two thirds of the temporal lobe (with 83:7). Scintigraphy proved to be more efficient in the fourth ventricle (with 1:3), the cerebellar hemisphere (with 21:9), the parieto-occipital region (with 43:8) and the occipitomedial region (with 19:3). In the diagnosis of recurrences, angiography was shown to be primarily valuable for tumors located in the frontomedial/parasagittal area and in the posterior two/thirds of the temporal lobe (with 15:1 each) and parietal area (with 12:1). The particular value of scintigraphy was evident for tumors located in the parietotemporal and temporo-occipital regions (with 3:2 each), in the Sylvian fissure (with 4:1), the anterior third of the temporal lobe (with 5:1), frontolateral regions (with 12:2), and the subfrontal/medial areas (with 6:1).

Comments

The detection rates of intracranial tumors by angiography in this analysis was remarkably high with positive results in 91,6% (752/821) of the cases, either as a space-occupying lesion (264 cases – 32,2%) or as a definite or suspected tumor (488 cases – 59,4%). In our opinion this high yield was due to the following two factors:

1. The technique: all lateral views in the angiographic series were made sterioscopically. This gives an impressive demonstration of the vascular courses within the skull and allows detection of vessel displacement or stretching, avascular areas, and structures with neovascularization with much greater certainty than the usual angiographic views. This empiric concept is based on many years of experience and has proven itself in the search for aneurysms, as well as for tumors.

2. The experience of the diagnostician, as based on the number of angiograms done. In the past several years an average of 1000 angiograms per year were done at our institute. This experience is augmented by a constant close association with the clinicians which allows for surgical or autopsy verification of the radiological diagnosis. In this manner, the angiographic diagnostic criteria could almost always be controlled and, if necessary, corrected.

Of the cases studied with radioisotopes, scintigraphy gave a definitely positive result in only 64% of the cases in this study. According to reports in the literature, this is a relatively low yield. The primary reason probably lies in the large variety of tumors studied by scintigraphy. It is well known that the uptake of many of these tumors is poor, as for example in astrocytomas, epithelial cysts, gliomas and medulloblastomas. On the other hand, meningiomas were detected in 82.1% (46/56), glioblastomas in 80.9% (55/68) and metastases in 69.6% (39/56) of the cases. This lies well within the usual limits. We believe that a closer comparison of scintigraphic results and diagnostic capabilities is only possible in cases with identical tumor histology. Differences in the fine structure of the tumors are frequently associated with variations in isotope uptake. That differences in tumor location are especially significant in regard to the effectiveness of diagnosis is self evident and need not be further emphasized. An analysis of the results seen in relation to tumor localization is not possible for our large number of cases within this study. It shall be the subject of a subsequent evaluation and report.

In as much as the angiographically and scintigraphically studied tumor groups were not identical, a valid comparison of the results can only be made in 256 cases. To arrive at a reliable result, and especially to afford a judgement concerning the possibilities of diagnosis in cases of tumors not recognized by one or the other methods of study, we believe that a comparison in the manner in which we have done it (Table 4) is essential. Only in this way is it possible to provide the clinician with a well founded concept regarding the optimal sequence of diagnostic studies. Simple tabulation of positive and negative results would not achieve this. The fact that significantly more scintigraphically negative tumors could be diagnosed by angiography than angiographically negative tumors by scintigraphy substantiates the high regard for angiography of our neurosurgeons. In contrast, however, the comparison still shows that scanning alone provided a positive diagnosis in 7% (17/256) of the cases studied.

The value of angiographic and scintigraphic results for the preoperative diagnosis of intracranial tumors is closely associated with the information (case history, clinical findings, other neuroradiological examinations, etc.) required by the neurosurgeon as an indication to operate. Therefore, the angiographic and scintigraphic results must first be integrated into the total available diagnostic data before the value of any one of these diagnostic procedures can be evaluated separately. Such an analysis can only be made retrospectively and only in a case material where the tumor diagnosis was formulated preoperatively or before death and could then be verified either by surgery or autopsy. Cases in which the tumor diagnosis was not established are therefore not contained in this study.

Our evaluation of the significance of angiography and scintigraphy is bases upon information given us by the neurosurgeons. Naturally, this is only valid for the diagnostic-surgical unit of the University of Zurich. All data used was taken from the neurosurgery charts. The neuroradiologic diagnoses used in this study were those given in the original radiology reports. With this, an objectivity has been attained which allows a comparison of results with those of other hospitals as long as the necessary information is available and comparable.

In many ways this analysis affords only a rough evaluation because the frequency with which the diagnostic procedures were performed, as well as their results, are given only in relationship to either the histology or localization of the lesions. In future reports, it will be shown that the capabilities of angiography and scintigraphy vary for histologically identical tumors depending on their localization.

Judging from the large number of patients referred to us for angiography with the suspicion of having an intracranial tumor, we may assume that the clinician was aware not only of the high percentage of positive results, but also of the relative safety associated with this examination. Not only were operable patients studied, but also patients in whom a surgical procedure was contraindicated from the start were examined for various medical reasons. The function of angiography in such cases was to confirm or rule out the suspicion of tumor, either primary, recurrent or metastatic, and thus explain the clinical situation. In addition, more exact information as to tumor type and location enabled the clinician in many cases to decide upon an appropriate nonsurgical mode of therapy. Today, however, we feel that the question is justified if this information may not otherwise be obtained. At least in cases of recurrence and metastases with the ever present possibility of multiple lesions, scintigraphy alone may suffice as long as the tumor is adequately demonstrated. It is probable that as sequence scintigraphy becomes more widely used, one may well do without angiography with increasing frequency.

Summary

The importance of angiography and scintigraphy in establishing the preoperative diagnosis in 1039 histologically confirmed intracranial tumors was analyzed and the following conclusions made:

1. The probability of diagnosing intracranial tumors independent of their histology and location is 91,6% by angiography and 64% by scintigraphy. These figures, however, are based on two partially overlapping tumor groups.

2. In the group of tumors examided by both methods, the angiography was positive in 86% and the scintigraphy in 68%. In 7% of the cases no diagnosis could be made, either by scintigraphy or by angiography. It was proven that the scintigraphically negative tumors could be more frequently diagnosed by angiography than could the angiographically negative tumors be diagnosed by scintigraphy.

3. Based on the number of significant results achieved by angiography and scintigraphy, a quotient can be derived. This quotient represents the relative efficiency of these two modes of examination and may be related to tumor histology and/or localization.

4. The analysis proves that angiography and scintigraphy complement one another in their efficiency. The larger number of angiographically positive results in our institute confirms our preference for angiography. But a brain scan has significance for the preoperative diagnosis, when the clinical symptomatology was not explained or was insufficiently clarified by angiography. Scintigraphy may also be of greater value in cases of recurrent tumor or suspected multiple or bilateral lesions.

Gegenüberstellung der Angiographie und Hirnszintigraphie in der Diagnostik von intrakraniellen raumfordernden Prozessen

E. Klaus, J. Kuba und M. Ševčík

Die Hirnszintigraphie hat zweifelsohne ihr volles Bürgerrecht in der Diagnostik von intrakraniellen Raumforderungen erworben und wird heute als Routine-Untersuchungsmethode laufend eingesetzt.

Den Kernpunkt unserer Abhandlung sehen wir in der Wertung der Bedeutung der Szintigraphie im weiten Rahmen der Diagnostik von Raumforderungen und in der Abwägung ihrer Aussagekraft gegenüber der Carotis- bzw. Vertebralisangiographie.

Die cerebrale Szintigraphie führen wir routinemäßig nach intravenöser Applikation von Radiopertechnetat, resp. ^{113m}In-EDTA mittels eines Magnascanners der Fa. Picker durch.

Die Kontrastfüllung der Carotis und Vertebralis nehmen wir perkutan, resp. durch Femoraliskathetrisation in schneller Bildfolge am AOT-Gerät vor.

Wir untersuchen seit November 1968 szintigraphisch insgesamt 573 Patienten. Bei 179 wurde ein intrakranieller raumverdrängender Prozeß nachgewiesen und zwar 166mal Tumoren, 7mal Abscesse und 6mal chronische subdurale Hämatome. Es hat sich erwiesen, daß sich der intrakranielle Prozeß in 90%, resp. 86% – wenn wir die Anzahl der Patienten subtrahieren, bei denen der Befund nicht eindeutig war – szintigraphisch darstellen ließ. Diese Resultate und die Erfahrungen anderer Untersucher lassen es berechtigt erscheinen, die Szintigraphie als routinen atraumatischen „screening test" bei Verdacht auf eine intrakranielle Raumforderung anzuwenden, wobei wir uns bewußt sind, daß ein positives Szintigramm nicht tumorspezifisch ist. Wir können zwar recht häufig, mit großer Wahrscheinlichkeit in Bezugnahme auf das klinische Erscheinungsbild auf den Charakter des szintigraphischen Herdes schließen. Dennoch werden wir immer in richtiger Wahl auch die Kontrastuntersuchung einsetzen. Ganz ausnahmsweise werden wir uns bloß mit dem szintigraphischen Resultat zufrieden geben.

Da die cerebrale Angiographie das expansive Substrat direkt durch Anfärbung oder durch arteriovenöse Kurzschlüsse nachweisen kann, diente uns deshalb diese Methode als Kriterium zur Beurteilung der Aussagekraft der Szintigraphie bei der Erfassung von Raumforderungen.

Die szintigraphische Untersuchung war im Vergleich zur Angiographie nur bei wenigen Patienten entscheidend. Der prozentuale Anteil bei supratentorialen Geschwülsten ist 3%, bei infratentorialen 16%, in der Gesamtaufstellung, bei der beide Untersuchungen vorgenommen wurden, 5%.

Nach dem Angeführten hat es den Anschein, als ob die Szintigraphie bezogen auf die Angiographie nur eine untergeordnete Rolle spielt. Die klinische Enddiagnose einer intrakraniellen Raumforderung hat aber von der Sicht des Neurochirurgen nicht nur die Topik, sondern ebenfalls die Ausdehnung und die vorausgesetzte Qualität zu enthalten. Die Angiographie kann uns diesbezüglich nur dann voll befriedigen, wenn es zur teilweisen oder kompletten Anfärbung des Neoplasma kommt. Dies war aber nur in 46% der Fall. In 48% waren bloß indirekte Raumverdrängungszeichen vorhanden und in 6% war der angiographische Befund unauffällig.

Als Beispiel einer direkten Tumordarstellung erwähnen wir die capilläre Anfärbung eines parasagittalen Meningeoms. Hier ist der szintigraphische Herd, was Größe und Form betrifft, spiegelbildähnlich.

Der typische Durastern eines Meningeoms ist im Arteriogramm ersichtlich. Das Szintigramm weist dann in gleicher Lokalisation und in derselben Ausdehnung einen gut umschriebenen homogenen Anreicherungsherd auf.

In beiden Fällen erbrachte die Angiographie ein Maximum von Information, während sich das Szintigramm nur vor Anwendung der Kontrastuntersuchung als wertvoller „screening test" bewährte.

Demgegenüber sahen wir bei einem anderen Fall das seitliche Arteriogramm einer frontotemporalen Raumforderung, ohne Zeichen von Anfärbung. Im Szintigramm kam es zu einer gut umschriebenen Herdanreicherung, die von der Sicht der Szintigraphie im Hinblick auf das klinische Zustandsbild als Absceß gedeutet wurde. Die Autopsie bestätigte die Diagnose.

Bei einem weiteren Fall war im sagittalen Vertebralisarteriogramm eine Raumforderung des rechten Kleinhirnbrückenwinkels ohne Zeichen von Anfärbung ersichtlich. Das dazugehörende Szintigramm ergab in der Seitenansicht einen runden ausgedehnten Herd derselben Lokalisation. Bei der Operation wurde ein pfirsichgroßes Meningeom entfernt.

Die letzten zwei Fälle zeigen, wie der szintigraphische Befund durch Festlegung der Größe, Lage und Form der Raumforderung bei nur indirekten Tumorzeichen im Angiogramm weitere wertvolle Fingerzeige geben kann.

Wir haben in unserer Aufstellung weitere 36 Kranke, das ist 20% des Gesamtkrankengutes, bei denen eine angiographische Untersuchung aus den verschiedensten Gründen nicht durchgeführt wurde. Hier gab es 28mal positive szintigraphische Bilder. In diesem Fall stellt die Szintigraphie eine wertvolle diagnostische Bereicherung dar. Werten wir die Aussagekraft der Szintigraphie bei allen isotopisch untersuchten Probanden, so kommen wir zu einem Prozentsatz von 55%, wo sie zur Enddiagnose beisteuerte.

Rückschlüsse auf die Art des vorliegenden raumfordernden Prozesses sind bei isolierter Wertung der konventionellen Szintigraphie nur selten zu erwarten. In dieser Hinsicht ist die cerebrale Angiographie derzeit der Szintigraphie überlegen. Außerdem hängt die Darstellbarkeit des Tumors im Szintigramm, wie gut bekannt ist, von seiner Lage, Größe und histologischen Qualität ab. Dafür sprechen zum Beispiel auch negative szintigraphische Befunde bei der Mehrzahl der Kranken mit Hypophysenadenomen und fehlende Herdanreicherungen bei kleinen Metastasen in unserem Krankengut, die sich angiographisch gut nachweisen ließen.

Abschließend können wir sagen, daß sich die Szintigraphie nicht nur als „screening test" mit hoher diagnostischer Treffsicherheit bei Patienten mit suspekter Raumforderung bewährt, sondern anhand unserer Vergleichsuntersuchungen im Rahmen einer komplexen Untersuchung zur Diagnosestellung tatkräftig beiträgt. In einem hohen Prozentsatz steuert sie zur Festlegung der genauen Lage, Größe und Form der Raumverdrängung bei. Für den Neurochirurgen ist sie wegen der plastischen stereoskopischen Abbildung der Hirngeschwulst ein vorzügliches Hilfsmittel.

Es besteht kein Zweifel, daß durch den kombinierten Einsatz der Errungenschaften der Nuklearmedizin und der herkömmlichen Kontrastmittelverfahren die diagnostische Ausbeute in der Neuroradiologie um ein Beträchtliches zu steigern ist.

Isotope Encephalography and Cerebral Angiography in the Diagnosis of Brain Lesions

J. H. M. VAN ECK and L. PENNING

In comparing cerebral angiography with isotope encephalography many authors have expressed the diagnostic reliability in a ratio of positive findings to total number of cases, and then jumped to conclusions on the value of both procedures.

Table 1 gives a survey of the pertaining literature. The reported percentages differ considerably, which is not amazing, as the material of various authors is as heterogenous as their criteria for a positive finding. Many of them disregard the intentional or unintentional selection of their cases, willing to ascribe a difference of a few percents to a special variant of the method designed and applied by themselves.

In spite of these objections, a survey like this one leaves a certain impression, viz. that the global accuracy of both methods is similar: angiography 55–100% (with an average of 82.3%) and isotope studies 62–96% (averaged 82.7%).

In our personal material we have ranged the results of each procedure in a five-point scale:

1. correct localization of a lesion.
2. correct lateralization but false localization.
3. correct lateralization without localization.
4. general disturbance without lateralization or localization.
5. negative finding, i.e. normal picture.

In a series of 1000 patients, the first 500 were examined by manual RIHSA-encephalography (Planiol) and the next 500 by technetium brain scanning. Intracranial expanding lesions were present in 316 patients, including supratentorial and infratentorial tumors, abscesses, haematomas and vascular malformations. All of these cases were studied with isotopes and 246 also by angiography. For the evaluation angiography was only considered if it had been carried out on the side of the lesion or, in case of infratentorial pathology, by way of the vertebral artery.

Table 2 shows that, also in this series, the number of exactly localized lesions was almost equal for angiography and for isotope studies: 76%. The angiogram, however, yielded an additional 11% of lateralized lesions and thus had less complete failures (14%) than the isotope test (21%).

Now it is important to know how often one method was positive and the other negative. Table 3 shows the angiographic findings in 66 patients with a negative isotope test, and the isotopic findings in 39 patients with a negative angiogram. It is clear that the diagnostic reaches of the two methods only partly overlap, which makes both indispensable. Table 4 gives a list of cases, where this situation occurred.

A normal angiogram was found rather frequently in cerebral metastases and in craniopharyngiomas, a normal isotope study more often in epidermoid cysts, arachnoidal cysts, neuromas, some haematomas and deep vascular anomalies.

Still this table does not tell anything about those cases, where both methods were positive, but one of them in a more convincing way or giving more information

Table 1. *Results of isotope studies and cerebral angiography in the literature*

Year	Authors	Isotope studies			Angiography		
		Number	Local.	Percentage	Number	Local.	Percentage
1956	Escobar	13	8	62%	11	9	82%
1961	Sweet *et al.*	202	182	90%	120	96	80%
1961	McAfee and Taxdal	71	52	73%	43	30	70%
1962	Aronow	298	286	96%	173	153	94%
1962	Wilcke	160	112	70%	130	97	75%
1962	Wilcke and Friedman	184	134	73%	670	521	77%
1963	Dugger and Pepper	34	31	90%	34	31	90%
1963	Wende	79	73	93%	79	65	82%
1963	Graban *et al.*	25	20	80%	25	19	76%
1964	McAfee and Taxdal	141	101	71%	95	70	74%
1965	Wende	239	208	87%	191	154	81%
1965	Brenner *et al.*	27	17	63%	14	14	100%
		69	54	78%	34	34	100%
1965	Spencer	28	24	86%	22	19	86%
1965	Paoletti *et al.*	100	86	86%	63	56	89%
1965	Afifi *et al.*	62	52	84%	36	33	91%
1965	Avioli *et al.*	51	39	76%	25	19	76%
1965	Bucy and Ciric	90	68	76%	80	44	55%
1965	Goodrich and Tutor	118	99	84%	85	70	82%
1965	Green *et al.*	41	31	73%	29	22	76%
1965	Kahn	61	46	75%	53	49	92%
1965	Overton *et al.*	100	84	84%	76	64	84%
1965	Takahashi	41	29	71%	17	5	29%
1965	Wang *et al.*	44	34	77%	36	25	69%
1965	Zimmermann and Bluestein	63	54	86%	42	31	74%
1966	McCormack and Newton	81	56	69%	68	54	79%
1967	Fontès *et al.*	60	54	90%	60	55	92%
1967	Planiol and Sachs	110	95	86%	110	102	93%
		214	204	95%	214	208	97%
1967	Loken *et al.*	141	109	78%	77	55	72%
1967	Witcofski *et al.*	92	75	81%	65	60	92%
1967	Allen *et al.*	65	51	78%	53	41	80%
1968	Koch *et al.*	110	86	78%	87	78	90%
1968	Wende	410	336	82%	298	238	80%
1968	Wilcke	220	178	81%	220	207	94%
	Total	3954	3269	82,7%	3435	2828	82,3%

Table 2. *Overall accuracy in a series of 1000 patients*

	Angiography		Isotope studies	
	Verified lesions (196)	All lesions (246)	Verified lesions (221)	All lesions (316)
Correct localization	152 = 77 %	74 % = 181	169 = 77 %	76 % = 241
Correct side (false local.)	11 = 6 %	6 % = 14	5 = 2 %	2 % = 5
Correct side (no local.)	9 = 5 %	5 % = 12	3 = 1 %	1 % = 3
General disturbance	2 = 1 %	1 % = 0	1 = 0 %	0% = 1
Normal picture	22 = 11 %	14 % = 36	43 = 20 %	21 % = 66

Table 3

Cases with negative angiogram (39)		Cases with negative isotope studies (66)	
Isotopes localizing	26	Angiogram localizing	24
Isotopes lateralizing	0	Angiogram lateralizing	5
Isotopes general disturbance	0	Angiogram general disturbance	1
Isotopes negative	13	Angiogram negative	13

Table 4

Isotope localization with normal angiogram (26):	Angiographic localization or lateralization with normal isotope encephalogram (29):
12 gliomas	10 gliomas
8 metastases	3 metastases
2 meningiomas	4 meningiomas
2 craniopharyngiomas	3 haematomas
2 unclassified tumours	2 carotid-cavernosus fistulas
	1 neuroma
	1 epidermoid
	1 arachnoidal cyst
	4 unclassified tumours

as to the exact site, size, nature or multiplicity of lesions. A careful analysis of individual case-histories led to the following impressions:

1. if there is a discrepancy in localization, isotopes mostly indicate the correct site of a lesion, unless a clear tumour stain is seen in the angiogram.

2. in manual gamma-encephalography the size of a lesion sometimes seems to be larger than its real size, but this occurs less often in scintigraphy.

3. multiplicity was detected as frequently by angiography as by isotope studies, but not always in the same patient. For this purpose, double or triple angiography is mostly required.

4. we regard the prediction of the nature of a lesion by isotope encephalography with all reserve. Using short-lived isotopes nobody has been able to do so successfully. With RIHSA it is possible in a number of cases, but often only after several repeated measurements. We found Planiol's criteria to be not quite satisfactory.

In a smaller group of 82 anatomically verified lesions we have made a retrospective blind study, reinterpreting all RIHSA-encephalograms and angiograms without knowing any personal or clinical data of the patients. The results are summarized in Table 5, which shows that the correct type of lesion was more often indicated by the G.E.G. (46%) than by the angiogram (20%). If we include those cases, where the angiogram suggested a malignant tumor (i.e. glioblastoma or metastasis) and those were the G.E.G. mentioned the correct type as second choice, the difference becomes smaller (57 vs. 44%).

Table 5. *Prediction of type of lesion by means of blind reinterpretation*

Gammaencephalogram				Angiogram	
57% = 47	25	38 = 46%	correct choice	16	20% = 16; 36 = 44%
	13		first choice[a]	0	
	9		second choide[b]	1	
	0		"malignant"[c]	19	
	18		wrong choice	9	
	2		no choice made	26	
	15		negative	11	

[a] Correct type of lesion indicated as first of two possibilities.

[b] Correct type of lesion indicated as second of two possibilities.

[c] Correct indication of "malignant tumour" without preference for glioblastoma or metastasis.

We wish to conclude our paper with the following remarks:

1. Cerebral angiography and scintigraphy may give complementary information in :

a) large cysts with small mural tumour (the extension of the cyst is often seen in the angiogram, the proper tumour in the scan).

b) large haematomas from small vascular malformations (here the scan shows the extension of the haematoma, the angiogram mainly the aneurysm).

c) infarctions with or without vascular occlusion (the angiogram shows the occlusion, if present; the scan shows site and size of the infarction, which may vary considerably from patient to patient).

2. Angiography is the method of choice in :

a) vascular malformations (small ones escape detection in isotope encephalography, and the scan blurs the structure of larger ones).

b) low-grade astrocytomas and epidermoid cysts, which often leave the blood-brain barrier intact.

As it is seldom known beforehand, which type of lesion is to be expected, isotope studies should be carried out before angiography, except in real emergency or in a patient with subarachnoid haemorrhage.

3. Isotope encephalography is to be preferred for:

a) cerebral metastases, the operability of which depends on the exclusion of multiplicity (in such cases isotope scanning or scintiphotography offers the best survey of the whole skull).

b) postoperative control, or the early detection of recurrent tumours (angiography may fail by the absence of shifted vessels in a non-staining tumour).

4. Although in several centres craniotomies are done on the sole base of a positive brain scan, most neurosurgeons want an angiogram for further orientation. In many non-surgical or inoperable cases, however, isotope encephalography can be said to have replaced cerebral angiography.

Summary

The results of isotope encephalography and cerebral angiography in a series of 1000 patients are reported and discussed. Intracranial mass lesions were present in 316 cases. Isotope studies were made in every such case, angiography was performed in 246. The diagnostic value of the two procedures was compared both by statistical elaboration and by analysis of individual case histories.

The overall accuracy of localization was some 75% for either method, but the angiogram yielded lateralization in another 12% and the scan in only 3%. In the individual patient, it was often seen that one procedure was positive and the other one negative. Occasionally the two tests gave complementary information on the site, size, type or multiplicity of lesions.

This complimentary aspect was most striking in large cysts with a small mural tumour, in haematomas from a small aneurysm, and in several infarctions. Isotope studies often are of more avail in multiple metastases and in recurrent tumours, whereas angiography is superior in vascular malformations and in low-grade astrocytomas.

Although most neurosurgeons want both scan and angiogram before proceeding to craniotomy, isotope encephalography has reduced the need of angiography in many cases not apt for surgery.

L'imprégnation des tumeurs cérébrales

Etude atériographique, scintigraphique et angioscintigraphique au pertechnétate de ^{99m}Tc de 100 tumeurs opérées

M. Akerman, E. Hertzog, Ch. Zilberberg et C. Koutoulidis

La valeur de l'artériographie et de la scintigraphie pour le diagnostic de tumeurs cérébrale sn'est plus à démontrer.

Notre travail porte plus particulièrement sur le mode d'imprégnation des tumeurs par le produit de contraste iodé de l'artériographie, d'une part, et par le ^{99m}Tc d'autre part. Son but est de déterminer les éléments qui permettent d'orienter le diagnostic de nature des tumeurs cérébrales.

Matériel

Font l'objet de cette étude les 100 dernières tumeurs cérébrales opérées dans le service du Prof. G. Guiot, avant juillet 1970 et qui ont été explorées à la fois par artériographie et par scintigraphie au ^{99m}Tc.

Le détail de ce matériel est donné sur le tableau 1. Il comporte peu de tumeurs de la fosse postérieure, car pour leur diagnostic, il a été fait davantage appel à l'encéphalographie gazeuse ou à la ventriculographie par moyen de contraste opaque.

Tableau 1. *100 tumeurs cérébrales opérées, explorées par artériographie et par scintigraphie*

Nature		Siège	
Méningiomes	31	Hémisphères cérébraux	74
Gliomes malins	22	Base du crâne	18
Gliomes à évolution lente	17	Fosse postérieure	8
Métastases	14		
Divers	16		

Méthodes

L'étude artériographique

Les angiographies carotidiennes ont été en grande majorité effectuées par ponction directe de l'artère. Aussi souvent que nécessaire, on procéda à une injection sélective des carotides interne ou externe. Quant au système vertébrobasilaire, son opacification fut obtenue soit à contre-courant par ponction de l'humérale, soit par cathétérisme selon la méthode de SELDINGER, soit quelquefois par ponction directe. La soustraction d'image a été utilisée dans la majorité des cas et toujours dans les cas litigieux.

Le produit de contraste habituel est l'Acétylamino-triodobenzoate de Méthylglucamine à 25% d'Iode (Vasurix 25).

Les explorations scintigraphiques

Elles ont été réalisées après injection intra-veineuse de 5 à 15 millicuries de ^{99m}Tc. sous forme de pertechnétate, avec un Magnascanner III ou avec une caméra à scintillations Digicaméra III, Nuclear Enterprises.

L'intensité de la fixation radio-active tumorale a été mesurée sur les scintigraphies en comparant la radio-activité tumorale à celle de la zone symétrique non pathologique sur les incidences frontales, ou à celle d'une zone saine quelconque sur les profils. Avec la caméra à scintillations ces mesures ont été faites à l'aise d'un analyseur à mémoire à 4.096 canaux.

Les résultats ont été classés en quatre groupes selon l'intensité de l'imprégnation radioactive. Ces groupes ont été définis sur le tableau 2.

Tableau 2. *Classification des résultats scintigraphiques*

$$F = \%\ \text{Fixation}^* = \frac{{}^*\text{Tumeur} - {}^*\text{Région saine}}{{}^*\text{Région saine}} \times 100$$

Groupe I:	Fixation nulle ou non significative	$F \leqslant 20\%$
Groupe II:	Fixation modérée	F: 20 à 50%
Groupe III:	Fixation intense	F: 50 à 80%
Groupe IV:	Fixation très intense	$F \geqslant 80\%$

Une étude dynamique de la vitesse de l'imprégnation radioactive a été réalisée dans 27 tumeurs et également dans 3 cas d'angiome. Cette étude dynamique est faite à la caméra à scintillations et comporte, après injection intra-veineuse rapide de Technétium, la prise de 6 photographies successives à 5 sec d'intervalle. Les photographies suivantes sont prises à quelques minutes d'intervalle, jusqu' à ce que soit atteint un maximum d'imprégnation de la tumeur.

L'analyseur à mémoire à 4.096 canaux, associé à un enregistreur sur bande magnétique, sert à réaliser des courbes dynamiques dans des régions sélectionnées du crâne.

Résultats

1. Les résultats globaux sont présentés sur le Tableau 3. Les pourcentages de résultats anormaux obtenus par artériographie et par scintigraphie sont équivalents. Les échecs de chaque méthode ne se recoupent pratiquement pas et 98% des tumeurs ont pu être mises en évidence en associant les deux techniques.

Tableau 3. *Résultats globaux*

	Artériographie	Scintigraphie	Artériographie + Scintigraphie
Positifs	90/100	91/100	98/100
Injection tumorale	30/100		

Une injection de la tumeur a été visible sur 30% des artériographies. Une délimitation précise de la tumeur est rendue possible par cette injection. La scintigraphie présente cependant une certaine supériorité sur l'artériographie dans la localisation exacte des tumeurs, car l'imprégnation radioactive correspond à la tumeur elle-même et permet une limitation plus précise dans tous les cas où l'angiographie ne montre qu'un refoulement vasculaire.

2. Il semble exister une relation entre l'intensité de la fixation radioactive et l'injection artériographique des tumeurs (Fig. 1).

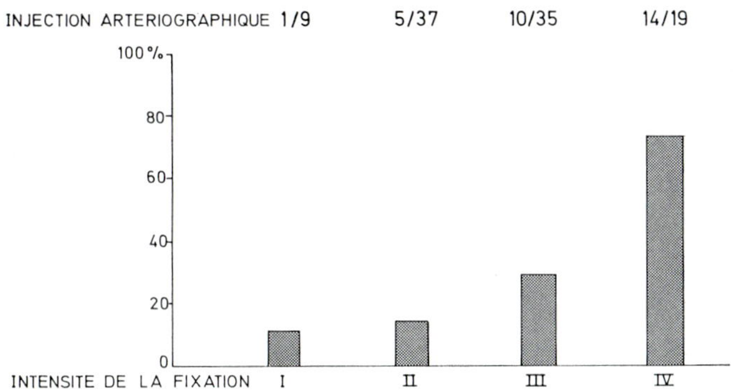

Fig. 1. Corrélation entre l'injection artériographique et l'intensité de la fixation radio-active tumurale

A mesure que la fixation radioactive augmente, le pourcentage des tumeurs injectées à l'artériographie croît.

Lorsqu'on considère les tumeurs selon leur nature (Fig. 2) ce parallélisme est particulièrement net dans les méningiomes et les glioblastomes. C'est dans ces tumeurs que le pourcentage d'injection artériographique est le plus élevé: 51% pour les méningiomes et 32% pour les glioblastomes.

Il est impossible, sauf dans de rares cas, d'établir un diagnostic de nature d'une tumeur uniquement sur l'intensité de sa fixation radioactive. On peut cependant noter que ce sont les méningiomes qui donnet le plus de foyers de fixation très intense. Dans les glioblastomes la fixation radioactive est le plus souvent intense. Elle est plutôt modérée dans les métastases. Dans les gliomes à évolution lente comme les astrocytomes on observe de très nombreux résultats normaux ou des foyers de fixation modérée.

3. Les renseignements les plus intéressants concernant la nature d'une tumeur semblent être donnés par *l'étude dynamique de leur vitesse d'imprégnation radioactive*.

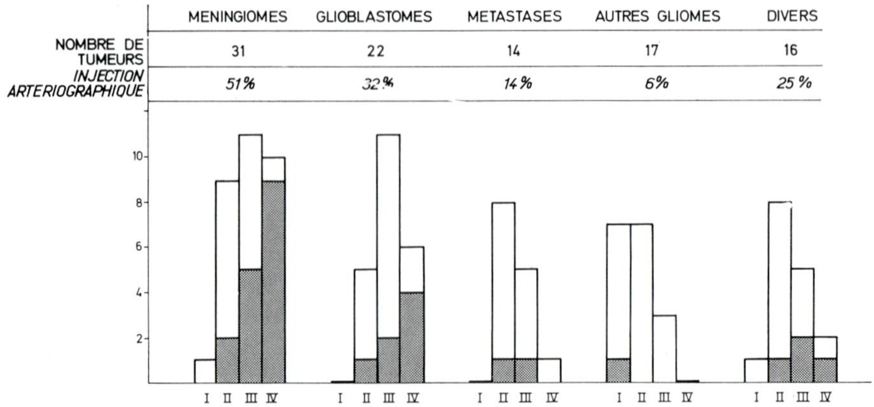

Fig. 2. Corrélation entre l'injection artériographique et l'intensité de la fixation radio-active selon la nature de la tumeur

Cette vitesse d'imprégnation est sous la dépendance de 2 facteurs essentiels: la richesse de la vascularisation tumorale et l'altération de la barrière hémato-encéphalique.

T. Planiol a montré avec la Sérum-Albumine marquée à l'Iode^{131} que l'on pouvait distinguer les tumeurs selon leur vitesse d'imprégnation, par des mesures successives faites au cours des 48 h suivant l'injection de ce composé radioactif.

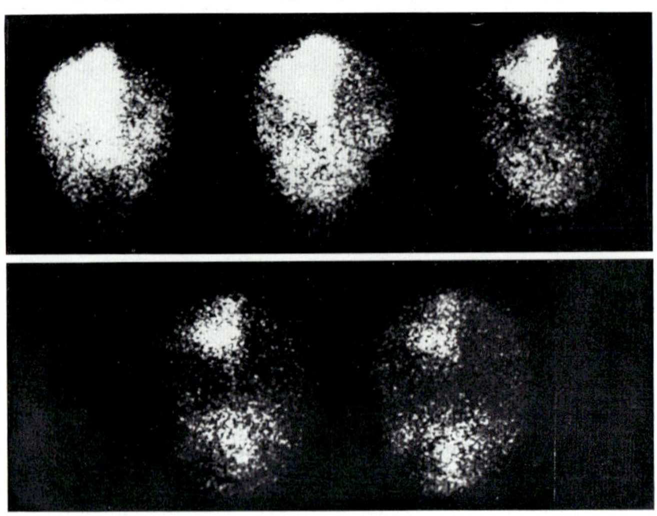

Fig. 3. Imprégnation radioactive immédiate (5 sec à 10 sec), puis rapidement décroissante, d'un angiome frontal interne droit

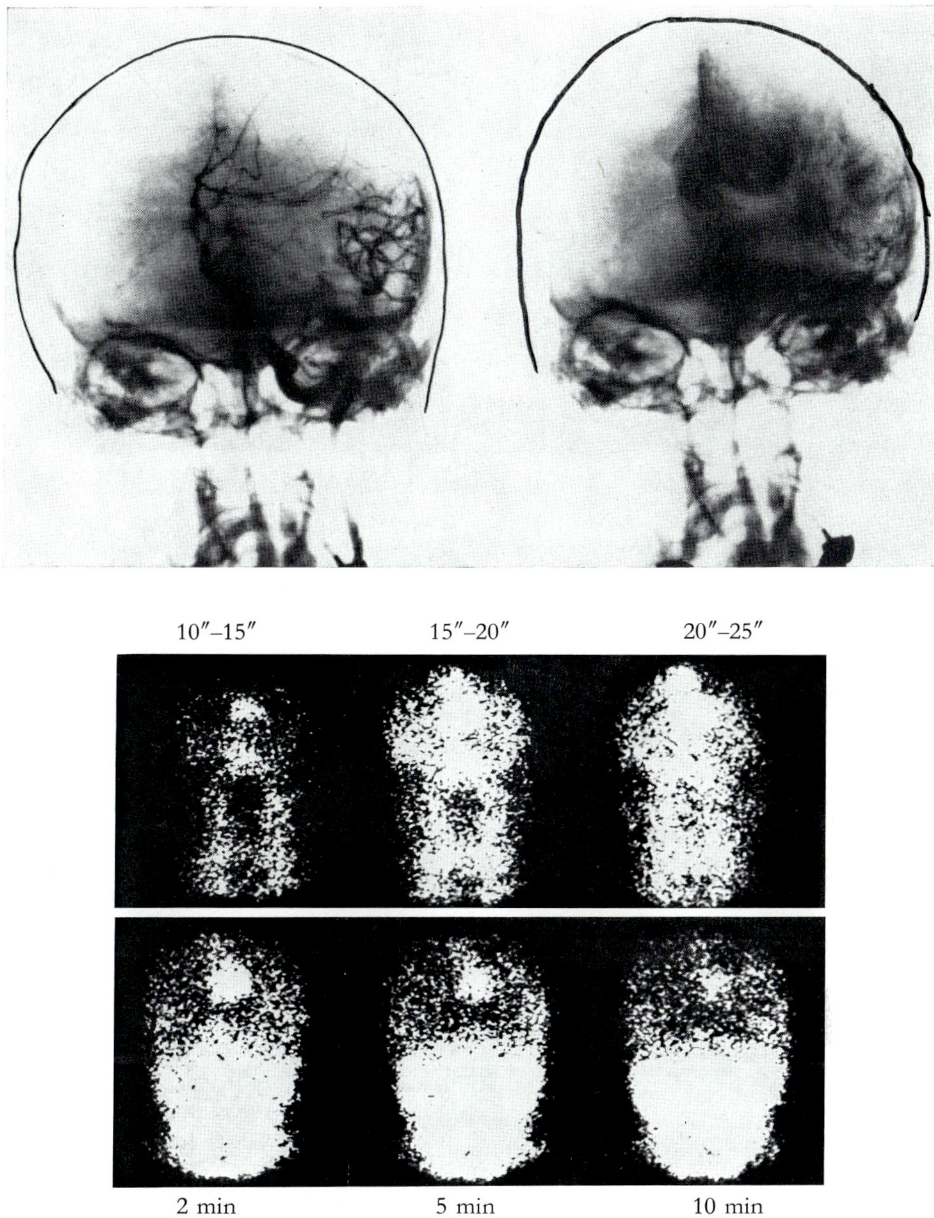

Fig. 4a et b. Méningiome de la faux du cerveau. a Images angiographiques. b Images scintigraphiques séquentielles: remplissage radio-actif maximum à la 25ème sec. Décroissance plus lente de la radioactivité tumorale

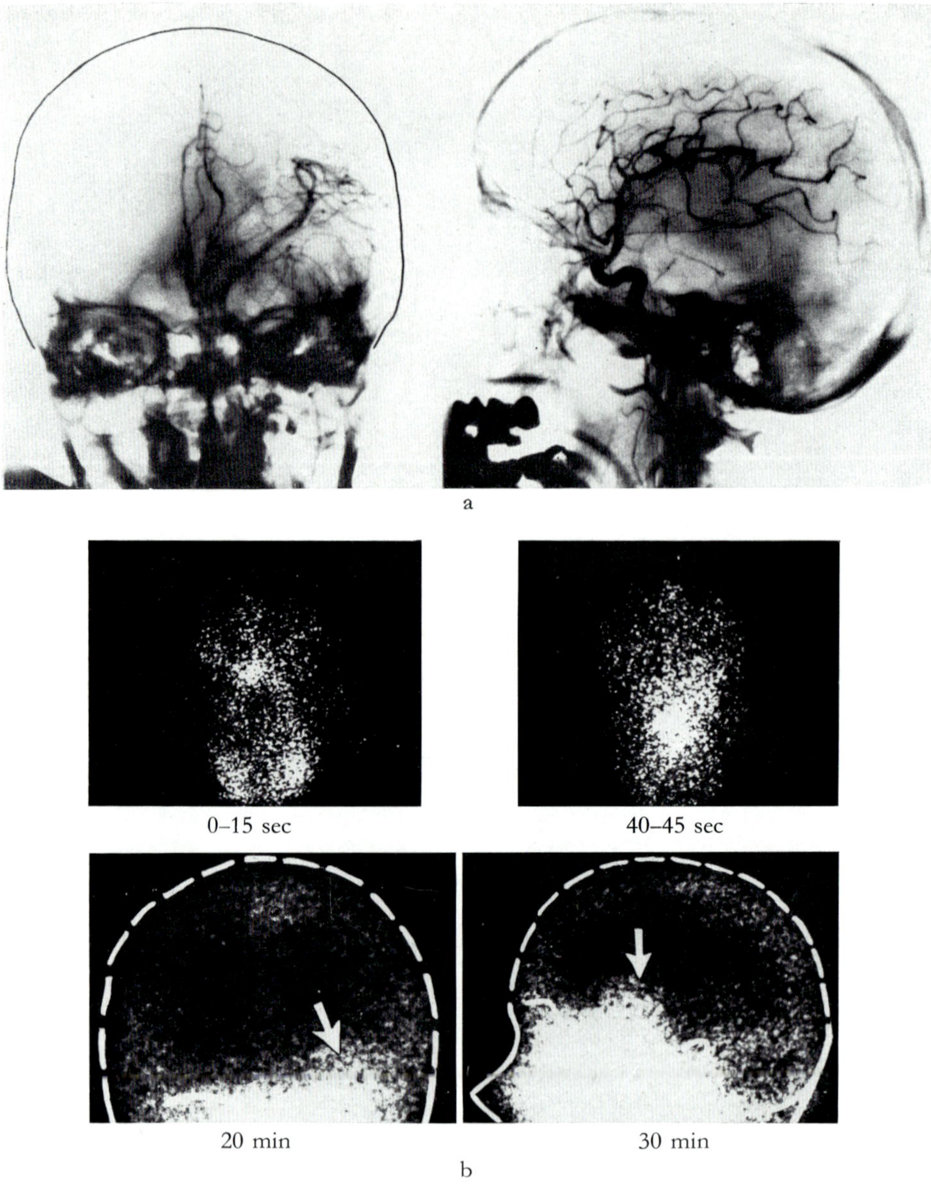

Fig. 5a et b. Glioblastome temporal gauche. a Image angiographique au temps artériel. De face, redressement du premier coude sylvien et refoulement de l'artère cérébrale antérieure. De profil, soulèvement de l'ensemble de l'artère cérébrale moyenne. b Images scintigraphiques. Entre 0 et 15 sec «angioscintigraphie»: les deux axes carotidiens et soulèvement de l'artère cérébrale moyenne gauche. De 40 à 45 sec: début d'imprégnation radioactive tumorale. A 20 et 30 min: foyer radioactif tumoral intense

Des phénomènes analogues peuvent être mis en évidence avec le pertéchnétate de ^{99m}Tc, mais dans un intervalle de temps beaucoup plus court, comme le montre le tableau 4 portant sur 30 explorations dynamiques.

Tableau 4. Étude dynamique de l'imprégnation des tumeurs par le pertechnétate ^{99m}Tc

	N	Imprégnation vasculaire		Imprégnation parenchymateuse	
		immédiate	progressive	1 à 20 min	> 20 min
Angiomes	3	3			
Méningiomes	10	2	7	1	
Hémangiomes	1		1		
Gliomes	8			7	1
Métastases	6		1	4	1
Divers	2			2	

Dans les lésions bénignes, richement vascularisées, comme les angiomes, les méngiomes, les hémangiomes, la lésion est imprégnée dès les premiers temps vasculaires de l'angio-scintigraphie réalisée à la caméra à scintillations. Dans les angiomes, le maximum d'imprégnation est immédiat, dès le premier temps artériel, pour décroître rapidement après (Fig. 3). Dans les méningiomes on note le plus souvent un remplissage progressif de la tumeur au cours des premières trente secondes (Fig. 4a et b).

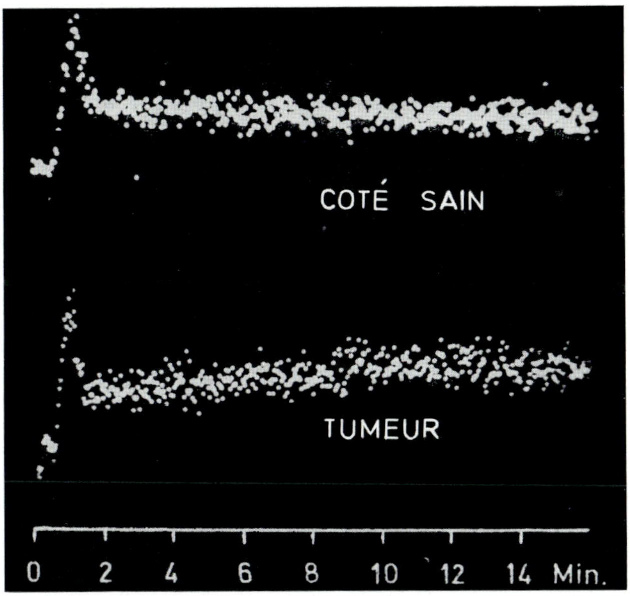

Fig. 6. Courbe d'imprégnation radioactive d'un glioblastome. Le maximum d'imprégnation de la tumeur est atteint à la 10ème min. Ces courbes sont obtenues sur l'analyseur à mémoire à 4096 canaux, à raison d'un point toutes les 0,5 sec

Dans les autres tumeurs, l'imprégnation radioactive est surtout liée à l'altération de la barrière hémato-encéphalique et elle se fait de façon plus lente et plus progressive au cours des minutes suivant l'injection du Technétium. Cette dynamique très différente de celle des angiomes et des méningiomes peut être illustrée par l'exemple d'un glioblastome (Fig. 5a et b). Elle peut être exprimée par des courbes comparatives des variations d'intensité radioactive à la fois dans la tumeur et dans la région saine homologue (Fig. 6).

Conclusions

1. Dans notre série de 100 tumeurs, dont la grande majorité était de siège sus-tentoriel, les pourcentages de tumeurs mises en évidence par artériographie et par scintigraphie au pertechnétate de ^{99m}Tc sont équivalents (90% et 91%).

2. L'association des deux méthodes a permis de mettre en évidence 98 des 100 tumeurs cérébrales étudiées.

3. Il existe une relation entre l'intensité de la fixation radioactive dans une tumeur et son injection à l'artériographie.

4. Il n'y a pas de corrélation étroite entre l'intensité de l'imprégnation radioactive et la nature de la tumeur.

5. Deux éléments peuvent contribuer efficacement à la détermination de nature d'une tumeur:

a) Son mode d'injection ou l'absence d'injection artériographique.

b) L'étude dynamique de son imprégnation radioactive á la caméra à scintillations.

La détection des métastases intracraniennes par scintigraphie et gammacisternographie

G. Galli, F. Simone, L. Troncone et G. de Rossi

Nous avons examinés 43 cas de métastases cérébrales, controlées par le cours clinique et les résultats opératoires et nécroscopiques.

Parmi nos cas, le carcinome poumonaire à été la plus fréquente source de métastases cérébrales (50%); suivent le carcinome mammaire et celui du rein (20% et 9%).

La métastase semblait unique dans le 55% des cas tandis que dans le 45% les foyers étaient multiples; c'est la tumeur pulmonaire qui nous a donné le plus élevé pourcentage de métastases multiples.

A la scintigraphie, les métastases peuvent présenter deux aspects:

1. le premier est celui d'une tache arrondie, à limite nette, avec captation intense et homogène;

2. l'autre est celui d'une zone de captation faible et hétérogène, de forme irrégulière et à limite estompée.

Les localisations néoplastiques assument l'un ou l'autre de tels aspects en rapport à divers facteurs; il y a une captation faible et une forme irrégulière lorsque les foyers sont petits ou nombreux; dans le cas d'hématome ou d'œdéme péritumoral; quand le foyer présente des zones necroticomalaciques; lorsq'il est enveloppé de couches de

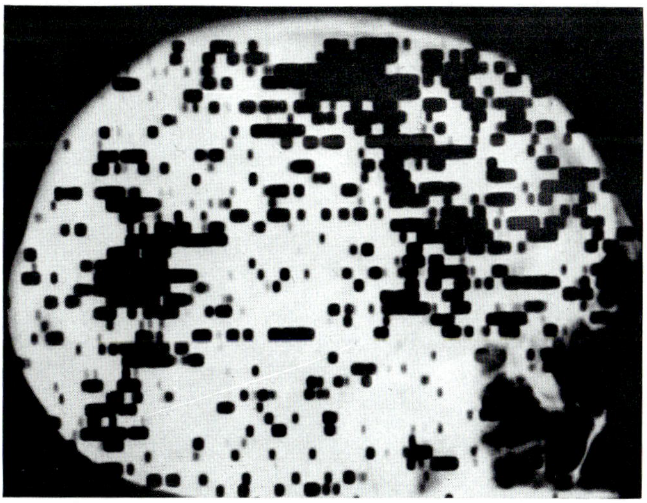

Fig. 1

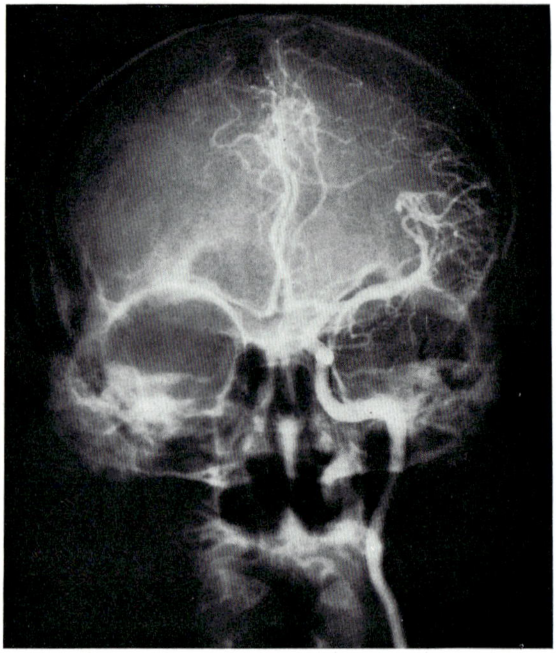

Fig. 2a

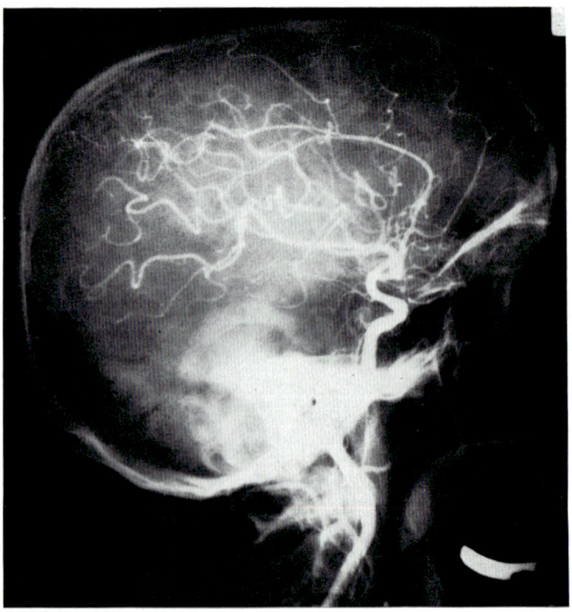

Fig. 2b

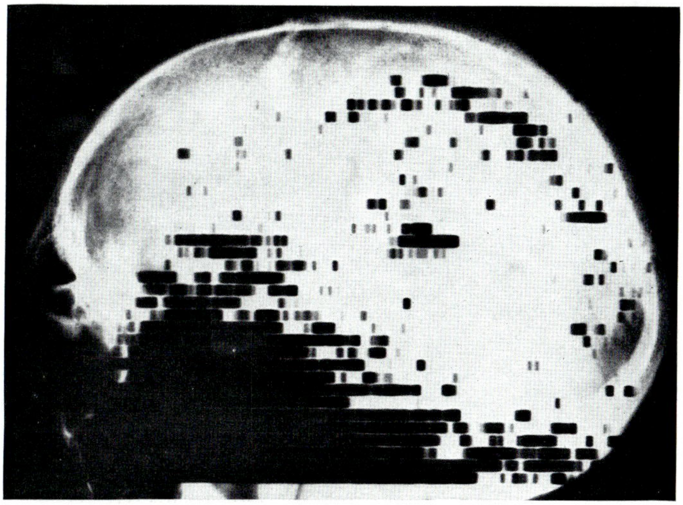

Fig. 3a

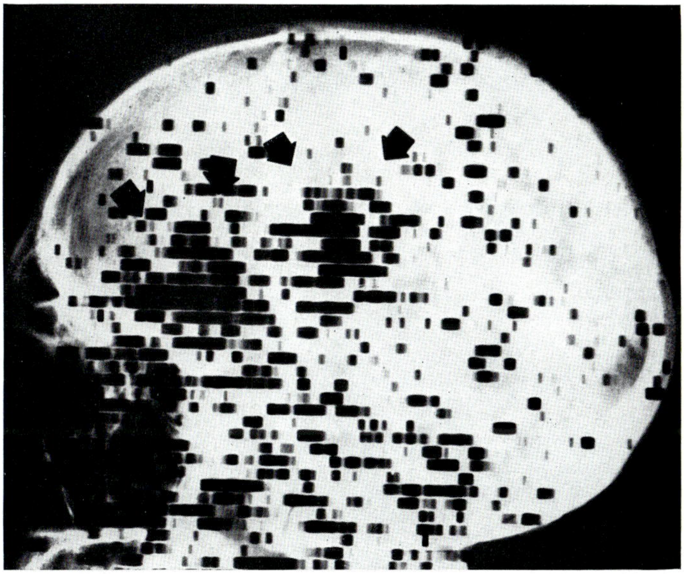

Fig. 3b

gliose réactive. Même le type de vascularisation a son importance; aux cadres scintigraphiques du Ier type correspondent souvent des aspects angiographiques caractérisés par une impregnation de la tumeur semblable à celle du méningiome; au 2 ème type des vaisseaux irréguliers et tortueux ou l'absence d'une vascularisation pathologique de la tumeur.

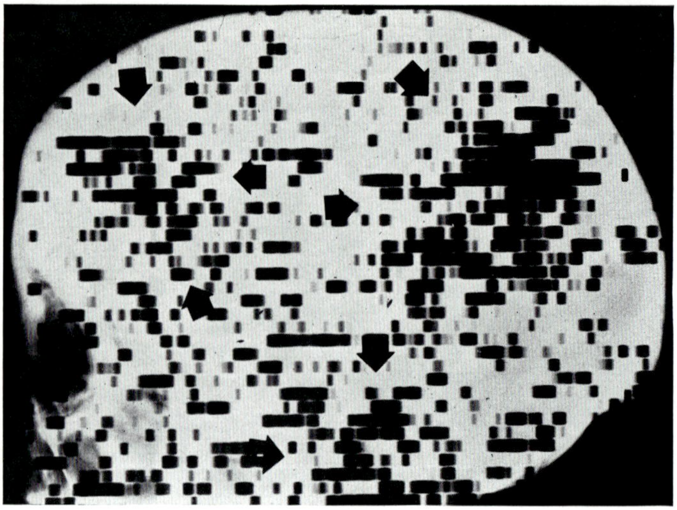

Fig. 4

Toutefois, en comparant la scintigraphie et l'angiographie, il faut souligner que la scintigraphie est bien plus efficace que l'angiographie dans la démonstration des métastases. Surtout les metastases petites et peripheriques, lorsque leur dissémination limite le déplacement des formations vasculaires, peuvent échapper à l'angiographie mais pas à la scintigraphie.

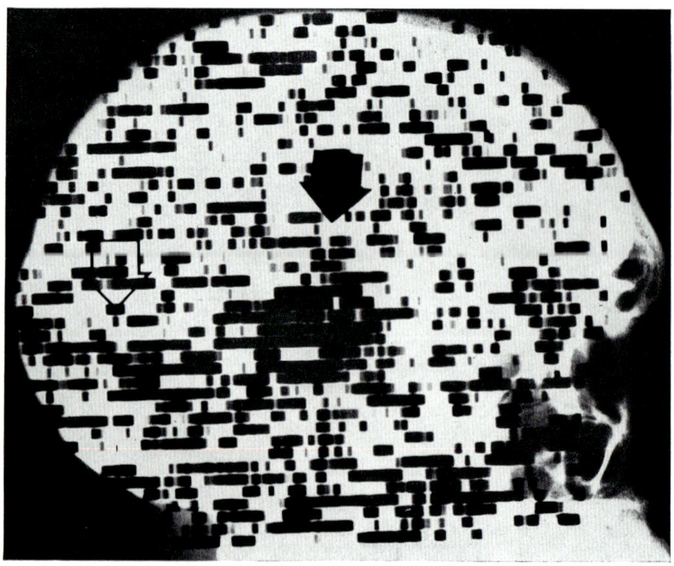

Fig. 5

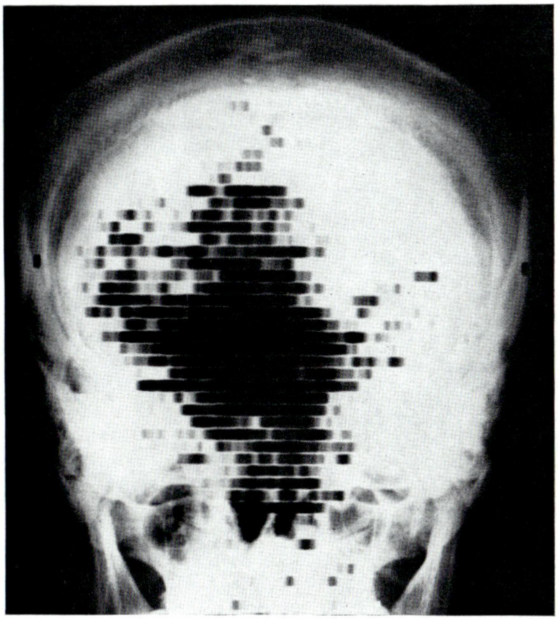

Fig. 6

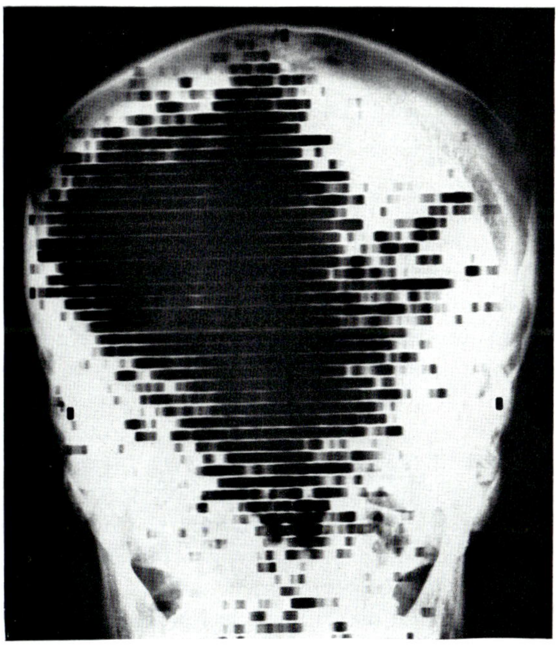

Fig. 7

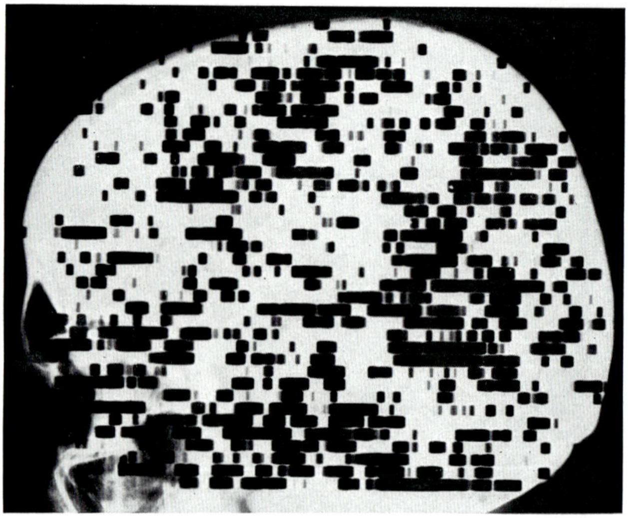

Fig. 8

La dissémination de métastases de la fig. 1 ne peut pas être soupçonnée, par example, à l'angiographie (Fig. 2a + b); même dans les temps capillaires et veineux il n'y avait pas des données significatives.

La valeur diagnostique de la scintigraphie est plus grande quand il y a la possibilité de la repéter le jour après l'introduction de la substance radioactive: avec la Chlormerodrin nous avons l'habitude de faire des observations à la Ière h et 24ème h et quelque fois 48ème h; avec ^{99m} Tc et ^{113m} In il est conseillable un contrôle entre la 4ème et la 6éme h. Sur 70% de nos cas, la métastase était mieux reconnaissable et souvent plus volumineuse dans le scintigramme à la 24ème heure; quelque fois, seulement cela permettait d'identifier l'altération ou de reconnaître la multiplicité des foyers pathologiques. Dans le cas de la figure 3a (Chloromerodrin ^{203} Hg) à la 1ère h la présence de métastases n'est pas sûre; mais dans le scintigramme à la 24ème h on peut voir deux grands foyers (métastases de t. poumonaire), (Fig. 3b).

Même la méthode scintigraphique a ses limites, surtout pour la possibilité que des foyers pathologiques d'autre nature simulent la presence d'une métastase; et il faut rappeler, à ce propos, que les malades avec une tumeur avancée sont exposés aux incidentes vasculaires cérébraux, comme des hémorragies et des tromboses.

Dans un des nos cas avec tumeur poumonaire l'histoire clinique et la symptomatologie faisaient soupçonner des métastases cerebrales; le scintigramme (Fig. 4) semblait le confirmer, mais à l'autopsie on a observé seulement des foyers multiples d'hemorragie.

Récemment, un autre examen radioisotopique se plaça aux cotés de la scintigraphie: la gamma-cisternographie. Nous avons été surpris en observant l'importance des alterations relevées par cet examen dans 8 cas de métastases cérébrales. Elles consistent dans une lente diffusion de la iodoséralbumine, dans l'amputation du »trident« Silvien, en de vastes défauts de remplissage des espaces sousarachnoidiens iusq' à une compléte absence d'activité dans un hèmisphère cérébral; on peut avoir aussi la pénétration de l'émetteur radioactif dans les ventricules cérébraux.

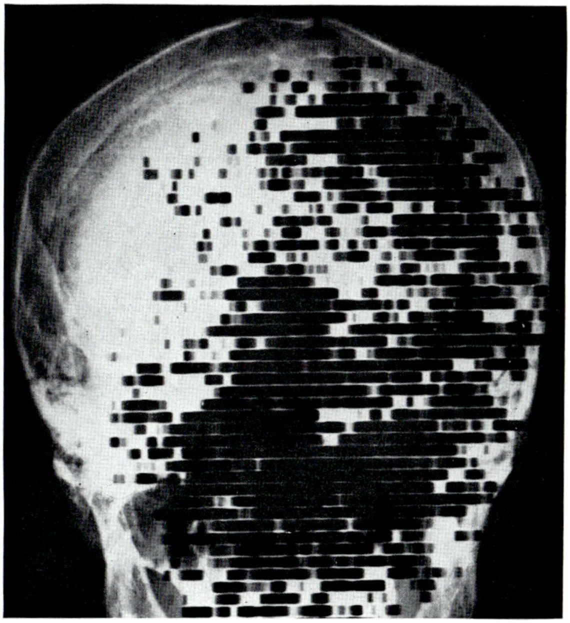

Fig. 9a

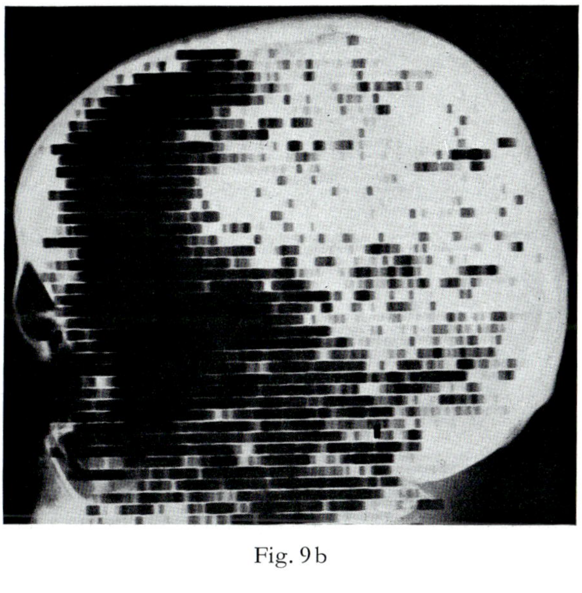

Fig. 9b

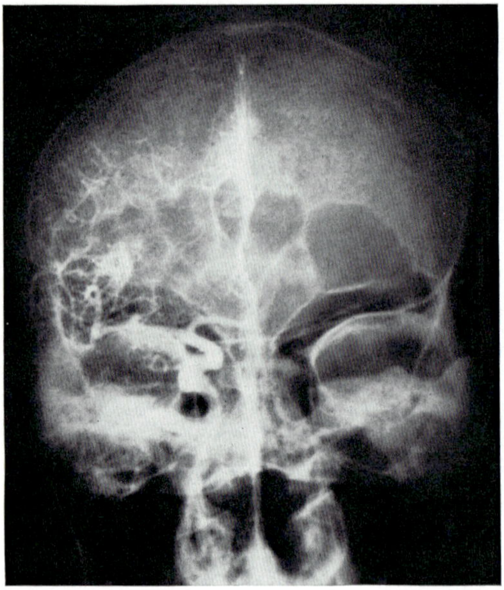

Fig. 10a

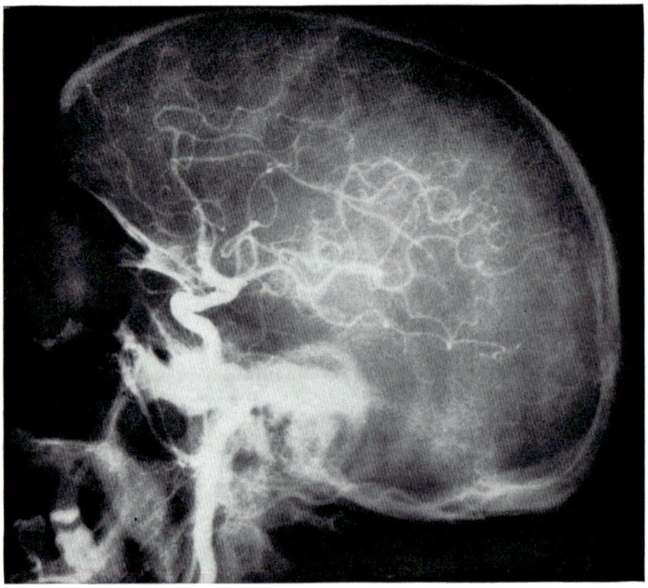

Fig. 10b

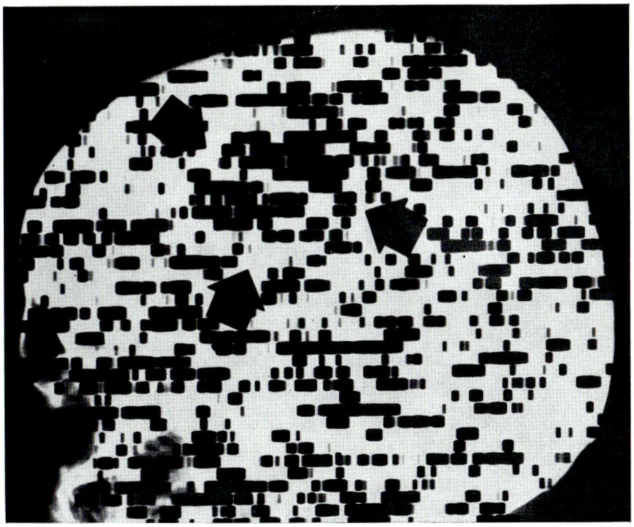

Fig. 11

Dans le cas de la figure 5 (T. mammaire) on voit à la scintigraphie deux métastases: la gamma-cisternographie (7ème h) (Fig. 6) montre l'amputation de la branche gauche du »trident« et le déplacément des structures moyennes. A la 24éme h est encore plus marquée l'absence de la iodoseralbumine dans une vaste zone des espaces sousaracnoidiens de la convexité cérébrale gauche; le traceur est présent dans le ventricul cérébral lateral droit (Fig. 7).

Dans un autre cas (t. poumonaire) le scintigramme (Fig. 8) fait soupçonner une disseminations de petites métastases mais les données de la gamma-cisternoscintigraphie sont bien plus éclatantes car il y a une absence de radioactivité dans presque tout l'hémisphère cérébral droit (Fig. 9a+b), tandis que l'artériographie (Fig. 10a+b) ne permettait pas d'imaginer la gravité des alterations.

Aussi dans le cas des figures 11+12 au pétit foyer métastatique frontal aperçu à la scintigraphie (Fig. 11) correspondent à la gamma-cisterno-scintigraphie (Fig. 12a+b) des larges défauts de remplissage radioactif des éspaces sousaracnoidiens.

On pourrait conclure que en cas de métastases cérebrales l'alteration de la circulation du L. C. S. est imposante; donc les données de la gammacisternographie sont – en géneral – plus éclatantes que celles de la scintigraphie, même si elles ne sont pas spécifiques. Voilà pourquoi nous pensons que avec la cisternographie il y a la possibilitè de surmonter certaines limitations de la scintigraphie. Biensûr, la cisternographie ne peut pas remplacer la scintigraphie: celle ci est toujours indispensable pour identifier les foyers pathologiques et pour les localiser de manière a justifier la symptomatologie, ou pour établir et controler la radiothérapie.

Toutefois la gammacisternographie, comme examen complémentaire, pourrait éclaircir des cas qui sont à la limite et confirmer la pertinence cérébrale des altérations, jusqu'a eviter d'avoir recours à des techniques laborieuses et plus dangereuses comme celles de la neuroradiologie.

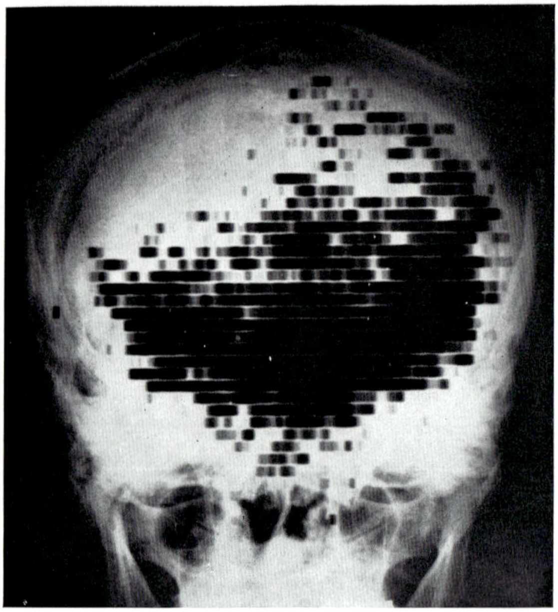

Fig. 12a

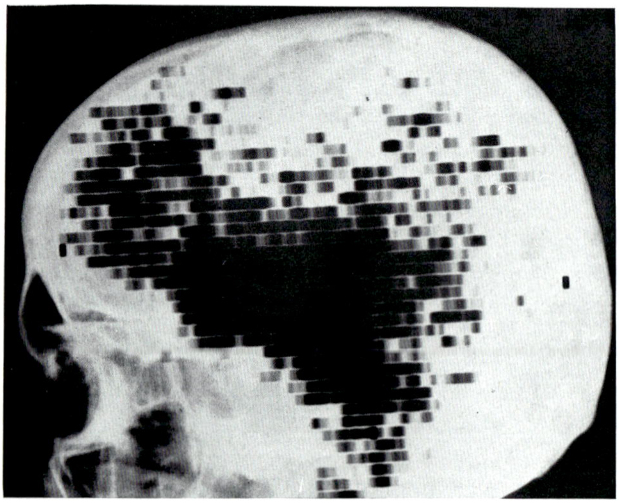

Fig. 12b

The Value of Diagnostic Procedures in Brain Tumor Identification

E. Schmidt-Wittkamp, U. Piepgras and F. Ohlmann

The positive effect of different investigations by the diagnosis of brain tumors is evaluated by the screening of a continous series of 2000 cases. All of these patients had the symptoms of brain disorders and were therefore brain scanned with different radioisotopes mainly with ^{197}Hg-Chlormerodrine and ^{99m}Tc Pertechnetate. The scanner used for these investigation was a PICKER-Magna Scanner V.

In these group of 2000 cases there were 278 patients who had a brain tumor. The histological diagnosis of these tumors is shown in Table 1.

Table 1

Tumors	Anzahl
Glioblastoma	68
Astrozytoma	14
Medulloblastoma	2
Oligodendroglioma	12
Spongioblastoma	2
Ependymoma	2
Unclassified glioma	15
Meningeoma	36
Neurinoma	8
Pituitary tumors	13
Pinealoma	1
Rare Primary Brain Tumors	17
Metastases	46
Tumors without Histological Diagnosis	42
Total	278

In the evaluation of the different methods of identification of brain tumors the percentage of the total cases has been determined and the results comparecd with other studies (Table 2).

The *X-rays of the skull* show in 38% of our cases that a brain tumor was present. Overton *et al.* (1965) and Goodrich *et al.* (1964) found a similar percentage in their studies of about 37% and 39%. About the same time, 1965, Afifi found only 17% of his brain tumor cases with the normal x-ray.

The *electroencephalogram* did not show a marked difference from the results of the other investigators. Previously, the *pneumoencephalogram* gave a positive indication

Table 2

	Overton *et al.* (1965)	Goodrich *et al.* (1963)	Loken *et al.* (1967)	McCormack and Newton (1966)	Afifi *et al.* (1965)	Own results
Normal-X-rays	37	39	—	—	17	38
EEG	71	67	—	—	60	61
Scan	84	85	78	68	48	82
PEG	91	80	76	85	86	79
Angiography	84	85	72	79	91	85

of brain tumor in most cases, and even today this process has a limited but worthwhile indication. We use pneumoencephalographic studies only if all other neuroradiological procedures give no clear picture of the brain lesion. In our series pneumoencephalography indicated that 79% of the studied cases had a brain tumor and located the exact area. In the series made by Loken *et al.* (1967) the results showed an identification percentage of 76%. Other authors reported a higher rate of identification: Overton 91%, Afifi 86%, McCormack and Newton 85% and Goodrich 80%.

Brainscanning has a positive result in 82% of our cases with brain tumors. In some cases the brain scann showed positive indications where before there was no suspicion of tumor. In other cases the brain scann supported the original diagnosis. Overton showed 84% and Goodrich 85% with a positive result and the investigations of Loken indicated 78%, which is not much different than the forementioned rates. Only McCormack and Newton had positive indications in 68% and Afifi in 48% of their cases.

Angiographic studies of the brain stand at the present as the most dominant process in the positive indication of a tumor. and the presurgical verification of the type of tumor. With a positive rate of 85% in our cases there is practically no difference between the findings of Overton, Goodrich, and McCormack. The difference in the percentage rates of the other authors is probably caused by the different characteristics and the nature of the case sent to the investigators for study.

In concluding this study one can say, that for the verification process of a brain tumor three methods, which are easily performed and which are completly unharmfull to the patient are of dominant importance. That is: X-rays of the skull, EEG and espially brain scanning. A wide spread use of these three methods will bring us to a diagnosis of brain tumors in an infant stage, so that immediate treatment can be initiated.

Vergleichende Untersuchungen zur Aussagekraft verschiedener szintigraphischer Untersuchungsverfahren und der Angiographie in der Hirntumorlokalisationsdiagnostik

U. Zeidler, S. Kottke, A. Seeberg und H. Hundeshagen

Es soll dargelegt werden, welche Indikationen für die Hirnszintigraphie sich aus unseren Untersuchungen ergeben haben. Voraussetzung hierfür ist die Kenntnis des diagnostischen Wertes der Szintigraphie.

Die diagnostische Aussage hängt dabei von der Lokalisation des Tumors ab. 92% aller Hemisphärentumoren konnten nachgewiesen werden. Nur 42% der basisnahen oder infratentoriell gelegenen Tumoren waren darstellbar. Auch die Abhängigkeit von der Art des Tumors ist evident: 10 der nicht erkannten Hemisphärentumoren waren Astrocytome (Kernohan I/II).

Bei der Angiographie zeigten nur 50% der wiedergegebenen Tumoren eine Kontrastmittelfärbung oder pathologische Gefäße. In den übrigen Fällen waren Gefäßverlagerungen durch avasculäre Massen erkennbar; in 10% der Fälle fand sich auch im Angiogramm kein Tumorhinweis. In neun dieser Fälle konnte eine exakte Lokalisation durch die Szintigraphie erfolgen.

Die Verlagerung der Gefäße kann gering sein, wenn der Tumor von größeren Gefäßen entfernt gelegen ist, insbesondere bei paramedianen Geschwülsten, oder wenn ein perifokales Ödem nur gering ausgeprägt ist. In diesen Fällen, die unter Umständen zusätzlich eine Pneumencephalographie erforderlich machen, kann statt dessen die Szintigraphie erfolgreich eingesetzt werden. Durch ihre Anwendung ist die Anzahl zusätzlich erforderlicher Pneumencephalographien bei Hemisphärentumoren reduziert worden. Die Szintigraphie ermöglicht zusätzlich eine gute Beurteilung bei vermuteter Balkeninfiltration und kann bei multiplen Prozessen dem Verfahren der Angiographie überlegen sein.

Das subdurale akute Hämatom und Gefäßmißbildungen, die nicht zu Blutungen geführt haben, sind keine Indikation für die Szintigraphie. Trotz nachweisbarer Erfolge ist die Methode wegen der schlechteren Auflösung der Tomo-Angiographie unterlegen. Auch die Serienszintigraphie kann diesen Nachteil nicht aufwiegen.

Artdiagnostische Hinweise erlaubt das szintigraphische Bild allein nicht. Durch Berücksichtigung anderer Momente wie Prädilektionsorte und Verlaufsuntersuchungen lassen sich gewisse hilfreiche Schlüsse ziehen.

Wesentlich für die Bewertung der Methode ist die Präsentation der Information für den Therapeuten. Wir unterstützen die Forderung der Neurochirurgen nach Darstellung in natürlicher Größe für den Vergleich zu angiographischen und pneumencephalographischen Befunden. Diese Information läßt sich bei dem heutigen Stand der Technik am besten und sichersten mit einem Scanner gewinnen. Dabei können Szintigramm und Röntgenbild auf dem gleichen Film aufgenommen werden.

Aufnahmen mit der Gammakamera bringen bei exakter Betrachtung nicht den propagierten Zeitgewinn und haben verminderte Nachweis-Sicherheit bei verschlechterter Lokalisation zur Folge. Wenn Schnelligkeit und Datenverarbeitung gewünscht werden, scheint unter Berücksichtigung des derzeitigen technischen Standes ein Szintigraphie-Gerät mit zwei Detektoren sinnvoll und anderen Verfahren, auch dem 10-Kristall-Scanner überlegen. Ein parietal gelegener Tumor konnte aus der Information beider Meßköpfe zusammen und nach Abzug der Information von der gesunden Seite dargestellt werden. Eine gleichzeitige Röntgenaufnahme des Schädels würde den Wert dieser Darstellung noch erhöhen.

Die Bedeutung der Szintigraphie ist nach unseren Befunden in der direkten Tumordarstellung zu sehen, die es ermöglicht, avasculäre raumfordernde Prozesse exakter einzuordnen und damit vor dem operativen Vorgehen eine noch größere Sicherheit in der Beurteilung von Lage und Ausdehnung des Tumors gewährleistet.

The Value of Brain Scintigraphy (Technetium-99m) in the Topographic Diagnosis of Space-Occupying Intracranial Lesions

H. Waldbaur, W. Walter, E. Krönert and F. Wolf

In a group of 260 patients where brain scintigraphy with ^{99m}Tc-pertechnetate was carried out, there were 148 brain tumor patients.

Table 1 shows a comparison of the scintigraphic and angiographic findings in cases of supratentorial tumor. In a series of 123 cases, there were 15 normal scintigrams, 18 questionable or inexactly localized findings and 90 patients (73%) where the localization and extent of the tumor could be demonstrated with accuracy. In the angiogram, the space-occupying lesion was localized largely on the basis of vessel displacement in 57 cases (46%) while another 48 patients (39%) revealed a tumor "shadow" which indicated the extent of the tumor. The highest degree of accuracy was achieved by scintigraphy in cases of glioblastomas (94%), whereas only 33% of the astrocytomas were found by this method. In cases of meningioma the percentage was 89% and in cases of carcinoma metastases, 70%. In 12 cases of recurrence, the topographic diagnosis was good in 10 cases, all 6 gliomas being among them. In this group, the histological picture of the recurrence generally revealed signs of malignant degeneration.

Table 2 demonstrates the significance of scintigraphy and angiography in setting the indication for operation. Among the 123 above-mentioned supratentorial tumors, the scintigram was decisive for setting the indication for operation in 6 cases, in another 23 patients the scintigram permitted a better topographical diagnosis than the angiogram, in 63 cases the results were identical, 21 times the results of the angiography was better, in 8 cases pneumoencephalography or ventriculography was performed in addition to the scintigram and the angiogram and in 2 cases the angiographic finding was complemented by the scintigram.

Of the 13 infratentorial tumors only 6 could be localized accurately with scintigraphy (Table 3).

To exemplify the cases where scintigraphy was the decisive method of all the investigations performed, the pictures of one patient are shown in whom the angiogram did not serve any localizing function while the scintigram showed a deep-seated, bilateral and thus inoperable tumor. At the autopsy of the patient, who died a short time later, a Hodgkin sarkoma was found which occupied the more caudal parts of the corpus callosum and of both lateral ventricles, as well as the brain stem.

How the results of angiography and scintigraphy can complement each other is demonstrated in the example of a parieto-occipital glioblastoma. Here the extent

Table 1. *Scintigraphic and angiographic findings in supratentorial tumours*

	Number of Pat.	Scintigraphy normal	Scintigraphy questionabl. or inexactly localized	Scintigraphy localisation and extension correct	Angiography normal	Angiography pathol. without localisation	Angiography localis. correct	Angiography localisation and extension correct
total without cases of recurrence	123	15	18	90 (73 %)	6	12	57 (46 %)	48 (39 %)
Glioblastoma	48	1	2	45 (94 %)	2	1	19	26
Astrocytoma	12	5	3	4 (33 %)		2	7	3
Oligodendroglioma	2	1		1			2	
Glioma with increased growth	6		2	4			4	2
Meningioma	19		2	17 (89 %)		3	6	10
Carcinoma metastases	10		3	7 (70 %)	1		6	3
Sarcoma	7		1	6	1	1	3	2
Epidermoidal tumours	3	2	1			1	2	
Other tumours	10	3	2	5		2	6	2
Tumours of brain stem	6	3	2	1	2	2	2	
Recurrences								
total	12	2		10 (83 %)		1	5	6
Glioma	6			6			2	4
Ependymoma	1			1		1		
Meningioma	4	2		2			2	2
Sarcoma	1			1			1	

Table 2. *Significance of scintigraphy and angiography for setting indication for operation [supratentorial tumours]*

	Number of Pat	Scintigram decisive for setting indication	better topical diagnosis by scintigraphy	identical results	Results of angiography better	additional examinations necessary	angiographic results completed by scintigram
total without cases of recurrence	123	6	23	63	21	8	2
Glioblastoma	48	2	9	33	3		1
Astrocytoma	12		1	3	7	1	
Oligodendroglioma	2		1		1		
Glioma with increased growth	6		3	1	2		
Meningioma	19	3	4	12			
Carcinoma metastases	10			8		2	
Sarcoma	7		2	4		1	
Epidermoidal tumours	3				2	1	
Other tumours	10	1	2	2	4		1
Tumours of brain stem	6		1		2	3	
Recurrences							
total	12	1	2	5	3		1
Glioma	6		1	3	1		1
Ependymona	1	1					
Meningioma	4			2	2		
Sarcoma	1		1				

was largely determined by the degree of vessel displacement in the angiogram. Only a portion of the affected area was depicted in the scintigram as a zone of increased activity. The suspicion that the remainder of the tumor was cystic, was confirmed at operation.

Table 3. *Scintigraphic findings in infratentorial tumours*

	number of Pat.	normal	questionable or inexactly localized	localisation and extension correct
Medulloblastoma	1	1	—	—
Spongioblastoma	3	1	1	1
Angioblastoma	1	1	—	—
Carcinoma-Metastases	7	2	1	4
Trigeminal Neurinoma	1	—	—	1
Total	13	5	2	6 (46 %)

^{57}Se-Scintigraphy in Differential Diagnosis of Benign and Malignant Cerebral Processes

E. NORDMAN and A. REKONEN

By using ^{99m}Tc in gamma scintigraphy it is possible to visualize different processes in the brain. However, malignant and benign cerebral lesions cannot be differentiated by means of ^{99m}Tc scintigrams. Some authors (CAVALIERI, PEREZ-MODREGO, FREDERIKSEN) have used sodiumselenite (Se-75) in the scanning of tumours situated in different parts of the body. They were able to visualize about $^{2}/_{3}$ of malignant tumours by using this isotope.

We have used ^{75}Se in tumor scanning for over a year, and the purpose of this work has been to study the tumour specifity of the sodiumselenite ^{75}Se and the value of this method in differential diagnosis of benign and malignant processes.

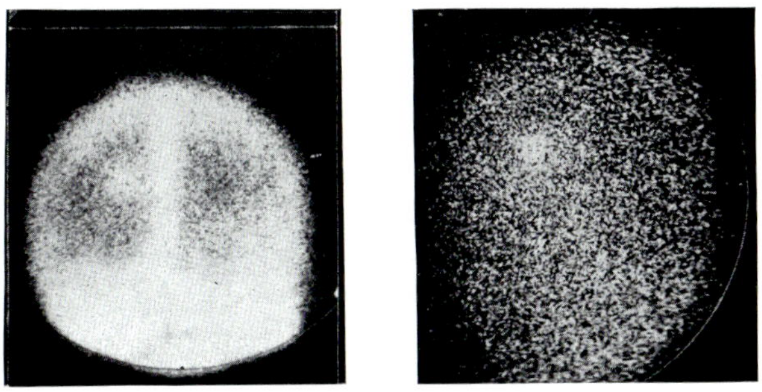

Fig. 1. ^{99m}Tc and ^{75}Se-scintigraphies of the metastasis of cutaneous melanoma in the brain

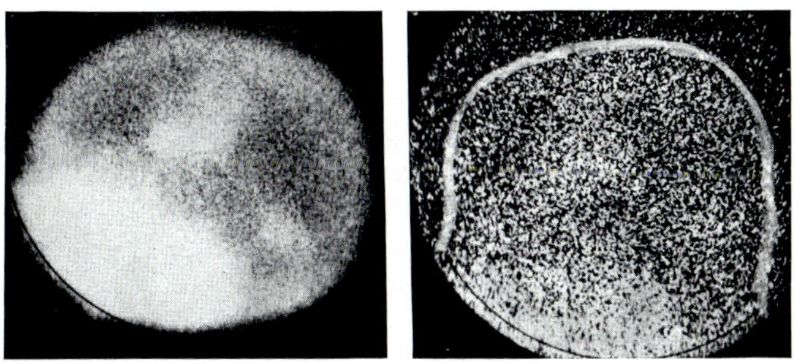

Fig. 2. Cerebral infarct pictured with ^{99m}Tc and ^{75}Se

The material is composed of about 50 patients with different brain lesions. The first gamma scintigraphy was performed by using of 10 mCi ^{99m}Tc and during the following day the patient was scanned with 300 μCi of ^{75}Se sodium selenite. Pictures were taken by a gammacamera Pho Gamma III. Positive findings were detected by us in about 80% in the malignant cases. Detectable accumulation was seen with selenite in 75% in the same cases. ^{75}Se accumulation diminished to a considerable amount or disappeared after radiotherapy. In the group of the benign brain processes the ^{99m}Tc accumulation was seen in all cases. A positive finding with selenite was seen only in 30% of the same cases, and in these the isotope accumulation was rather poor.

As examples brain scans of malignant and benign lesions are presented.

Differential Scintigraphic Diagnosis of Focal Brain Lesions

M. Sanguineti, G. Scopinaro, A. Gottlieb, S. Damiani and G. Grossi

The alteration of the blood-brain barrier, the presence of a stroma and the increased vascularity are the main conditioning factors of the radioactive material uptake in focal brain lesions. An active uptake of the indicator by the tumor cells has been recently demonstrated. The time course of the accumulation of radioactivity depends on the prevalence of one of the already mentioned factors; its space pattern is strictly related to the shape and extent of the lesion. We think it is possible to suspect the nature of the lesions by analizing the time course and the space patterns of the abnormally increased activity.

Analysis of Time Course of Radioactivity

In evaluating the scintigraphic activity of a lesion and the time needed for accumulation and elimination of the indicator it is useful to take the vascular area of vertex as a term of comparison. It is then possible to establish a semiquantitative ratio between pathological and vascular activity and, namely:

1. to judge on the single scan whether the abnormal area as compared with the vertex is hypo-, iso- or hyper-active;

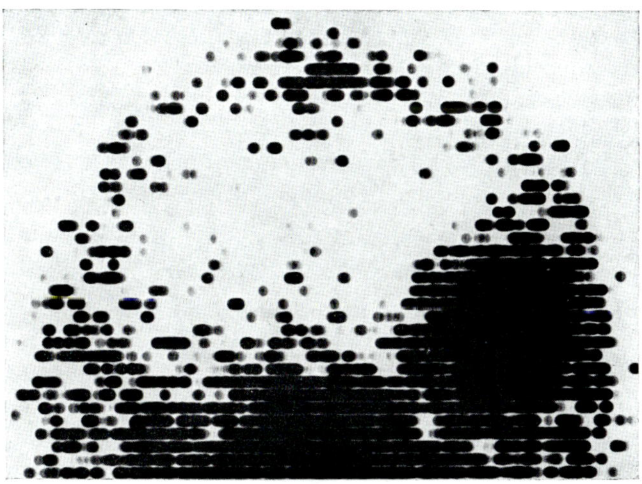

Fig. 1a

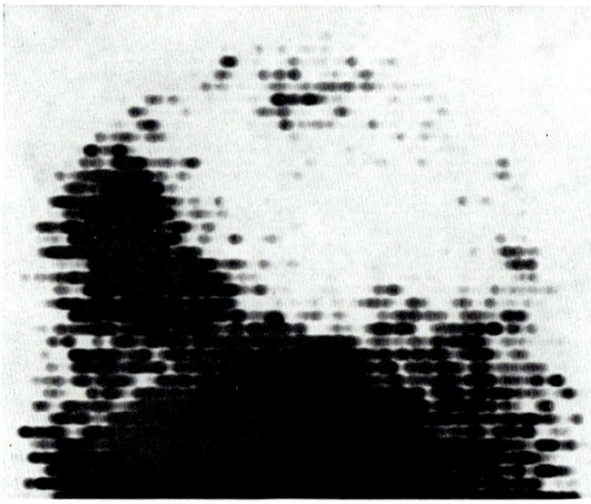

Fig. 1b

2. to evaluate with a series of scans, taken at different times, whether the accumulation of the tracer in the lesion takes place sooner or later than that at vertex and, chiefly, whether the activity of the lesion decreases before or simultaneously with the vascular one.

On the basis of our experience and of the data published by different authors we think it is possible to arrive at the following conclusions:

A. In considering the lesion to vascular area concentration ratio it may be stated that:

1. The activity of most of the tumors and brain softenings is higher than the vascular one (see Figs. 1 and 2).

2. In the intracerebral vasculopathic or post-traumatic hematomas the focal activity is equal or lower than the vascular one (see Fig. 2).

3. The subdural hematomas characteristically show in the antero-posterior and postero-anterior views an activity higher than that present at the vertex while in the lateral views the concentration is lower (see Fig. 3).

4. In craniotomies and in brain contusions the activity is always lower than that at the vertex (see Fig. 4).

5. In brain abscesses the activity may be higher or lower than at vertex, this variability being related to size and stage of the lesion (see Fig. 2).

B. In comparing the time behaviour of the activity of the lesion with that of the vascular activity at the vertex it may be stated that:

1. While in some tumors a captation cannot be demonstrated at all, in some others it can take place either early or very late. We think nevertheless that for a differential diagnosis between tumoral and non tumoral lesions it is usefull to observe wether or not the activity of the lesion decreases simultaneously with the vascular one. We can thus see that usually the activity of a neoplastic lesion decreases slower than that at vertex and that some tumors ar still highly active when the circulating activity is a negligible one (see Fig. 5).

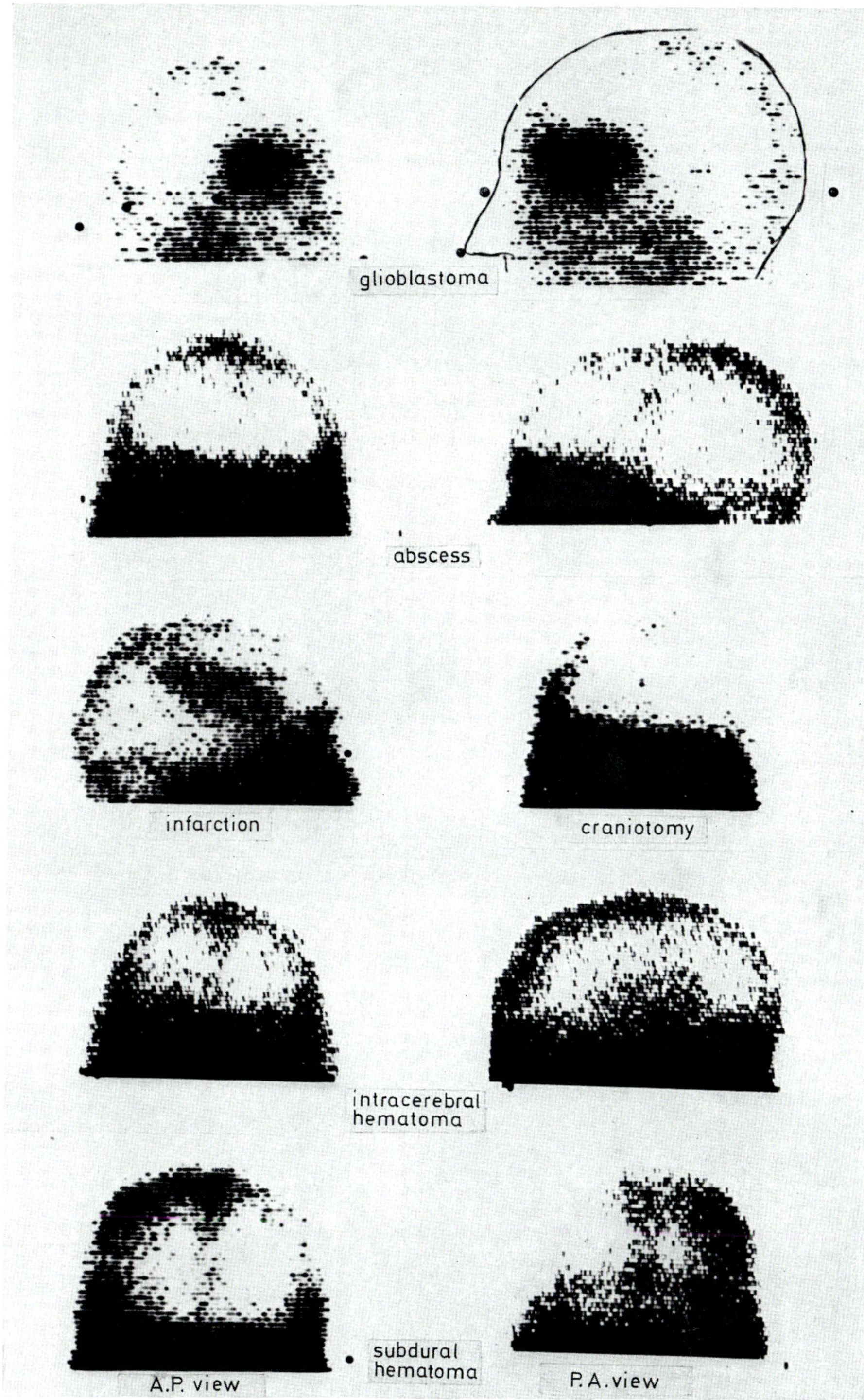
glioblastoma
abscess
infarction
craniotomy
intracerebral hematoma
subdural hematoma
A.P. view
P.A. view

Fig. 2

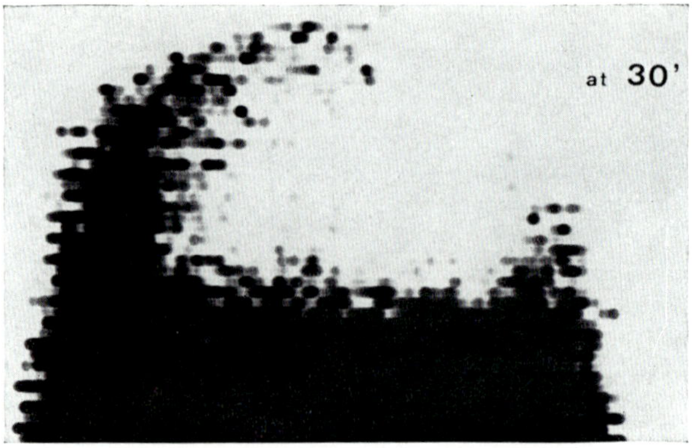

Fig. 3a

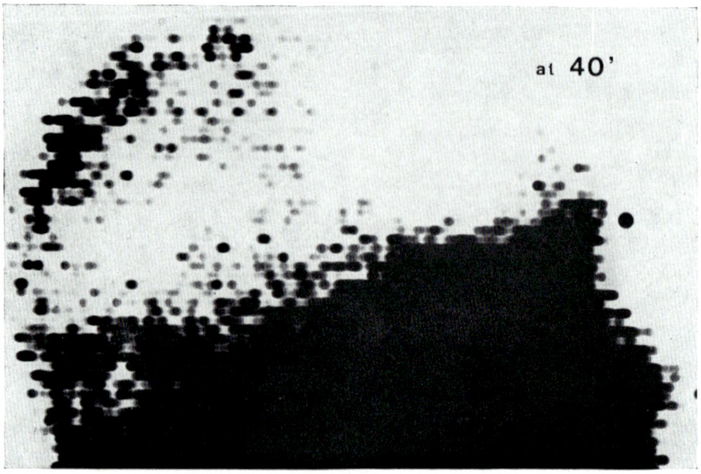

Fig. 3b

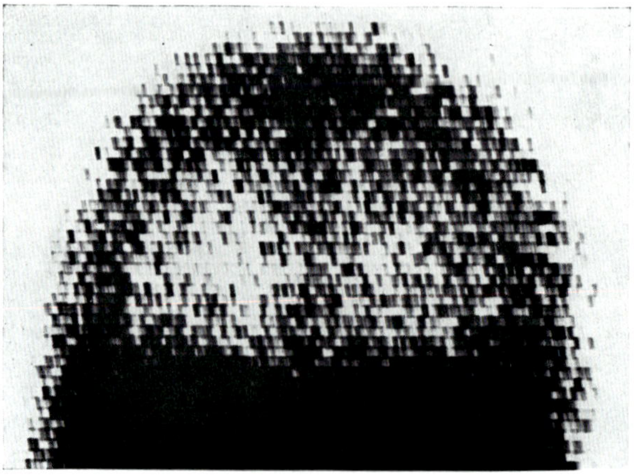
Fig. 4a

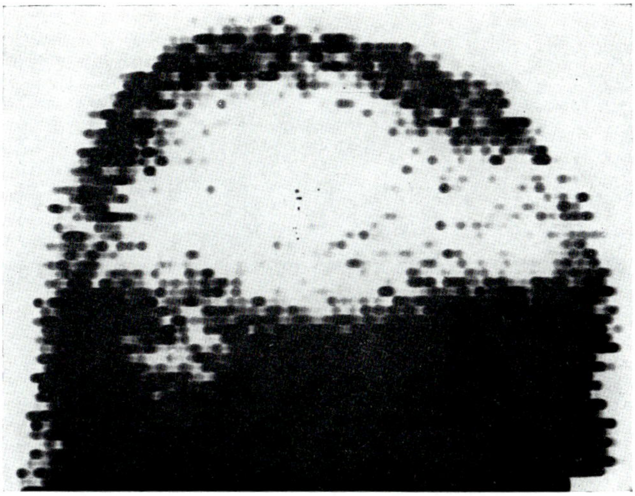

Fig. 4b

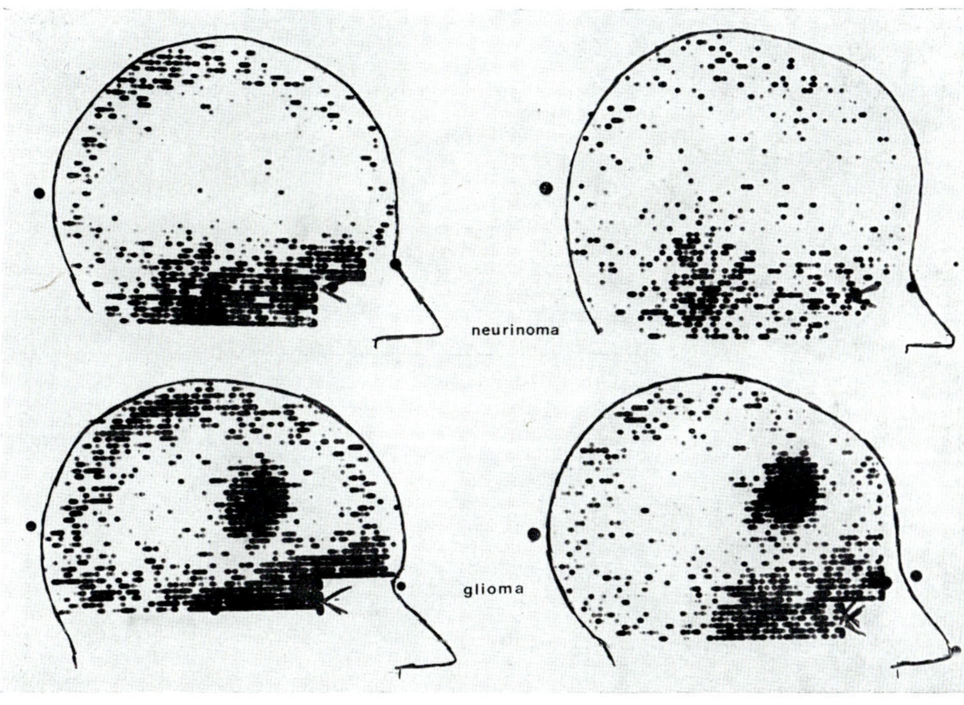

Fig. 5

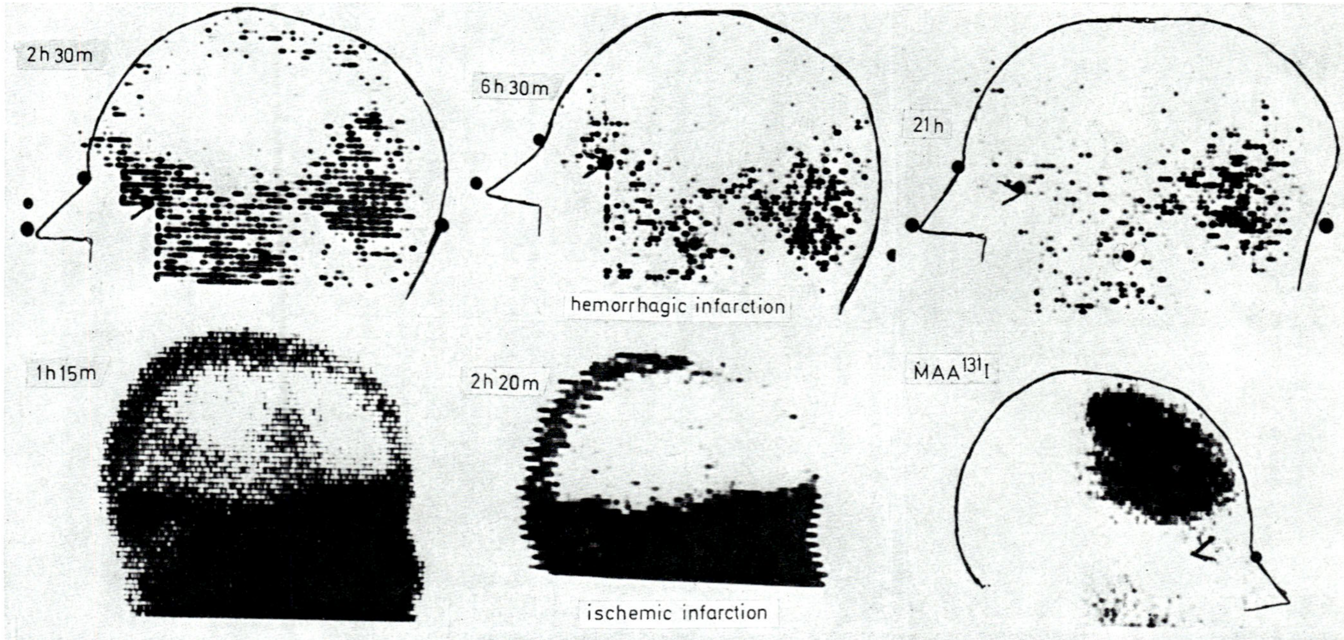
2h 30m
6h 30m
21h
hemorrhagic infarction
1h 15m
2h 20m
MAA ^{131}I
ischemic infarction

Fig. 6

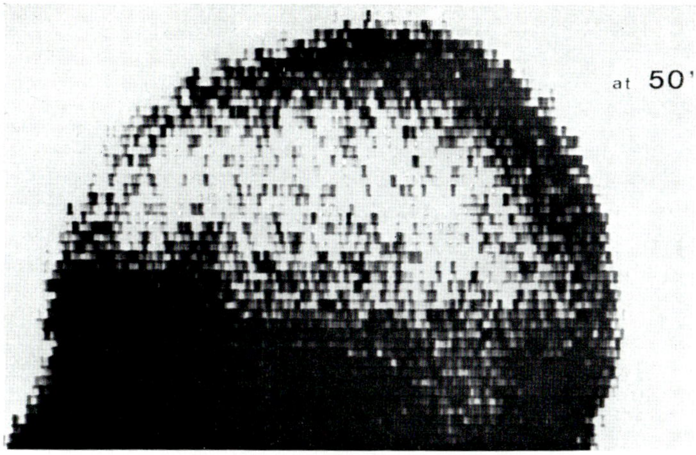

Fig. 7a

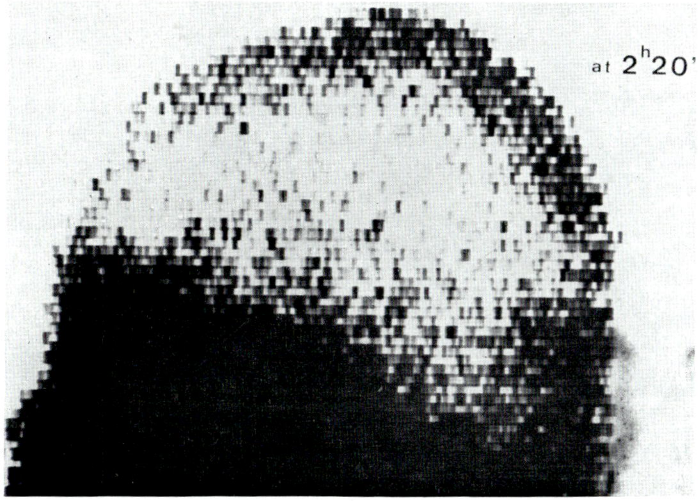

Fig. 7b

2. In the case of a brain softening a different behaviour is present according to the type of softening (ischemic or hemorrhagic). In the case of an ischemic softening the increasing vascularity around the lesion plays a leading role in determining the accumulation of the tracer and therefore the activity decreases almost simultaneously with the vascular one.

On the other hand, in the case of a hemorrhagic softening, the activity is chiefly related to the alteration of the blood-brain barrier so that the concentration is not only high but also its removal from the softened area takes place slowlier than from the vascular area (see Fig. 6).

3. In case of intracerebral vasculopathic hemorrhage the activity decreases almost simultaneously with that at the vertex (see Fig. 7).

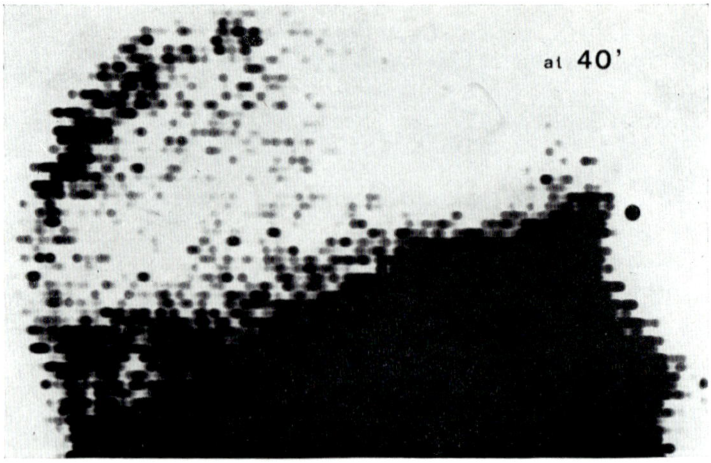

Fig. 8a

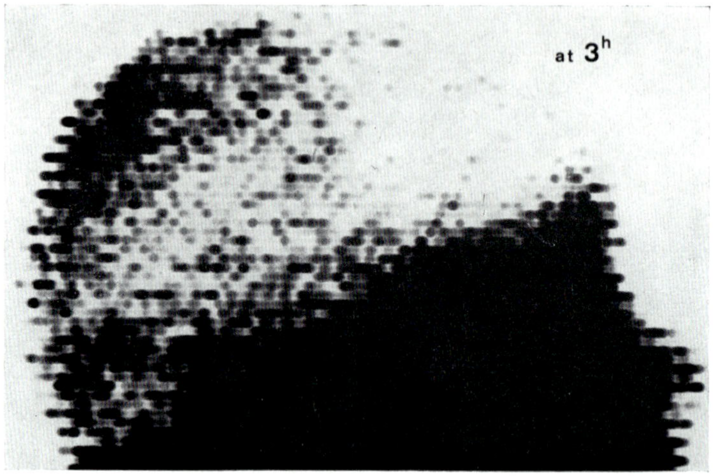

Fig. 8b

4. In case of subdural and intracerebral hematomas the activity decreases slowier than that at the vertex. (see Fig. 8).

5. In cases of aneuryms the activity-removal is related to the role played by the "vascular" component of the scanning positivity.

6. In brain contusions the activity decreases very soon.

7. In craniotomies the activity decreases simoultaneously with that of the vascular area.

Analysis of Space Distribution of Radioactivity

The space patterns which help in the differential diagnosis of focal brain lesions are: shape, borders of the pathological area, mode of distribution of the activity within the lesion.

Round or oval shapes are characteristic of tumors, abscesses and intracerebral hematomas; it must be stressed that such a shape may be seen both in anterior and lateral views.

A wedge shaped area in one of the two orthogonal views is characteristic of brain softenings.

In vasculopathic brain hemorrhages, aneurysms and brain contusions there is no typical shape.

A crescent pattern in the anterior and posterior views is typical of subdural hematomas. A similar shape is seen when the tracer accumulates in craniotomies (see Fig. 2).

In intracerebral vasculopathic hemorrhages, brain contusions, craniotomies or (only in lateral views) subdural hematomas the borders of the active area are irregular and the distribution of the activity within the lesion is inhomogeneous; the other focal brain lesions display well defined and regular borders and the distribution of the activity is homogeneous.

For what concerns the site of the active area in relation to the nature of the lesion we believe, in agreement with most of the other Authors, that a peripheral localization speaks against the tumoral nature of the lesion and that, among the vascular lesions, those located in the territories of anterior and posterior cerebral arteries are rarely shown with brain scanning.

Apport d'une technique de double marquage dans le diagnostic differentiel des lésions cétébrales

S. Askienazy, R. Di Paola, J. P. Constant, J. P. Chodkiewicz et M. Schlienger

Actuellement on demande de plus en plus à la gamma encephalographie de porter un diagnostic de nature sur les lésions décelées.

Dans ce but nous avons appliqué au domaine de la scintigraphie cérébrale la technique du double marquage.

Son principe réside en l'injection, à une demi-heure d'intervalle, de deux radioéléments très différents par leur spectrométrie et leur espace de diffusion, et en la réalisation simultanée des scintigraphies avec chaque isotope.

Deux critères essentiels peuvent être retenus afin de porter un diagnostic rapide de nature: La cellularité et la vascularité de la lésion, ce dernier caractère se rapprochant des signes apportés par l'angiographie carotidienne.

Deux isotopes à vie courte conviennent fort bien à cette détection simultanée: Le ^{99m}Tc et le ^{113m}In que l'on utilise soit sous forme de pertechnetate, ou d'In. DIPA, afin d'étudier la cellularité, soit sous forme de Serum Albumine Technetiée ou d'InPH4. afin d'étudier la vascularité de la lésion.

Deux associations sont donc possibles: – Soit le Tc et l'Indium PH4.

Resultats

A ce jour cent deux examens ont été réalisés, et une première analyse de la comparaison des images obtenues nous permet de distinguer quatre grandes catégories d'images scintigraphiques.

Les images purement vasculaires

L'espace vasculaire est imprégné par la seule albumine. On peut néanmoins noter l'existence d'une très discrète imprégnation par le produit à destinée cellulaire, celui-ci étant encore présent en très faible quantité dans l'espace vasculaire.

Le diagnostic ne fait aucun doute, et l'on peut être certain de la nature purement vasculaire de la lésion.

Les images a predominance callulaire

On obtient une image dont les dimensions cellulaires sont supérieures aux dimensions de l'espace vasculaire.

Elles sont caracteristiques de lésion peu vascularisées.

Les images a predominance vasculaire

Dù l'image vasculaire est de taille supérieure à l'image cellulaire. On les rencontre dans les hématomes chroniques et dans les tumeurs très hémorragiques.

Les images a vascularité et cellularité indentiques

C'est le cas de certains ménigiomes ou de certains métastases. Il est évident que ces seuls caractères ne suffisent pas et qu'il faut également considérer l'aspect morphologique de chacune de ces images, l'association de deux criteres étant nécessaire pour évaluer la nature de la lésion.

Nous n'avons encore qu'une très faible expérience des fixations respectives dans les accidents vasculaires, mais elles semblent extrêmement variables avec l'âge de l'accident.

Enfin cette technique est d'intêret considérable, dans la surveillance des malades opérés et irradiés.

En effet la réapparition d'une image cellulaire et vasculaire signifie la récidive, alors que la seule image cellulaire peut très bien n'être que la conséquence des actes thérapeutiques.

Critiques

Certes, il faut considérer les parts respectives des deux images avec certaines réserves.

En effet: l'indium ayant une énergie bien supérieure à celle du téchnétium, il sera bien mieux détecté dans les lésions profondes et il risque ainsi, de faire apprécier de manière erronée les concentrations respectives de deux éléments.

Le *spectometre* réglé sur le pic photo-électrique du technétium enregistrera les impulsions dues au rayonnement diffusé de l'indium, et par conséquent on notera toujours un aspect légèrement positif de l'image réalisée au technétium, si l'indium est lui, nettement positif, et cela indépendamment des cellularité et vascularité de la lésion.

Certes notre expérience encore très limitée dans ce domaine ne nous permets pas encore de tirer de plus amples renseignements que cette grossière classification qui est notre actuellement, mais une étude plus poussée des résultats en fonction de l'anatomopathologie, doit nous permettre d'être plus précis dans l'appréciation de la nature de la lésion.

Die Bedeutung des Abklingfaktors für die Artdiagnose intrakranieller Tumoren bei Untersuchung mit ^{203}Hg (Chlormerodrin)

G. Lausberg, F. Schepelmann und C.L. Geletneky

Aus der eigenen Kasuistik von 302 Untersuchungen mit ^{203}Hg (Chlormerodrin) wurde bei 68 histologisch gesicherten intrakraniellen Tumoren die allgemeine Abklingquote der Aktivität über der Schädelbasis mit der Abklingquote über dem Herd verglichen. Entgegen früheren Literaturmitteilungen, daß der für die Tumordarstellung günstigste Untersuchungszeitpunkt rund 4 Std nach der Injektion gelegen sei, haben wir an einer kleinen Nullserie festgestellt, daß die Ableitung innerhalb der ersten beiden Stunden die beste Aussage ergibt. Diese Erfahrung wurde am großen Kollektiv bestätigt. Die Kontrollableitung nach 24 Std kann zusätzliche Informationen zur Tumorart ergeben. Die allgemeine Abklingquote des Strahlers über der Schädelbasis stellt sich so dar, daß nach 60 min noch 71,6% der Aktivität als Durchschnittswert besteht. Nach 120 min beträgt die Aktivität noch 38,3% und nach 24 Std liegt der Wert bei 9,8%. Der Vergleich der Aktivitätsmessung über dem Herd mit dem Nullwert über der Schädelbasis innerhalb der ersten Stunde nach der Injektion läßt für die Meningeomgruppe die Höchstwerte mit durchschnittlich 196% erkennen, gefolgt von Glioblastomen mit 178%. An dritter Stelle liegen die Metastasen mit 139%. Oligodendrogliome, Astrocytome und Ependymome liegen in der Grundaktivität innerhalb der ersten Stunde unter 100% ohne sichere Gruppendifferenzen. Die gleiche Untersuchung nach 24 Std durchgeführt zeigt für die Gruppe der letztgenannten Tumoren eine relative Aktivitätserhöhung im Vergleich zur Schädelbasis auf 160%, während Meningeome mit 232% und Metastasen mit 208% etwas höher als die Werte der ersten Stunde gelegen sind. Die größte Streubreite zeigt die Glioblastomgruppe mit 94% bis 220% bei einem Mittelwert von 165%.

Die Ergebnisse der Untersuchung an 68 histologisch gesicherten Hirntumoren zusammengefaßt zeigt, daß die szintigraphische Untersuchung bei intrakraniellen Tumoren innerhalb der ersten beiden Stunden die besten Ergebnisse erzielt. Die Anreicherung des Strahlers über Glioblastomen, Meningeomen und Metastasen ist zu diesem Zeitpunkt relativ am stärksten im Vergleich zur Aktivitätsrate über der Schädelbasis. Die Kontrolluntersuchung nach 24 Std zeigt für die übrigen hirneigenen Tumoren eine deutliche Erhöhung der relativen Aktivität, währenddem die Relation bei Glioblastomen, Meningeomen und Metastasen keine zusätzlichen Aussagen vermittelt.

Impulssumme und Lage bestimmt. Die Aktivität der Punktionsstelle wurde ausgeklammert.

Die Variation der Ansprechwahrscheinlichkeit der Kamera auf Grund der verschiedenen Abstände der Aktivität von der Dedektorachse erforderte Wertkorrekturen der Impulssummen, die alle mittels Computer vorgenommen wurden.

1. Als Erstes wurde der nahezu konstante Kameraleerwert abgezogen.

2. Danach wurde die relative Ansprechwahrscheinlichkeit eines jeden der 4096 Kanäle für eine Punktquelle bestimmt. Zu diesem Zweck wurden die Ansprechwahrscheinlichkeiten über einer gedachten Ebene und zwar in einer sagittalen und einer horizontalen Achse des Patienten gemessen. Daraus wurden durch Interpolation die Werte für die einzelnen Kanäle errechnet, wobei das angewendete Verfahren auch einen Teil der Asymmetrie der Ansprechwahrscheinlichkeit um O, dem Punkt maximaler Empfindlichkeit, berücksichtigt (Abb. 2). ε_{ki} ist die auf den Ort maximaler Ansprechwahrscheinlichkeit bezogene relative Ansprechwahrscheinlichkeit des Punktes mit den Koordinaten, $_{i,k}$.

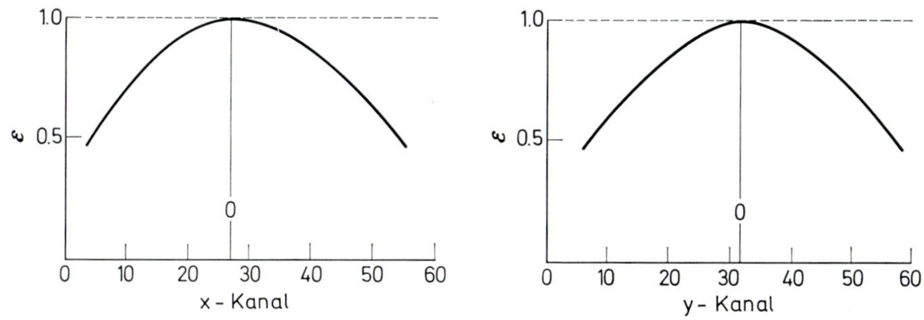

a

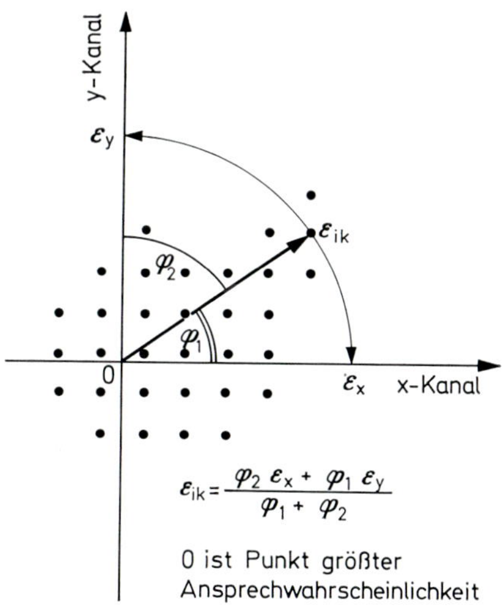

b

Abb. 2a–b. Interpolationsmethode. a Messung der relativen Ansprechwahrscheinlichkeiten in zwei zueinander senkrechten Achsen. b Berechnung der relativen Ansprechwahrscheinlichkeiten ε_{ik} aus den Meßkurven

Die Aktivität über der Lunge (Abb. 3, volle Kurve) wurde, der Größe dieses Areals wegen, durch eine konstante Aktivitätsverteilung gleicher Impulszahl ersetzt (strichlierte Kurve). Nach Anwendung eines Korrekturfaktors k_L ergibt sich die wahre Aktivität (punktierte Kurve). Der Korrekturfaktor wurde nach der Formel

$$k_L = F_L / \sum_{i,k} \varepsilon_{ik}$$

berechnet, wobei F_L die Zahl der Kanäle im Lungenbereich bedeutet und die Summation über die Kanäle des Bereiches zu erstrecken ist.

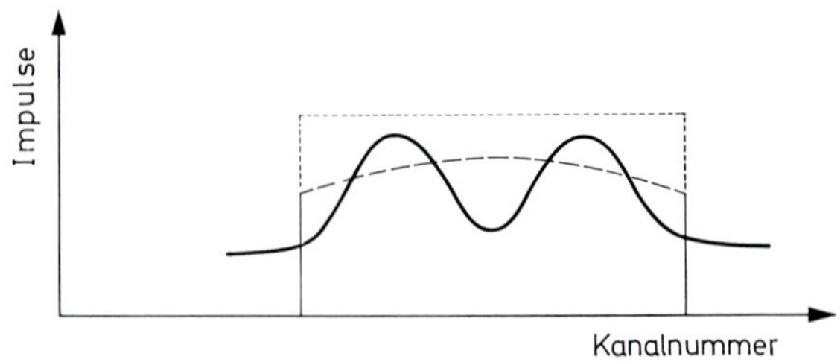

Abb. 3

Die Schädelaktivität wurde im Mittelpunkt des entsprechenden Bereiches zusammengefaßt gedacht, da sie einer zweidimensionalen Gaußverteilung mit geringer Halbwertsbreite entspricht. Daher vereinfacht sich der entsprechende Korrekturfaktor k_S zu

$$k_S = 1/\varepsilon_{i*k*}$$

wobei $_{i*k*}$ die dem Mittelpunkt der Schädelaktivität entsprechende Ansprechwahrscheinlichkeit darstellt.

War die Lungenaktivität so gering, daß sie nicht genau abgegrenzt werden konnte, so mußte sie auf eine mittlere Fläche normiert werden.

In gleicher Weise wie die Aktivität über der Lunge wurde die Körperleerwertaktivität behandelt.

Die Zuverläßigkeit dieser Vorgangsweise wurde an Phantomexperimenten überprüft.

Als Maß für die Größe der Kurzschlüsse des regionalen Hirnkreislaufes wurde aus den so korrigierten Werten ein Quotient: Aktivität über den Lungen zu Aktivität über der Schädelhälfte errechnet. Er ist von der verabreichten Dosis unabhängig.

Ergebnisse

Abbildung 4 zeigt die errechneten Lunge/Schädelquotienten von 24 Patienten in der Reihenfolge, in der sie untersucht wurden. Die Quotienten schwanken von 0,888 bis 0. Die histologischen Diagnosen sind aus dem operativ gewonnenen Material gestellt worden und sind ebenfalls aus Abbildung 4 zu ersehen. Es ergibt sich, daß die Quotienten bei den Meningeomen zwischen 0 und 0,015 bei den Metastasen zwischen 0,04 und 0,053 und bei den gliomatösen Tumoren zwischen 0,06 und 0,9 liegen, wobei die Glioblastome die größten Quotienten aufweisen.

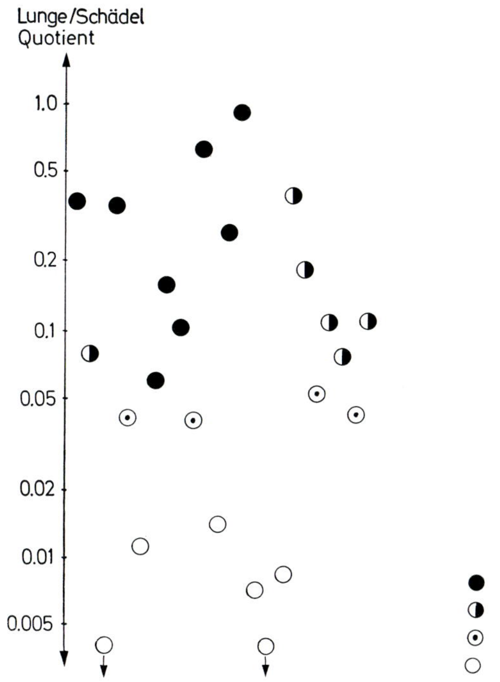

Abb. 4. Glioblastome, Astrocytome, Metastasen, Meningeome

Diskussion

Die präoperative Differentialdiagnose von Hirntumoren wird hauptsächlich aus dem klinischen Bild und den Serienangiogrammen gestellt. Von den nuklearmedizinischen Methoden hat sich in unserem Krankengut die Angioszintigraphie bewährt, welche eine Unterscheidung der Gliome von den Meningeomen gestattet. Die sichere Abtrennung der metastatischen Geschwülste sowie die Aufdeckung der infiltrativen Astrocytome – zwei Probleme von besonderem neurochirurgischem Interesse – hat aber auch das Angioszintigramm nicht zu lösen vermocht.

Mit dem hier beschriebenen Verfahren und aufgrund der bisherigen Ergebnisse scheint ein Weg gegeben, der auch diese Lücken in der Diagnostik und Differentialdiagnostik der Hirntumoren schließen könnte

Unabhängig vom diagnostischen Wert dieses Verfahrens zur Feststellung von Großhirnastrocytomen ist es noch interessant, daß diese Geschwülste alle erhebliche arteriovenöse Kurzschlüsse aufwiesen, was in den hohen Lungen/Hirnquotienten zum Ausdruck kam. Die Quotienten waren auch bei jenen Astrocytomen hoch gewesen, die histologisch einen Malignitätsgrad I–II aufwiesen – also relativ gutartig waren – und auch angiographisch nicht die Spur von frühen Venenfüllungen aufgewiesen hatten. Es scheint so zu sein, daß mit der hier beschriebenen Methode der Shuntbestimmung der Gliomcharakter selbst dieser „benignen" Astrocytome herausgefunden werden kann.

Femorocerebral Angiography: A New Technic Using Preformed Ducor Catheters

V. C. HINCK and M. P. JUDKINS

Less than three years ago the authors published an article describing a new technic for selective catheterization of cerebral vessels via the femoral artery using preformed catheters. Now popularly known as the headhunting technic, it has enjoyed very favorable reception in countless angiographic laboratories across the United States.

The preformed catheters, available commercially at home since 1968, have recently appeared on the European market. Eager to describe our method to you, we welcome the opportunity presented by the Angiography symposium of the European Association of Radiology.

Catheter Description

We use a seven or eight French polyurethane catheter within the wall of which is incorporated a braid of fine steel that imparts strength, resilience and a high degree of torsion control. These features, in combination with specially designed preformed head-hunting curves, make this catheter the implement of choice for most selective femorocerebral angiography.

There are three head-hunting curves. The first is used whenever an artery can be entered by *direct advance*. The second is used whenever a brachiocephalic branch issues from the aortic arch at a very acute angle. Direct advance is then impossible and the tip must be *hooked back* into the lumen from the opposite direction. The third head-hunter, used also for a hooking maneuver, is only indicated for entry of an innominate artery which originates low on the ascending side of a steeply sloping arch.

Technic

Percutaneous femoral puncture is performed using an 18-gauge arterial needle, a 0.038 in. guide wire, and a tapered 6 in., six or seven French, Teflon tube for dilating the puncture tract before introducing the catheter. Once introduced, the catheter is flushed intermittently to prevent intraluminal clotting.

For simplicity of presentation, let us consider the use of the first head-hunting curve in the selective catheterization of a patient with a normal aortic arch and undistorted brachiocephalic branches. The catheter is advanced from the distal aortic arch with its tip pointing laterally until it enters the left subclavian artery. After advancing a short distance, it is rotated to point medially and passed into the vertebral artery for selective injection.

Withdrawn to the arch and pointed toward the ascending aorta, it is advanced to innominate orifice, pointed cephalad and eased forward. In this manner it usually moves directly into the right common carotid artery although occasionally it will prefer the subclavian. In the latter instance, it can be advanced for selective entry of the vertebral artery.

As we have just indicated, the catheter traversing the innominate artery will show preference for either the carotid or the subclavian branch. In either event, to enter the alternate branch one may use one of two maneuvers:

a) Withdraw to the innominate artery and advance again *while applying torsion* to the catheter. Counterclockwise torsion will usually be helpful; or

b) Withdraw to the innominate artery and insert a guide several centimeters beyond the tip of the catheter. The guide tends to straighten the terminal curve and, in so doing, usually enters the other branch.

For entry of the left common carotid artery, the catheter is withdrawn to the proximal part of the innominate artery and rotated to bring the tip into the ascending arch. Then, after withdrawing the tip a few millimeters beyond the innominate orifice, counterclockwise torsion is slowly applied.

The tip will respond by sweeping gradually around the circumference of the aorta and, if at the correct "latitude", it will enter the left carotid lumen propelled by its own resilience (unless torsion has been too rapid). If not at the correct latitude, it will sweep a complete circle without entry; or it will reenter the innominate artery if not withdrawn sufficiently; or it will enter the left subclavian artery if withdrawn too far.

Success depends on *slow* rotation and withdrawal by *small* increments. If counterclockwise rotation fails, clockwise rotation sometimes brings quick success. It should be noted that the torsion maneuver described for left carotid entry is often used for catheterization of the innominate or left subclavian artery. Accordingly, though a catheter may traverse an artery by direct advance, a rotary maneuver may be required initially to gain entrance.

The hooking maneuver may best be exemplified by use of the second headhunting curve in a moderately tortuous arch. The catheter is inserted over a guide in the usual manner and flushed in the descending portion of the thoracic aorta. To regain the preformed curve, lost when the catheter was introduced over the wire, it can be rotated into the innominate artery, or failing this, reformed on the aortic valve. Reforming on the valve, the operator should be alert for catheter tip wedging in coronary orifices. Furthermore, should the tip inadvertently slip into the left ventricle, it must be withdrawn promptly. The maneuver may then be repeated.

With the catheter curve reformed and situated in the ascending aorta, it is rotated so that the tip points to the outer surface of the arch and withdrawn until it enters the innominate artery. If arch tortuosity is not severe, it can then be advanced into the carotid artery over a guide wire. Should tortuosity prevent futher advance, it may be necessary to inject from the innominate artery. Though less than ideal, we have sometimes managed to get satisfactory contrast of cerebral vessels from such a nonselective injection.

To go from the innominate to the left carotid artery, one may advance again to the ascending aorta and rotate the catheter tip so that it no longer points to the outer surface of the arch, withdraw it beyond the innominate orifice, and reverse rotation to point the tip cephalad. Further withdrawal will first hook the catheter into the carotid lumen and then advance it for firmer footing. Further entry over a guide wire is then usually possible. The maneuver just described is the same as that used for hooking the innominate artery with the third head-hunting configuration.

On several occasions, particularly in angiographic evaluation of glomus jugulare tumor, we have used the first head-hunting curve for femorojugular venography with uniform ease and success. On the other hand, the catheter tip has proven too large for selective injection of the inferior petrosal sinus.

Discussion

Evaluating the effectiveness of this technic, we performed an unselected series of 200 angiographic examinations on 193 patients, 80% of whom were over 40 years of age. The incidence of arteriosclerotic tortuosity was accordingly relatively high. Of 200 examinations, 125 included arch angiography and 100 were selective three-vessel studies. The series involved angiography of 475 cerebral arteries of which 91% were selectively catheterized. An additional 3% showed good contrast with non-selective injection. Overall success therefore was 94%. For three-vessel examinations the average procedure time was 64 min from time of injection of local anesthesia to withdrawal of the last catheter.

As to permanent complications, we recorded one death, two homonymous hemianopsias and one hemihyperesthesia. Dorsails pedis and posterior tibial pulses disappeared in one patient without treatment and without apparent sequellae. Two femoral clots were removed by use of Fogarty catheters.

At this writing, after about 500 patients and 1,200 cerebral arteries, results continue to be eminently satisfactory.

Cerebral vascular lesions

Optic Atrophy Due to Intracranial Aneurysms

H. Gökay

I would like to present two cases of primary optic atrophy produced by the compression of an intracranial aneurysm. Jefferson, in 1937, gave the first systematic account of the various interferences with the visual pathways which can be brought about by intracranial aneurysms. He made the analysis of 66 cases, collected through an extensive search of the literature. Although the aneurysms are not so rare, their treatment is still an interesting problem. This is especially true of the aneurysms in the chiasmal region, not only because of the variety of the visual defects which they produce but because of the problems that their successful handling entails.

In the literature one can find many writers, giving examples of neurological deficits, due to intracranial aneurysms.

Dandy for instance gave sparse accounts of 8 cases of aneurysms, but these were poorly documented. Direct contributions limited to the subject of visual defects are few.

Aneurysmal pressure on the chiasma blocks afferent retinal impulses, partly by direct pressure, but largely by anemia. The rapid improvement in vision, that carotid ligature brings in some cases suggests a vascular basis for most of the defects, though of course, if it is continued, atrophy of some fibers must follow. That happens with pituitary adenomas in the same circumstances. Blood supply to chiasma is carried on by a large number of short vessels,no one of which is dominant or can be regarded as an artery of major supply. It follows that pressure on any part of the chiasma or intracranial portion of the optic nerves leaves the vasculature of the rest undisturbed. The field defects caused by aneurysms are not always similar to the ones produced by pituitary tumors. These are usually symmetrical bitemporal defects.

Few of the aneurysms are wholly in the midline. Those that come nearest to occupying that position are those springing from the anterior cerebral artery usually at its junction with the anterior communicating artery. The internal carotid artery lies generally in or just behind the lateral chiasma angle. The main trunk leans a little away from the chiasma to continue into its main branch, the midle cerebral artery. In aneuryms of the internal carotid trunk in its intradural portion must come into contact with the chiasmal edge? Aneurysms of this part of the carotid trunk are very common especially at its anastomosis with the posterior communicating artery. These aneurysms usually cause an isolated oculo-motor palsy.

Occasionally an aneurysm will insinuate itself beneath the chiasma and cause much of the same effects as plain lateral compression or else a bitemporal effect.

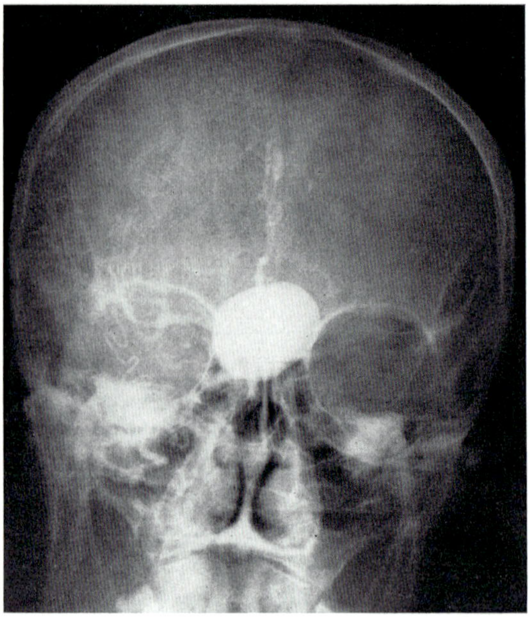

Fig. 1

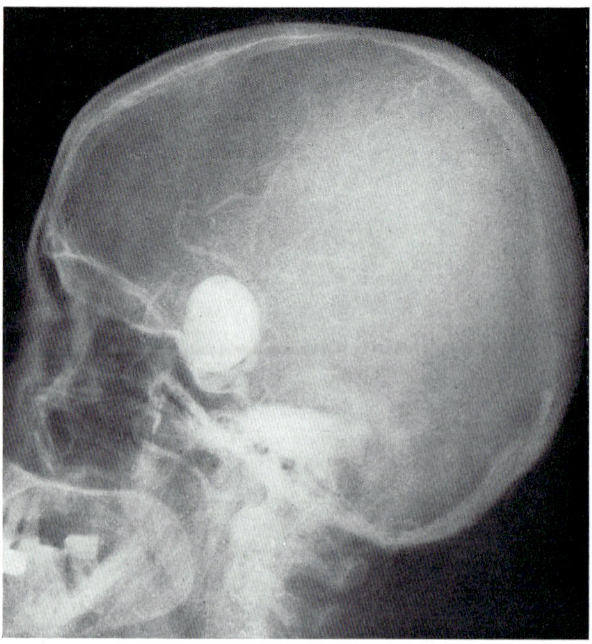

Fig. 2

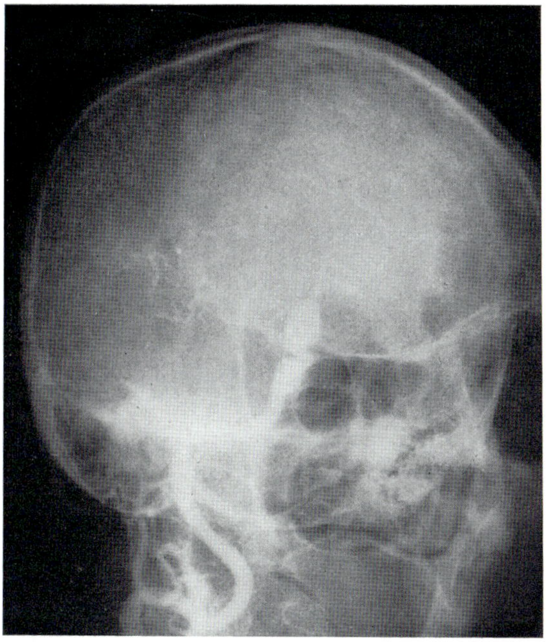

Fig. 3

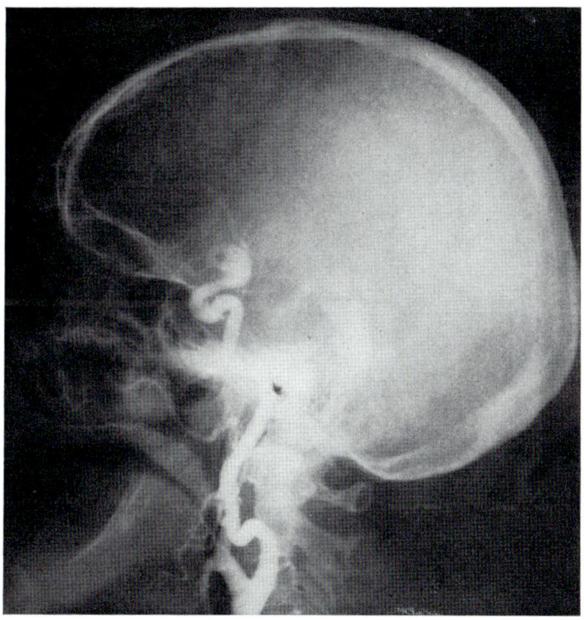

Fig. 4

Presentation of Cases

Case 1: M.A.Unit no: 003865, a 62 years old housewife was admitted to the Admiral Bristol hospital on April 28, 1969 with the chief complaint of blindness in one eye. The history obtained from the patient revealed that she began to notice some decrease in the vision of her right eye 5 years before her admission.

At the same time, she also experienced mild haedache. The vision in the right eye was lost completely in about 15 days. The diagnosis of glaucoma was made and treated accordingly by several ophthalmologits. She began to notice a gradual decrease in the vision of her left eye for the last 2 years. Just before her admission, a craniography was done and this revealed a questionable defect around the sella turcica. A neurosurgical consultation was asked. The examination revealed primary optic atroph in both fundi. The right eye was blind; there was no reaction to light in the right pupilla. There was a temporal defect in the left side. There was no other finding in the physical and neurological examinations. The laboratory examinations were within normal limits. A diagnosis of a possible tumor was made. A bilateral carotid angiography was performed on April 29, 1969 and this revealed a large aneurysm on the right internal carotid artery (Figs. 1 and 2).

On April 30, 1969 the right common carotid artery was ligated under local anesthesia. The patient tolerated the procedure well, but she complained of severe headache for 15 days. 6 months after the operation left vision was normal and she began to see light in the right eye. The vision in the right eye continued to improve gradually, up until the writing of this report.

Case 2: B. V. Unit no. 005484, a 68 years old housewife was admitted to the Admiral Bristol hospital on Nov. 9, 1969 with the chief complaint of difficulty in her vision. The history obtained from the patient revealed that she experienced a severe headache and lost the vision in her right eye one month before her admission. She consulted an ophthalmology out-patient clinic in a hospital. The diagnosis of a primary optic atrophy was made, and she was treated accordingly. The family of the patient was not satisfied with the diagnosis so they consulted another ophthalmologist who asked for a neurosurgical consultation. The examination revealed blindness in the right eye and a temporal defect in the left side. The craniography was normal, the patient had an arterial hypertension. The blood pressure was 180/100. The fundoscopic examination revealed primary optic atrophy in both sides. On Nov. 10, 1969 a carotid angiography was performed. This revealed a large, single aneurysm of the right internal carotid artery (Figs. 3 and 4). On Nov. 13, 1969, the right common carotid artery was ligated under local anesthesia. The patient tolerated the procedure well. She complaied of severe headache for about a month. In her last control examination on August 4, 1970 she still had her left temporal defect, but she had begun to see with her right eye.

Both of these cases were treated for primary optic atrophies, one due to glaucoma, the other due to arterisclerosios. They were diagnosed with the aid of cerebral angiography. This proves the importance of angiography in cases of primary optic atrophies of undetermined origin. Both cases were treated with ligature of the common carotid artery with good results. An intracranial approach was not used because of the size of the lesions and the age of the patients.

Radioisotopic Evaluation of Cerebral Vascular Lesions

M. K. Loken and L. Gold

It is the purpose of this communication to illustrate the use of techniques of Nuclear Medicine for the study of patients with cerebral aneurysms, arterial-venous malformations and occlusions. The results of these studies have been correlated with conventional angiography.

A scintillation (Anger) camera or rectilinear scanner is being used to obtain conventional brain scintiphotograms at approximately one hour after the intravenous administration of 10–15 mCi of ^{99m}Tc (pertechnetate) to a patient suspected of having a cerebral-vascular lesion. In addition, rapid sequential serial scintiphotography is carried out using a scintillation camera to visualize the radioisotope bolus as it traversed the major cerebral arterial and venous structure during its initial passage.

Case 1: Patient (C. O.) who experienced sudden onset of left hemiparesis, received 15 mCi technetium by intravenous injection with the camera directed toward

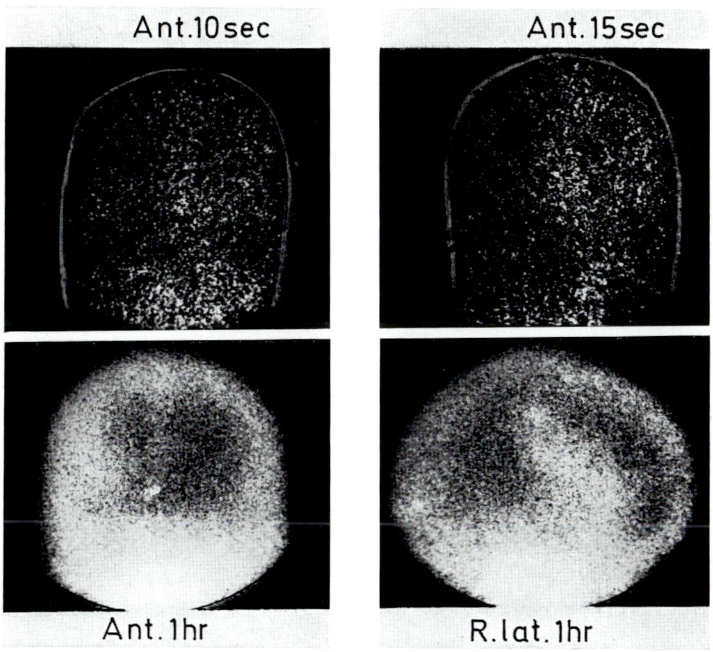

Fig. 1. Patient (C. O.) Diminished flow to right middle cerebral artery distribution with infarction pattern on delayed views

the anterior head. Scintiphotograms obtained at 10 and 15 sec after injection are shown in Fig. 1. There is evidence of decreased flow to the middle cerebral group on the right side. An anterior and right lateral scintiphotogram obtained one hour after injection shows a sharp focus of increased activity in the right parietal area corresponding to the region of increased blood flow. This finding is typical in patients with vascular occlusion and cerebral infarction. A cerebral angiogram showed almost total occlusion of all branches of the right middle cerebral artery.

Case 2: This 59 year old male, (W.M.), experienced a sudden onset of right hemisparesis after having been involved in a minor auto accident. 10 sec. after the administration of 15 mCi of ^{99m}Tc a scintiphotogram (Fig. 2) shows normal flow

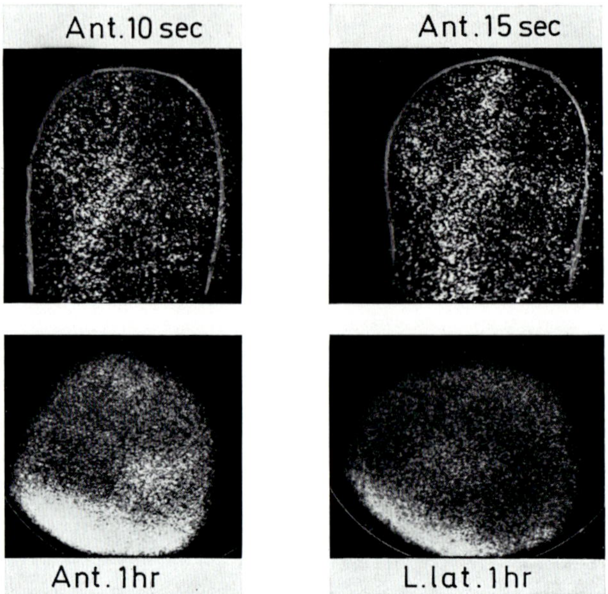

Fig. 2. Patient (W. M.) Occlusion of left internal carotid artery and diminished flow to left middle cerebral artery with infarction pattern on delayed views

in the right carotid artery with minimal flow on the left side. There is likewise evidence of slightly greater flow to the region of the middle cerebral group on the right than on the left. A scintiphotogram obtained 15 sec after injection shows similar findings with the radioisotope in the capillaries and proximal veins. An anterior and left lateral picture obtained in one hour show an accumulation of radioactivity in the frontal parietal region on the left side indicative of occlusion of the Sylvian branches of the left middle cerebral artery. A subsequent cerebral angiogram confirmed this impression (Fig. 3).

Case 3: Fig. 4 shows selected right lateral scintiphotograms obtained at 10 and 30 sec after intervenous administration of 10 mCi ^{99m}Tc intervenously into a 17 year old male (G. B.). The scintiphotogram on the left shows passage of the radioactivity via the right internal carotid artery into the brain. There is a sharp focus of abnormal activity seen at the base of the brain which persists through scintiphotogram No. 3

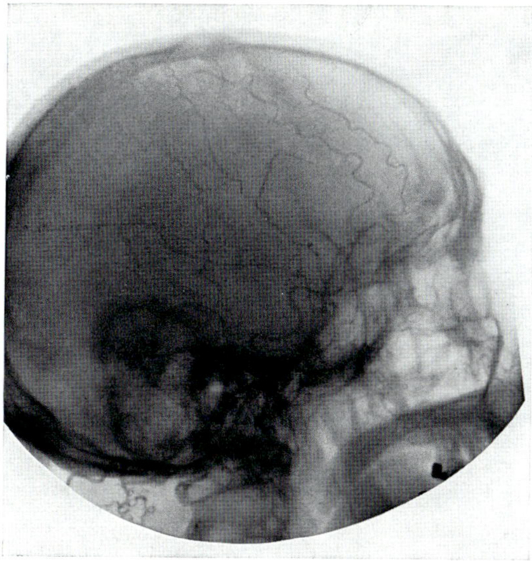

Fig. 3. Patient (W. M.) Angiogram showing occlusion of Sylvian branches of left middle cerebral artery

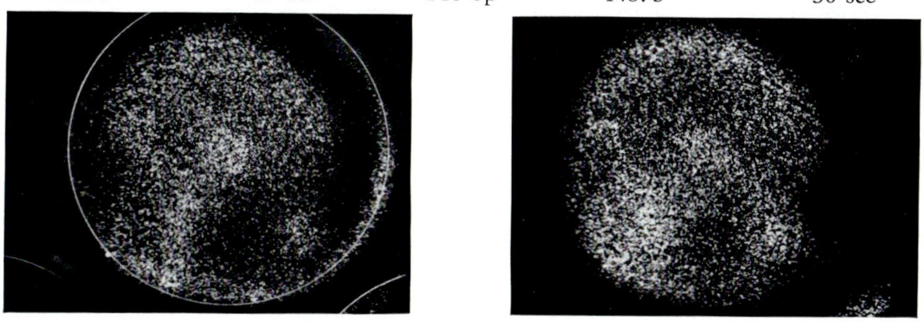

Fig. 4. Patient (G. B. Right) lateral ^{99m}Tc flow study showing abnormal collection (pool) of radioactivity in posterior temporal region

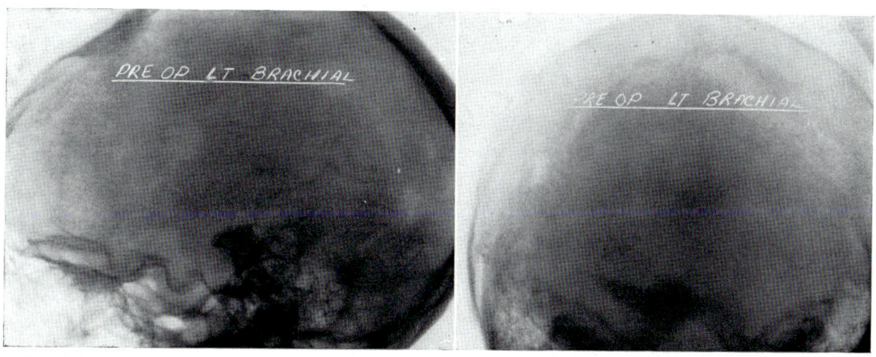

Fig. 5. Patient (G. B.) Angiograms showing aneurysm of the right posterior cerebral artery

No. 1 10 sec Post op No. 3 30 sec

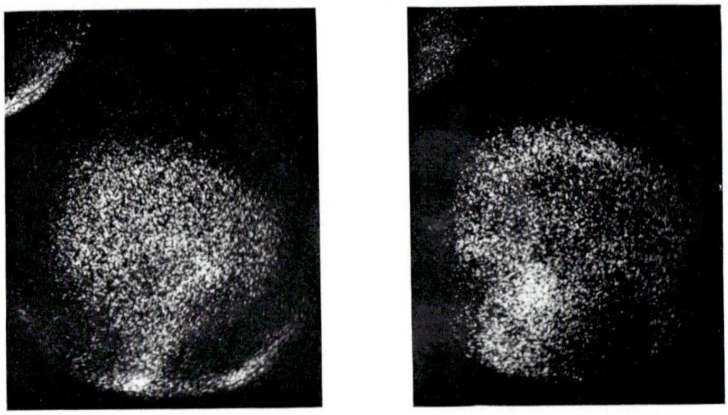

RT Lateral 15,000 cts RT Lateral 15,000 cts

Fig. 6. Patient (G. B.) Normal post-op ^{99m}Tc flow study

45 min Post op L 45 min RT

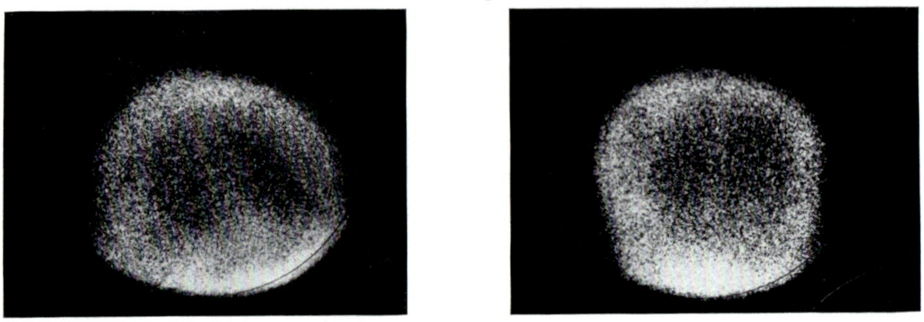

RT Lateral Posterior

Fig. 7. Patient (G. B.) Normal post-op brain scintiphotograms

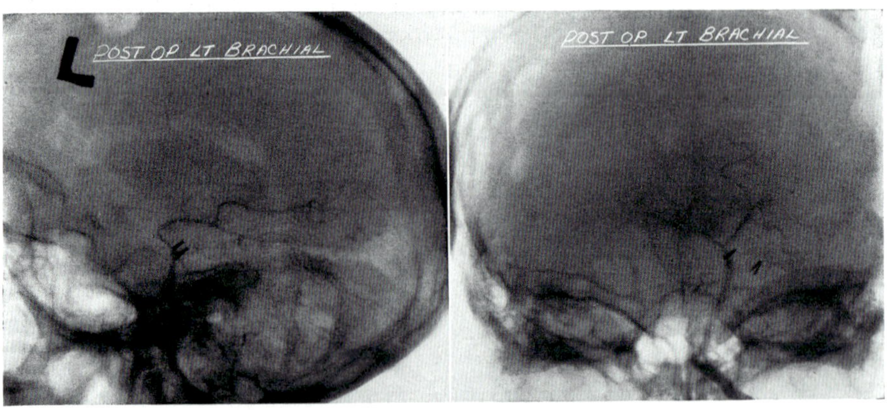

Fig. 8. Patient (G. B.) Normal post-op angiogram

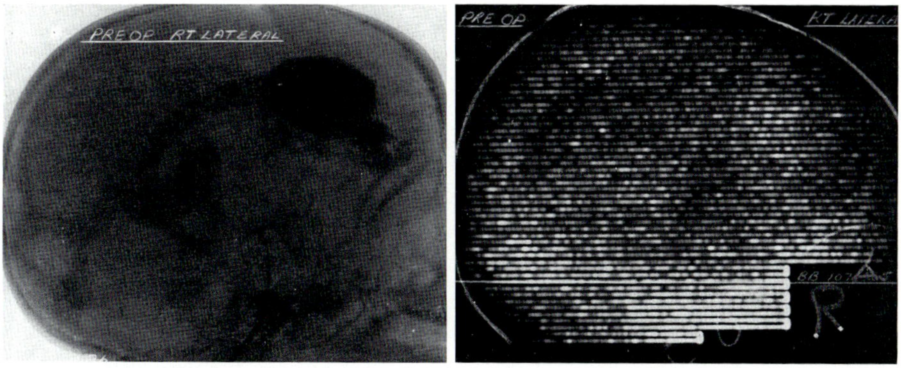

Fig. 9. Patient (B. B.) Scans showing abnormal focus of radioactivity in the frontal area

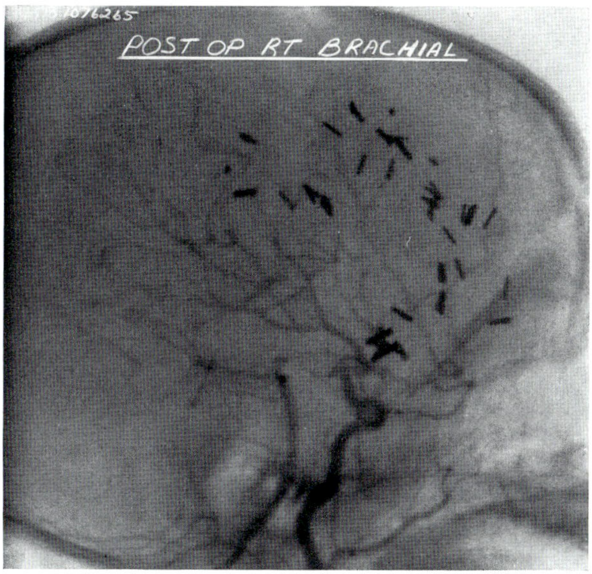

Fig. 10. Patient (B. B.) Angiograms showing large arteriovenous malformation

obtained at 30 sec. There is no evidence of early venous drainage. Two films selected from a left brachial angiogram performed on this patient are shown in Fig. 5. These films demonstrate the presence of a large fusiform aneurysm of the right posterior cerebral artery. This patient was subsequently taken to surgery and the aneurysm was clipped. Post-operative flow studies as well as conventional scintiphotograms were found to be normal (Figs. 6 and 7). Likewise a postoperative left brachial angiogram showed no evidence of abnormality (Fig. 8). Clips placed on the aneurysm at surgery are evident in these films.

Case 4: Fig. 9 shows a right lateral rectilinear scan and cerebral angiogram film of a 6 month old patient (B. B.). 7 mCi of ^{99m}Tc was administered 1 hr prior to the scan which shows an abnormal focus of activity in the frontal area which

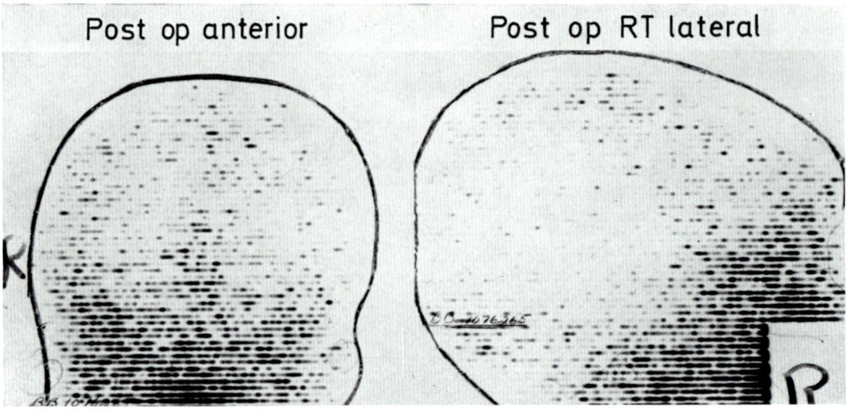

Fig. 11. Patient (B. B.) Normal post-op brain scan

corresponds to a large arterial venous malformation. This malformation is supplied by both anterior cerebral and left middle cerebral arteries as seen on the angiographic film. This arterial-venous malformation was successfully removed at surgery as may be appreciated in the post-operative right brachial angiogram (Fig. 10). Scans obtained post-operatively using ^{99m}Tc were normal (Fig. 11).

Case 5: Sequential scintiphotograms obtained during the first 30 sec after administration of 15 mCi ^{99m}Tc to a 63 year old patient (T. J.) are shown in Fig. 12. This patient had experienced episodes throught clinically to represent repeated subarachnoid hemorrhages. These 5 pictures show a sharp focus of activity in the midline which persists well into the venous phase of this study. This was felt to represent an aneurysm in the region of the Circle of Willis which may have been leaking slightly at the time of the arrival of the radioactive bolus. Confirmation of an aneurysm was obtained during cerebral angiography (Fig. 13). The lower set of pictures in Fig. 12 were obtained at 1 hr after the administration of the radioisotope and show no abnormality.

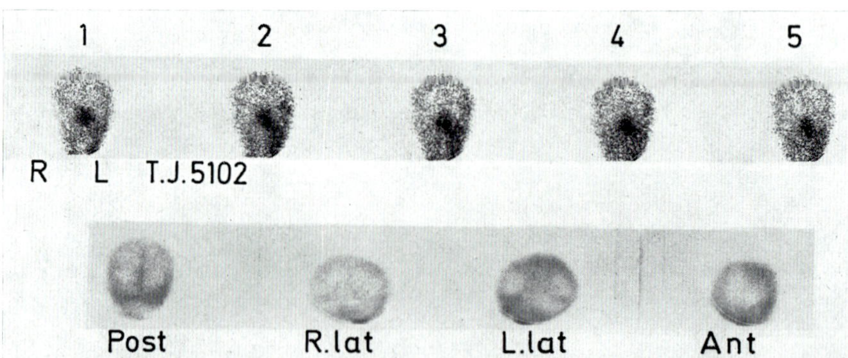

Fig. 12. Patient (T. J.) ^{99m}Tc flow study showing midline focus of activity near the Circle of Willis

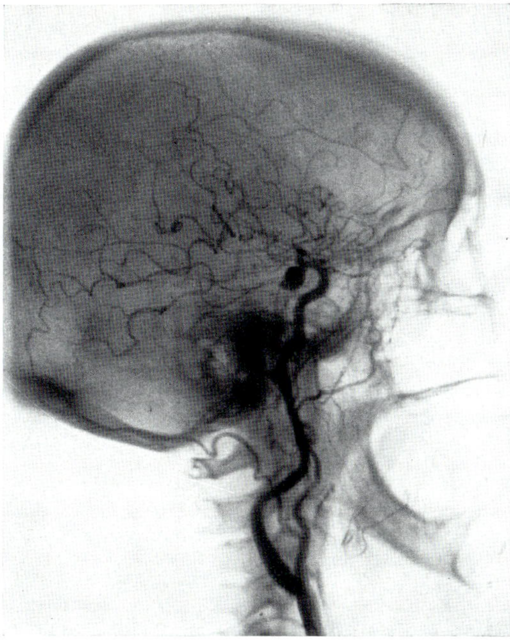

Fig. 13. Patient (T. J.) Angiogram showing aneurysm in the region of the Circle of Willis

Discussion

Neglibible amounts of ^{99m}Tc cross the blood-brain barrier during the first passage of this material into the cerebral circulation after its intervenous administration. Thus alterations from the normal distribution of radioactivity during this passage can be used to depict some vascular abnormality. Increased radioactivity indicates the presence of a cerebral aneurysm or arterial-venous malformation and a decrease in activity usually indicates cerebral infarction or the presence of an avascular mass such as a subdural hematoma. Rapid appearance of radioactivity in the sagittal sinus indicative of early venous drainage was observed in arterial venous malformations but not in aneurysms.

Excellent correlation of the dynamic and static scintiphotographic studies with cerebral angiographic studies performed both pre-operatively and post-operatively was found in all of our patients studies. Sequential scintiphotograms obtained immediately after radioisotope injection have accurately defined both the location and the character of cerebral vascular lesions.

The Determination of Cerebral Death by Cerebral Angiography

E. BÜCHELER and C. KÄUFER

In view of a sensible reanimation and considering organ transplantations the determination of death is unanimously oriented on the irreversible loss of function of the brain as the decisive criterium. Clinical signs and isoelectric-EEG do not allow the diagnosis of cerebral death with reasonalbe certainty. According to our experiences this can, however, be verified more reliable by cerebral angiography. As cerebral death is understood as the irreversible functional loss of cortex and brain stem, bilateral carotid – and vertebral angiography are necessary to fulfill this definition.

In comparative investigations with needle puncture, cerebral panangiography and transfemoral selective catheterangiography we found the latter to be the optimal method and carried it out in 23 patients in a total of 45 brain death determinations. It also appears to be advantageous to be able to carry out an angiogram of the donor organs with the same catheter. Before cerebral angiograms are carried out an isoelectric-EEG has to be present. Intracranial circulatory interruption leads to irreversible anoxic damage depending from the time. After the reanimation time of the brain has been exceeded, the irreversible loss of function can be proved by cerebral angiography.

An interruption of contrast medium in the internal carotid artery with normal filling of the external carotid artery prove cerebral death in the carotid angiogram (Fig. 1). In the vertebral angiogram a circulatory arrest in the basilar or vertebral artery suggest loss of cerebral functions (Fig. 2). The stop is typically localised at the siphon level for the internal carotid artery and at the atlanto-occipital level for the vertebral artery. If the circulatory arrest in these vessels occurs in the cervical region organic vascular occlusions have to be considered in the differential diagnosis. Selective angiography of the four leading cerebral arteries clarifies the anatomical and functional situation.

If initial areas of the medial and posterior cerebral artery have a rudimentary filling or the circulation is slowed down exceeding 15 sec not showing a venous phase, the interpretation of the findings for a cerebral death are more critical, as the fact of complete interruption of circulation is not present, althought no sufficient circulation for brain function should exist in this extreme slowness of blood flow.

The question is whether in such cases minimal cerebral flow is present in these arteries or whether this phenomenon is produced by the unphysiological increased injection pressure which presses the contrast material into the arteries. The latter appears to be correct as the contrast material can be demonstrated in the arteries over a longer period of time. Furthermore, we were unable to obtain such findings with

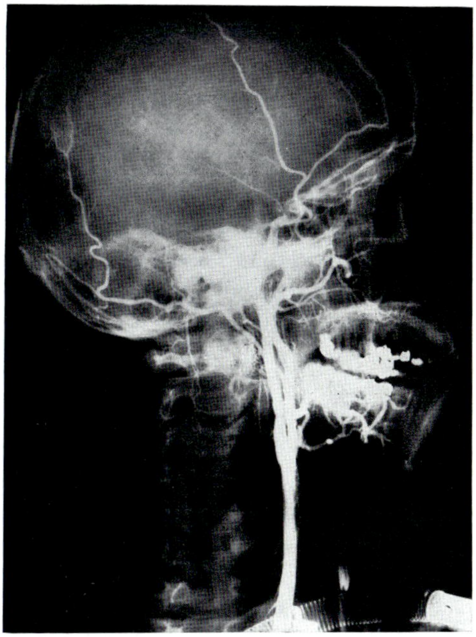

Fig. 1. Right carotis angiogram. Stop of the contrast medium on the basis of the skull

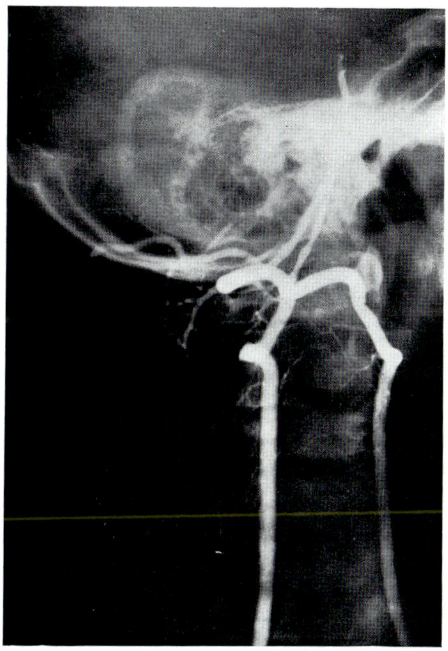

Fig. 2. Right vertebralis angiogram: Stop of the contrast medium in the arteria basilaris

cerebral panangiography carried out for comparison. As a minimal cerebral flow cannot be excluded in these cases with absolute certainty, we regard this finding because of the difficult problems involved as a transitional stage and so far not as absolute proof for cerebral death.

According to our investigations blood circulation in the bed of the basilar artery stops later than in the internal carotid. In some cases where an interruption of circulation was demonstrated in the internal carotid arteries, we observed a contrastation of the posterior fossa arteries and a filling of the carotid siphon via the posterior communicating artery in the vertebral arteriogram. Diagnosis of cerebral death can therefore not be limited to the circulatory interruption in the carotid arteries, but also has to include the distribution area of the basilar artery.

For the certain diagnosis of irreversible cerebral death therefore the timing of angiography is of paramount importance. Considering the time interval between circulatory arrest in the internal carotid arteries and the basilar artery the vertebral angiography according to our experiences appears to be of primary importance in the determination of cerebral death. Angiography should not be performed immediately upon obtaining an isoelectric-EEG, since an intracranial blood flow may still be present at this stage via the vertebral arteries.

The interruption of cerebral circulation demonstrated in stages by serial angiography in the internal carotid and vertebral arteries may be regarded as definite proof for the irreversible loss of brain functions, since restitution is impossible following such permanent cerebral anoxia and brain death has definitely occurred.

Correlation of Angiography and Angioscintigraphy in Diffuse Cerebral Vascular Lesions

E. Deisenhammer and B. Hammer

In more than 100 patients angioscintigraphy has been performed immediatly after carotid angiography. Using the same needle, in adults 50 μCi of human albumin makroaggregates (MA) with a diameter of 5–50 μ have been injected during 20 sec. With this method no side effects were observed.

Excluding focal cerebral lesions including vascular ones there remained 100 cases with either a normal angiogram or the so called signs of a diffuse cerebral vascular lesion. In these it seemed worthwhile to correlate the angiograms with the results of angioscintigraphy. The following observations have been made:

1. Normal angioscintigrams. The distribution of the MA corresponded to the area of the brain supplied by the branches of the internal carotid artery. The maximal rate of activity was in the center of this region due to the approximately spherical spatial distribution.

2. Normal variations. In some cases the area of the brain supplied by the contralateral anterior cerebral artery or by the ipsilateral posterior cerebral artery was visible in the scan. This distribution of the MA could be seen in cases, in which these vessels were well outlined also in the angiogram. Cases with poor angiographic visibility of the contralateral anterior cerebral artery or the ipsilateral posterior cerebral artery respectively seldom showed such a scintigraphic pattern.

3. In nonrecent large vascular lesions the angioscintigram showed a cold spot correlated to the infarcted region due to the lack of transport of MA to this region.

4. In three cases angioscintigram was done during the period in which the technetium scan is positive and shows the extent of the malacic tissue. This accumulation of a tracer is probably due to the vascular reactions in the infarcted tissue at this time. These cases showed a partial or even complete trapping of MA in the region approximately marked by the high uptake of ^{99m}Tc Pertechnetate. The angiograms showed the signs of luxury perfusion.

5. A definitively abnormal configuration of the distribution of the MA was seen in a large number of cases. These were characterized by the irregular intensity of uptake of MA. Spots of different size with more or less high uptake were seperated by regions with very low uptake. There was no correlation to the clinical picture or to angiographically visible thrombosis of vessels. In a high percentage these angioscintigrams showed a correlation to the angiographic picture of the so called diffuse cerebral vascular process, which is characterized by the presense of widening, kinking and varying diamter of vessels and rarefication of small vessels in the angio-

gram. A correlation between angiogram and angioscintigram could be found in 79% of the cases.

These results indicate a correlation between the organic lesion in the cerebral vessels visible in the angiogram and the abnormal angioscintigram. The latter demonstrate a disturbance at the level of the capillaries, the nature of which is still uncertain. The diminished uptake of MA could be due to thrombosis of small vessels unseen in the angiogram or it might be a hemodynamic effect consequent to the vascular lesion.

In three cases a high uptake of MA could be seen to correspond to the region of an infarct demonstrated by the positive technetium scan. These region might represent small infarcts in a phase of vascularisation.

Our results demonstrate the possibility of correlating vascular alterations seen in the angiogram with pathological changes at the capillary level as expressed by pathological angioscintigraphic scans.

Application of the Anger Camera in the Evaluation of the Permeability of Pudenz Valves

Evaluation of a New Method

F. Arnaiz Bueno, R. Carrillo Yagüe, J. L. Chamorro Romero and J. Ortiz Berrocal

Introduction

In spite of the numerous and diverse operations for the surgical treatment of hydrocephalia, from 1956 onwards the procedure of CSF derivation into the cardiac cavity, regulated by means of valves, has become popularin the neurosurgical field.

The systems frequently utilized Spitz-Holter or Pudenz-Heyer comprise, essentially, a proximal tube leading into the lateral cerebral ventricle, a distal tube that is introduced through the jugular vein until its extremity lodges in the right auricle, and an intermediate device to which both are connected, placed under the skin of the head. This intermediate device can be exteriorly pumped to activate the flow of CSF trough the system or to ascertain its permeability.

The most frequent complications in this type of derivative interventions are infections (endocarditis, meningitis and for septicaemia), and obstruction of either extremity.

Fundamental principle for the correct function of these derivations is that the distal or cardiac and be correctly sited in the right auricle; if it is placed in a lower position – in the ventricle –, the risks of endocarditis are great; if placed in upper position – superior cava –, there is a trend to thrombosis and obstruction of the tube. Though at surgery the system remains perfectly placed, later on (especially in babies), because of growth, it slips to an upper position, and when it is about to slip out of the auricle, it must be lengthened by a simple intervention in the neck, for if it gets thrombosised obstructed the intervention can become extraordinarily difficult, and it is impossible, in most of the cases, to reach the heart but through another jugular vein.

Nulsen, one of the pioneers of this type of surgery, in 1960 began to perform prophilactic lengthening prior to the obstruction of the distal tube. As an average, when the valve was installed in the first month of life, the first revision is made at four months, the second at seventeen, the third at forty-two months and so on.

After ten years of world-wide experience and thousands of Holter and Pudenz valves placed, it has been possible to reduce the number of complications, but without eliminating all of them. Several authors have contributed technical modifications to obviate the difficulties and better the results.

The object of this communication is to present a method that, with the help of radioactive materials, allows us to detect in time a badly functioning Pudenz valve when there is a partial obstruction in its distal end, at the same time orienting us about its situation. It is part of a more ambitious project to verify and quentify the whole bypass system.

In the "Clinica Puerta de Hierro", we always use of Pudenz valves, which, in our opinion have more advantages and less inconveniencies than Holter valves. During the intervention we use an electrocardiographic method to make sure of the correct placement of the distal end in the right auricle, and then we try to control the situation by thorax-penetrating radiography (the most caudal portion, where a valve that prevents the return flow of blood is lodged is made of radio-opaque material). Anyhow it is very often impossible to visualize it in a radiography due to its small size (particularly when using the thinner pediatric terminal) and to its continuous movement within the blood; in these cases, not knowing the situation, we cannot safely plan the prophylactic lengthening. The transcutaneous pumping mechanism of the intermediate device is very useful to discover a total obstruction in any of the two tubes; if it is the proximal one, after pressing the central valve, it will collapse, if the obstruction is in the distal tube, the valve cannot be depressed. The difficulty arises when the obstruction is partial, regarding the distal end, its is possible to depress the valve, though it will offer a certain resistence, more or less influenced by the subjectiveness of the operator. It will be understood that the evaluation of this resistance throug skin and subcutaneous connecting tissue is very difficult, and subject to the subjective influence of the operator.

As the reservoir or intermediate device of the Pudenz valve is made of silicon, it can be punctured from the exterior with a very thin needle, without any damage. Therefore we have thought to inject through it a certain quantity of radioactive material and perform a photoscan with the Anger camera on the distal portion of the system in order to obtain almost immediately its morphologic representation; then we pump the reservoir a number of times and we perform another photoscan, testing the permeability of the system in an objective way and without and discomfort for the patient. As we can see, with only one test of easy realization we can ascertain situation, morphology and permeability of the bypass system.

Materials and Methods

Any sort of radioactive material that can be detected from the exterior and has a physical and biological half-life rendering its use harnless may be employed (we must consider that most patients are babies).

The radiocompounds we have used have been ^{99m}Tc and ^{113m}In for their special characteristics of physical half-life of 6 and 1.7 h, respectively, and their adequateness for external detection. We have used generators of 50 mCi of ^{99}Mo and ^{113}Sn in order to get an eluate of high specific activity that would allow us to administer doses from 300–500 μCi in a volume smaller than 0.5 ml.

The detection and registration apparatus has been an Anger camera (Pho-gamma III), with a thallium-activated INa crystal of 0.6×11" and 19 photomultiplicators, using a low energy collimator of 4,000 square holes (if we were using ^{99m}Tc) or a collimator of 771 circular holes of medium energy (if we were using ^{113m}In). The recording system has been in polaroid, after having prefixed 150,000 computations in the first exploration (about 120 sec) and after prefixing times in the remaining explorations. Likewise we have checked the record with a multiparametric visualization system of 4,096 chanels fitted to the camera. To control the situation of the catheter we have used three radioactive indicators, each one containing 9,5 μCi of ^{57}Co placed in jugulum, IV right costo-sternal articulation and above the breast mamilla.

The radioactive material was injected directly in to the subcutaneous reservoir of the bypass system through the skin, with an insulin needle.

Before applying our method to patients, we determined the capacity of the Pudenz valve reservoir and the volume expelled in each pumping stroke. The reservoir has a capacity of 0.5 ml and in each stroke 0.1 ml are expelled trough the distal end; therefore, if the valve is permeable, in five strokes all the liquid contained in the reservoir will have disappeared. We can verify this fact experimently filling the reservoir with 0.5 ml of radioactive material and placing the distal and proximal ends in containers full of water; in these conditions we take a photoscan, ascertaining that there was radioactive material in the reservoir and in the distal tube. Then after five pumpings in the central reservoir, we have taken another photoscan observing that the radioactive material had disappeared from the reservoir and from the distal tube and appeared exclusively in the container of the distal outlet. In no case did we encounter a passage of radioactivity to the container communicating with the distal tube (Fig. 1).

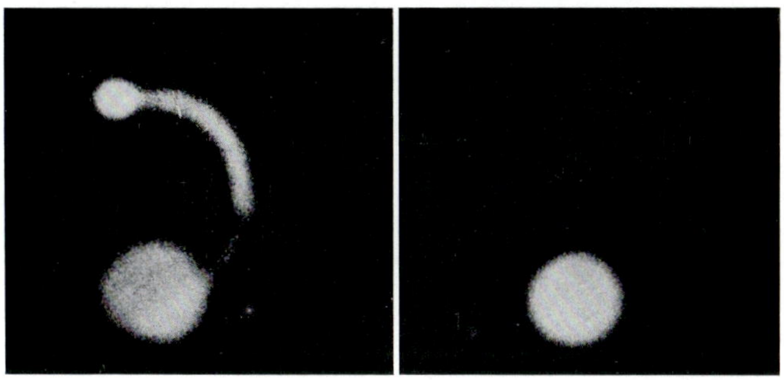

a b

Fig. 1a. Photoscan of a phantom of Pudenz valve, after injecting 0.5 ml of ^{99m}Tc solution in the central reservoir. b The same phantom after five strokes in the central reservoir. Notice the disappearance of radioactive material from the valve and its appearance in the drainage container

The valve we have used has always been Pudenz's, which, in our opinion, offers certain advantages when compared with Holter's. It consists of a chamber or reservoir that is placed under skin of the head and from which issue two tubes: one, the proximal, leads into the lateral cerebral ventricle, and the distal empties into the right auricle. In the reservoir there is a membrane valve that obstructs the passage of liquid to the ventricular system, but it allows passage towards the cardiac cavities; at the end of the distal tube there is another valve (of radio-opaque material) to prevent the passage of auricular blood to the interior of the catheter. It has over the Holter valve the great advantage that the central reservoir can be punctured with a thin needle from the exterior as many times as it is necessary, an almost impossible manoeuver in that type of valve.

Results

We shall analize the results in permeability and situation studies, both in normal and pathological cases.

Studies of Permeability

Normal Cases

We have studied 10 patients between 7 and 15 days following the placement of the bypass system and that did not show any clinical symptomatology. In all of them, after the introduction of the material in the reservoir, we took the first photoscan, observing the morphology and situation of the distal end of the system; afterwards, and after ten strokes on the chamber and having prefixed the time used to get the first photo, we got a second photoscan. In all the cases we were studying, the radioactive material of the catheter had completely disappeared and it was distributed all over the body, particularly in the thyroid glands (indirect sign that the indicator had passed to the general circulation). We never needed more than 10 strokes Figs. 2 and 3).

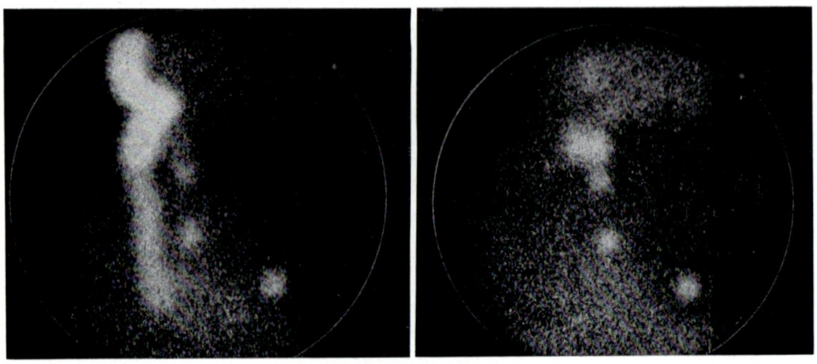

a b

Fig. 2a and b. Photoscan of the distal end of a Pudenz valve working correctly on a hydrocephalic patient. a Distal end of the bypass system in basal situation. b After ten strokes in the central reservoir, the radioactive material of the bypass system has disappeared and can be seen in the thyroid glands

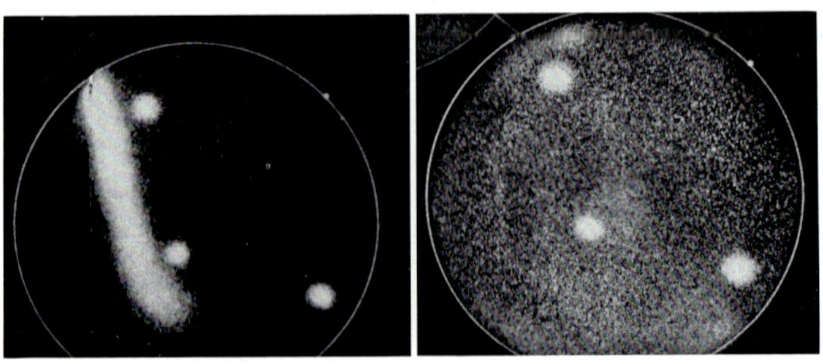

a b

Fig. 3a and b. Photoscan of a Pudenz valve in perfect working order. a Basal situation. b After 10 strokes in the central reservoir

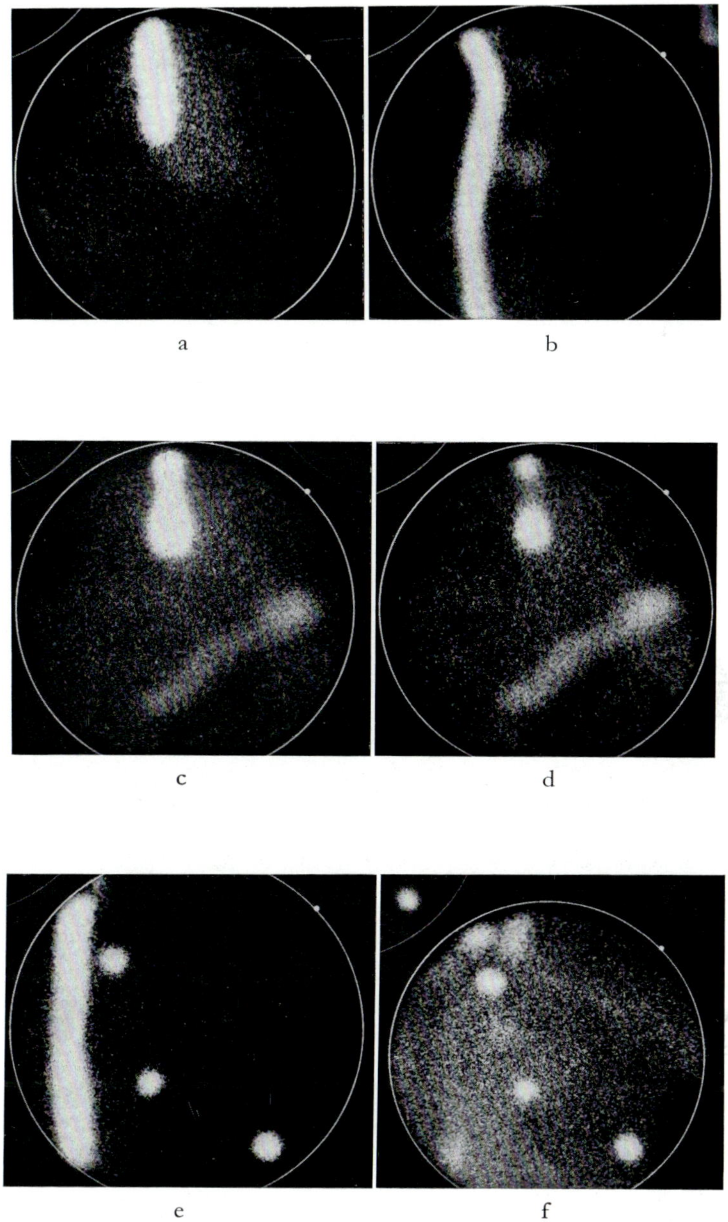

Fig. 4a–f. Photoscan of the distal end of a Pudenz valve in a patient with obstruction of the bypass system. Before the operation: a Distal end of the Pudenz valve in basal situation. b View of the catheter along the neck and the thorax in basal situation. c After twenty stroke in the central reservoir the radioactive material persists in the terminal portion of the bypass system. d After a further one hundred strokes the radioactivity still persists in the terminal portion. After the operation: e Distal end of the Pudenz valve in basal situation. f After ten strokes in the central reservoir the radioactive material has completely disappeared; the thyroid gland can be seen

We have not studied in this context any cases of complete obstruction of the distal end, as this possibility can be easily detected by simple pression in the valve chamber.

We have performed the study on four cases of partial obstruction of the distal system, clinically suspected; we have needed from 40 to 120 pumpings to force the indicator out of the catheter (Fig. 4). We have diagnosed two cases of partial obstruction of the system in patients that had no symptomatology and on whom we were performing study as routine control; the clinical symptomatology appeared, respectively, at 2 and 4 months after the scan discovery, as certaining the obstruction in the reintervention. We have also had one case in wich a partial obstruction of the distal tube and the necessity of a reintervention were clinically suspected; the photoscan study was absolutely normal, and we delayed the intervention awaiting its evolution; at present it is now 3 months since we performed the exploration and the patient feels perfectly well, without any necessity of surgical reintervention; the new control photoscan studies are still normal (Fig. 5).

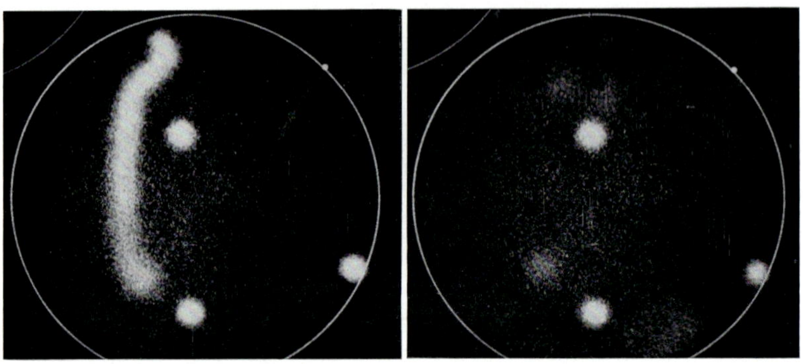

a b

Fig. 5 a and b. Patient with clinical suspicion of partial obstruction of the distal tube of the bypass system. The photoscan study was completely normal, for which reason delayed the intervention; three months later the patient was feeling perfectly well, without any necessity of surgical reintervention; the new control photoscan studies are still normal. a Pudenz valve in basal situation. b After ten strokes there is no radioactive material left in the bypass system; the thyroid gland can be seen

Studies of Localization

We perform the studies of localization comparing the situation of the catheter full of radioactive material to reference points placed in the external jugulum, IV right costo-sternal articulation, and breast mamilla. They are of a certain interest in those cases in which the radiographic visualization of the distal end of the catheter is difficult or impossible; notwithstanding, we think they are less interesting than the permeability studies, since that the alteration in the situation produces at the same time alterations in the permeability of the system.

Discussion

At present there are very few methods to study the situation and permeability of the CSF bypass systems, with the further disadvantage that they are all based on indirect findings.

The usual localization studies consist fundamentally of: a) performing an electrocardiogram during the operation as the catheter advances from the jugular vein to the heart until the apparition of a *P* wave shows it has reached the auricle; this method cannot be used for a later control, since that it can be employed only during the operation. b) localization of the distal end of the catheter through thorax-penetrating radiography; it is not always visible, due to its small size and continuous motion in the blood flow. With radioactive material we can demostrate in a simple and elegant form the catheter situation.

The methods presently used to study the permeability of the bypass system are indirect too, and moreover they have the disagreeable inconvenient that the substances must be injected either into cerebral ventricles or into lumbar subarachnoideous space.

Al these methods employ also radioactive materials and are based on the measurement of the radioactivity either in the plasma or in the blood at time intervals after the lumbar o intraventricular injection. If the radioactive materials are found in colloidal solution, some authors measure the hepatic uptake by Küpffer cells between 2 and 6h after the injection.

It is evident that these methods are liable to many errors and present two fundamental disadvanteges: a) necessity of either intraventricular or lumbar subarchnoideous space injection, with discomfort for the patient, and b) lack of direct information.

As we have previously said, our method avoids these two disadvantages since that we get a morphologic and graphic representation of the system and the means of administration of the radioactive materials is a simple subcutaneous injection. We only have to be careful not to perforate with the needle the membrane inside the central chamber of the system, otherwise all the radioactive material would penetrate into the ventricles. So far such an incident has not happened in our researches.

Conclusion

We present a method for the study of the situation and permeability of Pudenz valves by radioactive materials; it has the advantage, over the conventional methods previousely used, that it enables us to demostrate in a direct and objective way the working of the bypass system and that it is absolutely innocuous and practically free of trauma for the patient. This study is only part of a wider project in wich we will try to quantify the amount of the CSF through the valve system.

The Use of Angiokinematography in Diseases and Closures of Cerebral Vessels

E. M. Klausberger

The evaluation of the flow of blood in the area of the A. carotis and A. vertebralis requires the preparation of the morphological conditions in the areas of the trunks and branches of these vessels. Modern technical equipment and contrast media most recently developed guarantee secure information on the condition of the vessel walls and the alterations of diameter.

Functional results and information about the passagetime in the trunks and branches as far as the capillary area are provided by angiokinematography with the high-speed-camera.

Gamma-camera and multi-canal-accumulator are used, too, in measuring the complete and regional cerebral flow of blood in the hemispheres.

The arteriosclerotic plaque and the generalised alterations of the vessel walls show a diminution of the calibres with a circumscribed dilation of the vessels or the calibre-strong trunks with tiny branches. Due to the cerebral angiokinematography controlled by the heart-rhythm delayed passage in the vascular sections with larger diameters can be shown. As a manifestation of the more insufficient process of nutrition this delay of the flow of blood, on the whole, is in agreement with the pathological standard of the Xenon-measure of the cerebral flow of blood.

In case of a closure of the A. carotis interna or the A. cerebri media there is often no sufficient involution of the clinical symptoms, though in the serial angiogram calibre-strong collaterals are displayed. The cerebral angiokinematography directed by the cardial rhythm can prove the blatant delay of passage in the extensive collateral ways. The deficient clinical involutions of these sections is explained by the bad condition of nutrition.

Alterations of the vessel walls and closure of the cerebral vessels can be localised by serial angiography. Angiokinematography controlled by the heart-rhythm with the high-speed-camera (75 pictures/sec) analyses the passage time in circumscribed vessel-sections and collaterals. Thus diagnostic, prognostical and therapeutic results to a greater extent can be gained.

The Value of Brain Scintigraphy (Technetium-99m) in the Differential Diagnosis and Follow-Up of Cases of Cerebro-Vascular Disease

H. Waldbaur, W. Walter, F. Wolf and W. Schiefer

In a group of 360 patients in whom brain scintigraphy with ^{99m}Tc-pertechnetate was performed, there were 25 patients with cerebral infarction or an intracerebral hematoma due to diffuse vascular disease. Scintigraphy was found to be a very valuable method of investigation here, especially in regard to the differentiation between cerebrovascular diesease and brain tumor. In agreement with the data in the literature, we found little or no increase in activity in the first few days after the onset of neurological deficits, maximum activity after 2 weeks and normasisation in the course of subsequent weeks.

A few cases will now demonstrate our observations:

1. 48-year-old female patient, previous history unremarkable, normal blood pressure. Relatively acute onset of headache, rapidly progressing left-sided hemiparesis without loss of consciousness. On admission, complete left-sided hemiparesis, bulbar voice, awake and oriented, echoencephalographic displacement 3,5 mm to the left, EEG showed right precentral focus.

The angiogram indicated a precentral lesion, and the brain scintigram performed 2 days after onset of illness showed a somewhat diffuse focus of activity in the parietal region. 1 week after onset of the disease the focus is considerably more marked and it becomes less again in the scintigram performed after 3 weeks. 5 weeks later the activity has disappeared and the neurological deficits have subsided. This is an unequivocal case of encephalomalacia.

2. 23-year-old male with a traumatic carotid-cavernous fistula. Neurological examination unremarkable. The aneurysm appeared in the angiogram and the scintigram was unremarkable. At operation, the common carotid artery is first ligated and at the subsequent operation, the internal corotid artery in the neck is tied. Following discharge, the patient had a wild night followed by right-sided hemiparesis and aphasia, which normalized at the new admission. The slight increase in activity in the left temporal area was observed 5 days after the onset of hemiparesis and a more marked focus after 14 days. The increase in activity had completely disappeared 4 weeks later at which time the neurological deficits had also normalized.

3. 21-year-old male, acute right hemiparesis following alleged slight head injury. On admission complete hemiparesis on the right and complete aphasia. Normal echo-finding, severe changes in the EEG. The angiogram revealed a rare case of carotid occlusion at the level of the siphon with meningeal anastomoses coming from the posterior cerebral artery, and the scintigram showed a massive increase of activity in the region of the middle cerebral artery corresponding to the neurological deficits (14 days after onset of the disease).

The subsequent course was seen in control brain scintigrams. 3 weeks after the onset of the disease, the activity decreases and 8 days later the amount of activity has again decreased. 7 weeks after the onset of the disease, there ist little activity present. The neurological deficits underwent a corresponding improvement although the angiographic control showed no change in the circulation.

Zur Differentialdiagnose früh abführender Venen im Carotisangiogramm

H. Hacker

Früh abführende Venen und diffuse Kontrastmittelansammlungen oder -anfärbungen sind als charakteristische Befunde bei Tumoren und Gefäßmißbildungen bekannt. Ähnliche Befunde sind 1958 von Woringer u. Mitarb. bei entzündlichen Hirnerkrankungen beschrieben und 1966 von Ferris und Mitarb. bei cerebralen Gefäßerkrankungen. Lassen fand 1967 bei der Messung des regionalen cerebralen Blutflusses mit der ^{133}Xenon-Clearance einen erhöhten shuntähnlichen Blutfluß in der Umgebung infarzierter Hirnregionen. Dieses Phänomen ist unter der Bezeichnung „Luxusperfusion" bekannt geworden, man spricht heute von Vasoparalyse. Folgende pathophysiologische Regulation wurden aufgeklärt: Im Bereich einer mangelnden Blutversorgung führt der Sauerstoffmangel zur Anreicherung von Milchsäure. Diese Übersäuerung erweitert im Grenzgebiet zum normalen Gewebe die kleinen Gefäße maximal, der Blutfluß ist stark erhöht. Angiographisch haben wir das Bild einer Anfärbung mit früh abführender Vene. Gleichzeitig kann sich in der Infarktzone ein Ödem ausgebildet haben, das als Raumbeschränkung Arterien und Venen verlagert. Die Unterscheidung zwischen Tumor und Gefäßprozeß ist dann gelegentlich schwierig.

Verlaufsuntersuchungen des cerebralen Blutflusses mit Xenon bei Gefäßprozessen haben jedoch einen wesentlichen Hinweis gegeben. Die Vasoparalyse in der Randzone von Infarkten ist eine temporäre Erscheinung, die bis zu 24 Std nach einem Gefäßverschluß einsetzt und nicht länger als 7–14 Tage nachzuweisen ist. Das heißt, daß auch im angiographischen Bild eine Hyperämie mit früh abführender Vene nach 14 Tagen verschwunden sein muß. Ist dies nicht der Fall, so kann mit großer Wahrscheinlichkeit die Diagnose eines Tumors oder einer Gefäßmißbildung gestellt werden.

Für die Praxis muß daher bei Patienten mit früh abführender Vene im Angiogramm, bei denen typische Zeichen für ein Neoplasma oder einen Gefäßprozess fehlen, die Angiographie nach 14 Tagen wiederholt werden. Dann ist eine sichere Diagnose möglich.

Es sollte dabei beachtet werden, daß nach 2 Wochen dehydrierender Behandlung Gefäßverlagerungen völlig zurückgegangen sein können und eine Raumbeschränkung nicht mehr diagnostiziert werden kann. Das schließt nach unseren Erfahrungen jedoch das Vorliegen eines Tumors nicht aus.

Das hier beschriebene Vorgehen zeigt, wie die angiographische Diagnostik durch Erkenntnisse, die durch Isotopenmethoden gewonnen wurden, weiter verbessert werden kann.

Opacification des veines de l'orbite au cours de l'angiographie carotidienne externe

G. Salomon, G. Giudicelli, P. Castan et D. Mitard

Depuis la publication du travail de Hacker, nous connaissons les phénomènes *d'opacification* de la *veine ophtalmique supérieure* dans l'angiographie cérébrale.

Elle s'opacifie dans le sens antéro-postérieur au cours de l'artériographie carotide externe. Elle peut s'opacifier occasionnellement dans le sens postéro-antérieur au cours l'angiographie carotidienne interne.

Nous avons constaté de même la très grande fréquence de l'opacification de la veine ophtalmique supérieure au cours de l'artériographie carotidienne externe où elle apparait dans plus de 8 cas sur 10. Nous devons préciser que tous nos examens ont été réalisés sous anesthésie générale.

Cette fréquence de l'opacification de la veine ophtalmique nous amène à insister sur deux points précis:

a) d'une part, ainsi que l'a précisé Hacker, il est vraisemblable que la veine ophtalmique supérieure représente *une voie de drainage de la muqueuse des cornets*. Nous n'avons cependant pas retrouvé le même parallélisme entre l'importance de l'opacification de cette muqueuse et la visibilité de la veine ophtalmique supérieure.

Aussi il nous semble que la veine ophtalmique supérieure constitue de plus la voie de drainage physiologique *des parties molles extra-crâniennes* de la partie antérieure de la *voûte* qui sont vascularisées par *l'artère temporale superficleile*. Le sang veineux atteint la veine ophtalmique supérieure par l'intermédiaire des *veines frontales* et de la *veine angulaire*.

Ceci peut expliquer que l'on puisse voir les deux veines ophtalmiques supérieures droite et gauche alors que les muqueuses des fosses nasales ne sont opacifiées que d'un seul côté.

b) d'autre part, la très grande fréquence de l'opacification de cette veine ophtalmique supérieure au cours de l'angiographie de la carotide externe nous a conduit depuis quelques années à utiliser l'artériographie carotidienne externe chaque fois qu'une exploration des veines de l'orbite est nécessaire.

Nous avons pû constater que non seulement la veine ophtalmique supérieure est visible, mais aussi quelquefois les *veines absidales antérieures et postérieures*.

L'étude des *processus expansifs intra-orbitaires* peut être réalisée ainsi dans la même séance par artériographie carotidienne interne afin de voir l'artère ophtalmique et ses branches et par artériographie carotidienne externe afin de voir le *courant veineux supérieur*.

Nous précisons que toutes ces données ont été établies à partir d'angiographie sélective de l'artère carotide externe.

Pathalogical Processes of the Spinal-Canal

L'arteriographie médullaire

R. Djindjian

1. L'exploration angiographique de la moëlle semblait difficile du fait :

a) du calibre étroit de ses vaisseaux,

b) et de la multiplicité d'origine de ses artères nourricières.

Un pas en avant a été réalisé par l'aortographie que nous avons préconisée en 1961. L'artériographie sélective des artères intercostales a transformé depuis 1966 l'exploration angiographique de la moëlle car elle a permis:

c) d'obtenir des images de face et de profil de qualité incomparable, améliorées encore par la soustraction.

2. La technique utilisée est la suivante :

a) cathéter à extrêmité recourbée introduit par voie fémorale.

b) l'extrêmité du cathéter est introduit dans l'ostium de chaque intercostale avec injection de 3 à 4cc de produit de contraste et prise de cliché sur chaque artère, car les artères médullaires sont invisibles sur l'écran de télévision.

c) pour la région cervicale, nécessité d'opacifier la sous-clavière gauche et droite et leurs branches vertébrales et cervicale profonde.

3. Un bref *rappel anatomique* est nécessaire pour la compréhension de la vascularisation de la moëlle.

Celle-ci est assurée par un axe artériel spinal antérieur nourrissant les $^3/_4$ antérieurs de la moëlle et 2 axes artériels postéro-latéraux irriguant une faible portion postérieure.

L'axe spinal antérieur est nourri par 3 ou 4 artères radiculo-médullaires issues de l'artère sous-clavière et des artères intercostales, la plus volumineuse étant l'artère d'Adamkiewicz irriguant à elle-seule la moëlle dorso-lombaire; une lésion à ce niveau entraînerait une ischémie médullaire. Les axes postérieurs sont nourris à l'opposé par de nombreuses artères radiculo-médullaires et de ce fait leur ligature n'entraîne pas d'ischémie, et ainsi apparaît cette notion chirurgicale capitale: à savoir que l'on peut sacrifier sans risque les artères postérieures, alors que les artères antérieures doivent être respectées.

4. L'artériographie médullaire permet une étude *in vivo* de la vascularisation normale de la moëlle.

a) L'artère d'Adamkiewicz en épingle à cheveux avec une branche ascendante grêle et une branche descendante volumineuse.

b) La branche dorsale, d'aspect identique mais plus grêle, naissant de la 2°, 3°, ou 4° artère intercostale.

c) L'artère du renflement cervical plus volumineuse dont la branche ascendante rejoint l'artère spinale antérieure issue de l'artère vertébrale.

d) L'artère spinale postérieure est plus grêle, elle présente un aspect en épingle à cheveux plus étroite. Elle est en position para-médiane.

Ainsi l'artériographie normale va nous permettre de mieux comprendre l'artériographie pathologique que nous envisagerons dans les angiomes, les tumeurs, l'ischémie médullaire.

Les angiomes médullaires

L'artériographie dans les angiomes médullaires est la plus spectaculaire. 70 cas ont été opacifiés par l'artériographie.

L'artériographie sélective est le seul examen valable: elle permet:

a) d'affirmer la malformation et sa nature artério-veineuse avec une artère nourricière, une masse angiomateuse, une veine de draînage.

b) elle précise le volume de l'angiome.

c) surtout elle précise le nombre et le siège des pédicules nourriciers. L'artériographie médullaire est donc le seul examen permettant d'établir un bilan pré-opératoire précis. En effet:

d) Les angiomes rétro-médullaires nourris par les artères spinales postérieures sont seuls justiciables d'une exérèse complète.

e) Les angiomes intra-médullaires nourris par les artères spinales antérieures sont actuellement inopérables.

f) Les angiomes mixtes peuvent bénéficier de l'exérèse ou de l'embolisation des seuls pédicules postérieurs.

L'artériographie dans tumeurs vertebro-médullaires

Elle peut fournir des renseignements que n'apporte pas la myélographie. En effet elle présente un double avantage:

1. situer l'origine de l'artère d'Adamkiewicz pour éviter de la blesser lors des interventions responsables de certaines paraplégies post-opératoires.

2. lorsque la tumeur est opacifiée permettre un diagnostic étiologique: comme dans un cas:

a) de neurinome en sablier (image artériographique de tumeur bénigne).

b) de métastase (avec artériographie de tumeur maligne).

c) d'un angio-réticulome intra-médullaire.

d) de tumeurs osseuses comme les angiomes vertébraux.

L'artériographie dans les ischemies médullaires

La vascularisation de la moëlle a ceci de particulier qu'il s'agit d'une vascularisation de territoire; chaque territoire est irrigué par une seule artère et l'obstruction ou la lésion d'une de ces artères suffit à déterminer un foyer myélomalacique dans ce territoire.

Le siège et les causes de l'obstruction peuvent se situer à différents niveaux:

1. au niveau de l'axe artériel spinal antérieur par une tumeur intra-médullaire ou nue hernie discale médiane qui refoule l'artère d'Adamkiewicz.

2. au niveau des artères radiculo-médullaires, par des néoformations épidurales, des radicotomies, des cyphoscolioses.

3. au niveau de l'aorte: clampage temporaire, ligature d'artères intercostales en chirurgie thoracique, lésions athéromateuses surtout: sténose ostiale et sténose de l'artère intercostale nourrissant l'artère d'Adamkiewicz. Ces lésions sont en tous points superposables aux sténoses carotidiennes ou vertébrales et sont responsables à notre avis d'un grand nombre de paraplégies sans causes.

Scintigraphie

La poursuite de l'analogie de l'artériographie médullaire avec l'artériographie cérébrale nous a conduit à utiliser d'autres méthodes d'exploration, à savoir l'injection de produits radio-actifs:

1. soit injection des macro-agrégats marqués à l'iode-131 ou au technécium-99.

a) dans une artère intercostale opacifiant l'hémi-vertèbre et la côte ou.

b) dans une artère intercostale nourrissant l'artère d'Adamkiewicz (opacification vertébrale et médullaire).

c) application dans les tumeurs vertébro-médullaires (un cas de métastase).

2. soit injection de Xenon-133 dans l'artère intercostale nourrissant l'artère d'Adamkiewicz avec établissement de clearance médullaire qui permettra d'apprécier le débit médullaire.

En conclusion : L'artériographie médullaire se révèle être un examen:

a) indispensable au diagnostic et au traitement des angiomes.

b) nécessaire à la compréhension de l'ischémie médullaire.

c) complémentaire pour le diagnostic des tumeurs.

The Significance of the Magnetic-Tape Recording of Myelographies with Duroliopaque for the Diagnosis of small Space-Narrowing Processes in the Cervico-Thoracic Region of the Spinal Canal

H. HERRSCHAFT and F. GLEIM

Myelographies of space-limiting processes in the cervicothoracic region of the vertebral canal which are not yet great and extended enough to produce a higher degree of narrowing of the spinal subarachnoid space have been most difficult to perform by means of the hitherto available methods of examination. Thus a considerable number of spondylopathies and myelopathies, among which especially extradural, degenerative and traumatic pathological processes originating from the vertebral disks and ligamentous apparatus of the cervico-thoracic parts of the spinal column, could not be clearly diagnosed. In the past 3 years we succeeded in developing a new method of examination, characterized by the use of magnetic-tape recordings and the instillation of a recently developed contrast medium insoluble in water. This new method allows an optimal opacification of the cervico-thoracic cerebrospinal-fluid spaces. A detailed description of this method and a report on employment and efficiency of the continuous televisionband recording in total spinal-canal myelography have already been formulated in other publications[1].

Method

The myelographies are carried out with a „Magister" (C.G.R. Paris), a distant-control X-ray apparatus (Figs. 1 and 3). During television screening a fully transistorized television recorder, the „Ampex" model VIDEOTAPE-RECORDER 7003, *continuously* shoots the process of examination. Magnetic-tape recording allows to reproduce in full details the dynamic course of the examination, to repeat this course as many times as desired, and to stop it at any moment in order to carefully study and assess the image sector in question. Since the picture quality of the tape recording nearly equals that of radiographs serial spot films of the different spinalcanal segments as otherwise would be necessary are superfluous. Instead of the X-ray films the magnetic tapes are used for documentation. In safe keeping the durability of these tapes is nearly unlimited. They may be filed in archives in the same way as X-ray films.

---

1 HERRSCHAFT, H., GLEIM, F.: Klinische Erfahrungen mit der kontinuierlichen Fernseh-Bandaufzeichnung von Duroliopaque-Myelographien. Der Radiologe *11*, 8–14 (1971).

HERRSCHAFT, H.: Die kontinuierliche Fernseh-Bandaufzeichnung bei der Gesamtspinalkanal-Myelographie. Röntgenblätter *25*, 10–21 (1972).

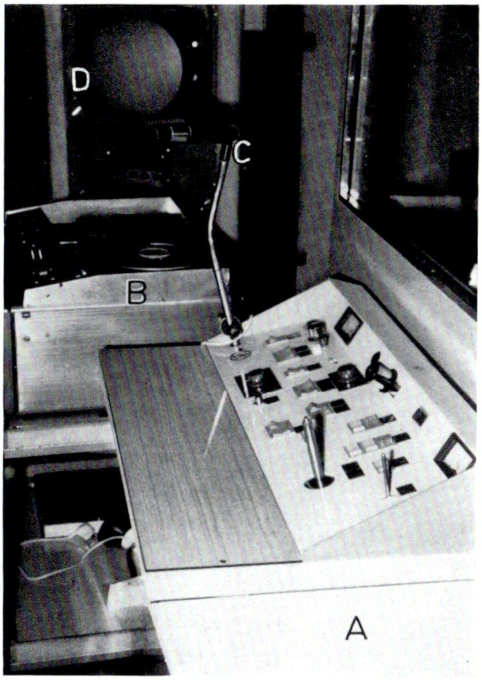

Fig. 1. Equipment for the Magnetic-Tape Recording of Myelographies. A = Control desk for the distant-control-x-ray apparatus ("Magister", C.G.R., Paris – Koch & Sterzel, Essen). B = Television recorder ("Ampex"-model: Videotape-Recorder 70003). C = Microphone, necessary to take up a comment during examination. D = Apparatus for television-screening

In normal myelography with Duroliopaque of the entire spinal canal the process of recording takes 15 minutes. On a Video tape examinations of totally 4 myelographies may be recorded. When selecting for documentation only the pathological findings and those normal findings which are necessary for excluding a space-giving or space-narrowing process in the spinal canal the number of myeolographies to be recorded on one tape may be readily increased to 10. By means of an electronic cutting-technique among the total of registered phases of examination only diagnostically relevant sections are selected and transmitted on a tape meant for the archives.

The contrast medium used is Duroliopaque, an ethyl monoiodostearate. Due to its low viscosity Durolipaque in an amount of 12 to 20 ml may be instilled without pain, and postradiologically may be removed again from the spinal-fluid spaces without difficulties. With this new contrast matter, for the first time, it is possible to fill the whole spinal canal with an uninterrupted stream of radiopaque substance. Thus it meets the requirements for a continuous recording of the course of examination.

As concerns the process of examination it is to say that under fluoroscopic control, following lumbar puncture and instillation of the contrast medium, the patient in sitting position (Fig. 2), and without moving himself is brought first into left lateral position by tilting the examination table toward his head (Figs. 3 and 4) and subse-

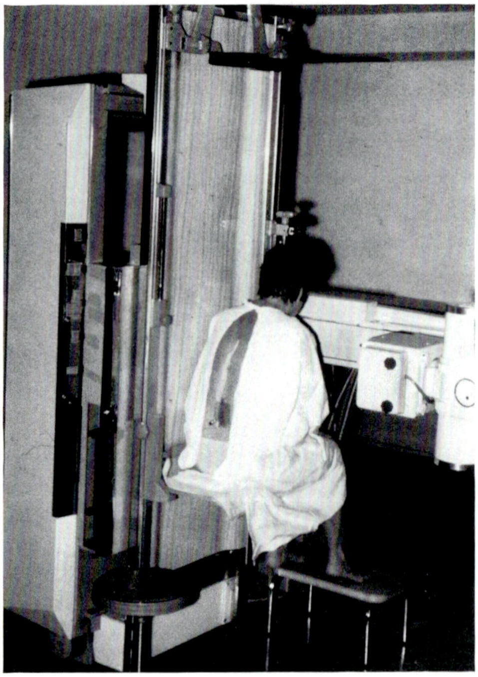

Fig. 2. Position I. Patient sitting on the foot-stay of the vertical tilted examination table. Lumbar puncture and instillation of the contrast medium are performed

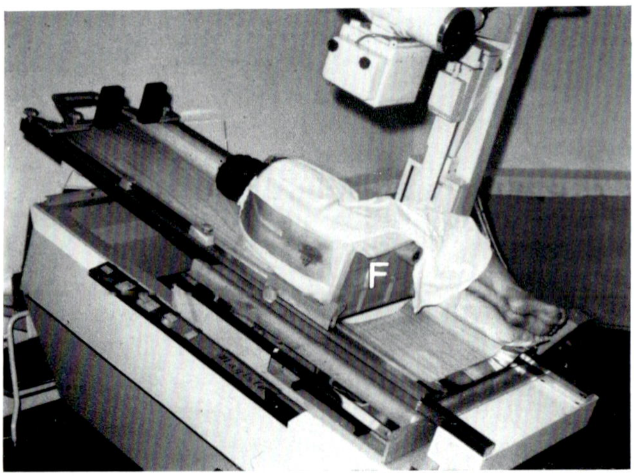

Fig. 3. Position II. Patient in lateral position. Examination table tilted toward his head. Foot-stay still in "sitting-position"

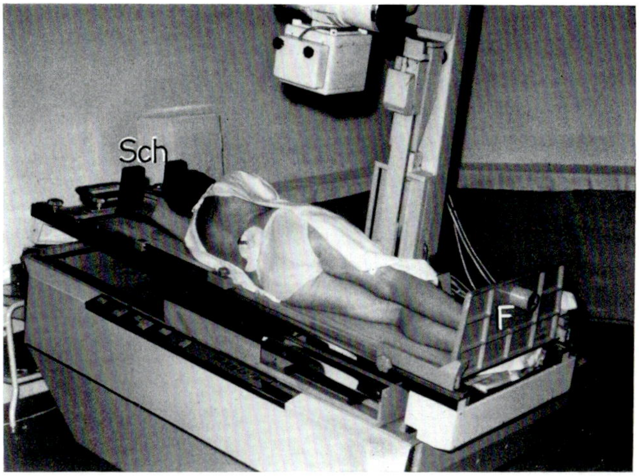

Fig. 4. Position III. Patient in left lateral position. Foot-stay (F) moved to the end of the examination table. Sch = shoulder support not yet applied

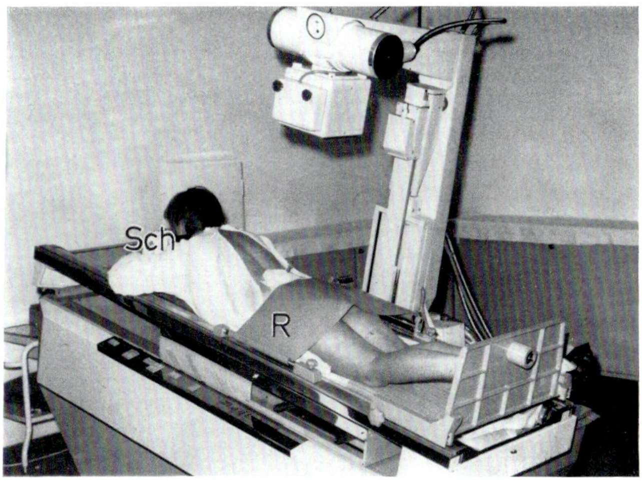

Fig. 5. Position IV. Patient in prone position. Shoulder support (Sch) and back strap (R) applied

quently into prone position by turning him around the longitudinal axis of his body (Fig. 5). The patient keeps this position for the rest of the examination. In order to prevent a sliding off when the head is lowered a shoulder support and a back strap are applied. The subsequent examination is performed under continuous television-screening. With the head lowered, successively lumbar, thoracic and cervical parts of the spinal canal are explored, whereby the quantity of contrast medium used (12 to 20 ml) ensures the ventral wall and the lateral limitations of the spinal canal including root ventricles to be completely reproduced. Following the examination of

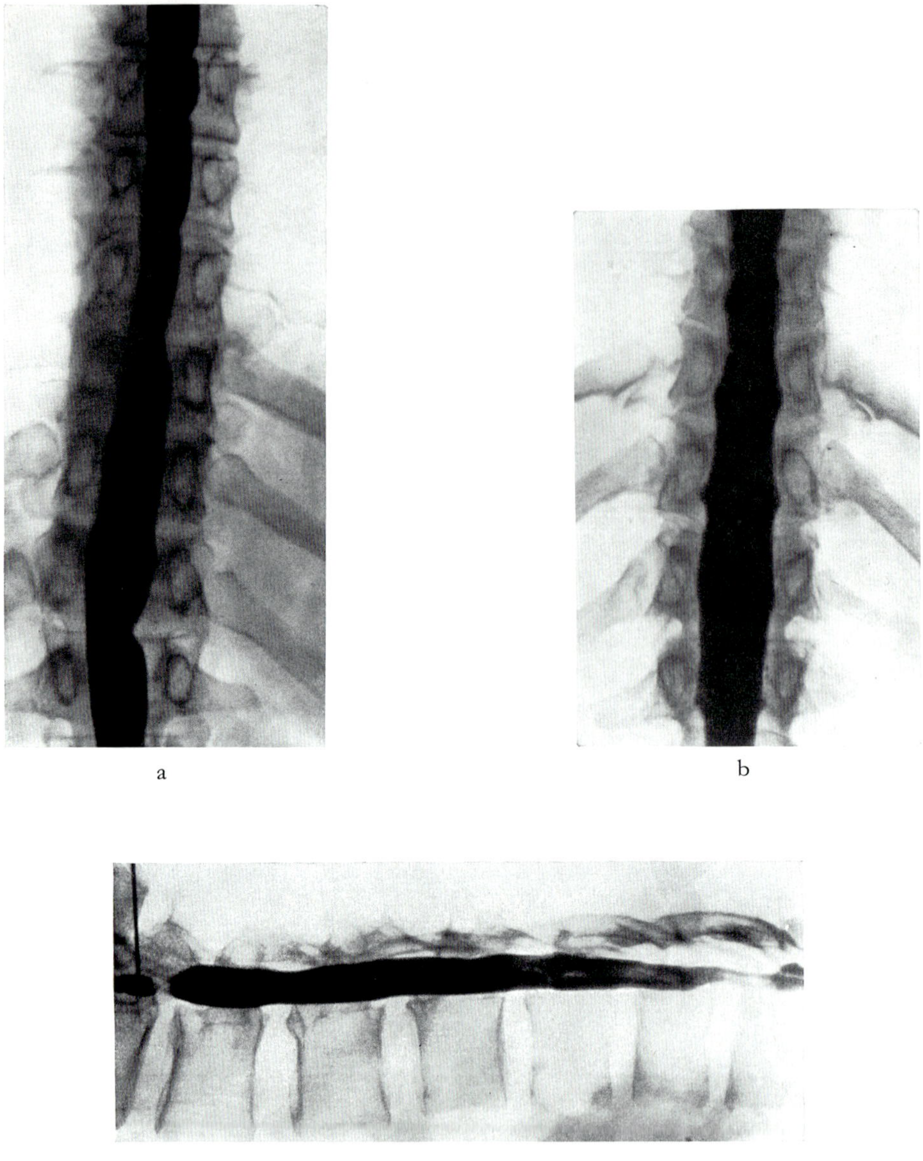

a b c

Fig. 6a–c. Normal thoracic myelograms. a and b. Postero-anterior ray path. c. Horizontal ray path

the cervical parts of the spinal canal the table with the patient is slowly brought back into its normal position so that the reflux of the contrast medium to the conus terminalis of the subarachnoid space can be observed and recorded, again under fluoroscopic control. Immediately after ending of the myelography the contrast medium is removed with the puncture canula kept over the examination.

Only in rare cases it is necessary to deviate from the examination scheme above described. Despite the safety measures such as shoulder support and back strap the patient has enough freedom of movement so that under pathological circumstances not only a screening in the p.a. ray path but also in oblique and lateral position may be performed without difficulty. For radioascopy in horizontal ray path a second tube is necessary.

Under normal circumstances the above examination method allows a complete and clearly interpretable opacification of the cervico-thoracic regions of the spinal canal (Figs. 6 and 7).

In contrast to Duroliopaque the iodine esters insoluble in water and which up to now had been used for visualization of the thoracic part of the spinal canal (Pantopaque, Ethiodan, Myodil) as a rule do not allow to obtain a reliable and clearly

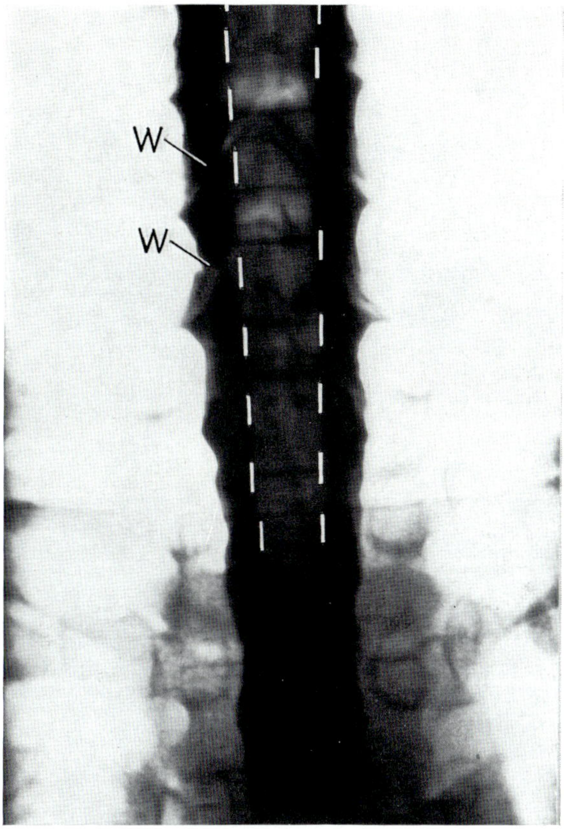

a

Fig. 7a and b. Normal cervical myelograms. x-ray films in the postero-anterior ray path. Patient in prone position. Examination-table in head down position. Tilting angle 60 degree. In the closed column of contrast medium breadth an limitations of the cervical subarachnoid space including root ventricles (W) are recognizable as well as localisation and outlines of the cervical medullar, which in the middle of the contrast column is to be seen at reduced opacity (punctured line). c. X-ray in horizontal ray path. Patient in prone position.

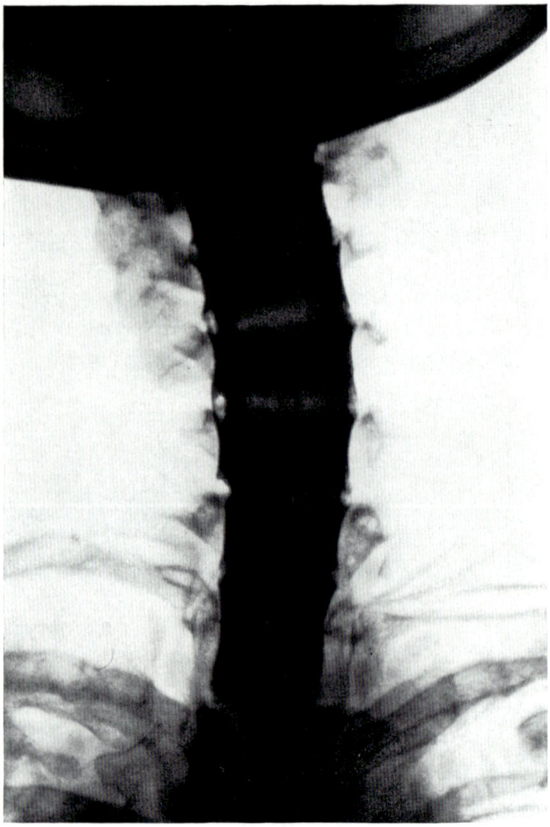
Fig. 7b

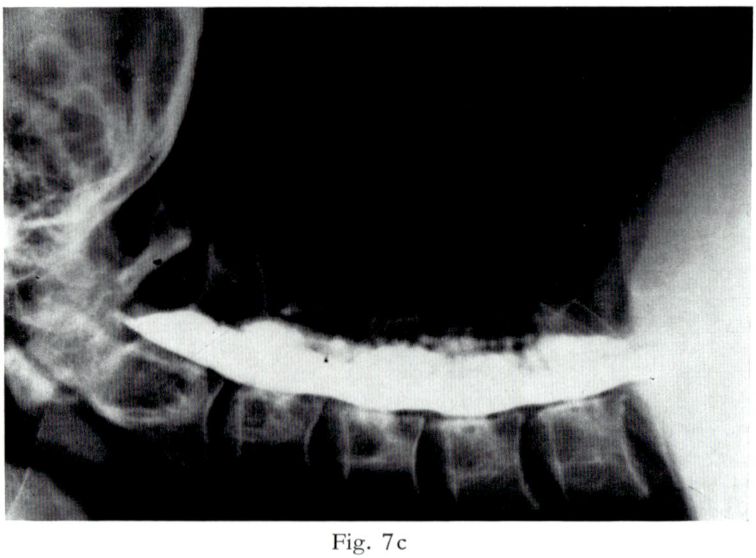
Fig. 7c

interpretable myelogram. Due to the ascending displacement of these contrast media irregularities in the contrast-medium column generally occur after the lumbo-dorsal passage in form of round or oval blancs of different size, sand-glass-shaped narrowings and unilateral concave defects of the contrast medium (Fig. 8). Often the contrast-matter column is even totally disrupted to radiopaque spots of various size scattered over a great number of segments of the thoracic spinal column (Fig. 9).

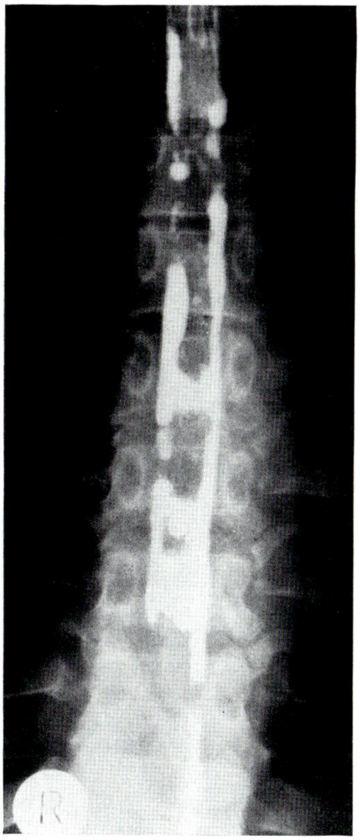

8

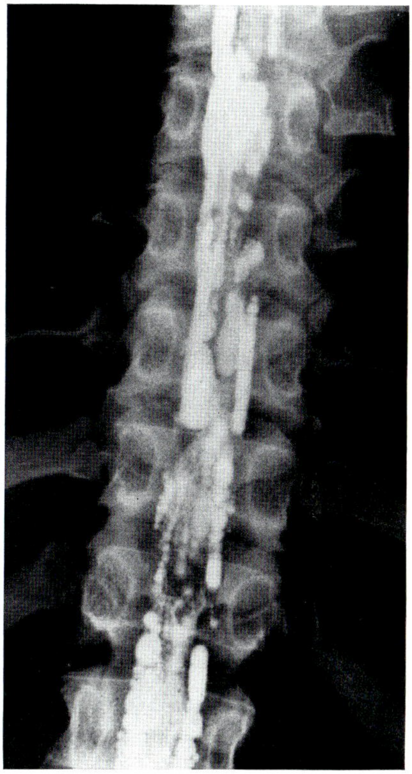

9

Fig. 8 and 9. Technical contrast-medium artefacts in the thoracic part of the spinal canal, produced by one of the iodine esters insoluble in water, which up to now have been used for visualization of the cervico-thoracic subarachnoid spaces. 8. Irregularities in the contrast-medium column in form of round or oval blacs of different size and sand-glass shaped narrowings. 9. Contrast matter column totally disrupted to radiopaque spots of various size, scattered over a great number of segments of the thoracic part of the spinal canal

Because of these irregularities in many cases it has not yet been possible to distinguish in the thoracic part of the spinal canal between pathological alterations and technical contrastmedium artefacts which morphologically are very similar. As a rule physicians had to content themselves with noting the passability of the spinal canal. Small and some mediumsized space-requiring processes which did not yet visibly obstruct the passage remained unrecognized or were detected only as pathological alterations without any possibility of a closer assessment.

With Duroliopaque in more than 90% of all cases the contrast medium can be channeled as an uninterrupted column even through the thoracal part of the spinal canal. Breadth and limitations of the thoracic spinal-fluid spaces including root ventricles are accurately visualized. The thoracic region of the spinal cord appears as a less opaque line in the middle of the contrast column. In a similar way the cervical subarachnoid spinal-fluid spaces are visualized. In order to make the contrast medium completely fill the cervical region of the spinal canal, in lowering the head, a tilting angle of 40–50 degree is generally sufficient. Only in exceptional cases a greater tilting of the examination table is necessary. In head-down position, as well as in the subsequent horizontal position of the patient the contrast medium completely fills the cervical part of the spinal canal and the adjacent regions of the upper thoracic spinal column. Breadth and limitations of the cervical subarachnoid space (including root ventricles) as well as localisation and outlines of the cervical medullar, which in the middle of the contrast column is to be seen at reduced opacity, are well recognizable and interpretable (Fig. 7a).

Constant blancs of contrast medium within this normally uninterrupted, homogenous contrast band are always to interpret as indicating a circumscribed space-reducing process. Our examinations have shown that blancs in the contrast-medium column are always associated with a circumscribed obstruction of the contrast-medium flow in that region. When the course of examination is continuously recorded nature, form and duration of the passage obstruction may be accurately ascertained.

In the same way as contrast-medium blancs, not or only insufficiently filled root ventricles frequently occuring in connection with contrast-medium blancs but sometimes also independently must be interpreted as pathological. Size and seat of the contrast-medium defect indicate the extent and segmental localisation of the space-narrowing process. The nature of the space-requiring process, however, is not clearly shown by myelography. Particularly the nature of small space-reducing processes is very hard to diagnose. In the following figures (Fig. 10a–c.) you will find 3 contrast-medium defects which show the same morphological pattern, and had been diagnosed by operation as space-narrowing processes: one case of intradural meningeoma, antother of sequestrated disk prolapse and a thrid one of intramedullary metastasis.

The evaluation of 60 magnetic-tape recordings of myelographies with Duroliopaque in the presence of space-narrowing processes in the thoracic and cervical regions of the spinal canal reveals that on the basis of parameters such as size, form, segmental localisation of the codntrast-medium blanc and nature of the obstructed passage only in a restricted number of cases it is possible to localize the space-requiring process with respect to the spinal cord and its membrane. In a complete stop ($^1/_5$ of our patients) the limitations of the contrast-medium column, as a rule, do not allow conclusions about the exact seat of the space requirement in respect to the spinal cord and its membranes. In these cases by tape recording only the complete obstruction of the contrast-medium flow can be found out. This is quite different in cases where the cerebrospinal-fluid spaces are only partially obstructed or when the present contrast-medium blancs are associated only with light obstructions of the passage ($^4/_5$ of this series of patients). In these cases television-tape recording performed with Duroliopaque as contrast-medium is more helpful than the hitherto usual methods of examination. When using this new method the well-known cir-

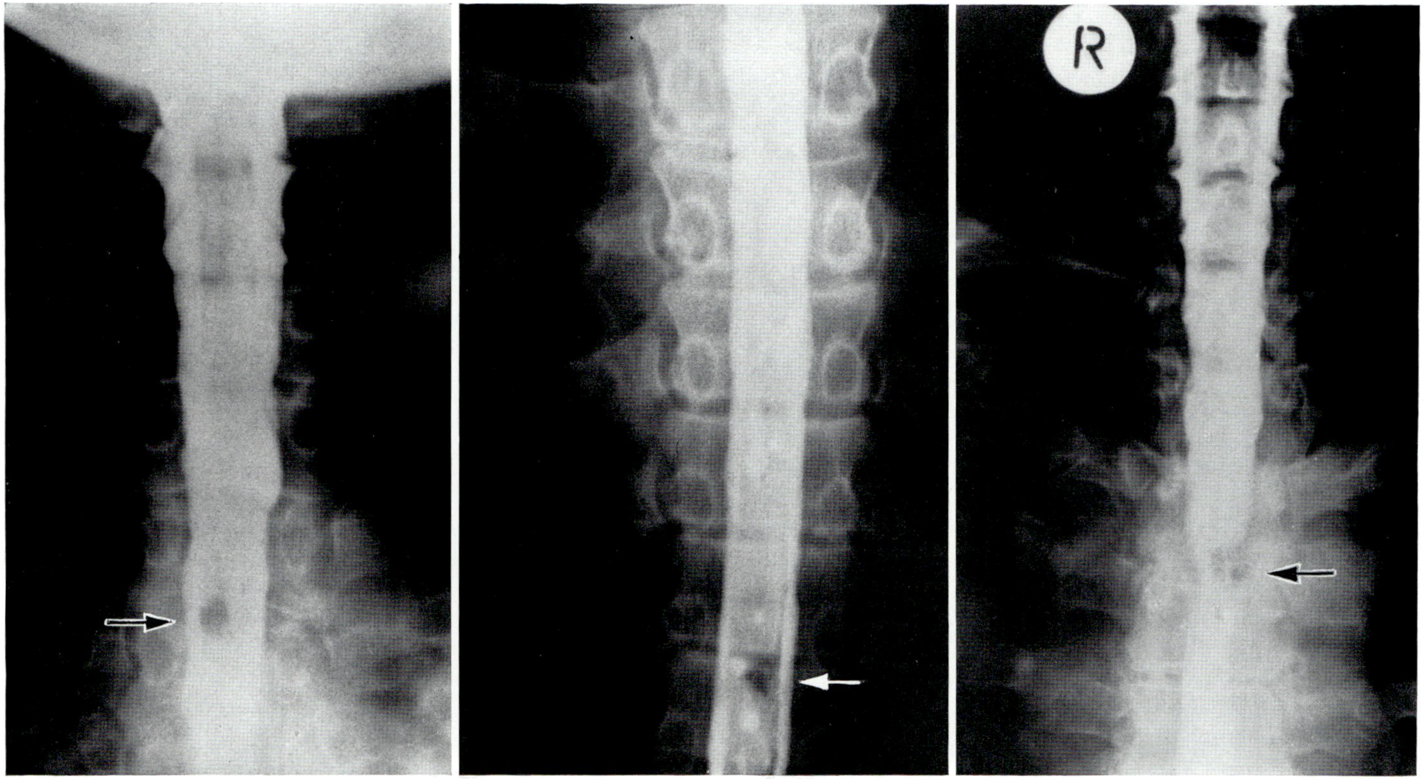

a b c

Fig. 10a–c. Duroliopaque – myelograms of three small space-occupying processes in the thoracic part of the spinal canal. (Arrows). a Sequestred disk prolapse Th_3/Th_4. b Intradural meningeoma. c Intramedullary metastasis. All three cases verified by operation teria for distinguishing between intramedullary and extramedullary-intradural and extradural space-narrowing processes are enlarged by the parameter of "dynamics of the contrast-medium passage". Thus the criteria considerably gain in clearness.

The continuous tape recording of myelographies with Durodiopaque helps to distinguish between small spacenarrowing processes and technical contrast-medium artefacts. A comparison of the results obtained with the hitherto usual method – screening in alternation with serial spot films and Pantopaque as contrast medium – with those realized due to the continuous tape recording of myelographies with Duroliopaque reveals a decrease at about 30% in the number of myelographs which cannot be clearly interpreted or which are falsely negative. Falsely positive findings have not been established during the totally 160 tape recordings.

The value of this examination method may be best proved by the tape recordings themselves. Therefore I will end up with the demonstration of a film showing a myelography of the entire spinal canal. The examination had been carried out in a patient with a small disk prolapse in the cervical region which in the meantime could be verified and removed by operation.

Space Occupying Processes of the Spinal Canal and their Diagnosis through Intraosseous Spinal Venography

H. VOGELSANG

The angiographic diagnosis of space occupying processes of the vertebral column and spinal canal has been steadly increases and technically perfectionized in the past few years. When we consider the fact that an arteriography of the spinal canal as diagnostic method for localizing a space occupying process has to be complemented through further examinations, we can perhaps consider as the best method of examination at the present time the transosseous phlebography. She can be excercised first through a vertebral body (cervical portion), or secondly through a vertebra spine (thoracic or lumbar portion). Considering the anatomic construction of the spinal column's and spinal canal veinssystem, it is only natural that the phlebographic examination the best method is for finding epidural localized tumours. For example the hourglass formed Neurinoma can be exposed, with the possibility of a deposition in regards to a paravertebral or intraspinal course of tumour. (Fig. 1): A negativly

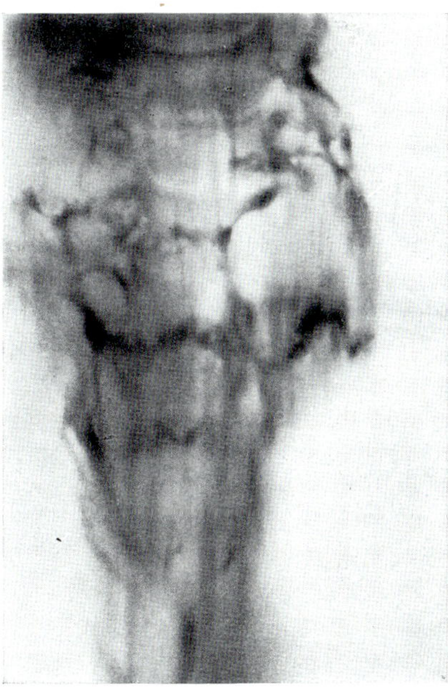

Fig. 1

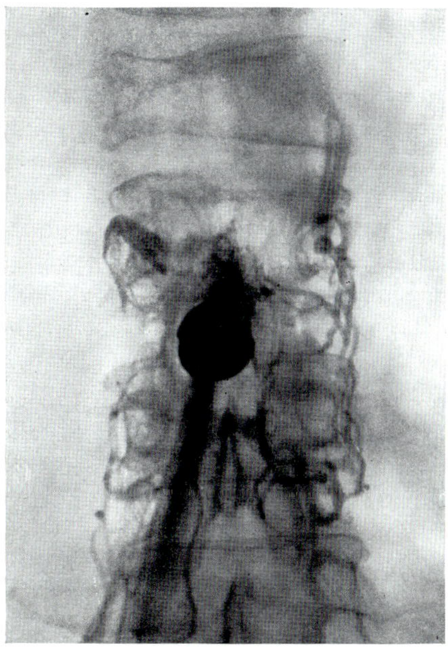

Fig. 2

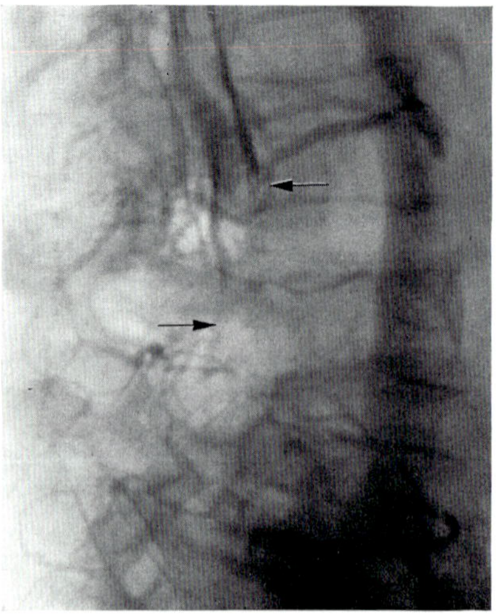

Fig. 3

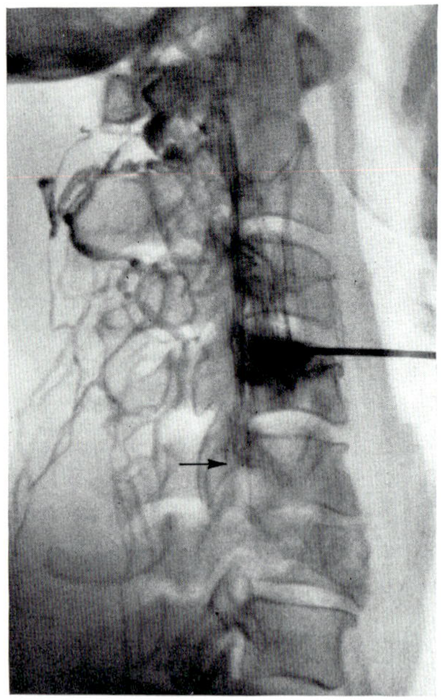

Fig. 4

displayed tumor, with it's course of grown in a paravertebral direction). By metastatic growth it is very important to prove the true direction of growth in the spinal canal and it's surrounding soft parts (Fig. 2: Transverse lesion of the spinal cord due to distruction of the first lumbar vertebra body. One segment lower we can observe an obstruction of all veins; Fig. 3: Ischialgia through a Granuloma as a result of chronic myelosis. Phlebographia showing obstruction of the anterior component of the epidural plexus at the lower border of L 3, and of the posterior component only from the middle of L 4; Fig. 4: Benigna Osteoblastoma of the sixth cervical vertebra body with an incompleted transverse lesion. It further shows an obstruction of the epidural veins one segment higher). By intradural space occupying tumours lying juxta or intramedullary (Meningioma, Ependymoma, Glioma) there has to be a tumour as well as a local diagnosis made when the expansure of the growth results in a compression and obstruction of the epidural veins. With exception of the Neurinoma and Metastasis the changes on the veins themselves are not specific. Due to the fact that all the examined and bioptic cleared tumour cases – over 70 – positively show changes on the blood vessels themselves, it is safe to say that the intraosseous spinal venography can be used as a complementary as well as a competative Examination in regards to the myelography.

Diagnosis by Scanning in Pathological Processes of the Spinal Canal (Intravenous Myelo-Scanning)

U. PIEPGRAS and P. VOETS

The myelo-scanning following *intrathecal* administration of radioisotopes has become an important method of investigation, developed in particular by the basic studies of ZEITLER and DIETZ. Another method to vizualize the spinal canal, its content, and its nearer vicinity by scanning is performed by injecting *intravenously* the radioactive substance, as it is done in brain scanning. The technique of myelo-scanning after intravenous administration of radio-nuclides was introduced into neuroradiology by FAZIO and coworkers and was described for the first time in 1968. We have used myelo-scanning for about one year (PIEPGRAS and VOETS, 1970).

Technique and Range of Application

1. Normal intravenous myelo-scintigram (Fig. 1)[1]:
Scanning 60 min after intravenous injection of 5 m Ci ^{99m}Tc pertechnetate. The thyroid is blocked by 400 mg sodium perchlorate, as it is normally done, 30 to 60 min before the injection of technetium. The blockade of the thyroid ist necessary particularly if a special vizualization of the cervical area is intended. The most important condition to obtain optimal results if investigation requires a careful covering of the paravertebral area with lead strips leaving free a zone of 4 to 5 cm over the spinal canal. The scan velocitiy is 60 to 80 cm per minute, the distance of the lines is 0.1 cm. This example demonstrates the typical *normal distribution of activity* with a low concentration in the cervical an lumbar regions and an increased concentration in the thoracal region. The maximum of concentration is regularly found between the fourth and the minth thoracal vertebra in a normal case. The exceeding accumulation of isotopes in this region is due to an increased concentration of radio-nuclides in the heart and the thoracal aorta, as it was also demonstrated by FAZIO. An increased accumulation in the caudal scan zones corresponds with the technetium concentration in the rectum.

2. Detail of intravenous myelo-scintigram of a 66 year-old patient with a radiculoneurinoma at C2/3 right which was operatively and histologically[2] verified

1 All scintigrams are black and white reproductions of colour scintigrams. They render only insufficiently the colour shading.

2 We wish to thank Prof. Dr. LOEW, director of the Department of Neurosurgery and Professor Dr. DHOM, director of the Department of Pathology, University of Saarland, Homburg-Saar, for reports of their operative and histological findings.

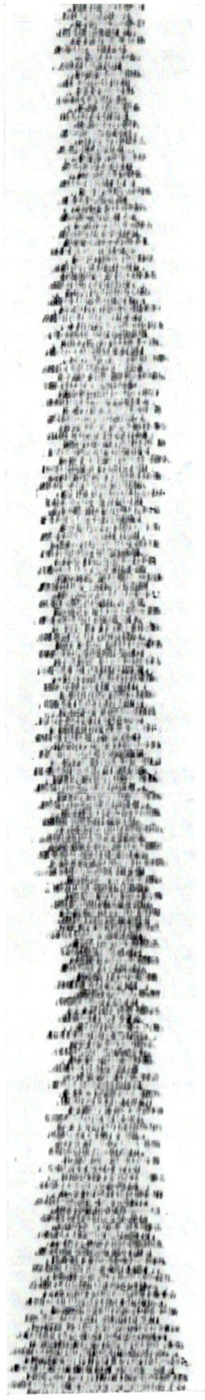

Fig. 1. Normal intravenous myelo-scintigram

Fig. 2. Intravenous myelo-scintigram of a radiculo-neurinoma (→) at C2/3 right (detail)

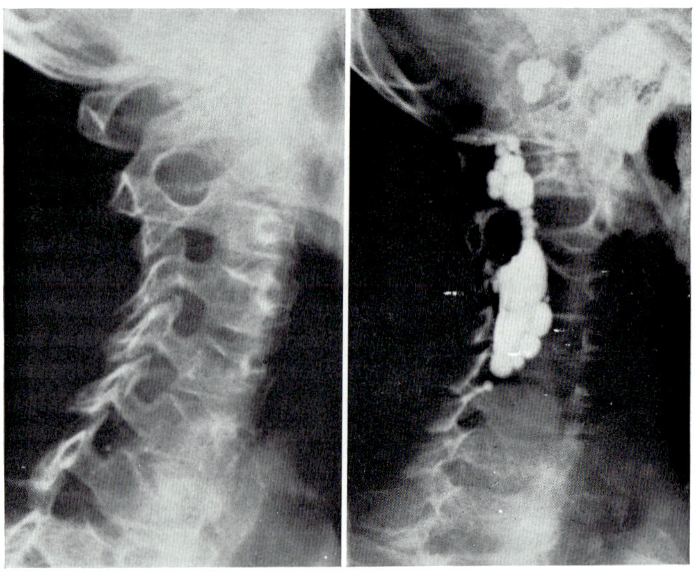

Fig. 3. The same case as in Fig. 2. Extension by pressure of the intervertebral foramen at C2/3 right by a radiculoneurinoma. Extrusion of the contrast-medium by the intraspinalpart of the tumour

Fig. 4

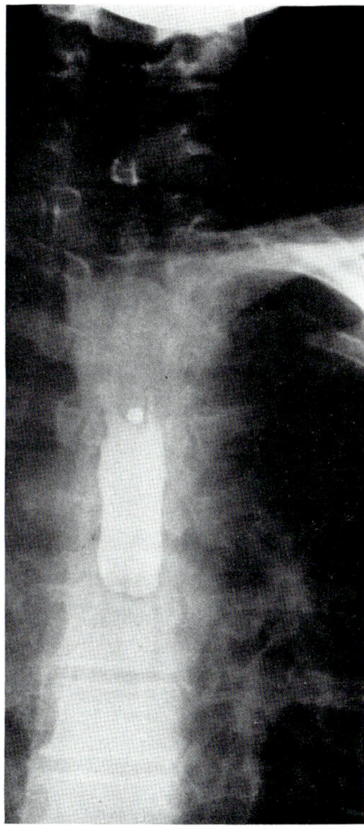

Fig. 5

Fig. 4. Osteochondroma at Th2 and Th3 with intensive accumulation of activity in the intravenous myeloscintigram (→)

Fig. 5. The same case as in Fig. 4. Myelogram with Duroliopaque++ : Completely blocked passage of the contrast-medium in the area of the lower pole of the spinal space-occupying lesion (the lead-mark corresponds with the lower demarcation of the scan focus)

(Fig. 2). A localized pathological concentration can be demonstrated in the tumour zone. The focus can be correlated in its localization with the pathological transformations in the radiograph (Fig. 3). A typical extension by pressure of the intervertebral foramen at C2/3 is found in the radiograph. In the myelogram with Duroliopaque[3], no blockade of passage can be detected, however, a distinct extrusion of the contrast-medium by the intraspinal part of the tumour.

3. Intravenous myelo-scintigram with an extensive pathological focus producing an intensive central accumulation at Th2 and Th4 (Fig. 4). A total blockade of the contrast-medium passage in ascending direction is identical – as shown in the contrast-medium myelogram (Fig. 5 – with the lower pole of region of increased activity in the scan. In this case, the cause of the radiological and clinical symptoms is a large osteochondroma, proven by operation and histological examination – extending far into the intraspinal space, a type of tumour which shows, according to

3 Byk-Gulden, Konstanz/Germany.

our investigations, an extremely high concentration of technetium. This example demonstrates that intravenous myeloscanning does not only indicate the pathological process itself, but also provides additional informations which are of importance particularly if the diagnostic value of contrast-medium is reduced by a complete compression of the spinal subarachnoid space. In our case, the intravenous myelo-scanning has indicated a spinal lesion extending into cranial direction, and it has saved the patient as well as the investigator an additional descending myelography with suboccipital puncture.

Summary

The intravenous myelo-scanning is a new technique to examine the spinal canal and its content by administration of radioisotopes. The new technique can be easily performed without any inconvenience for the patient. First results show that the intravenous myelo-scanning is able to enlarg considereably the diagnostic possibilities of neuroradiology in pathological processes of the spinal canal.

Möglichkeiten und Grenzen der Rückenmarkszintigraphie

E. Zeitler

Die *Myeloszintigraphie*, das heißt die szintigraphische Darstellung des spinalen Liquorraumes mit radioaktiven Isotopen, hat sich seit 1964 durch systematische Anwendung in einigen Zentren als eine wertvolle Ergänzung und Bereicherung der neuroradiologischen Darstellungsverfahren des Rückenmarks und seiner umgebenden Hülle erwiesen. Sie wurde bisher dort nicht angewandt, wo entweder entsprechende apparative Voraussetzungen fehlten, die organisatorischen Probleme einer Zusammenarbeit zwischen Neurologen, Neurochirurgen, Neuroradiologen und Nuklearmediziner größer waren als die Absicht dieses Verfahren einzuführen oder die vielleicht zu hohe Einschätzung von Darstellungsverfahren mit positivem oder negativem Kontrastmittel der Einführung dieser nuklearmedizinischen Methode im Wege standen. An dieser Einstellung ändert die von Joseph u. a. betonte Tatsache nichts, daß die Liquorraum-Szintigraphie eine der mühsamsten und zeitraubensten nuklearmedizinischen Methoden ist. Sie steht hier zum Vergleich gegen die Myelographie mit Luft, die durchaus ebenfalls einen hohen ärztlichen und apparativen Einsatz erfordert, will man zu brauchbaren Ergebnissen kommen. Gestatten Sie mir daher hier eine Randbemerkung an die Nuklearmediziner: Am ärztlichen, also auf anatomische und physiologische Besonderheiten ausgerichteten Bemühen um die Diagnostik wird sich erweisen, ob die Nukelarmedizin neben dem, die apparative Seite viel besser beherrschenden Physiker, als selbständige klinische Disziplin positiv im Sinne des Patienten dauerhaft wirken kann.

Meine folgenden Ausführungen stützen sich auf die Ergebnisse, welche in den Jahren von 1964–1967 gemeinsam mit dem Neurochirurgen Dietz, dem Physiker Wolf und mir im Institut für Klinische Strahlenkunde der Universität Mainz an mehr als 200 Patienten gesammelt werden konnten.

Seit der ersten Anwendung von RIHSA-J-131 zur Myeloszintigraphie durch Bauer und Yuhl 1953 sowie von Perryman (1958) und Bell (1959, 1962) in den USA vergingen einige Jahre bis auch in Europa diese Methode aufgegriffen wurde. Ja, sie wurde sogar in den Instituten der ersten Anwendung durch Arbeitsplatzwechsel des Inaugurators wieder verlassen. In der Zeit wurde in der Sowjetunion von Krupin und Liass Radon und ^{133}Xenon in Anlehnung an die Gasmyelographie erprobt. Das ^{222}Radon hat wegen seiner relativ hohen Strahlenbelastung auch in der SU keine weitere Anwendung gefunden und ^{133}Xenon hatte keine Vorteile gegenüber dem RIHSA J-131. Den intensiven Studien und Bemühungen von Di Chiro seit 1961 in den USA und den Arbeitsgruppen in Turin (Baggio i. a. 1963), Straßburg (Gros, Wackenheim u. a. 1964) und Mainz (Dietz, Zeitler und Wolf, 1964) ist die sich etwas schleppend vollziehende Weiterverbreitung und die heutige

Kenntnis über die Möglichkeiten und Grenzen des Verfahrens zu verdanken. *Wesentliche Weiterentwicklungen* stellen die Einführung der *Kameraszintigraphie* durch ASHBURN u. a. 1968, die Phantomstudien durch JOSEPH u. a. 1969 und die Erprobung anderer *kurzlebiger Radionuklide*, welche die Verwendung höherer Dosen bei besserer Photonenausbeute ermöglichen, dar. So haben DI CHIRO und AKHTAR ^{99m}Tc-Pertechnetat; HODAK, DICHIRO ^{99m}Tc-Human Serum Albumin; TOUYA kolloidales Indium 113 m und zuletzt WAGNER und JOSEPH mit Mitarb. Ytterbium 169-DTPA in ersten Einzelversuchen erprobt.

Die größten Erfahrungen liegen heute mit RIHSA-J-131 vor und die Erstellung von ^{99m}Tc-Humanserumalbumin ist vielleicht mit einem neuen „kit" in Zukunft etwas erleichtert (COOPER u. a.). Dieses Präparat würde einer breiteren Anwendung im Rahmen der Differentialdiagnose des Hydrocephalus bei Säuglingen und Kleinkindern verhelfen, für die Lokalisation von Tumoren mit Kontrollszintigraphien nach 24 und 48 Std wäre es jedoch weniger geeignet.

Das noch wenig erprobte Ytterbium-169-DTPA mit einer physikalischen Halbwertzeit von 32 Tagen würde eine wirtschaftliche Vorratshaltung ermöglichen, zumal der Komplex über Wochen stabil bleibt (JOSEPH). Da es glomerulär filtriert wird besteht eine biologische Halbwertzeit von 10 Std und die Strahlenbelastung wird von WAGNER mit dem Fünffachen derjenigen für ^{99m}Tc-Humanalbumin errechneten angegeben.

Die szintigraphische Darstellung der spinalen und endokraniellen Liquorräume kann sowohl mit dem Linearscanner, als auch mit der Kamera erfolgen.

Bei der RIHSA-J-131-Myelographie werden in Einzelampullen beziehbare Mengen von 100 mikro-Curie Aktivität in 1 ml Lösung verwendet. Der Eiweißgehalt pro Ampulle beträgt 1–2 mg entsprechend einer spezifischen Aktivität von 50–100 mikro-Curie pro mg Eiweiß. An den Tagen vor der Anwendung ist eine Blockierung der Schilddrüse durchzuführen. Zur Vermeidung unerwünschter Nebenwirkungen, für die im wesentlichen das Humanalbumin verantwortlich sein dürfte, hat sich die von uns vorgeschlagene intrathekale Prämedikation von 50 mg Prednisolon durchgesetzt und früher beobachtete Nebenreaktionen wie Kopf- und Rückenschmerz, Meningismus und Brechreiz sind selten.

Da es die Aufgabe der Szintigraphie ist neben dem Nachweis eines pathologischen Substrates auch dessen Lokalisation zu bestimmen um diesen einer gezielten chirurgischen Behandlung zugängig zu machen ergibt sich die Aufgabe, dem schwarzweißen oder farbigen Strichbild anatomische Bezugspunkte zuzuordnen.

Zwei Möglichkeiten stehen hierfür zur Verfügung: die einfachere ist die Markierung anatomischer Bezugspunkte an der Körperoberfläche, wie sie die Punktionsstelle, die Dornfortsätze, der Beckenkamm und Narben darstellen. Die etwas schwierigere besteht darin, daß das Photoszintigramm auf einen unter gleichen geometrischen Bedingungen belichteten Röntgenfilm geschrieben wird. Eine exakte Superposition beider Belichtungen ist nicht einfach. Derartige Photoszintigramme können jedoch eine exaktere Zuordnung zu Wirbelabschnitten verhelfen.

Durch Anfertigung eines Scan sofort nach intrathekaler Injektion des Radionuklides kann immer eine Region mit abruptem Aktivitätsabbruch dargestellt werden, da noch keine gleichmäßige Ausbreitung im Spinalkanal eingetreten ist. Die Anfertigung von Serienszintigrammen nach der Injektion haben Aufschluß über die Liquordynamik erbracht und uns bei Verwendung markierten Humanalbumins gezeigt, welche Zeitpunkte für die anatomische Dokumentation der Liquorräume am geeignetsten sind.

Nach lumbaler Injektion ist, falls kein Austritt großer Aktivitätsmengen mit dem Liquor in den Periduralraum stattgefunden hat, der gesamte Spinalkanal im Scan darstellbar. Eine weitere Voraussetzung hierfür ist, daß keine Liquorpassagestörung besteht. Daraus ergibt sich, zumindest bei allen unklaren Befunden am ersten Tag die Notwendigkeit einer Szintigraphie am Tag nach der Injektion. Zu diesem Zeitpunkt ist bei Verwendung von ^{131}J die Impulsrate oft nicht mehr sehr hoch. Neben dem Spinalkanal gelingt es jedoch nach 24 Std die extracerebralen endokraniellen Liquorräume darzustellen. Manchmal kommt es auch zur Aktivitätsansammlung im Ventrikelsystem, selten kann ein Hirnscan geschrieben werden. Nach *subokzipitaler* Applikation der Aktivität ist die Cervikal- und Thorakalregion bereits nach 4–6 Std gut darzustellen. Der lumbale Abschnitt wird jedoch erst nach 24 Std erfaßbar. Für die Darstellung der lumbalen Spinalräume ist daher auch die lumbale Injektion vorzuziehen. Auf die endokranielle Ausbreitung brauche ich im Rahmen dieses Referates nicht eingehen, muß aber darauf hinweisen. daß es nach 24 Std trotz versuchter Blockade der Schilddrüse in 30–40% der Patienten zu einer unterschiedlich starken Aktivitätsanreicherung in ihr kommen kann.

Daraus resultieren einige Möglichkeiten der Fehlinterpretation. Die Verbreiterung des Aktivitätsbandes an der zerviko-dorsalen Übergangsregion ist in der Regel eher eine Aktivitätsansammlung in der Schilddrüse, als ein pathologischer Befund. (Das mittlere Szintigramm welches in Seitlage angefertigt wurde soll dies eindeutig belegen.) Weiterhin kann sowohl auf dem ersten, als auch auf weiteren Szintigrammen eine erhöhte Aktivitätsansammlung am Ort der Punktion bestehen. Es ist nicht von Vorteil in diesem Bereich das Maximum und die Höhe der background-Unterdrückung vorzunehmen. Außerdem ergeben sich am ersten Tag sehr leicht Zonen verminderter Aktivität allein aus der mangelnden Aktivitätsausbreitung. Daraus ergibt sich, daß es *immer besser ist*, *einen Scan auch am Tag nach der Injektion* auszuführen. Spätere Kontrollen sind nur selten erforderlich. Ihre Information wird durch den steigenden background und die Aktivitätsabnahme im Spinalkanal zusätzlich geringer, da bereits eine Abwanderung in das Blut stattgefunden hat.

Untersuchungen mit dem ARMAC-Unterarmzähler haben gezeigt, daß bereits 1 Std nach Applikation Aktivität im Blut nachweisbar ist und das 48 Std später ein Maximum der Blutaktivität besteht bei Verwendung von RIHSA-J-131. Die mittlere Eliminationszeit aus dem Liquor liegt nach unseren Untersuchungen zwischen 36 und 72 Std. Die *Strahlenbelastung des gesamten Liquorraumes* liegt, bei Annahme eines Liquor-Volumens von 150 ml, bezogen auf eine effektive Halbwertzeit von 12 Std, zwischen *3 und 6 rad.*

Die Mehrzahl der Patienten wurden untersucht wegen Verdacht auf intraspinale Raumforderung bedingt durch einen Tumor oder einen Bandscheibenvorfall. Danach kommen die Fälle mit Verdacht auf eine Arachnitis und schließlich in gleicher Häufigkeit P. mit Verdacht auf eine craniale Liquorfistel, einen posttraumatischen Zervikalen Wurzelausriß und spinale Missbildungen. Hinzu können noch Fälle kommen mit Verdacht auf Myelitis oder Haematomyelie und wie im Material von Joseph, Herrmann, Graul u. a. (1970) bei „cervikaler Myelopathie“ infolge degenerativer Veränderungen der Halswirbelsäule. – Die Zysternographie schließlich ist bei Verdacht auf Liquorzirkulationsstörung in der hinteren Schädelgrube gleich welcher Ursache indiziert.

Gelegentlich tritt Aktivität in mehr oder minder großer Menge durch den von der *Punktionsstelle geschaffenen Stichkanal* in den Periduralraum aus. Kleine Extravasate stellen sich kaudal der Injektionsstelle in Form von Knospen oder Haken dar, die an anderen Stellen – abseits der Injektionsstelle – für eine krankhafte undichte Stelle der Hüllen des Rückenmarkes gedeutet werden können. – Kommt es zu größeren Aktivitätsaustritten, so ist die szintigraphische Darstellung der Periduralräume unbeabsichtigt möglich. Wenn man dies nicht richtig beurteilt kommt es zu Fehlinterpretationen wie: Megakauda oder Cauda spinalis duplex. Trotz dieses Austrittes der Aktivität in den Peridualraum kann ein Bandscheibenvorfall, wie im mittleren Bild erkennbar, als Aktivitätsaussparung erkannt werden.

Das entscheidende Symptom bei allen pathologischen Veränderungen im Myeloszintigramm ist der *Aktivitätsausfall* bzw. die *Liquorpassagestörung* unabhängig von der Art des pathologisch-anatomischen Substrates. Unabhängig vom Ort der Applikation und dem anatomischen Befund zeigt die Szintigraphie allein die Aktivitätsaussparung am Ort der Obstruktion an. Sie ist in den meisten Fällen nicht so komplett, daß nicht doch eine geringe Aktivitätsmenge diffundieren könnte. Dadurch erlaubt die Myeloszintigraphie nach Punktion nur an einem Ort *häufiger die kraniale und kaudale Begrenzung der Obstruktion* anzuzeigen, als die Myelographie mit positivem Kontrastmittel.

Infolge der geringen Nebenreaktionen und keiner Gefahren hinsichtlich einer Spätschädigung kann die szintigraphische Darstellung der Liquorräume auch zur *Kontrolle nach operativer Behandlung* erneut ausgeführt werden.

Während die Lokalisation pathologischer Veränderungen bezogen auf das Achsenskelet relativ exakt bestimmbar ist, kann die Myeloszintigraphie bisher nur selten Hinweise für eine *Seitenlokalisation* erbringen. Die relativ geringen Sicherheiten hinsichtlich einer Seitenlokalisation treffen natürlich auch für die Lokalisation innerhalb des Spinalkanals ventral oder dorsal lokalisierter Befunde zu. Profilszintigraphie und Computerszintigraphie dürften jedoch in der Lage sein hier noch weitergehende Informationen zu liefern.

Bei der *Arachnitis spinalis* sind 2 Formen szintigraphisch zu unterscheiden: die proliferierende, als deren extremster Vertreter die kalzifizierende Pachymeningitis hypertrophicans anzusehen ist. Die zweite Form ist die fibrosierende, die zu einer Verschmälerung des Subarachnoidalraumes führt und diesen nicht vollständig verlegt. Ihr charakteristisches Bild ist die Verschmälerung des Aktivitätsbandes, welches dem Subarachnoidalraum entspricht und auch eine quantitative Aktivitätsminderung, die im Farbszintigramm (rechts) deutlich erkennbar wird. Dies entspricht den gleichförmigen Veränderungen in allen Abschnitten der Arachnoidea in derselben Höhe. Auch hier, so meine ich, könnte die Computerszintigraphie noch wesentlich differenziertere Informationen liefern. Dies vor allem zur Unterscheidung von Variationen, wenn im Computer die normale Variationsbreite als subtrahierbarer Wert mit eingegeben würde.

Die Leistungsfähigkeit der Myeloszintigraphie wurde schon mehrfach an der Objektivierbarkeit des *Bandscheibenvorfalles*, der häufigsten intraspinalen Raumforderung geprüft. Dabei besteht Übereinstimmung in allen Publikationen, darin, daß Massenprolapse gut nachgewiesen werden können. Das Frühszintigramm zeigt häufig dabei nicht mehr als die Kontrastmittelmyelographie: einen totalen Stop. Erst spätere Kontrollen erlauben in derartigen Fällen die Differenzierung von 1 oder 2 benachbarten Nukleus pulposus-hernien. Auch in der jüngsten Publikation auf der Tagung in Hannover vor 14 Tagen berichteten JOSEPH u. Mitarb. darüber, daß sie von 20 Patienten mit Bandscheibenvorfall 16 – das sind 80% – nachweisen konnten.

Die Grenzen der Methode mit unseren derzeitigen Möglichkeiten werden jedoch besonders deutlich, bei dorsolateralen kleinen Bandscheibenhernien, die auch mit der Kontrastmittelmyelographie nur bei schräger Projektion durch Kompression der Wurzelscheide erkannt werden. Jedoch gibt es, besonders im Segment L5/S1 auch eine Reihe von Bandscheibenhernien, die infolge des physiologisch größeren Abstandes zwischen Wirbelhinterkante und ventraler Begrenzung des Duraschlauches oft nicht myelographisch nachgewiesen werden können. In einer früheren Mitteilung haben wir zur Klärung dieser Frage die Kontrastmittelmyelographie und die Isotopenmyelographie simultan durchgeführt. (DIETZ u. a.). Die Analyse bei 100 Fällen dieser Gruppe ergab, daß die Kontrastmittelmyelographie in 74% und die RIHSA-Myeloszintigraphie nur in 41% einen eindeutig pathologischen Befund erbrachte. Hinzu kommt, daß bei weiteren 36 Fällen in denen die Kontrastmittelmyelographie einen eindeutigen Befund gab, der Befund der Myeloszintigraphie nur fraglich, negativ oder nicht verwertbar war. Dem stehen in dieser Gruppe nur 3 Fälle gegenüber, bei denen die Isotopendiagnostik allein für die Erkennung des Bandscheibenvorfalles erfolgreich war. Daraus resultiert, daß Bandscheibenhernien mit dorso-lateraler Lokalisation, die sehr klein sind, mit der Myeloszintigraphie nicht oder nur ausnahmsweise mit der jetzigen Technik erfaßbar sind.

Zur Diagnostik der unterschiedlichen Formen von *Mißbildungen* im Bereich des Spinalkanals ist es empfehlenswert immer auch einen seitlichen Scan anzufertigen. Von großer praktischer Bedeutung ist die DD von paravertebralen Verschattungen im Röntgenbild des Thorax. Die Szintigraphie nach intrathekaler Gabe von einem Radionuklid klärt, ob diese Verschattung mit dem Spinalkanal in Verbindung steht, durch die Ansammlung der Radioaktivität innerhalb der Verschattung. Im Gegensatz zu Neurinomen und Sympathikustumoren kann auf diese Weise einfach eine intrathorakale Meningocele nachgewiesen werden.

Vor Einführung der Myeloszintigraphie konnte der Nachweis eines *zervikalen Wurzelausrißes* nur durch die Injektion von Pantopaque subokzipital geführt werden. Dabei ist eine Lagerung des P. auf die Seite der neurologischen Schädigung erforderlich. Im Pantopaque-Myelogramm kommt es dann zu der bekannten kugelförmigen Ausweitung der Wurzeltaschen und selten tritt das ölige Kontrastmittel in das umliegende Gewebe aus. Mit der Myeloszintigraphie gelingt es wesentlich einfacher den Ausriß durch den Defekt der Arachnoidea nachzuweisen. Nach subokzipitaler Injektion von RIHSA-J-131 und Lagerung des Patienten in Bauchlage zeigt die 1 oder 2 Std später geschriebene Szintigraphie deutlich eine örtliche begrenzte zipflige Verbreiterung des Aktivitätsbandes in Höhe der ausgerissenen Wurzel des Plexus cervikalis. Zusätzliche Strahlenbelastung durch lange Durchleuchtungszeit entfällt hierbei völlig.

Obwohl auch der Nachweis *rhinogener* und *otogener Liquorfisteln* mit dem Prinzip der Myeloszintigraphie, nach Applikation von radioaktiven Stoffen lumbal oder subokzipital in den Liquorraum geführt wird, kann ich auf dieses so erfolgreiche

Gebiet der nuklearmedizinischen Diagnostik der Liquorräume nicht näher eingehen. Es sei nur gesagt, daß ihr Nachweis und ihre Lokalisation, wie schon in einer früheren Mitteilung von uns dargelegt wurde, mit keiner anderen Methode so sicher und exakt gelingt. Ihr Nachweis ist sowohl durch Szintigramme bei seitlicher Projektion des Schädels als auch bei frontaler Projektion erkennbar. Die Beziehungen zur Schädelanatomie sind durch Überprojektion mit Übersichtsaufnahmen und Tomogrammen des Schädels relativ klar darzustellen.

Die diagnostischen *Möglichkeiten* der Rückenmarkszintigraphie sind besonders *günstig* hinsichtlich eines Nachweises und der Lokalisation von intraspinalen Veränderungen die eine Liquordiffusion behindern und eine Einengung des Subarachnoidalraumes direkt bewirken. Sie sind *gering* bei Veränderungen, die nur den Peridualraum einengen und auf die Nervenwurzeln und deren Scheiden einen Druck ausüben. Derartige Nukleus-pulposus-Hernien sind ohne Änderung der Untersuchungstaktik und größere apparative Aufwände nicht nachzuweisen. Der Nachweis eines zervikalen Wurzelausrisses, von spinalen Mißbildungen wie Mengiocelen, von Liquorfisteln und der Arachnitis spinalis jedoch ist ohne Gefahr für eine Schädigung mit keiner anderen Methode so leicht und so sicher zu führen wie mit der Szintigraphie des Spinalkanals. Dabei ist bis jetzt RIHSA-J-131 noch das geeigneteste Radionuklid und die neuen Präparate bedürfen noch eingehender Prüfung.

Ein Vergleich mit der diagnostischen Leistungsbreite der Angiographie des Spinalkanals ist meines Erachtens noch nicht möglich, da die arterielle Angiographie bisher nur vereinzelt und dann besonders bei der Fragestellung nach intraspinalen Angiomen angewandt wurde. Bei der Diagnostik der Bandscheibenvorfälle erscheint jedoch die Ossovenographie (VOGELSANG) eine größere Sicherheit zu besitzen, als die Myeloszintigraphie. Vergleichsserien hierüber fehlen jedoch noch in gleicher Weise wie gegenüber der noch immer besten Methode zum Nachweis der Bandscheibenhernien: der lumbalen Kontrastmittelmyelographie.

A Comparison of Myeloscintigraphy, Myelography and Discography in Detection of Spinal Block Lesions

H. Otto, J. Sauer, O. Fiebach and W. Bettag

The Myeloscintigraphy is considered as a proved method nearly without any risk for pathological changes in the spinal canal. Various authors inform of good results about the diagnostic of space occupying processes, lesions of nerve roots, miscellaneous and inflammatory alterations. With the aid of selected cases we examined the efficiency of myeloscintigraphy in comparison with the radiological methods. Especially we asked after the value of the myeloscintigraphy for the neurosurgeons.

First of all the myeloscintigraphy was effected by an injection of $100 \mu Ci$ ^{131}J-HSA; lately we used exclusively 1–3 mCi ^{99m}Tc-Pertechnetat in istotonic solution. We chose the localisation of the injection according to the clinically suspected position of the process. We preferred the suboccipital injection when a process of the cervical region could be expected. After an hour we examined using the scintilation camera whether the activity has reached the suspected block in the passage when the patient was placed accordingly. In demonstrating the discovered process we made use of characteristic anatomical points and marked the lesion on the surface of the body.

In this paper we discuss the results of examinations of 21 selected patients. All of them were examined as well by myeloscintigraphy as by radiological methods such as myelography and discography. In 8 cases it concerns a spinal cord tumor and in 12 cases a cervical disk hernitation. Merely in one case we carried out the myeloscintigraphy at a lumber disk prolaps. While judging the single methods we tried to find out, whether the space occupying process could be recognized, whether its localization and in case of a tumor the extension could be found out. Furthermore we questioned, whether it was possible to say something about the nature of the process. Finally we dealt with the indication for operation.

In the range of the tumors we could find out that the block lesion in question could be recognized by means of the myeloscintigraphy in all cases, in addition to this fact the extension of the tumor could be fixed in 2 cases. The myelography with Pantopaque allowed equally the localization of the tumor and furthermore gave differential diagnostic signs to the kind of the process in question. For the reasons above mentioned the myelography with Pantopaque was conclusive for the indication of the operation in all our cases.

We found in 7 cases of our patients with cervical disk herniation which were operated upon a low activity over the cervical region in the myeloscintigram because of abnormal narrows of the cervical spinal canal. However, this diagnosis was not sufficient for the indication and choice of the way of operation. On the one hand this is caused by the small resolution of the detectors, on the other hand errors are possible caused by the physiological narrows in the cervico-thoracal region.

The myelography with a positive contrast medium or with air and the discography gave conclusive indication for the surgeon in most of the cases. However, in the cervical region it is not always possible to make a clear diagnosis despite this methods. Therefore a space occupying process could be excluded only by laminectomy in one of our patients. In the five not operated patients myeloscintigraphy showed 3 times an abnormal narrow in the spinal canal the myelography showed a partial stop in 4 cases. The discography of the above mentioned patients was conclusive for a conservative treatment.

Our material shows that the myeloscintigraphy is suitable to indicate a space occupying process in the spinal canal. As to the diagnosis of tumors it can be stated the extension of the process in individual cases in which the myelogram shows a complete stop. As to the cervical disk herniations the diagnostic results of the method is not sufficient for the neurosurgeon. So far the myelography and the discography are not to be replaced.

Thyroid Lesions

A Study of the Parameters Influencing the Clinical Use of Iodine-123*

H. N. Wellman, J. F. Mack, E. L. Saenger, R. E. Goldsmith and V. J. Sodd

A number of reports have suggested the wider use of Iodine-123 as the ideal radioisotope of iodine because of its theoretical advantages. A short Half-life of 13,3 h, a primary gamma photon of 159 keV of high abundance and absence of beta particle emission result in a dose reduction variously estimated at 30–100 fold over commonly used Iodine-131. In addition, the low energy 159 keV gamma and a lesser abundant 28 keV X-ray offer promise of improved imaging resolution utilizing low energy high resolution collimators.

These promising characteristics have led to a program to promote the development and clinical evaluation of Iodine-123 in the laboratories of the Bureau of Radiological Health and the University of Cincinnati.

We have previously reported on both the development of techniques for Iodine-123 production and also on preliminary clinical experiences, primarily evaluating the maximum possible thyroid dose reduction feasible in substituting Iodine-123 for Iodine-131. The preliminary conclusions suggested that Iodine-131 was still superior when the two radioisotopes were compared on an equal count rate basis. Most techniques used to produce Iodine-123 also result in a small percent of Iodine-124 contamination. Since the previous studies utilized a low energy collimator, excess collimator penetration by the higher energy gamma photons (603 and 723 keV) of Iodine-124 was proposed as a possible explanation for the less satisfactory results of Iodine-125 thyroid imaging. Goolden and Rhodes have also alluded to potential disadvantages of Iodine-123 contamination with Iodine-124.

The studies reported herein were undertaken to elucidate further the factors involved in attempting optimal thyroid scanning with Iodine-123. The protocol (Table 1) of the present studies departed from that previously reported in that a higher mean dose of about 300 μCi of Iodine-123 was employed, and the 31-hole high energy collimator utilized for Iodine-131 was used with Iodine-123, in addition to the 1045 hole, low-energy, high-resolution collimator. As seen in the protocol, both 6 and 24 h, 159 keV scans were performed utilizing the two collimators and Iodine-123 in an attempt to evaluate the possible collimator penetration of higher energy contaminants. Gamma camera images with a single pin-hole collimator were optional. After completion of Iodine-123 scans on day 2, a conventional Iodine-131 thyroid scan was obtained with 100 μCi administered dose to each patient. A total

* Supported in part by PHS Contract 86-67-212

Table 1. *Comparison of* ^{123}I *with* ^{131}I

Day I administer 300 μCi ^{123}I *p.o.*		
Rectilinear scans & collimators	6 h	24 h
1. 31 and 1045 hole	28 keV	28 keV
	159 keV	159 keV
2. Optimal gamma camera	159 keV	159 keV
3. 24 h uptake		
Day II administer 100 μCi ^{131}I *p.o.*		
1. Rectilinear scan – 31 hole collimator	—	364 keV
2. 24 h uptake		
Totals: 25 Patients with all rectilinear scans and some camera images		
9 Patients with some rectilinear scans		
Mean dose: 290 μCi		
Summary		
1. Total 9 rectilinear scans	Complete protocol	
2. 2 Optional gamma camera images		

of 34 patients were studied, with 25 patients having the 9 essential rectilinear scans used for intercomparisons. Most of this latter group also had gamma camera images. As seen in (Table 2) an attempt was made to perform all scanning modes at a constant information density of about 600 counts/cm^2.

However, this was only possible when using the 31-hole collimator since the Maximum speed of the scanner limited scanning with the 1045 hole collimator to a higher information density (about 1000 counts/cm^2) at the dose of Iodine-123 used in the study.

Table 2. *Mean information densities (counts/cm^2) on rectilinear thyroid scans*

	^{131}I	^{123}I							
Time hour	24	6	6	6	6	24	24	24	24
Energy keV	364	28	28	159	159	28	28	159	150
Collimator hole	31	31	1045	31	1045	31	1045	31	1045
Mean information density	590	620	1040	580	1020	550	960	490	860

Iodine-123 used in the study was principally produced by the direct Antimony-121 (α, 2n) Iodine-123 reaction and was administered to 29 patients. The mean Iodine-124 contamination at time of use was about 1.5%. The Iodine-123 was usually administered in approximately one half-life from time of production. Iodine-123 produced directly by Tellurium-122 (d, n) Iodine-123 and indirectly by Tellurium-122 (α3n) Xenon-123 $\xrightarrow[2.1\,h]{B^+}$ Iodine-123, containing negligible Iodine-

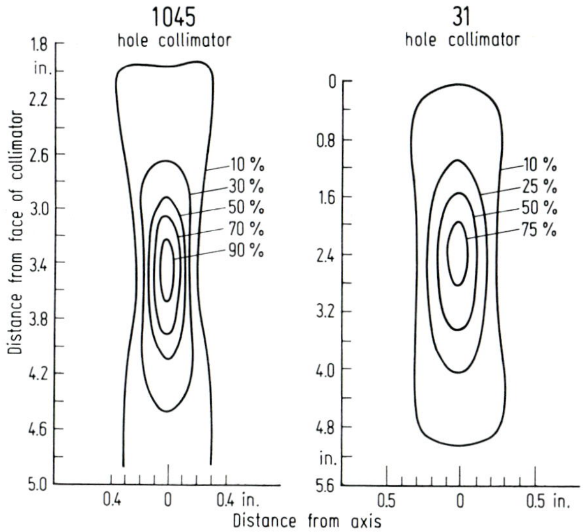
1045
hole collimator
31
hole collimator
Distance from face of collimator
1.8
in.
2.2
2.6
3.0
3.4
3.8
4.2
4.6
5.0
0
0.8
1.6
2.4
3.2
4.0
4.8
in.
5.6
10 %
30 %
50 %
70 %
90 %
10 %
25 %
50 %
75 %
0.4
0
0.4 in.
0.5
0
0.5 in.
Distance from axis

Fig. 1

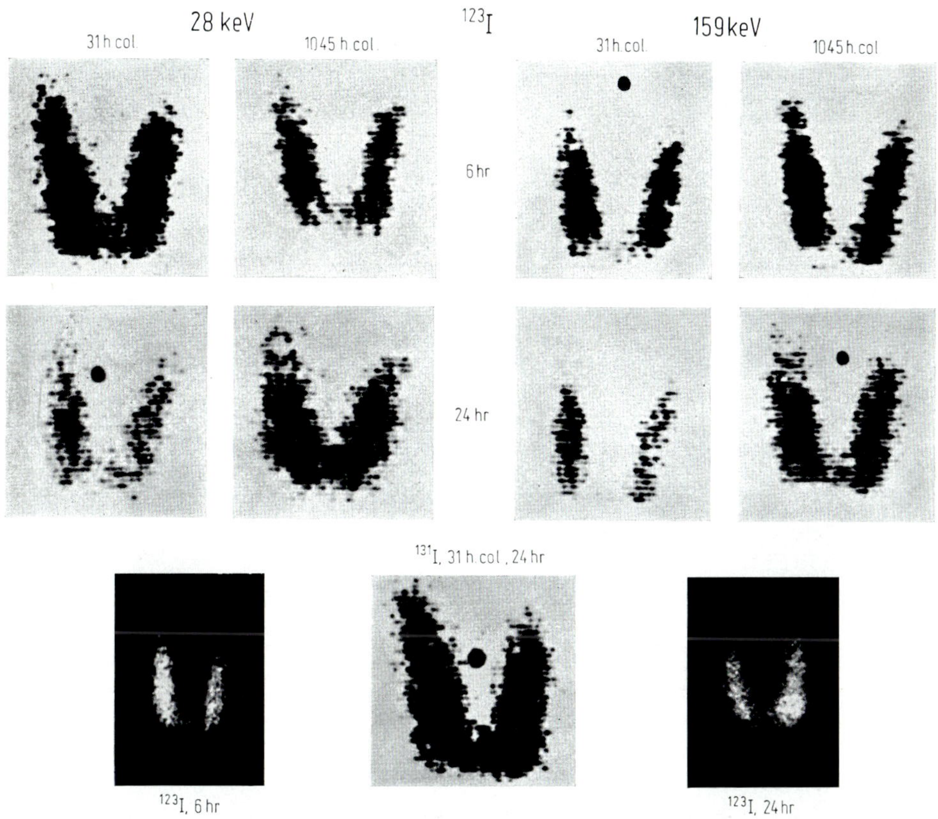
28 keV
123I
159keV
31 h col.
1045 h col.
31 h col.
1045 h col.
6 hr
24 hr
131I, 31 h col., 24 hr
123I, 6 hr
123I, 24 hr

Fig. 2

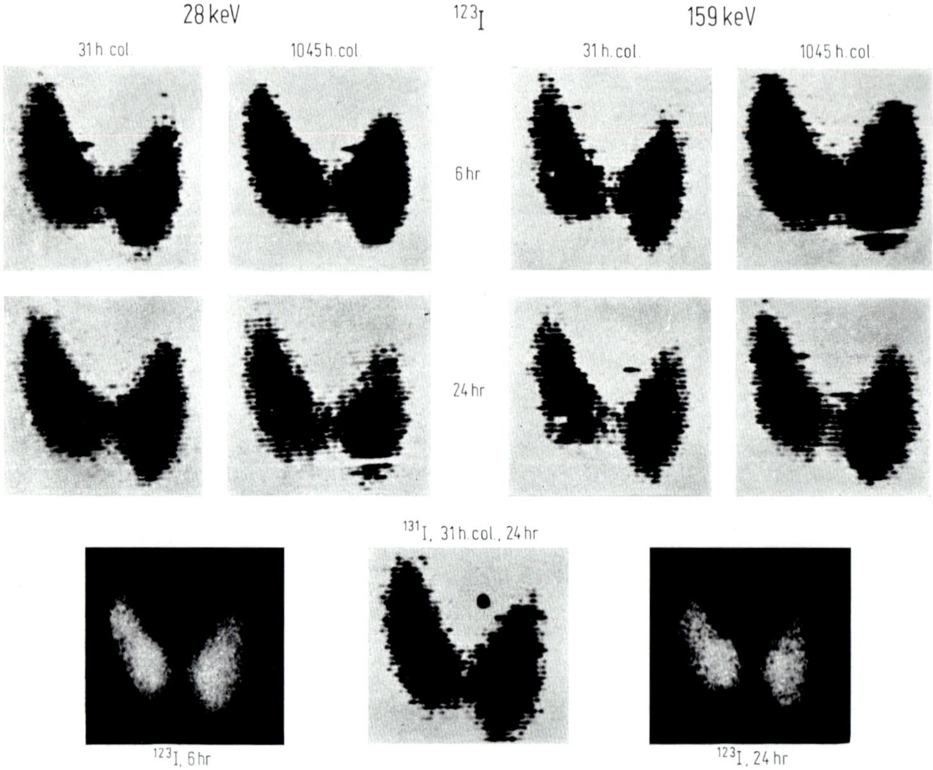
28 keV
^{123}I
159 keV
31 h. col.
1045 h. col.
31 h. col.
1045 h. col.
6 hr
24 hr
^{131}I, 31 h. col., 24 hr
^{123}I, 6 hr
^{123}I, 24 hr

Fig. 3

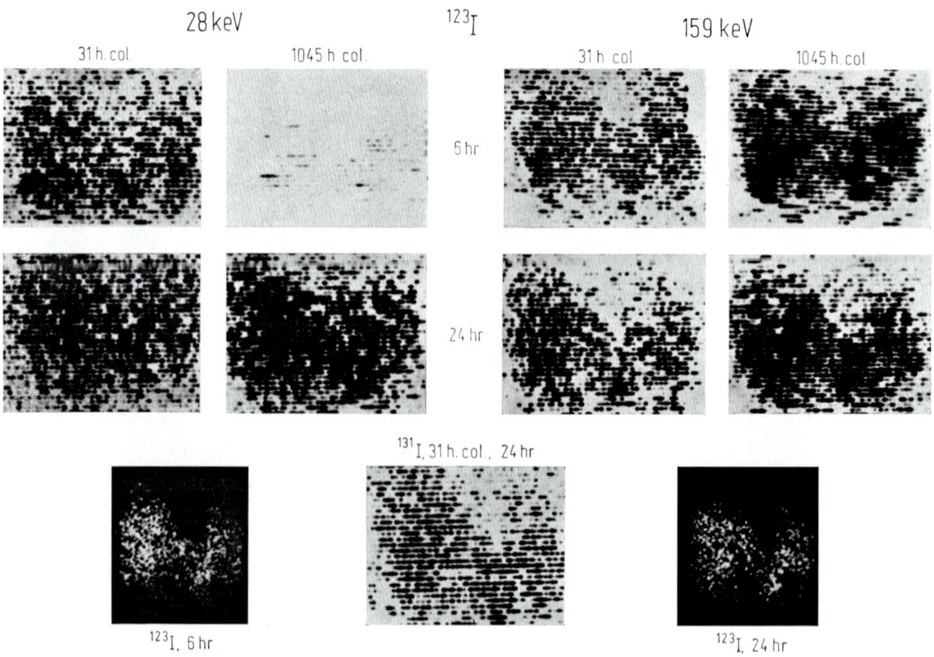
28 keV
^{123}I
159 keV
31 h. col.
1045 h. col.
31 h. col.
1045 h. col.
6 hr
24 hr
^{131}I, 31 h. col., 24 hr
^{123}I, 6 hr
^{123}I, 24 hr

Fig. 4

124, was given to 5 patients – too few to satisfactorily evaluate the elimination of Iodine-124.

The 31-hole collimator as used for Iodine-131 has approximately an eight mm, resolution at the 364 keV photon energy. However, the same collimator has a 5,5 mm resolution at 140 keV, the approximate energy of the principle Iodine-125 gamma, as seen in (Fig. 1) this compares very closely to the 5,75 mm resolution of the 1045-hole collimator.

The resultant nine scintiscans in each of 25 patients were all performed at the same line spacing and with the same light pipe to avoid observable scintigraphic difference. The 225 thyroid scans plus available gamma camera images were coded and grouped by patient. The scans were then read independently by four experienced physicians and ranked in order of preference as well as evaluated for clinical impressions of size, shape, homogeneity, presence of nodules and adequacy for interpretation. These readings were decoded, summarized and statiscally evaluated.

Results

The sequence of scans and gamma camera images to be used in some illustrative cases is seen in the normal patient in (Fig. 2). The 28 keV and 159 keV 6 h series

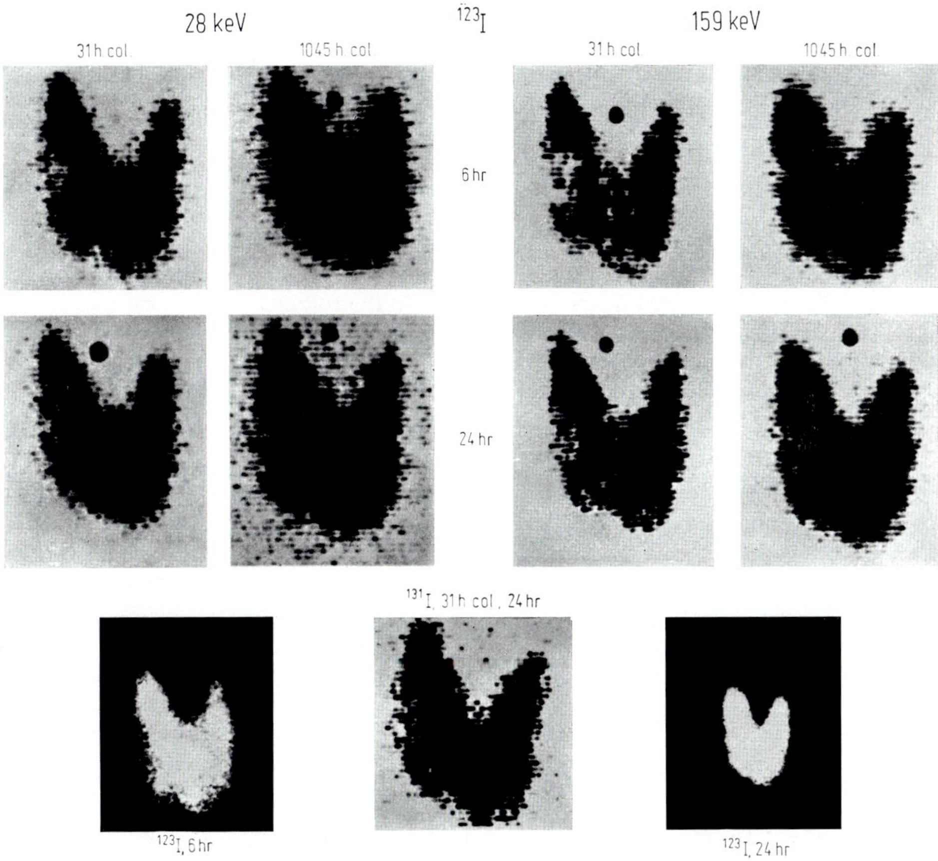

Fig. 5

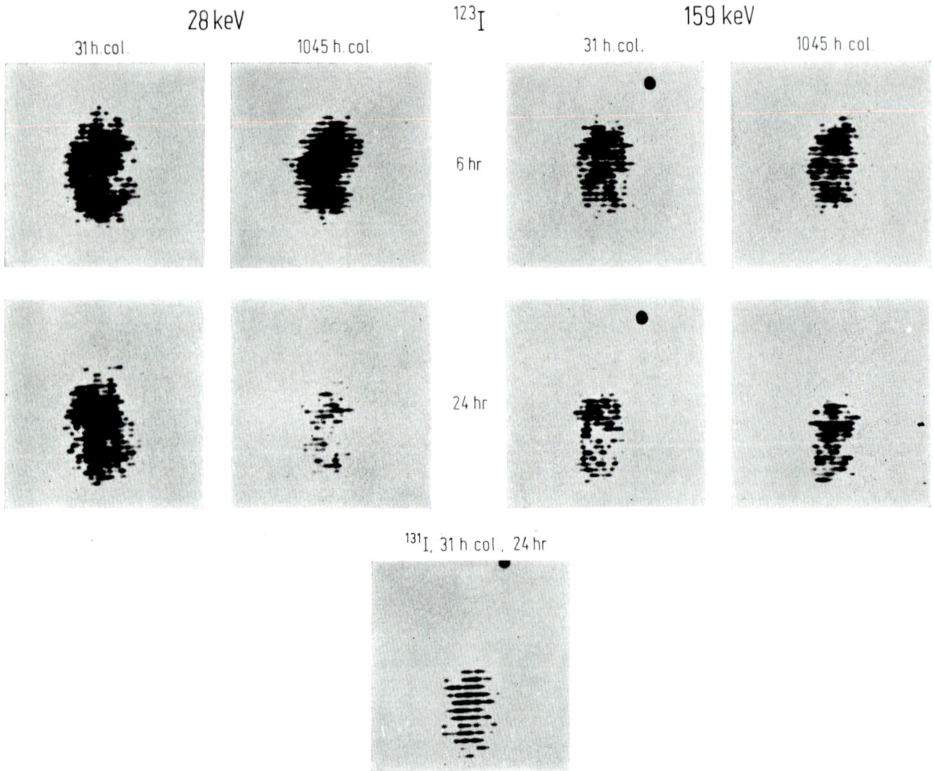

Fig. 6

is seen at the top with the same studies at 24 h in the middle. Gamma camera scintiphotos and the 24h Iodine-131 scan are at the bottom. A patient with GRAVES' disease is noted in (Fig. 3). Next, (Fig. 4) is the heterogeneous uptake seen in a multinodular goiter. This can be compared (Fig. 5) to a single cold nodule which is particularly well demonstrated in the 159 keV scans. Lastly, (Fig. 6), an autonomous nodule is depicted. These five examples give an opportunity to sample the intercomparison of Iodine-123 with Iodine-131. Also of interest (Fig. 7) is the case of a hypothyroid child with a congenital goiter. The low uptake made it undesirable to administer Iodine-131 and scans were only obtained utilizing Iodine-123, representing one of the nine cases not having undergone the complete protocol of scan studies.

The ranking scores by the observers (Table 3) are tabulated in decreasing order of preference with the 24 h, 159 keV, 1045-hole collimator Iodine-123 scans being first and the 24 h, 28 keV, 1045-hole Iodine-123 scans last. A similar ranking technique was reported in the previous study, when Iodine-131 was clearly preferred by all observers over all other treatments. In the present study, however, Iodine-131 is not clearly superior to the Iodine-123 scans. As seen in the bottom of the table, no significant difference was observed between observers, ner as was the case also in the previous study. The analysis of variance of the pooled data suggest a slight significant difference between the treatments that are compared, only at a level of

Table 3. *Analysis of variance by two-way classification*

Order of preference									
treatment	24 h 159 keV 1045 h. col. ^{123}I	24 h 159 keV 31 h. col. ^{123}I	6 h 159 keV 31 h. col. ^{123}I	6 h 28 keV 31 h. col. ^{123}I	6 h 159 keV 1045 h. col. ^{123}I	24 h 364 keV 31 h. col. ^{123}I	6 h 28 keV 1045 h. col. ^{123}I	24 h 28 keV 31 h. col. ^{123}I	24 h 28 keV 1045 h. col. ^{123}I
Observer									
I	135	144	151	123	126	101	125	129	90
II	151	150	135	116	115	123	108	116	105
III	140	136	137	121	116	122	115	111	104
IV	144	109	114	123	119	125	122	114	133
Total rank score	570	539	537	483	476	471	470	470	432

Results :
Accepting that data are likely to have normal distribution :
A) Observers $F(.95)_3.\ 24 = 8.64$ $F(\text{test})_3.\ 24 = 1.47$
No significant difference between observers
B) Treatment $F(.95)_8.\ 24 = 3.12$ $F(\text{test})_8.\ 24 = 3.27$
Significant Difference with level of risk >0.05

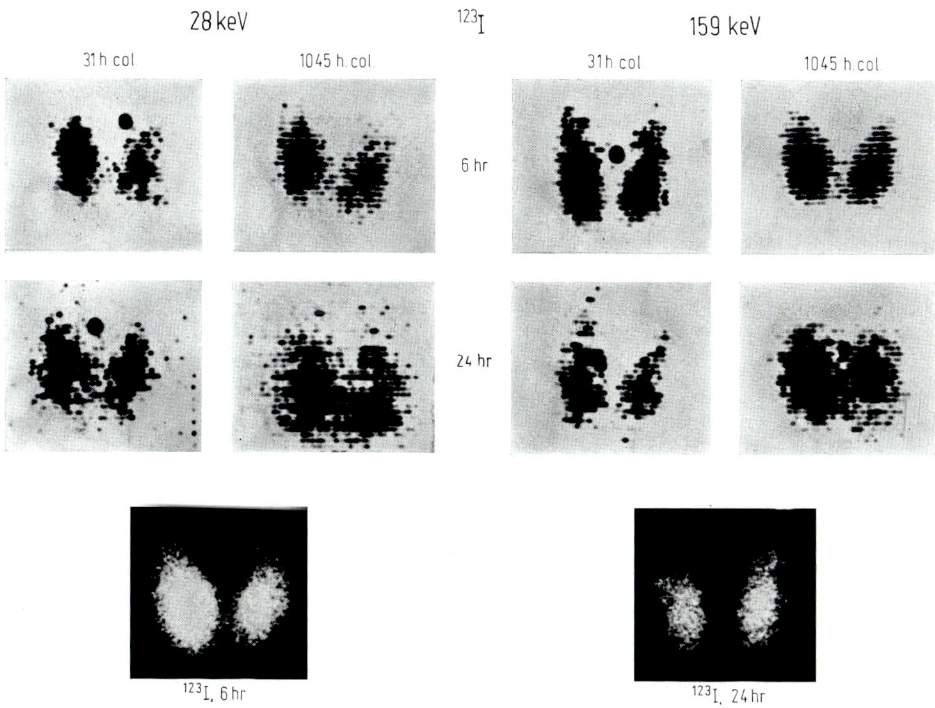

Fig. 7

risk less than 0.05. Furthermore, no significant difference could be found when component treatments were analyzed as pairs, especially the first ranked 24 h, 159 keV, 1045-hole collimator Iodine-123 scans versus the Iodine-131 scans. This also corresponded to the general opinion of the observers that in most cases there was very little difference between scan treatments in this study. Although gamma camera images were not correlated direcctly with scans, because of the bias inherent in their differing presentation from scans, it is interesting to note that gamma camera images were usually preferred to the scintiscans! Also, 28 keV scans were consistently ranked lower than other treatments, results similar to those of the previous study. In most cases, 3 of 4 observere usually agreed well on their impression of size, shape, homogeniety, presence of nodules, diagnosis and adequacy for in terpretation of the scans. A small number of 28 keV scans were considered inadequate for interpretation. Overall in both studies, 28 keV scans have been of little value, probably because of their high content of scattered higher energy photons.

Discussion

The results reported in this study then do not show any significant difference between scans done with Iodine-123 and Iodine-131 under the conditions tested. Use of a larger dose of Iodine-123 and/or the 31-hole collimator eliminated the previous superiority seen with the Iodine-131. However, Iodine-123 was not shown to be superior to Iodine-131. As noted above, the 31-hole collimator, although having only approximately 16% of the sensitivity of the 1045-hole collimator, has approximately the same resolution at the 159 keV energy of Iodine-123. All scans with Iodine-123 and Iodine-131 using the 31-hole collimator had approximately equal information densities. Thus the Iodine-123 scans should have some advantage because of the higher resolutions, but that effect was not clearly seen. The 1045-hole collimator Iodine-123 scans, on the other hand, had nearly twice the information density of the 31-hole scans with theoretically a high resolution of about 5 mm. and thus should have been superior, they were not.

It is probable, as suggested by other data from our laboratories, that there is a significant degradation of resolution when using the low energy collimator, due to the higher energy Iodine-124 contamination, which is at a level of approximately 5% at the time of a 24 h scan. The observers, in evaluating the scan treatments above, probably balanced resolution on the one hand with high information density so that they expressed a subjective impression that all scan treatments were similar. The gamma camera treatments were preferred over scan treatments, because septal penetration and scatter is a minimum problem with the contaminant scatter energy and high information densities can be obtained.

One could tolerate the presence of Iodine-124, but higher energy collimators would be necessary reducing markedly the sensitivity. This could be compensated for by utilizing larger doses of Iodine-123 than were used in the present study. However, very large doses of Iodine-123, on the order of 2 mCi, needed to reduce scanning time to approximately 10 min, would negate the dose reduction potential of Iodine-123, especially when contaminated with Iodien-124. Iodine-124, at 5% level of contamination, results in 3–4 times the absorbed thyroid dose as that produced by pure Iodine-123 alone.

Specially designed collimators and crystal systems on scanners can optimize these conditions to that small amounts of Iodine-124 contamination could be tolerated as well as the small amount of higher energy gamma (500 keV) of Iodine-123. Another alternative might be the utilization of the gamma camera-pin hole collimator combination as a partial answer to the use of contaminated Iodine-123, obtaining high resolution, high information density thyroid images in a reasonably short study time. The indirect production of pure Iodine-123 is feasible through the high yield Tellurium-122 (α3n) Xenon-123 reaction and still appears to us to be the best solution to the optimal utilization of the dose reduction and high resolution potentials of Iodine-123.

Die kombinierte Angio- und Szintigraphie in der Schilddrüsendiagnostik

U. Feine, H. Schmidt und K. Hoffmann

Die szintigraphische Untersuchung des Schilddrüsenparenchyms ist eine vielgeübte Methode zur Darstellung von Formveränderungen des funktionstüchtigen Parenchyms der Schilddrüse. Neben normal jodaufnehmenden Schilddrüsengebieten kann eine Vergrößerung und Verlagerung des Parenchyms Hinweise auf eine Schilddrüsenerkrankung geben.

Das Angiogramm der Schilddrüse, ausgehend vom Aortenbogen, wurde erstmals von Schmitt u. Mitarb. 1967 eingehender beschrieben. Verlagerungen von Gefäßen, Kaliberschwankungen und Gefäßverschlüsse können bestimmte Hinweise auf Schilddrüsenerkrankungen geben.

In den genannten 2 Untersuchungen stehen sich also Methoden zur Darstellung der funktionellen Morphologie des Parenchyms bzw. der Durchblutung des Organs gegenüber. Welcher Stellenwert in der Schilddrüsendiagnostik beiden Untersuchungen zukommt, soll hier kurz aufgezeigt werden.

Das Szintigramm der normalen Schilddrüse kann als bekannt vorausgesetzt werden. Das normale Arteriogramm der Schilddrüse ergibt eine Darstellung der 4 Arteriae thyreoideae mit ihrem Abgang aus den Trunci thyreocervicales bzw. den Arteriae carotides externae.

Die kombinierte szintigraphische und angiographische Untersuchung wurde an 45 Patienten bei insgesamt 60 angiographisch (transfemorale Aortenbogendarstellung mit Ödmann-Katheter nach Seldinger) untersuchten Patienten durchgeführt. Es handelt sich um 31 Frauen und 14 Männer, die zwischen 19 und 78 Jahren alt waren.

Tabelle 1 gibt die Liste der histologischen Diagnosen der benignen und der malignen Veränderungen bei den operierten Patienten wieder.

Als Kriterien für die diagnostische Beurteilung des Angiogramms werden Kaliberdifferenzen, Verlagerungen von Gefäßen, unregelmäßige Gefäßverteilung mit Anfärbungen und Aussparungen in der parenchymatösen Phase sowie Venenverschlüsse, angesehen. Aus diesen Symptomen lassen sich im allgemeinen Lage und Ausdehnung des Schilddrüsengewebes nicht so eindeutig entnehmen wie aus dem Szintigramm. So war in dem hier untersuchten Patientengut mehrfach die im Szintigramm abgebildete Struma im Angiogramm nicht eindeutig nachzuweisen. Dagegen ist es umgekehrt möglich, daß szintigraphisch kalte Bezirke einer Struma im Angiogramm charakteristische Strukturen erkennen lassen, die zur Diagnose beitragen können. So kann das Angiogramm zu einer weiteren Differenzierung

Tabelle 1

Benigne Veränderungen	
Kolloidreiches Schilddrüsengewebe	1
Struma colloides	2
Struma colloides nodosa	24
Struma colloides nodosa mit Adenomknoten	4
	31
Maligne Veränderungen	
Struma Langhans und Plattenepithel-Ca.	1
Schilddrüsen-Ca.	1
Teils drüsiges, teils solides Ca.	2
Solides Ca.	3
Plattenepithel-Ca.	1
Papilläres Ca.	1
Sarkom	1
Haemangio-Endothelio-Sarkom	1
	11
3 Kranke wurden nicht operiert	

kalter Bezirke führen. Unter den 25 Patienten mit kalten Knoten wurde bei 6 angiographisch untersuchten die Diagnose eines malignen Tumors gestellt. Bei allen diesen Patienten handelte es sich um einseitige Kompressionen bzw. Verschlüsse der Vena jugularis interna. Durch die Operation wurde die Malignität histologisch bestätigt. Bei 3 weiteren Patienten wurde wegen derselben, nicht so deutlich ausgeprägten Symptome angiographisch der Verdacht auf das Bestehen einer bösartigen Geschwulst ausgesprochen, der in zwei Fällen histologisch postoperativ bestätigt wurde. Bei 16 Fällen fand sich im Angiogramm kein Hinweis auf das Vorliegen eines malignen Tumors im Bereiche der szintigraphisch festgestellten kalten Knoten. Bei 2 Patienten wurde operativ doch noch ein maligner Tumor festgestellt, bei den übrigen 14 Kranken, die sämtlich operiert wurden, handelte es sich um knotige Kolloidstrumen. Die Tabelle 2 gibt im Vergleich die Ergebnisse der Szintigraphie und der Angiographie im speziellen Hinblick auf die Diagnose der malignen Struma wieder.

Eine diffuse Kontrastmittelanreicherung im Strumaparenchym ließ sich bei den 45 angiographisch untersuchten Patienten 17 mal erkennen, z. T. als Anfärbung der gesamten Struma, z. T. als lokalisierte Anfärbung einzelner Knoten. Es handelte sich hierbei um Patienten mit kolloidreichem Schilddrüsengewebe, mit Struma colloides nodosa mit und ohne Adenomknoten sowie 3 mal um Carcinome. Dabei färbten sich 7 mal kalte Knoten an, 2 mal heiße oder warme Knoten und 4 mal eine homogen speichernde Struma. Die Parenchymanfärbung kann also weiterhin Hinweise auf das Vorliegen kalter, im Szintigramm nicht dargestellter knotiger Hyperplasien der Schilddrüse geben, die sich nicht selten auch einmal dem Tastbefund entziehen können.

Tabelle 2. *Vergleich der szintigraphischen und angiographischen Untersuchungsergebnisse mit histologischem Befund*

Szintigraph. Befunde →	homog. Speicherung	kalter Knoten	heißer Knoten	Gesamtzahl	o. B.	Str. ohne Mal.-Zeichen	Str. m. fragl. Mal.-Zeichen	Struma m. Mal.-Zeichen	Gesamtzahl	Angio-graph. Befunde ←
Kolloidr. Schilddr.-Gew.	1			1	1				1	
Struma colloides	1	1		2		1	1		2	
Str. coll. nodosa	11	12	2	25	4	21			25	
Struma coll. nod. mit Adenomen	1	1	1	3		3			3	
Str. Langhans + Ca.		1		1		1			1	
Schilddrüsen-Ca.		1		1				1	1	
Drüsiges/solides Ca.		2		2				2	2	
Solides Ca.		3		3			1	2	3	
Plattenepithel-Ca.		1		1			1		1	
Papilläres Ca.		1		1				1	1	
Sarkom		1		1		1			1	
Haemangio-Endothelio-Sa.		1		1				1	1	
	14	25	3	42	5	27	3	7	42	

Zusammenfassend kann festgestellt werden, daß die Kombination von Szintigraphie mit angiographischer Darstellung des Struma eine weitere Differenzierung, vor allem der kalten Knoten bringt, so daß präoperativ über die Möglichkeit des Vorliegens maligne entarteter Strumaknoten eine bessere Aussage gemacht werden kann. Dies bedeutet einen wesentlichen Fortschritt, wenn man bedenkt, daß kalte Knoten je nach Statistik der einzelnen Untersucher in wenigen Prozenten bis zu 20% und höher später histologisch als maligne befunden werden.

Thyroid Angiography

P. Rossi

In the last two decades angiography has become a routine method of investigation of diseased organs. Although thyroid angiography has been known for many years it has not become popular or used to full advantage. Despite the relative use of palpation, scanning and clinical investigation, many lesions of the thyroid and parathyroid are best studied by angiography.

The technique consists of selective transfemoral route approach transfemoral catheterization of both the superior and inferior thyroid vessels using the Femoral-Cerebral I, French 7, or a modified coronary Cordis catheter. In cases where selective catheterization of the thyroid arteries is not possible via the femoral approach due to tortuosity of the vessels, the axillary puncture is performed and a French 5 polyethylene catheter is advanced and selectively placed within the inferior thyroid artery. This catheter is preshaped according to the anatomy of the patient. The amount of contrast injected in each single vessel varies from 3 to 5 cc and films are taken for approximately 15 sec in AP, oblique and lateral projections if needed. Subtraction technique is used almost routinely for detection of small lesions.

The superior thyroid artery is usually the first branch of the external carotid artery and may occasionally arise from the common or rarely from the internal carotid artery. Anatomically there are several smaller branches from the superior thyroid artery not directly related to the thyroid namely the infrahyoid, superior laryngeal and cricothyroid, which may be identified only with selective injections and subtraction technique.The important branches of the superior thyroid artery are the sternocleidomastoid artery and the two main arteries which supply the thyroid gland: The ventral medial and the dorsal lateral branches. The ventral medial branch is usually larger and anastomoses with the corresponding vessel of the opposite lobe forming a concave arch along the superior aspect of the isthmus which can be visualized following injection into either superior thyroid artery.

The inferior thyroid artery is usually a branch of the thyrocervical trunk, however, can originate from the subclavian vertebral arteries and the aorta. When it arises from the subclavian artery it usually takes off at the level of the internal mammary artery distal to the takeoff of the vertebral artery. The thyrocervical trunk usually divides in three branches, the inferior thyroid, the transverse scapularis and ascending cervical. The inferior thyroid artery courses medially and upward and passes posteriorly to the carotid sheath at the level of the 6th cervical vertebral body where it forms a sharp downward bend. This curve is called the cranial loop. From here the artery has a straight downward course, distributing small branches to the thyroid gland. At the level of the lower pole of the thyroid gland, the artery forms a second upward curve which is called the caudal loop. Anatomic variations may occur where the cranial and caudal loops are formed by two separate branches of the inferior thyroid artery either in one or both lobes. Other branches of the inferior thyroid artery are the esophageal, tracheal, inferior laryngeal, muscular branches and the parathyroid artery. The parathyroid arteries according to Halsted and Evans are supplied by a single artery. In practically every case the artery to the lower parathyroid gland arose from a prominent branch of the inferior thyroid artery. The upper parathyroid gland invariably has a short supplying artery which may arise from one of the main branches of the inferior thyroid or from anastomoses joining the superior and inferior thyroid arteries along the dorsal lateral portion of the thyroid. The thyroides are classically drained by three paired veins, the superior, middle and inferior veins, which anastomose and form a complex venous plexus throughout the entire thyroid bed. The superior and middle thyroid veins can be seen to drain directly into the internal jugular vein. The inferior thyroid veins drain into the respective ipsilateral innominate veins close to their junction. The superior thyroid vein can either be a single vessel or part of a trunk formed by the thyroid, lingual and facial trunk. In many cases, a large central vertical vein is seen to cross the isthmus, anastomosing with large ascending branches along the medial margins of each lobe. In some cases, the inferior thyroid vein may form the thyroidea ima.

Cases

1. Parathyroid Adenoma. A 16-year-old white female who sought medical attention because of thinning of hair. Routine laboratory investigation revealed unsuspected elevated calcium levels. Visualization of a large artery leading to the parathyroid adenoma with abnormal vascularity. Opacification of the whole parathyroid adenoma. Late phase visualization of staining with draining into the inferior thyroid vein.

2. Parathyroid Carcinoma. A 52-year-old white male presenting with a pathological fracture of the left humerus and multiple other lytic areas throughout the skeletal system and a palpable mass in the right paratracheal area. The calcium level was markedly elevated – 17 mg. percent. Right Subclavian Angiogram: Abnormal vascularity and the hypertrophy of the inferior thyroid artery with displacement of the cranial and caudal loops, absence of homogeneous cascularization of the tumor and in the capillary phase. Selective inferior Thyroid Angiogram: Selective injection into the costocervical trunk results in visualization of parasitic blood supply to the tumor with staining of a large mass.

3. Thyroid Adenoma. A 29-year-old man with thyroid adenoma was admitted with progressive paralysis of the lower extremities and a large right thyroid mass displacing the trachea to the left. Angiography was performed to see whether there was any relationship between the mass and the paralysis. Right Inferior Thyroid Arteriogram showed large displaced inferior thyroid artery and a dense stain at the periphery with avascularity in the center. Right Superior Thyroid Arteriogram – Good visualization of the right thyroid lobe displaced.

4. *Reticulum Cell Sarcoma of the Thyroid* A 53-year-old white female presenting with a right subclavicular mass, jauntice and weight loss. Inferior Thyroid Arteriogram: Staining of the large mass with diffuse staining throughout, displacement of the cranial and caudal loops of the inferior thyroid artery.

Superior Thyroid Arteriogram: Hypertrophy of the superior thyroid artery with visualization of homogeneous staining of the tumor.

Pulmonary Vascular Lesions

Comparison of Pulmonary Arteriography with Lung Scintigraphy in the Diagnosis of Pulmonary Emboli

K. Ranniger

Pulmonary scanning is easy to perform, has a low complication rate and causes only minimal discomfort to the patient. Therefore, pulmonary scanning often is done in preference to pulmonary arteriography. The question is whether such approach is justifiable or whether pulmonary scanning and pulmonary arteriography complement each other.

The advantage of pulmonary perfusion scanning is its easy application and the possibility of repeated scans to follow up the course of pulmonary emboli. Pulmonary scanning supposedly detects peripheral pulmonary emboli not seen on angiograms, even after superselective contrast material injection. Its disadvantage is that a scan is not specific. In the presence of pulmonary infiltrates, in emphysema and asthma, the scan shows a perfusion defect identical to that resulting from a pulmonary embolus. Furthermore, sometimes a scan is difficult to interpret. Especially, apical or small peripheral areas of decreased isotope activity might be misdiagnosed as perfusion defects. If larger branches of the pulmonary arteries are partially occluded, the scan might be negative because the isotope bypasses this occlusion and reaches the periphery.

The pulmonary arteriogram has the advantage that it localizes the embolus anatomically and rarely gives positive erroneous results. During the arteriogram, one can easily measure the pressure within the pulmonary artery and the right heart. The catheter can be left in place for follow-up measurements and urokinase can be injected through it. A pulmonary arteriogram is disadvantageous because it is less comfortable to the patient than a pulmonary scan, is a more complicated procedure, and carries a slightly higher risk. Even after superselective injection, small pulmonary vessels cannot be identified easily; therefore, emboli in these vessels might be missed.

During the last three years, we examined 135 patients with suspected pulmonary emboli by both arteriograms and pulmonary scans (Table) These studies usually were performed within 3 hours of each other; occasionally the time difference was as high as 24 hours, but never exceeded this time. In 84 cases – that is, 62% – an agreement between both studies existed and in 51 patients – that is, 38% – the results of the techniques were in disagreement. Both tests were positive in 54 patients and negative in 30.

It is worthwhile to look at the conflicting results a little closer. In a reltaively high number, the scan was positive while the angiogram was negative. Most of these

Table. *Findings in 135 patients examined by pulmonary scan and pulmonary arteriogram*

Number of patients	scan	arteriogram
54 (= 40 %)	+	+
30 (= 22 %)	–	–
39 (= 29 %)	+	–
12 (= 9 %)	–	+

positive scans showed small peripheral perfusion defects. Scintigraphically, it is not proven whether these defects are the result of true pulmonary emboli, whether they are caused by other pulmonary pathology, or whether they are misinterpreted scans in normal lungs. Often the clinical findings to not aid in differentiating these possibilities. Therefore, it will be difficult to evaluate the efficiency of either technique in this group of patients and one must conclude that a positive scan with a normal arteriogram does not necessarily indicate that an embolization was missed by the angiogram, although we know that small peripheral emboli might escape detection by angiography.

In 12 patients, the scan was negative while the pulmonary arteriogram showed evidence of an embolism. In the majority of the cases, a larger branch of the pulmonary artery was only partially occluded by the embolus, thus permitting the isotope to pass into the periphery, creating the impression of normal perfusion.

We believe that the pulmonary arteriogram and the pulmonary scan have their distinct indications:

The pulmonary scan should be performed if clinically questions are raised of small pulmonary emboli without severe systemic findings.

The pulmonary angiogram is indicated if massive pulmonary emboli are suspected clinically and embolectomy or caval ligation is a consideration. Furthermore, a pulmonary arteriogram should be available if a pulmonary infiltrate or pulmonary emphysema is present which will make the interpretation of a scan difficult or if the results of a scran are inconclusive.

Summary

Pulmonary scanning and pulmonary arteriography have distinct indications. It is not necessary to perform both studies routinely on the same patient.

The main discrepancy in the results of pulmonary arteriography and pulmonary scanning exists in the group where pulmonary scans are positive but angiograms are negative. Although smaller pulmonary emboli might not be detectable by arteriography, in most of the cases there is no proof that the perfusion defect indeed represented a pulmonary embolus, since a positive scan can have a variety of causes.

An angiogram is easier to interpret. Occasionally vessels can be narrowed secondary to endarteritic processes or by extrinsic compression. Decreased segmental supply in pneumonia and other infiltrates can be misdiagnosed as embolus. Broncho-pulmonary arterial communications following inflammatory processes might be present as peripheral ischemia. Often a superselective contrast material injection can resolve these problems.

Scintigraphy in Screening Pulmonary Emboli–Prospective Comparison with Angiography

H. N. Wellman, J. F. Mack, D. W. Romhilt, J. C. Holmes, P. Gandel, H. B. Spitz and J. C. Fenton

Since Ernst first demonstrated the possibility of pulmonary perfusion scanning with ^{198}Au absorbed on charcoal particles a little more than a decade ago, lung scanning has become an extensively used diagnostic procedure. Its routine clinical application did not become practicable, however, until Taplin perfected the use of labelled macroaggregated human serum albumin (Iodine-131 MAA). Unfortunately, somewhere along the way, the procedure has been widely misrepresented as a potential replacement for pulmonary angiography, rather than a complement are to it since the two are in no way competitive.

Emphasis has been placed on the utilization of lung scanning as a screening procedure in a prospective report of Moser *et al.* on 10 patients. Most reported studies suffer in part in that they are retrospective and often do not have entirely satisfactory studies on individual patients.

Over the last two and a half years, a prospective comparative study of pulmonary angiography and lung scanning has been carried out at the University of Cincinnati Medical Center in order to test the hypothesis that lung scanning is a satisfactory screening test in pulmonary embolic disease.

Methods

Patients were selected for this study on the basis of clinical probability of having pulmonary emboli. The clinical criteria utilized were the sudden onset of dyspnea, sometimes associated with syncope or hypotension and the symptoms of pulmonary infarction, namely sudden onset of pleuritic chest pain, dyspnea, and sometimes cough or hemoptysis. All but two of the studies were performed within 7 days of the onset of symptoms. In addition, 3 studies were on patients that had pulmonary angiograms at the time of cardiac catheterization and did not have any symptoms of pulmonary embolism. Each patient underwent pulmonary arteriography and lung scanning so that the findings of one did not bias the decision to perform the other. Scanning and arteriography were successively alternated as the initial procedure insofar as possible. In 25 studies, pulmonary angiography was performed first, and in 35 the lung scanning was done first. The procedures were interpreted independently. Both procedures were completed in all but one patient within 6 h of one another.

Lung Scanning

Lung scans were performed utilizing administered activities of 300 μCi of commercially available Iodine-131 MAA which were injected intravenously with the patient in the recumbent position. 35 perfusion studies were performed on the Gamma Scintillation Camera[1] and 25 on an Ohio Nuclear 5″ NaI crystal single probe rectilinear scanner with either collimator D or E. Aminimum study on both imaging systems consisted of anterior and posterior views. In only one study were just anterior views accepted because of the massive impairment of perfusion and the extremely critical condition of the patient. In most instances using the Gamma Scintillation Camera, all oblique views were also obtained, which aid considerably in delineating perfusion abnormalities. Lateral rectilinear scans were not performed because of the inherent difficulty of interpretation and the problems of patient immobilization. No complications occurred subsequent to lung scanning.

Pulmonary Arteriography

After a test dose for drug sensitivity and catheter positioning, a rapid injection of 50 ml, of Hypaque-75 at a pressure of 500 psi was made into the main pulmonary artery. Serial films were obtained with a rapid film changer. A second injection was sometimes necessary in an oblique position to delineate the pulmonary arterial tree satisfactorily. In two patients, arteriography could not be completed because of atrial wall perforation in one and severe venous spasm in the other.

Interpretation

All lung scan studies were coded and read independently by two of the authors (H. W., J. M.) as to location (upper, middle and/or lower third of the lung) and the extent of the lesions (decreased or absent perfusion). Disagreement between observer's interpretations of scans was noted in only 5% of the lesions. Pulmonary arteriograms were read independently by one author (H. B. S.). Criteria analogous to those used for scans were employed regarding location of lesions by thirds of a lung field and magnitude of lesions by assessing absent or decreased flow. Independent pulmonary scan and angiogram results were then correlated.

Results

60 complete studies of arteriograms and scans were accomplished in 49 patients. The 60 studies were divided into 4 groups: The criteria for group I were a positive arteriogram and negative scan: for group II: positive angiogram and positive scan: group III: negative angiogram and positive scan: group IV: negative angiogram and negative scan (Table 1). None of the studies fell into the group I category.

In group II, the total number of defects was quite similar in both the arteriograms and scans; however, when the flow or perfusion was classified as absent or decreased, the majority on the scans were described as absent and on the arteriogram

1 Nuclear Chicago Pho Gamma II or III

Table 1. *Pulmonary angiogram – scan intercomparison*

Group	Angiogram	Scan	Number of studies
I	Positive	Negative	0
II	Positive	Positive	24
III	Negative	Positive	28
IV	Negative	Negative	8
Total			60

as decreased. When an area of absent flow was present on the arteriogram, absent perfusion was always seen on the scan. However, there was some variance in the reading of decreased perfusion or flow in 6 of 44 defects on the right and 8 of 41 on the left; that is, decreased flow identified on the arteriogram, but normal perfusion on the scan. This variance occurred in about 15% of the total defects. Also, there was an almost equal number of perfusion defects identified on scans that were not noted on arteriograms. All instances of lesion variance were in patients who also

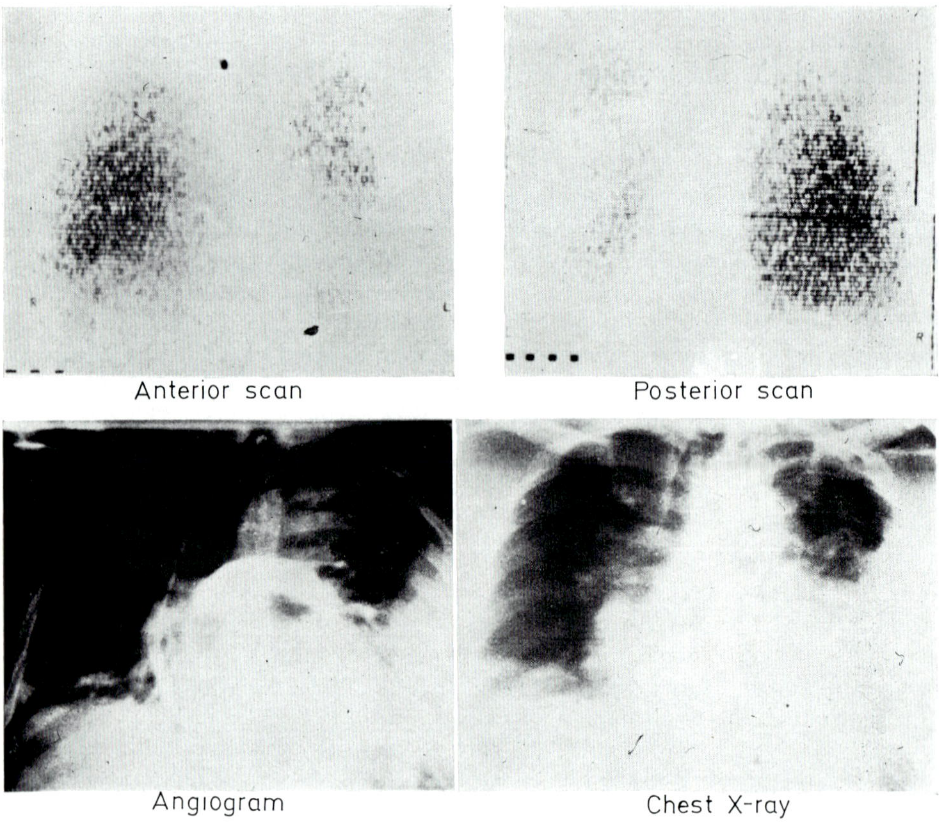

Fig. 1

had correspondence of flow and perfusion lesions in other areas of their lungs. 18 of the 24 (75%) studies in group II showed bilateral defects. It is interesting to note that no definite preponderance of emboli was seen between the upper, middle and lower thirds of the lung, except perhaps for an increase in the left lower third.

The 28 studies in group III with negative arteriograms and positive scans are presented in Table 3. There were fewer defects in group III, and, again, as in group II, the defects were nearly evenly distributed between thirds of the lung, both left and right. The majority of perfusion defects on the scans in this group were interpreted as decreased rather than absent. Also, defects were again seen bilaterally in about the same proportion (19 of 28 studies, 68%).

Some of the studies in group III had pulmonary emboli as illustrated by the following two examples. The first is a 40 year old man with a long history of venous insufficiency, admitted with a 4 day history of marked dyspnea, postural hypotension, and left pleuritic chest pain and hemoptysis on the day prior to admission. The lung scan revealed large perfusion defects in addition to the defect from a large left pleural effusion even though the arteriogram was interpreted as showing no definite emboli (Fig. 1). Despite adequate heparin therapy, the patient died 3 days later, and the autopsy showed old organizing pulmonary emboli in the left upper and lower lobar arteries and recent emboli in the right upper lobe artery.

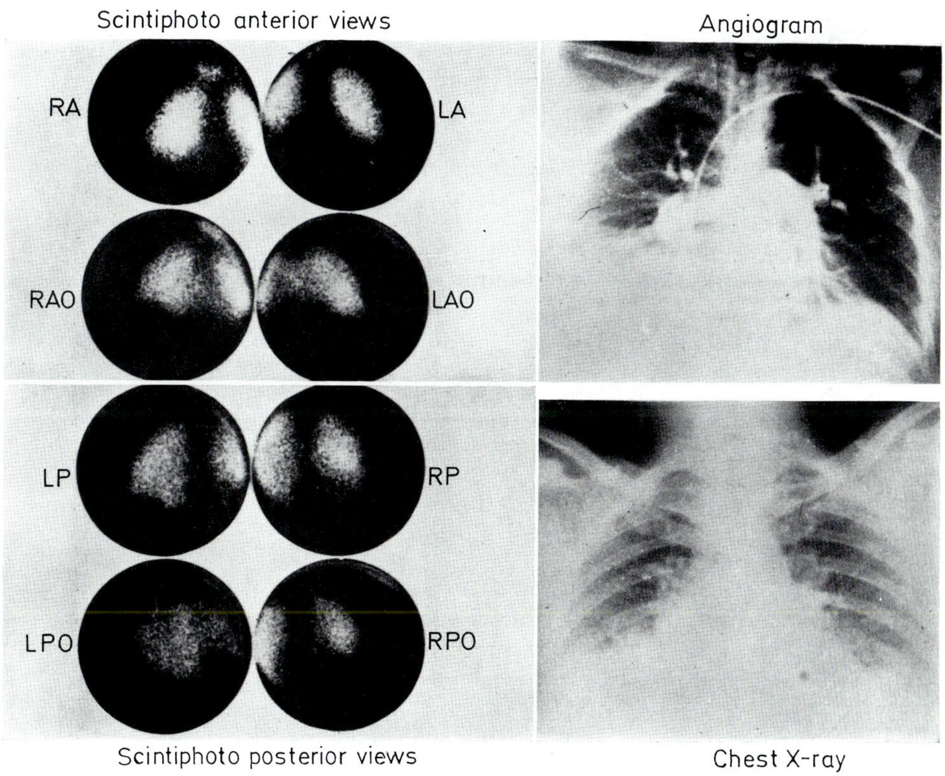

Fig. 2

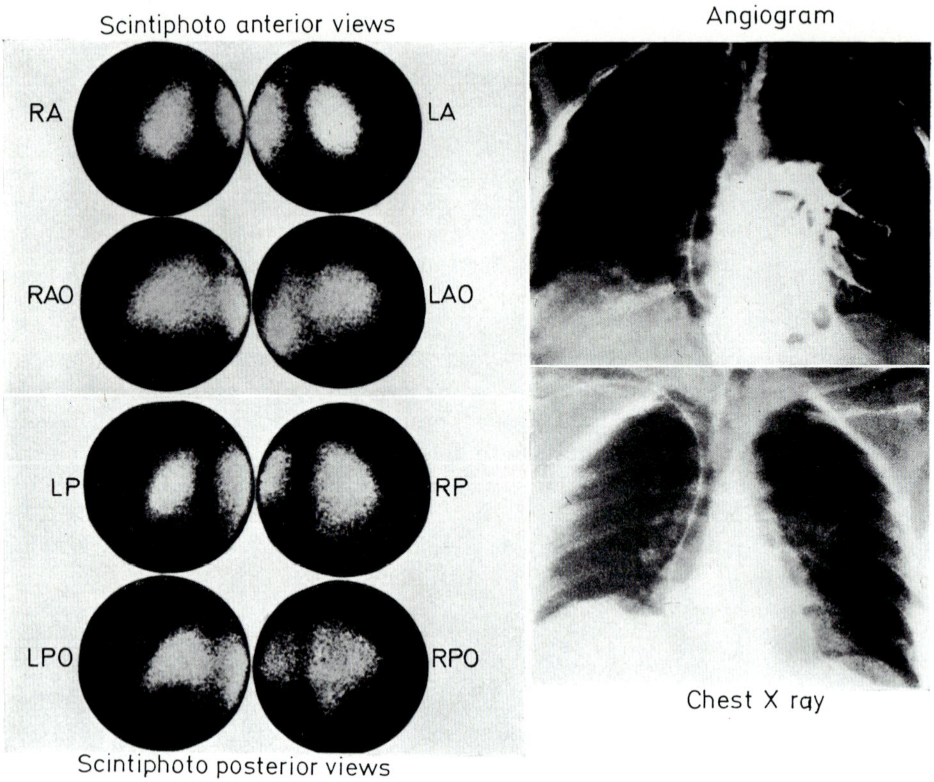

Fig. 3

The second patient had a positive scan and negative arteriogram on her first study (Fig. 2). 2 weeks later this patient had another episode of dyspnea and chest pain, and, at this time, both the scan and the arteriogram were positive (Fig. 3)

8 studies in group IV had both negative arteriograms and scans (Table 1). None of the patients in these 8 studies have been found subsequently to have pulmonary emboli.

Discussion

Emboli have no predilection to any lobe except for perhaps a slightly higher frequency in the left lower lobe (Table 2). This observation is in agreement with the findings of POULOSE *et al.* Also, we found that emboli seen on angiogram were bilateral about 75% of the time.

In the 60 studies comparing lung scans and angiograms, there was no study that had major arterial obstructive defects with absent perfusion on the angiogram that was not present on the scan, although there was some variance in the description of decreased perfusion in individual patients. Areas of absent perfusion on the scan were more likely to be associated with positive angiograms than areas of decreased perfusion. These observations support the hypothesis that the lung scan is a sensitive screening test which can be relied upon prior to pulmonary angiography, since the incidence of false negatives is low and associated with minor lesions.

Table 2. *Defect analysis-group II*

Defects		Angiogram (Positive)		Scan (Positive)	
		Right	Left	Right	Left
	Upper	17	13	17	9
Location	Middle	14	11	16	19
	Lower	18	24	13	21
Extent	Decreased	44	41	27	15
	Absent	5	7	19	34
	Total	49	48	46	49

Table 3. *Defect analysis-group III*

Defects		Angiogram (Negative)		Scan (Positive)	
		Right	Left	Right	Left
	Upper	—	—	15	15
Location	Middle	—	—	14	16
	Lower	—	—	11	19
Extent	Decreased	—	—	34	34
	Absent	—	—	6	16
	Total	—	—	40	50

The frequenc of false positives, in the sense of false positive for pulmonary embolism is difficult to ascertain. The lack of a positive angiogram in group III patients makes the determination of false positives difficult by virtue of the design of this study since we elected to compare lung scans to angiograms. Yet in the 28 studies in group III, we have presented two studies in which the angiogram was negative and the presence of pulmonary emboli was confirmed indicating the scan to be more sensitive. Additionally, in one other positive scan series, the patient had pulmonary emboli demonstrated on a subsequent angiogram. However, 4 studies in group III definitely had false positive scans. They were as follows; 1 patient had no emboli on post mortem examination 3 days later, but had fibrosis and tuberculosis in the apices where perfusion defects were present on the scan; the second patient had a carcinoma of the left main stem bronchus on bronchoscopy and post mortem examination and the scan was positive on the left; the third was one of the patients without any symptoms of pulmonary embolism undegroing cardiac catheterization for mitral stenosis who previously had undergone a lobectomy of the right upper fobe and the perfusion defect corresponded to the absent right upper lobe; the fourth patient had emphysema and apical blebs and the perfusion defects were noted in both apices. Of the remaining 21 studies: 6 were in patients with pleuritic chest pain, dyspnea and hemoptysis (3 also had thrombophlebitis); 8 were in patients with pleuritic chest pain and dyspnea (1 had thrombophlebitis); 2 were in patients with dyspnea only; and 5 were in patients with pleuritic chest pain only (2 had thrombophlebitis). Four of the patients had an elevated lactic dehydrogenase with a normal glutamic oxaloacetic transaminase, while none of the patients had any of the commonly associated electrocardiographic changes of pulmonary embolism as described by CUTFORTH and ORAM. In a clinical review of these patients, it is felt that at least half had definite pulmonary emboli.

To evaluate further the problem of false positives, we analyzed the potential diagnostic categories of the lung scan combined with the clinical history and chest film (Table 4). Categories A (positive scan and negative chest film) and B (positive

Table 4. *Diagnostic categories*

Category	Clinical history	Chest film	Lung scan	Likely result
A	Suggestive of emboli	Negative	Defects	Pulmonary emboli
B	Suggestive of emboli	Infiltrate(s)	Defects in different areas	Suggestive of emboli
C	Suggestive of emboli	Infiltrate(s)	Defects in same areas as infiltrates	Indeterminate
D	Equivocal history for emboli	Infiltrate(s)	Negative	Not pulmonary emboli

Table 5. *Evaluation of diagnostic categories*

Group	Studies	Categories			
		A	B	C	D
II	24	7	13	4	0
III	28	8	18	2	0

scan and chest film in which the infiltrate is in an area different than the defect on the scan) would be expected to have a high incidence of pulmonary embolus. This impression is borne out by distributing group II (positive scan and angiogram) into these categories (Table 5). Group III (negative angiogram: positive scan) is also distributed into these categories in Table 5 and has a similar breakdown. Since the distribution of the studies is similar in comparing groups II and III, and since the sensitivity of the scan is well established in group II, it seems quite reasonable to assume that the positive lung scans in group III are, to a large extent, caused by pulmonary emboli even in the absence of a positive arteriogram. Thus, the true incidence of false positives, although present, cannot be accurately estimated, and it appears that the lung scan when correlated with the chest X-ray and clinical findings is more sensitive than the angiogram in the diagnosis of pulmonary embolus. This seems to be particularly true in the smaller peripheral lesions. Lastly it must be emphasized that it is far more important for a screening test to have a low incidence of false negatives in contrast to false positives, a condition which the lung scan satisfies well. Angiography should be performed prior to pulmonary embolectomy or vena cava ligation. An angiogram will also be needed for a definitive diagnosis when the defect on the scan is in the same area as the infiltrate on the chest film. Pulmonary embolism is still a difficult diagnostic problem; however, the lung scan is a valuable addition to screen patients for this frequently encountered entity.

Abstract

In a prospective study, pulmonary angiography and scintigraphy have been evaluated and compared to determine the efficacy of the lung scan as a screening procedure in the diagnosis of pulmonary emboli. 60 studies in 49 patients were completed in 6 h of each other and interpreted independently. There was no study that had a positive angiogram and negative scan. Also, there was no study with major arterial obstructive disease and absent flow on the arteriogram that was not present as a defect on the scan. However, within these patients who had correspondence of lesions, there was a 15% variance in other areas of the lung between the scan and the angiogram when decreased flow was present. It is concluded that the lung scan is a reliable screening test in the diagnosis of pulmonary embolus.

Acknowledgments

Investigation supported in part by Grants HE-5776 and HE-5445 and Contract PHS 86-67-212.

Radiographic, Angiographic and Scintigraphic Findings after Relapsing Pulmonary Embolism

E. Nägele, H.G. Lasch, E. Wick, S. Grebe, D. Nolte and U. Schoen

In the acute major pulmonary embolism it is generally either too late to perform angiographic and scintigraphic examinations or the patient's very grave condition prohibits such examinations. In smaller, relapsing pulmonary embolism the situation is totally different. They are much harder to diagnose, in particular when the occlusion of a vessel does not lead to a pulmonary infarctation. An infarctation of the lungs, however, does not even occur in half of all pulmonary embolisms. These are the cases which we consider an indication for the performance of angiography and scintigraphy. Scanning, being the less complicated method, should be applied first.

I want to explain this by following example:

A couple of months after a delivery a 34-year-old patient fell sick of slowly progressing dyspnoea. We diagnosed a marked cor pulmonale with corresponding electrocardiographic findings and pulmonary function tests. As the case history – the parturition – and our X-rays supported a pulmonary embolism, we performed a scintigram with ^{131}J alb. It showed obvious defects of accumulation in particular in the right middle and the left lower area.

These findings caused us to pass a catheter to the right heart and to perform an angiography of the A. pulmonalis dextra. The pressure of the right ventricle and in the pulmonary artery was significantly elevated to 80 mmHg systolic. The arteriography proved that numerous major pulmonary arteries of all three lobes were occluded. The vascular deficiency was much more extensive than expected after the scanning.

In spite of the treatment with streptokinase and marcumar the patient's condition grew worse and 4 months later the young woman died of a failure of the right heart. The dissection confirmed our diagnosis "relapsing pulmonary embolism".

I would like to draw your attention to radiographic findings that have always impressed us in such cases.

If one compares scintigrams, angiograms and findings of post-mortem examinations, one can see the expected discontinuance of the A. pulmonalis and its branches in the angiogram. The fact, however, that a vessel or a whole vascular region disappears in a radiograph is amazing, for in the radiograph, a vessel gives the same density of the shadow, be it filled with blood or thrombotic material. The absorption of rays is practically the same in both cases. How, then, do the shadows of the vessels disappear?

First, it could be caused by a spastic contraction of the concerned pulmonary arteries, especially in recent cases. I refer to LAUR's observations.

In our chronically relapsing and only slowly progressing pulmonary embolisms the mechanical obstruction by the thrombus and, in particular, the cicatrized shrinkage of the vessels seem to be the main cause.

As the vessels are grossly dilated central to the discontinuance of the vessel, the impression of a break-off or amputation of the hilus is markedly increased.

Indications respectives de la scintigraphie et de l'angiographie dans l'embolie pulmonaire

M. Bory, J. F. Dumon, P. Djiane et A. Serradimigni

Nous voulons rapporter l'expérience acquise depuis 2 ans dans le diagnostic de l'embolie pulmonaire par la scintigraphie et l'angiographie.

Matériel d'etude

Parmi 70 malades explorés, nous n'avons retenu que ceux qui présentaient une embolie pulmonaire certaine, soit 43 malades. Tous les examens ont été pratiqué en période aigue.

14 malades ont eu simultanément les 2 examens.

19 malades n'ont eu que l'angiopneumographie.

10 malades n'ont eu que la scintigraphie.

Au total nous avons étudié:

33 angiopneumographies.

24 scintigraphies pulmonaires.

Les résultats

1. La comparaison des deux méthodes dans les 14 cas où il a été possible de les pratiquer simultanément, nous a montré que la répartition des images pathologiques intéressaient:

- les mêmes territoires sur les 2 examens dans 7 cas.
- des territoires plus étendus sur la scintigraphie dans 4 cas.
- des territoires plus étendus sur l'angiographie dans 3 cas.

Il ne semble donc pas, sur ces premiers résultats, qu'une méthode soit supérieure à l'autre pour dèpister l'embolie pulmonaire. Aussi avons-nous poussé notre analyse plus loin en étudiant les images scintigraphiques et angiographiques.

2. Les images angiographiques sont de plusieurs types:

– l'image de défaut de remplissage (Fig. 1). Elle traduit la présence de caillot comme le prouve notamment la vérification chirurgicale ou nècropsique (Fig. 2). Elle n'a jamais été retrouvée sur 150 angiopneumographies de sujets indemnes d'embolie, c'est dire sa spécifité.

– les images d'amputation ou de gracilité artérielle sont moins spécifiques car retrouvées dans d'autres affections pleuro-pulmonaires. Elles sont, toutefois, évocatrices dans le contexte.

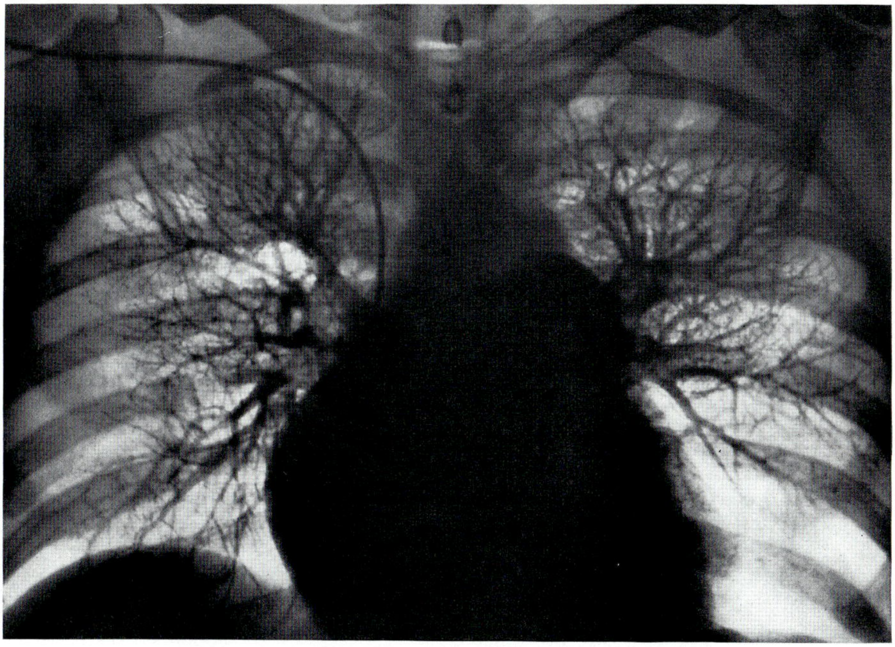

Fig. 1. Angiopneumographie d'embolie pulmonaire grave. Les images claires de caillot, visibles dans toutes les artères lobaires droites, sont pathognomoniques de la maladie

Ces images sont très fréquentes:
- les images de caillot = 21 fois.
- les images évocatrices = 11 fois.
- une seule fois, une image normale a été observée.

Ce tableau nous donne aussi les limites de l'angiopneumographie puisque les images sont 11 fois sans spécifité et 1 fois normale. Ces limites sont liées:

a) à la labilité du caillot (Fig. 3). Les images disparaissent à des examens successifs, il faut donc pratiquer l'angiopneumographie le plus tôt possible. L'image de défaut de remplissage existe 12 fois chez 15 malades le 1 er jour.

b) à la taille du caillot qui est difficilement reconnu au-delà des branches segmentaires.

c) à la superposition possible des images, d'où l'intérêt dans les cas douteux de pratiquer des injections sélectives sous différentes incidences.

Ces faits expliquent la possibilité d'angiopneumographie normale devant une embolie authentique. Mais cela est en définitive, exceptionnel et cet examen permet 2 fois sur 3 d'affirmer avec certitude l'embolie pulmonaire aigue.

3. Les images scintigraphiques:

Sur 24 scintigrammes, nous avons rencontré 1 cliché normal et 23 clichés pathologiques. Deux types d'images ont été observées:
- les images d'amputation.
- les images d'hypofixation (Fig. 4).

Les premières ont été notées 14 fois, les deuxièmes 16 fois. Elles sont associées chez 7 malades.

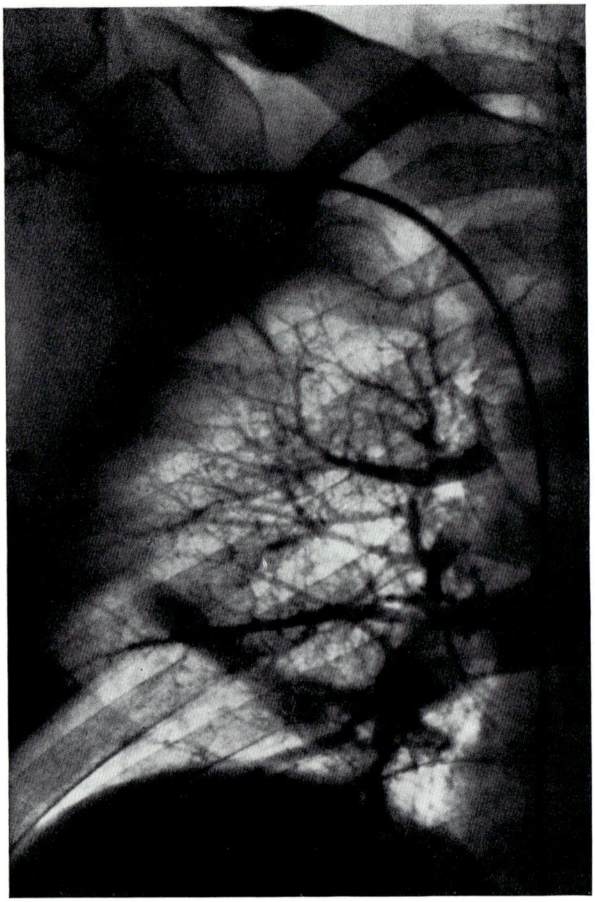

a

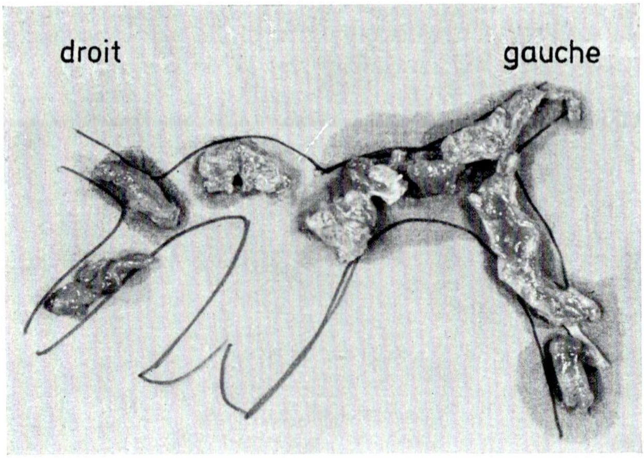

b

Fig. 2a. Angiopneumographie d'embolie pulmonaire aigue grave. b Constatation chirurgicale

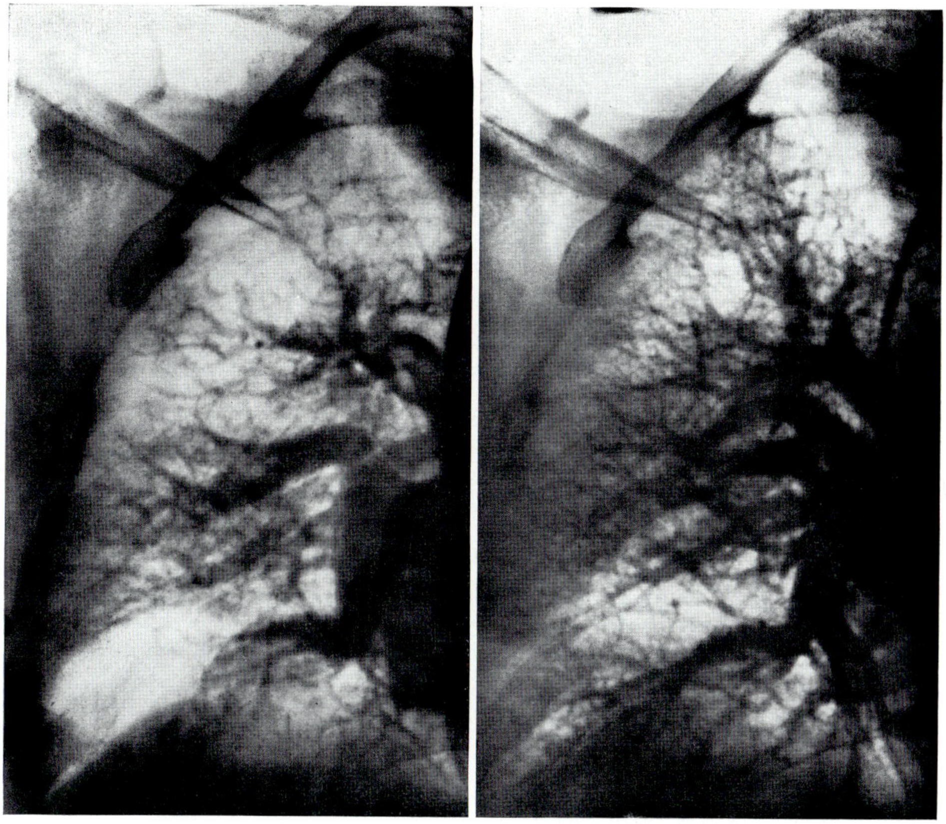

a b

Fig. 3a et b. Angiopneumographies itératives dans l'embolie plumonaire. a Image de caillot dans la lobaire supérieure droite. Amputation de la branche de Nelson. Amputation des branches para-cardiaque et externe de la lobaire inférieure droite. b 15 jours apres, toutes les images pathologiques ont disparu

Malheureusement ces images, si elles sont presque toujours présentes, ne sont pas pathognomoniques puisque nous les avons retrouvées sur 160 scintigrammes pratiqués chez des malades atteints d'affection pleuro-pulmonaires diverses. BRYANT les a aussi observées sur les scintigrammes des post-opérés indemmes d'embolie. Cela rend la scintigraphie bien imprécise. Néanmoins, chez 6 malades la répétition à la phase chronique des clichés scintigraphiques et angiographiques a permis de constater que les évolutions scintigraphiques et radiologiques étaient parallèles: l'amélioration (2 fois), la stabilisation (3 fois) ou l'aggravation (1 fois), se retrouvent simultanément sur les 2 examens.

En d'autres termes, la scintigraphie initiale ayant été étalonnée par l'angiographie, les scintigraphies ultérieures seront suffisantes à elles-seules pour apprécier l'évolution de la maladie embolique.

a

b

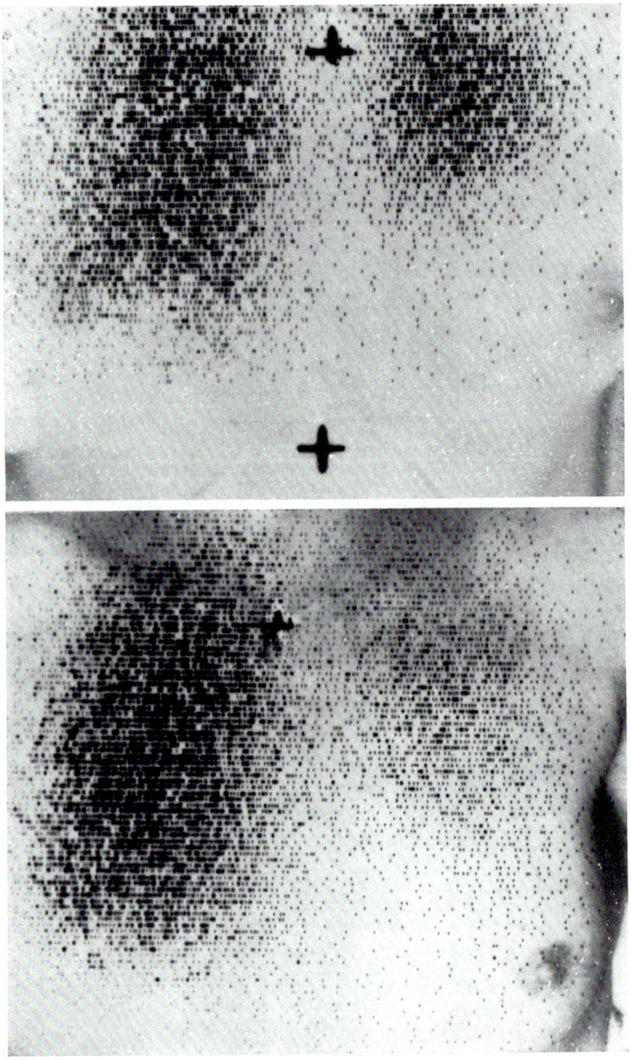

Fig. 4a et b. Scintigraphies pulmonaires par voie veineuse d'embolie pulmonaire aiguë. a Image d'amputation du lobe inférieur gauche. b Image d'hypo-fixation de toute la plage pulmonaire gauche. Ces images sont toutefois sans spécificité

Les indications

Elles seront déduites de l'analyse des avantages et inconvénients des 2 méthodes. L'appareillage est complexe dans les 2 cas. La réalisation et la répétition de l'examen est évidemment beaucoup plus facile lorsqu'on s'adresse à la scintigraphie. L'innocuité de la méthode, nulle lorsqu'on utilise la scintigraphie, est mineure lorsqu'on emploie l'angiographie.

En ce qui concerne la valeur des images, la scintigraphie ne saurait soutenir la comparaison avec l'angiographie qui est le seul examen à apporter un signe pathognomique et ceci dans $^2/_3$ des cas.

En définitive, pour le diagnostic l'angiopneumographie est la meilleure méthode, mais étant donné les difficultés de sa réalisation, elle n'est impérative que lorsqu'elle est indispensable à la conduite thérapeutique:

- contre-indication relative aux anticoagulants.
- embolie pulmonaire grave.

On ne fera appel à la scintigraphie que lorsque l'angiographie est contre-indiquée (insuffisants rénaux).

Pour suivre l'évolution de la maladie embolique, les 2 examens sont valables, mais la facilité d'obtention de tracés iteratigs, milite en faveur de la scintigraphie. L'idéal, toutefois, est d'associer initialement les 2 méthodes, puis de suivre ensuite la maladie par les scintigrammes.

Über den quantitativen Nachweis von Durchblutungsstörungen der Lungen, über deren Ursache und Ausmaß bei Patienten mit einer cavernösen Silikotuberkulose

H. SCHRÖDER und S. CH. PLECHL

Eine Komplikation der Silikose ist die cavernöse Tuberkulose. Zur Ermittlung quantitativer Durchblutungsstörungen der Lungen im Rahmen der cavernösen Silikotuberkulose wurden ein 3 Zoll-Magna-Scanner mit einem Triprober der Fa. Picker gekoppelt. Jede Scanzeile wurde in der Mitte unterteilt, die integrierten Impulsraten auf je einen getrennten Kanal gespeichert. Am Ende jeder Scanzeile wurden die gesammelten Informationen ausgedruckt. Die Auswertung der Meßergebnisse erfolgte unter Bildung von Verhältniszahlen der integrierten Impulse zwischen der rechten und der linken Lunge, sowie zwischen dem rechten und dem linken Oberfeld. Die Signifikanzberechnung wurde nach der T-Verteilung vorgenommen.

Zur Klärung der Frage nach der Ursache der Verteilungsstörungen von Jod-131-Albumin-Partikeln wurde ein Spezialkollimator unter Vorlage des Röntgenbildes bei 10 Patienten über dem Herzen aufgesetzt und der Aktivitätsdurchfluß von Technetium-99-Humanalbumin und von Jod-131-Albumin-Partikel gemessen.

Bei weiteren 10 Patienten wurden außerdem vor der Injektion der Albumin-Partikel Kollimatoren über den entsprechenden Lungenabschnitten aufgesetzt und der Einstrom der Aktivität in Kurvenform aufgenommen. Die hiermit gewonnenen Kurven sprechen nach unserer Ansicht für eine echte Minderdurchblutung des dem Fixationsausfall entsprechenden Lungenabschnittes.

Zur Klärung der Frage, ob Unterschiede in der Lungendurchblutung in Abhängigkeit von der Lage und Größe der Cavernen zu finden sind, wurden 17 Patienten mit rechtsseitigen Oberfeldcavernen ohne röntgenologisch nachweisbare Hilusbeteiligung und 7 Patienten mit röntgenologisch nachweisbarer Hilusbeteiligung untersucht und mit einem Normalkollektiv von 21 Patienten verglichen, bei denen die Lungen klinisch und röntgenologisch unauffällig waren. Hierbei zeigte sich ein signifikanter Unterschied zwischen den lungenkranken und den lungengesunden Patienten. Ein signifikanter Unterschied bestand ferner zwischen den Patienten, bei denen eine periphere und eine zentrale cavernöse Silikotuberkulose bestand.

Zusammenfassend dürfen wir feststellen:
Die Untersuchungsergebnisse sprechen nach unserer Ansicht für eine echte Minderdurchblutung der entsprechenden cavernösen Lungenabschnitte, wobei das Ausmaß der Durchblutungsstörungen davon abhängt, ob der Prozeß peripher oder zentral liegt bzw. den Lungenhilus durch sekundäre Schrumpfprozesse einbezieht.

Analysis of the Function of the Pulmonary Vascular System

R. Felix, H. J. van de Weyer, J. Assheuer, E. Bücheler and C. Winkler

The only task of the lung is to oxygenise the whole venous blood completely. This presumes that in all normally ventilated parts of the lung a normal blood flow exists and that in all parts of the lung, which are not ventilating, blood flow is reduced ore terminated. Thus hypoventilation must be followed by reduced circulation.

During normal breathing the number and the diameter of lung vessels are the same on both sides. (Fig. 1a). After taking angiogram and scintigram of both

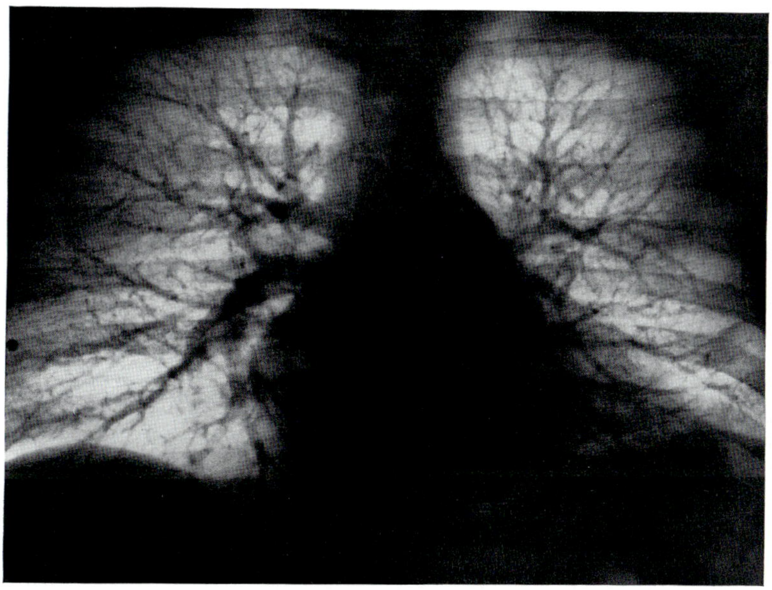

Fig. 1a

lungs under normal conditions the air passage of both lungs was separated by a so called Carlen's tube so that the respiratory gas mixture could be changed in each lung independantly. Unilateral hypoventilation of one lung can be simulated without disturbence of the airway dynamics by giving one lung a gas mixture corresponding to the partial gas pressures of venous blood (7 Vol.% CO_2, 5 Vol.% O_2, rest N_2; rebreathing of this mixture for 10 min). By this gaseous exchange terminates in this side and consequently the oxygenation of the passing blood.

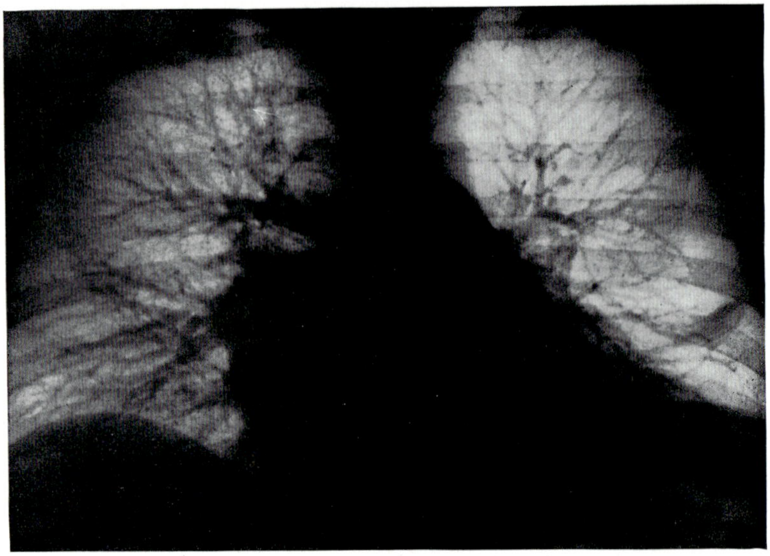

Fig. 1b

Figure 1b shows the same lung vessels as Figure 1a. But the left lung was hypoventilated as described above. The number and the diameter of the vessels of the left lung are functionally diminished compared to the right. The left lung is therefore hyperlucent.

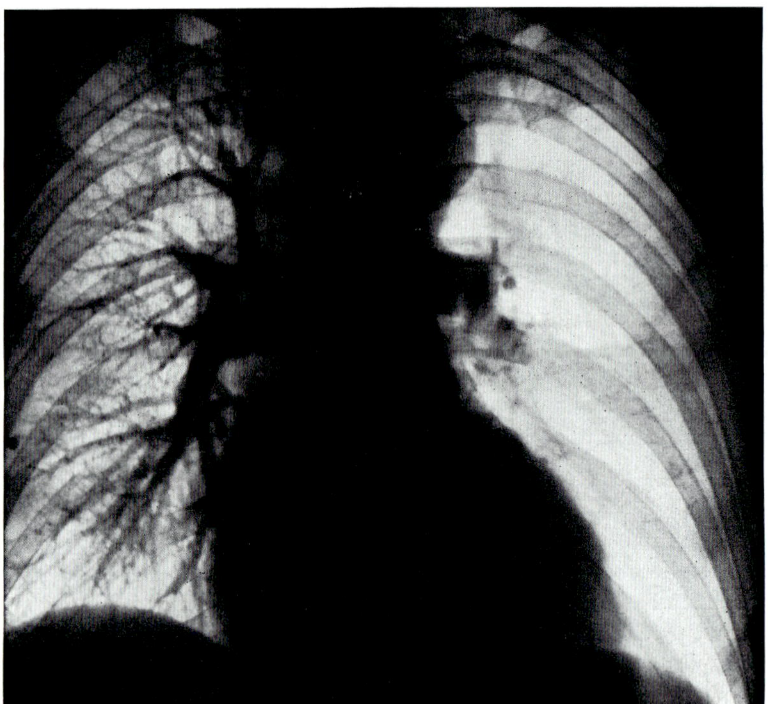

Fig. 2a

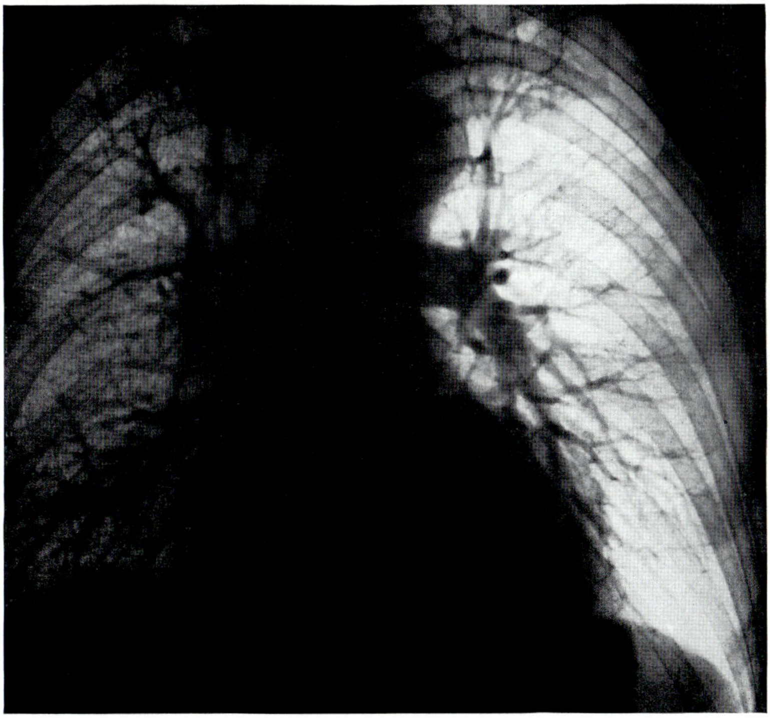

Fig. 2b

Normally the blood flow velocity in the vessels of both lungs is quite equal. But during unilateral hypoventilation (left lung in Fig. 2a) the blood flow velocity is decreased in the hypoventilating lung compared to the normally ventilating one. In Fig. 2a the blood stream on the right side has already reached the peripheral arteries while on the left the opacified blood is seen only in the main pulmonary artery. Fig. 2b shows the same lung 3 sec later. On the right side the contrast material passes already the pulmonary veins, whereas in the same time on the left side the arteries are still visible. Fig. 2c gives the same lung 3 sec later than Fig. 2b. Only the veins of the left side are still opacified. The diameters of the veins are very small. In the same time the passage of the contrast material on the right is finished.

These observations allow the following conclusion: in hypoventilating lungs the blood flow velocity and the diameter of blood vessels are reduced. Also the number of the perfused vessels in the hypoventilating lung is diminished.

The quantitative significance of these reactions is of deciding importance. Blood gas analysis does'nt give exact information about the regulation of these lung circulation and the distribution of the blood flow in the lungs.

Therefore we are dependent on computerscintigraphy for quantitative data of the distribution of blood flow and the regulation capacity in lung circulation. The relation if activity distribution between the right and the left lung (using intravenously applied macroaggregates [MAA], labeled with radioactive isotopes) represents the distribution of blood flow between the two lungs. Two different radioisotopes

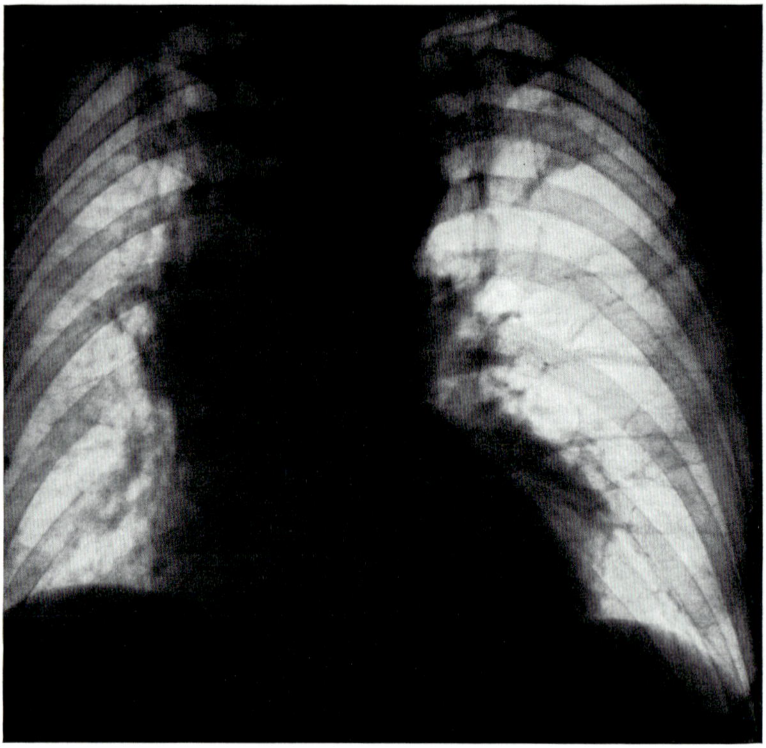

Fig. 2c

^{99m}Tc and ^{131}J) have to be applied for these measurements because two different conditions of the lung circulation have to be "fixed" (see the following). So-called polaroid-scintiphotos were taken with a gamma camera and for quantitative evaluation of activity distribution we used a computer.

Figure 3a represents the polaroid-scintiphoto of a 27 years old male patient, who suffers from a tuberculous cavity in the right upper lobe. The patient breathes normally. The relation of the activity distribution respectively of the perfusion distribution between the right and the left lung is corresponding to 55:45. This is a normal relation. In Figure 3b the right lung is hypoventilating with the gas mixture described above. The relation of perfusion distribution between the right and the left lung corresponds to 33:67 now. Because of this right sided hypoventilation 22% of the cardiac output are shifted from the right to the left lung.

Dependent on unilateral hypoventilation 24% of the cardiac output are shifted to the normally ventilating lung (mean value of 5 persons aged about 30 years with normal lung function). In normal persons there will be no elevation of the mean pulmonary arterial blood pressure during these redistributions of cardiac output due to unilateral hypoventilation. If the pulmonary vascular system is diminished on one side by emphysema or other diseases hypoventilation of this side loses its influence on the perfusion distribution.

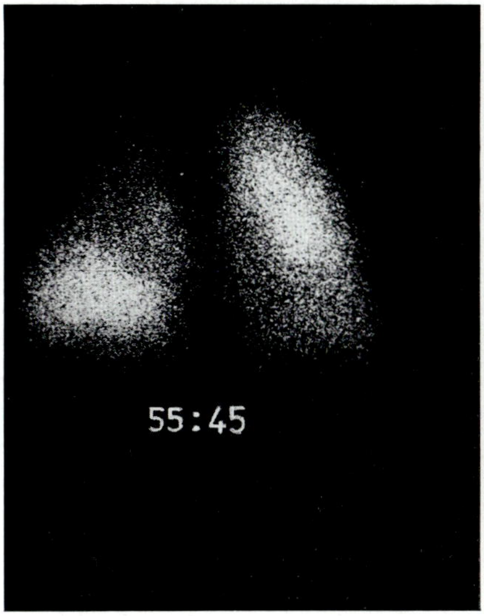

Fig. 3a

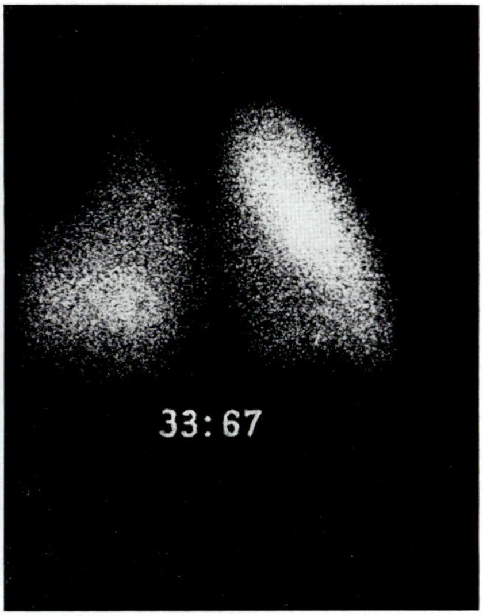

Fig. 3b

Figure 4 represents the relation of perfusion distribution during normal breathing in a 23 years old female patient suffering from a productive and cirrhotic tuberculosis with cavity in the left upper lobe. Consequently the relation of perfusion distribution right: left during normal breathing corresponds to 63:37. The circumscribed impairment of perfusion in the left upper lobe can be seen (Fig. 4a). In Figure 4b the left lung is hypoventilating with the gas mixture described above. In contrast to Figure 3b only 2% of the cardiac output are shifted from the left to the right lung in dependence on left sided hypoventilation. This phenomenon, i.e. the very little redistribution of cadiac output due to hypoventilation of the lung with impaired vascular system, can be seen regularly.

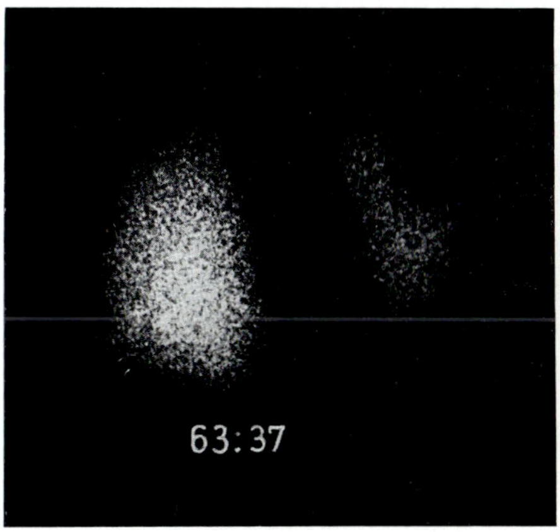

Fig. 4a

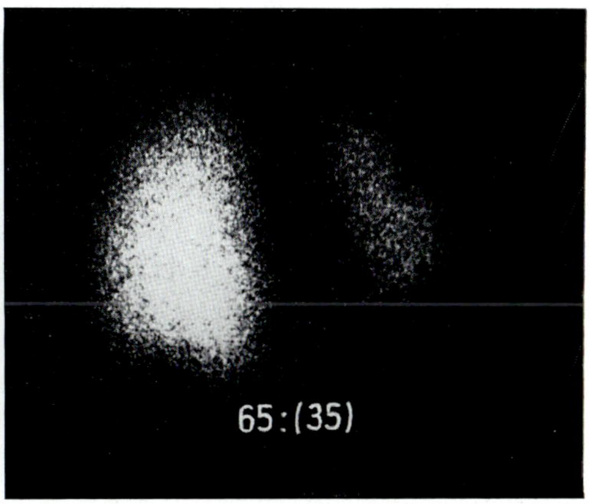

Fig. 4b

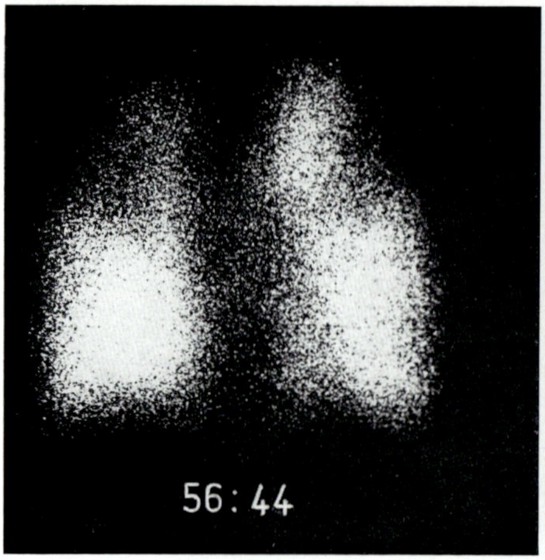

Fig. 5a

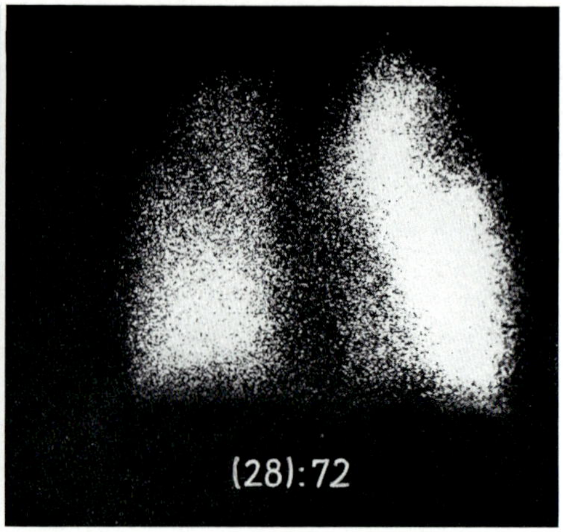

Fig. 5b

The question has to be claryfied wether ore not in patients with impaired unilateral ore bilateral vascular system unilateral hypoventilation may cause pulmonary hypertension.

Figure 5a represents the relation of perfusion distribution during normal breathing in a 26 years old female patient with productive and cirrhotic tuberculosis in left and right upper lobe. The relation of perfusion distribution right: left during normal breathing corresponds to 56:44. This is a normal relation. In Figure 5b the polaroid-scintiphoto during hypoventilation of the right lung can be seen. The relation of perfusion distribution between the right and left lung is now corresponding to 28:72. Because of the right sided hypoventilation 28% of the cardiac output are shifted from the right to the left lung.

The momentary load of the left pulmonary vascular system by 28% of the cardiac output causes an elevation of the mean pulmonary arterial blood pressure from 15 to 25 mmHg because the impaired vascular system of the left lung has not sufficient capacity for the additional blood volume per unit time.

The question wether ore not unilateral hypoventilation may cause pulmonary hypertension can be answered as follows:

The cross-sectional area of the unilateral pulmonary vascular system will be diminished by hypoventilation of this lung even then if the contralateral vascular system has not sufficient capacity for the additional blood flow per unit time. Under these conditions unilateral hypoventilation causes pulmonary hypertension.

If mean pulmonary arterial blood pressure will not be elevated during unilateral hypoventilation this furthermore gives evidence about the capacity of the contralateral pulmonary vascular system for additional blood flow per unit time (in % of the cardiac output), i.e. the maximum of this capacity can *not* be evaluated if mean pulmonary arterial blood pressure is *not* raising.

If mean pulmonary arterial blood pressure will be elevated during unilateral hypoventilation this gives evidence that, for instance in Figure 5, the capacity of the contralateral (left) pulmonary vascular system for additional blood flow per unit time is not as big as 28% of the cardiac output. These results may be important before pneumonectomy and for estimating the risk of a postoperative pulmonary hypertension with cor pulmonale.

Summaring radiological methods may contribute the following facts to the functional analysis of the pulmonary vascular system:

1. Unilateral hypoventilation diminishes the radius of the pulmonary arterial blood vessels as well as the number of the prefused arteries in this lung.
2. Unilateral hypoventilation diminishes the blood flow velocity in this lung.
3. Unilateral hypoventilation in about 30 years old individuals with normal lungs causes a shifting of about 24% of the cardiac output to the normal ventilating contralateral lung.
4. Unilateral hypoventilation ceases to influence blood flow distribution if impairments of the pulmonary vascular system on the same side are caused by pulmonary diseases (i.e. emphysema and others).
5. Unilateral hypoventilation may cause pulmonary hypertension if the contralateral vascular system has not sufficient capacity for the additional blood flow per unit time.

Semiquantitative and Planimetric Investigations of Pulmonary Scintiscans for the Estimation of Functional Disturbances of Lungs after Lymphography

H.-J. Fernholz and W. Dihlmann

It is well known that oil embolism takes place in some part of pulmonal capillaries after lymphography, and causes reduction of the ventilation and capacity of diffusion of lungs. Ventilation, diffusion and perfusion of lungs synchronize each other, so when oil embolism occurs in the pulmonal capillaries, disturbances of pulmonal blood flow will be occured. We carried out our investigations to prove these disturbances by use of pulmonary scintiscanning.

Lymphography was performed with injection of 8–24 ml contrast medium. Before and after lymphography, pulmonary scintiscans were carried out on constant conditions with use of ^{131}J-labelled macroaggregated human serum albumin for 19 patients. According to Feine's method we measured the accumulated activity and the distribution was calculated. Furthermore the accumulating area of lungs was calculated by planimeter.

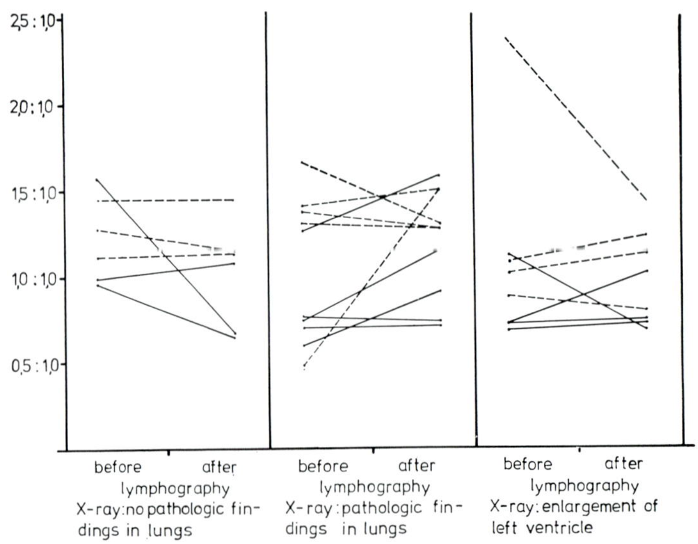

Fig. 1. Results of semiquantitative calculation of lung scans. The curves show the relations of distribution of activity between upper and lower segments of right and left lung before and after lymphography

Our method is not suitable to find out the absolute rate of reduction of pulmonal perfusion. Concerning to quantity and localisation we didn't observe any constant change of patterns of blood flow in lungs after lymphography. As well we didn't see displacement of blood volumes from lower pulmonal segments to upper segments as mentioned by LANGE and coworkers. But in patients with pathological pulmonal changes or enlargement of the left ventricle on X-ray we found displacement of blood volume from pathological to nonpathological or noncompressed pulmonal segments (Fig. 1).

It must be considered that the different reactions reflect the individual regulation of intrapulmonal blood distribution. There with, it will be possible that partial compensation of disturbance of diffusion is obtained.

Moreover, enlargement of pulmonal area after lymphography was planimetrically measured. This enlargement is most remarkable in patients with normal lungs on X-rays, and less remarkable in patients with pathological pulmonal findings or left ventricular enlargement. Also it is recognized that enlargement of pulmonal area depends on volume of applied contrast medium. That is, the more contrast medium is injected, the more the lung area is enlarged (Table).

Table. *Change of size of the perfused areas of lungs after lymphography detected by scintiscans of lungs*

	<10 ml contrast medium	>10 ml contrast medium
X-ray: normal lungs	$+ 13{,}2$ cm^2 ($n = 3$)	$+ 39{,}6$ cm^2 ($n = 5$)
X-ray: pathologic findings in lungs	$- 5{,}5$ cm^2 ($n = 2$)	$+ 8{,}7$ cm^2 ($n = 4$)
X-ray: enlargement of left ventricle	$+ 10{,}6$ cm^2 ($n = 3$)	$+ 20{,}9$ cm^2 ($n = 2$)
average increase	$+ 7{,}6$ cm^2 ($n = 8$)	$+ 24{,}9$ cm^2 ($n = 11$)

It is considerable that after lymphography elevated pressure in lung circulation which was established by FABEL and his coworkers causes opening of pulmonal reserved areas, where by it will be able to compensate the restriction of active pulmonal tissue. There are no relations between changes of pattern of blood flow and enlargement of perfused pulmonal areas.

All these changes of pulmonal perfusion, detected by scintiscanning, must be considered as a procedure of compensation, and with this, organism attemps to compensate alveolo-capillary block which is caused by oil embolism.

Perfusionslungenszintigraphie bei primär vasculär pulmonaler Hypertonie

K. Koppenhagen, H. Ernst, H. Meinhold, H. Paeprer
und H.W. Liebenschütz

Die Häufigkeit der primär vasculären pulmonalen Hypertonie hat in den letzten Jahren insbesondere mit der Einnahme von Appetitzüglern zugenommen. Die sichere Diagnose dieses Krankheitbildes gelingt lediglich durch pulmonal-arterielle Druckmessung. Untersuchungen an 34 Patienten mit Appetitzüglereinnahme (Aminorexfumarat) und davon 15 durch Druckmessung gesicherten pulmonalen Hypertonien sollen die Perfusionslungenszintigraphie zur Diagnose und Beurteilung dieses Krankheitsbildes prüfen.

Die Aufzeichnung der Lungenszintigramme erfolgte mit dem Picker-Dynapix. Zur sicheren und quantitativen Beurteilung auch diskreterer Perfusionsstörungen wurden alle Szintigramme vom Magnet-Speicher mit steigenden Subtraktionsraten erneut dargestellt. Zur Lungenszintigraphie verwendeten wir ^{131}J-markiertes Eiweißmakroaggregat in einer Teilchengröße zwischen 10–50 μ und einer Dosierung von 200μ Ci, das am liegenden Patienten bei ruhiger Atmung i.v. injiziert wurde. 27 von 34 Patienten wiesen eine deutliche Perfusionsstörung auf. Bei 2 Patienten konnte die Perfusionsminderung durch die Anamnese sowie cardiologisch-pulmologische Untersuchungen auf eine Bronchitis und Emphysem zurückgeführt werden. 25 Patienten (=70%) mit Aminorex-Einnahme zeigten nicht durch andere Krankheiten erklärbare Perfusionsstörungen. Wegen des Schweregrades klinischer Symptome und der Perfusionsausfälle wurde bei 15 Patienten der pulmonale Druck gemessen. In allen Fällen konnte eine primär vasculäre pulmonale Hypertonie gesichert werden. Die übrigen 10 Patienten mit leichteren Beschwerden und geringgradigen Perfusionsstörungen lehnten eine Pulmonalis-Druckmessung ab.

Unauffällige Lungenszintigramme haben wir beim Bestehen einer pulmonalen Hypertonie nicht registriert. Zwischen dem Schweregrad der nachgewiesenen Perfusionsstörungen und den gemessenen pulmonalen Drucken besteht eine annähernde Korrelation. Bei deutlichen Druckerhöhungen zeigen sich schwere, bei geringgradigen leichte Perfusionsstörungen. 12 von 15 Patienten mit gesicherten pulmonalen Hypertonien wiesen eine beidseitige Perfusionsstörung auf. 2 Patienten hatten einen Perfusionsverlust einer ganzen Lungenhälfte. Neben „mottenfraßähnlich" über beide Lungenhälften verteilten Perfusionsstörungen imponierte bei einigen schweren pulmonalen Hypertonien nur noch ein mantelförmiger Aktivitätssaum in den Randpartien der Lunge. Bei einigen Patienten fiel eine perihiläre Perfusionsminderung auf. Auffallend häufig ist das linke Lungenuntergeschoß betroffen, obwohl nicht in allen Fällen eine Herzverbreiterung nach links verantwortlich gemacht werden konnte. 8 Kontrollszintigraphien ergaben nach 5–12 Monaten nahezu den gleichen Befund, ein Patient wies eine mit den Druckverhältnissen parallel gehende Verschlimmerung auf.

Als Ursache der bei der primären pulmonalen Hypertonie beobachteten Perfusionsstörungen sind letztlich die zur Lumeneinengung bzw. vollständigen Verlegung führenden proliferativen oder durch funktionelle Engstellung bedingten Prozesse der Arteriolen und der kleinen muskulären Arterien anzusehen. Ein primär embolisches Geschehen ist auf Grund des Verteilungsmusters der Partikel unwahrscheinlich und erst als sekundäre Folgeerscheinung bei Perfusionsverlust einer gesamten Lungenhälfte anzunehmen. Perfusionsstörungen anderer Herz-Lungen-Erkrankungen können zumeist durch die üblichen cardiologisch-pulmologischen Untersuchungsmethoden abgegrenzt werden.

Bei der primär vasculären pulmonalen Hypertonie wird klinisch ein wahrscheinlich nur durch Gefäßspasmen ausgelöstes funktionell-*reversibles*, von einem durch organische Gefäßveränderungen hervorgerufenem, *irreversiblen* Stadium unterschieden. Zum Nachweis beider Schweregrade führten wir eine bereits zur Differenzierung des chronischen Asthma bronchiale vom destruktiven Lungenemphysem entwickelte „2-Phasen-Szintigraphie" durch. Durch zweimalige Szintigraphie mit unterschiedlich im Energiespektrum liegenden Radionuklid-Eiweißpartikeln (^{99m}Tc-und ^{131}J-Eiweißmakroaggregat) vor und nach Verabfolgung eines gefäßwirksamen Pharmakons (0,96 g Aminophyllin) kann man die durch das Medikament eintretenden Veränderungen der bei der ersten Untersuchung nachgewiesenen Perfusionsstörungen unmittelbar in einem Untersuchungsgang registrieren. 4 Patienten mit deutlicher pulmonaler Druckerhöhung zeigten mittels dieser Methode keine, 2 mit leichter pulmonaler Hypertonie eine sichere Perfusionsverbesserung. Im ersten Fall handelt es sich nach unserer Auffassung um ein therapeutisch schwer anzugehendes, organisch-obstruktives, im zweiten Fall um ein auf Medikamente gut ansprechendes funktionell-konstriktives Stadium.

Zusammenfassung

Die Perfusionslungenszintigraphie ist als leicht durchzuführende Untersuchung im Sinne eines Suchtests bei Patienten mit Appetitzügler-Einnahme und abzuklärender primär vasculärer pulmonaler Hypertonie einsetzbar. Zwischen dem Schweregrad der Perfusionsstörung und der Höhe des pulmonalen Drucks besteht eine abschätzbare Korrelation. Mittels der „2-Phasen-Szintigraphie" sind funktionell-reversible von organisch-irreversiblen Perfusionsstörungen zu trennen. Diese Untersuchung erscheint zur Beurteilung des Schweregrades und der Therapiemöglichkeit der primär vasculären pulmonalen Hypertonie bedeutungsvoll.

Angiography and Scintiscanning in Preoperative Assessment of Congenital and Acquired Lung Diseases

D. Novak, H. Frenzel and H. Wieners

Spirometry and blood gas analysis are feasible examination methods for evaluation of total lung function. In assessing regional functional disturbances both methods are applicable only under certain conditions. Diagnosis and evaluation of pathological changes of lungs from morphological as well as from functional point of view are domain of lung angiography and scintiscanning. These methods allow semiquantitative evaluation of extension and degree of lung parenchymal destruction. Loss of lung parenchyma in congenital and acquired lung diseases is demonstrated in angiogram as reduction and/or morphological abnormalities of lung vasculature. On the other hand, the localisation and relative amount of poorly perfused lungs are displayed in the pulmonary perfusion scan.

Methods

For the pulmonary angiography the catheter was placed in the main pulmonary artery and 30–40 ml of Angiographin were injected at a pressure of 4–6 kg/cm^2 by means of the Gidlund injector. Serial films were obtained with Elema-Schönander automatic film changer.

Perfusion lung scanning was performed after intravenous injection of 250 μCi of ^{131}J-macroaggregated albumin. Photoscans were produced by a scanner with a 5 in. crystal and a 19 hole collimator. After performing lung scanning, measurement of count rate over 6 defined lung sections was performed, using the same scanner and with the patient in supine position.

Semiquantitative Evaluation of Lung Angiograms

The destruction of lung parenchyma demonstrated by means of angiography was classified according to the proposal of Grill in 4 grades. This classification is based on visual evaluation of the degree of reduction of lung vasculature (Table).

Semiquantitative Evaluation of Lung Perfusion

The distribution of intravenously injected ^{131}J-macroaggregated albumin representing regional perfusion of lungs, was evaluated by the following two procedures:

a) Visual evaluation of lung scans and estimation of the degree of perfusion.

b) Measurements of radioactivity over 6 defined lung regions under constant geometrical conditions. This procedure was performed as follows: After termination of lung scanning with the patient in supine position, the longitudinal axis of each lung lobe as seen in the scan was drawn and divided in three sections of same length. The detector of the scanner was centered in the middle point of each lung section and the count rate was recorded (Fig. 1). The registered count rate was multiplied with a correction factor (F) allowing for the different anatomical diameters of various parts of lungs. The correction factor (F) was calculated using the measurements in a control group of 7 normal volunteers.

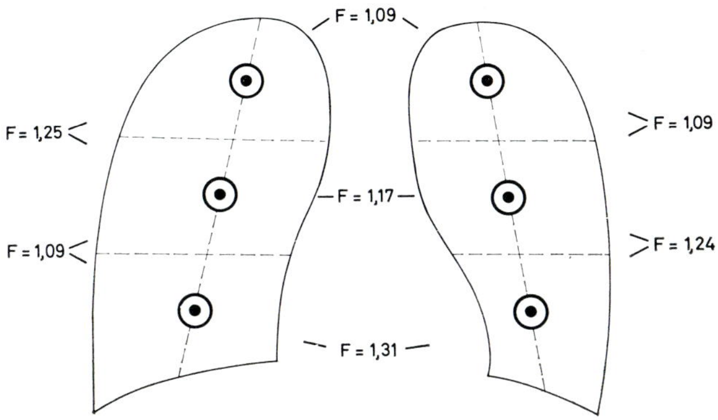

Fig. 1. Semiquantitative evaluation of lung perfusion based on measurement of count rates over 6 defined lung sections. The correction factor (F) considers the anatomical differences between various parts of the lungs and was calculated in a control group of 7 normal volunteers

The degree of decreased regional perfusion was expressed in per cent of deviation from highest count rate registered ($R_{max} = 100\%$). Calculation was performed using the following formula:

$$P_a = 100 - \left(\frac{R_a \times F_a \times 100}{R_{max}} \right)$$

P_a = perfusion of a lung section "a" in per cent of deviation from the norm ($R_{max} = 100\%$)
R_a = count rate measured over a lung section "a"
R_{max} = highest count rate measured over one of six lung sections
F_a = correction factor for lung section "a"

Case Reports

The validity of angiography and lung scanning in the assessment of patients with localized pulmonary parenchymal destruction is illustrated by demonstration of radiological findings in two cases.

Case 1

The roentgenogram (Fig. 2a) of a 47 year old male with dystrophy of the lung shows a distinct reduction of lung vasculature in the right lung. The angiogram (Fig. 2b) confirms this finding. The pathological changes demonstrated in the angiogram correspond to grade IV of the proposed classification (Table). The

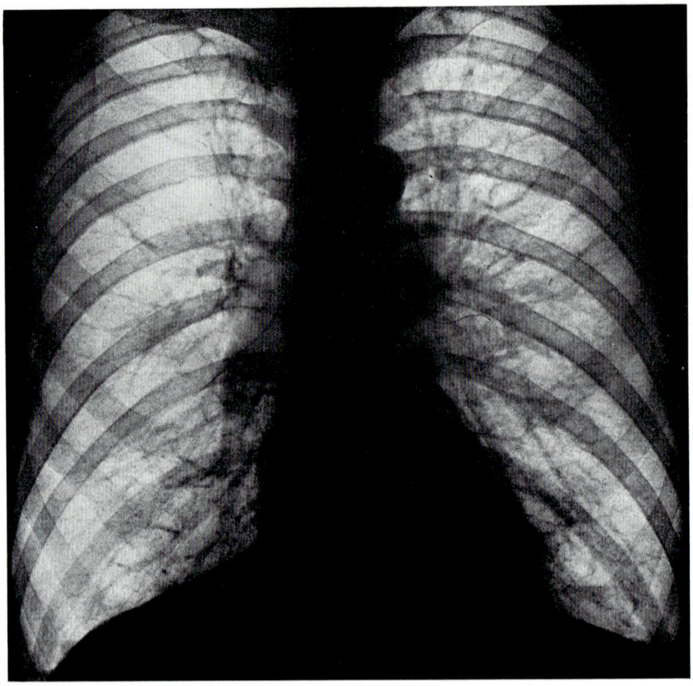

Fig. 2a

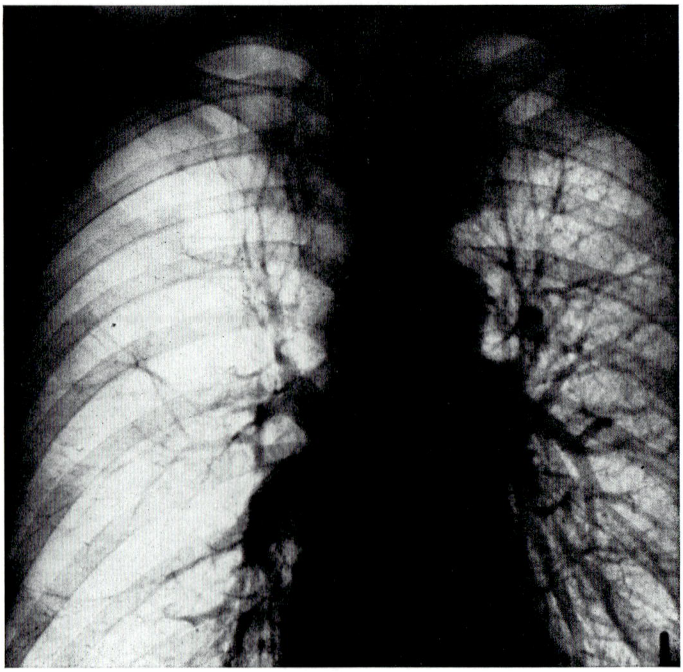

Fig. 2b

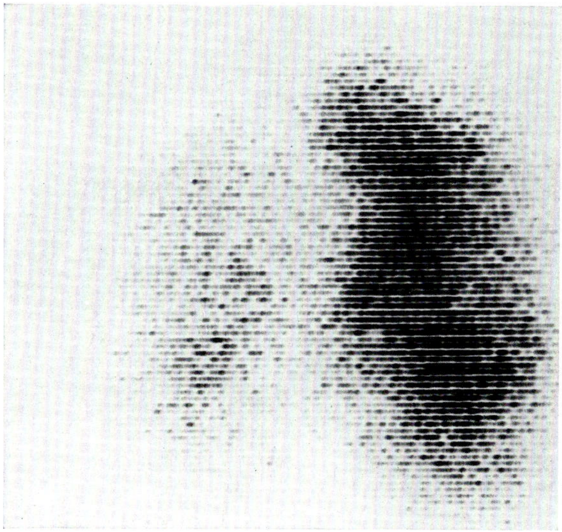

Fig. 2c

Fig. 2. 47 year old male with lung dystrophy. Roentgenogram. a shows a reduction of lung vasculature of right lung. Angiogram. b demonstrates a rarefication of lung vasculature corresponding to grade IV. Lung scan. c reveals only scanty perfusion of the right lung (grade IV) and decrease of perfusion of left lung (grade I)

lung scan (Fig. 2c) shows only scanty perfusion of right lung. Reduction of perfusion attains about 80 per cent of the normal corresponding to grade IV. The left lung shows a reduction of perfusion too, according to grade I.

Table. *Semiquantitative evaluation of angiographic and scintigraphic findings in lung diseases with localised destruction of lung parenchyma*

Grade of destruction of lung parenchyma	Reduction of lung vasculature as seen in angiogram	Reduction of regional perfusion based on lung scan and on count rates measured over 6 lung sections
I	under 25 %	under 25 %
II	25–50 %	25–50 %
III	50–75 %	50–75 %
IV	over 75 %	over 75 %

Case 2

Roentgenogram (Fig. 3a) of a 51 year old male with bullous emphysema of lungs. The angiogram (Fig. 3b) demonstrates a high degree of diminished vasculature in both upper lobes corresponding to destruction of lung parenchyma grade IV on the left and grade III on the right. In agreement with the angiographic findings the lung scan (Fig. 3c) shows extensive reduction of perfusion in left upper

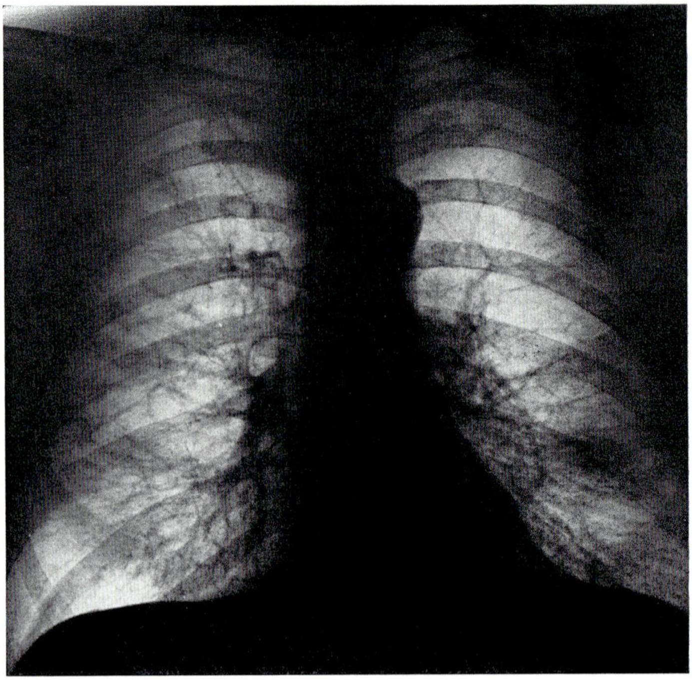

Fig. 3a

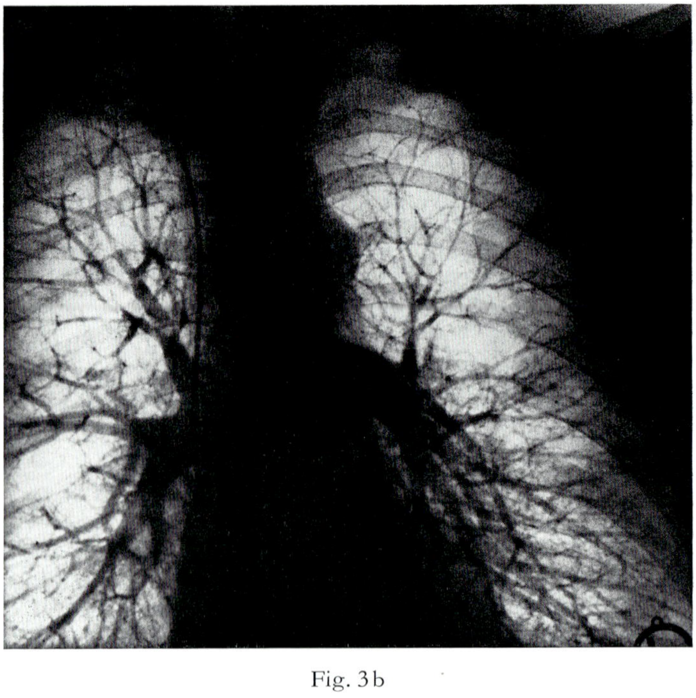

Fig. 3b

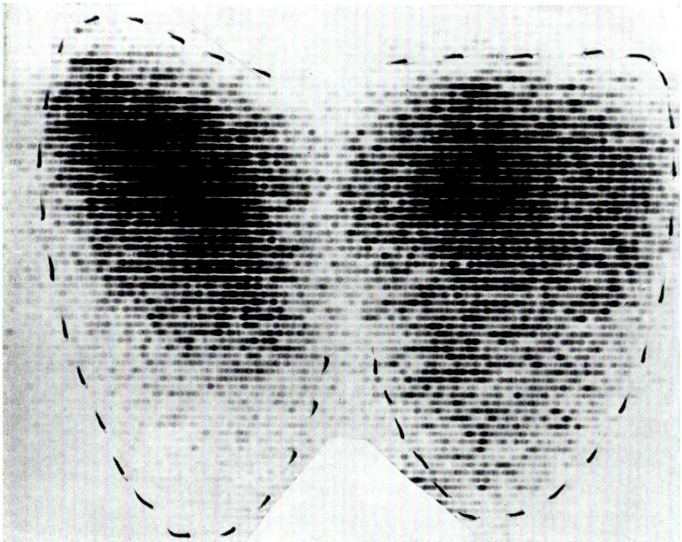

Fig. 3c

Fig. 3. 51 year old male with bullous emphysema. Roentgenogram. a demonstrates large emphysematous bullae in both upper lobes. Angiogram. b shows extensive rarefication and destruction of lung vasculature in the left upper lobe (grade IV) and in the right upper lobe (grade III) as well as compression of lung vessels in adjacent lung segments. Lung scan. c reveals decrease of perfusion in the left upper lobe (79% = grade IV) and in right upper lobe (56% = grade III)

and right upper lobe. Measurements of radioactivity over 6 defined lung section revealed reduction of perfusion of 79 per cent over the left upper lobe (grade IV) and of 56% over the right upper lobe (grade III).

Discussion

For about 25 years surgery of localised lung diseases, e.g. localised bullous emphysema, localised bronchiectasis, cystic disease of the lung, localised forms of lung dystrophy, is performed frequently and with encouraging results. Preoperative evaluation of morphological changes as well as of functional status in localised destructive lesions of lung parenchyma therefore is mandatory. For assessment of lung function spirometry and blood gas analysis are used. But for evaluation of the regional function in locally diseased lungs both methods are of limited value.

Roentgenological methods yield information of morphological but not of functional changes. The roentgenogram in bullous emphysema e.g. demonstrates the localisation and extension of emphysematous bullae as well as the degree of lung fibrosis in adjacent lung segments, whereas perfusion and reexpansion capability of lung after the resection of bullae cannot be evaluated. Compression and dislocation of segmental and lobar lung vessels, due to expansion of emphysematous bullae, can be evaluated angiographically to good advantage. Evaluation of capillary vasculature is a domain of lung scanning. Lung scanning is the method of choice in evaluation of regional lung perfusion. The results of lung scanning show a high correlation with findings of lung angiography. Therefore by angiography and lung scanning the assessment not only of localised destruction of lung parenchyma but also of the adjacent lung structure is possible. Use of both methods allows prognosis of postoperative pulmonary reexpansion. Reexpansion capacity of lungs depends not only on lung elasticity but also on condition of lung vasculature.

The validity of lung scanning could be increased using a semiquantitative method of interpretation. Various degrees of reduction of perfusion are to be expressed in defined order of magnitude. The presented method of measurement of activity over 6 lung sections is a simple and reproducible procedure for a semiquantitative evaluation of lung perfusion. This procedure affords equivalent results as densitometry of lung photo-scans, summing up all counts registered on a line of the scan, and counting of „dots" over a scan quadrant. But these three methods require additional instruments and are time consuming.

Use of computer and quantitative interpretation of lung perfusion will very probably lead to better diagnosis and evaluation of regional functional status in localised congenital and acquired lung diseases.

Conclusions

Lung angiography and scanning are very suitable methods for evaluation of pulmonary parenchymal destruction in localised congenital and acquired lung diseases. Both methods allow semiquantitative assessment of destruction of lung parenchyma using the proposed classification of pathological changes. Angiography and scintiscanning are complementary rediological methods. The domain of angiography is evaluation of lung vasculature. Lung scanning demonstrates reduced regional perfusion of diseased lungs. Therefore in preoperative assessment of lung status in localised lung diseases, e.g. bullous emphysema, cystic disease of the lung, bronchiectasis and localised congenital lung anomalities, both methods should be performed. Using the semiquantitative method of interpreting angiographic and scintigraphic findings, indication for operation and decision regarding the degree of resection can be defined more precisely.

Comparative Study of the Pulmonary Perfusion as Determined by Different Scintigraphic Techniques and by Angiography

R. Pauwels, K. Schelstraete, L. Verhaeghe, J. Tasson, M. Kunnen, M. van Vaerenbergh and F. Barbier

The physiopathological disturbances of pulmonary emphysema are mostly due to alterations in the ventilation-perfusion ratio. In most cases, the emphysematous lesions, responsible for these alterations, are at the alveolar and lobular level and are distributed throughout both lungs. Sometimes however these lesions can affect limited regions of the lungs. These cases may constitute a serious diagnostic problem since conventional X-ray often fails to demonstrate such localised lesions. It is the purpose of these paper to compare the diagnostic value of several specialized techniques.

Pulmonary angiography, pulmonary scintigraphy with Iodine-131 macroaggregated albumin (MAA scanning) and a Xenon-133 study of the ventilation and perfusion distribution were performed in 6 patients with known emphysema.

The following techniques were used:

1. *Angiography*: by percutaneous puncture or cutdown, a catheter was introduced in an antecubital vein and advanced into the main stem of the pulmonary artery. After injection of 40–50 ml of contrast medium (Isopaque 60%) serial X-rays were taken at a rate of three frames per second. A total number of 36 X-rays were taken per patient.

2. Anteroposterior *lung scan* was made in recumbent position, following the injection of 500 μCi of Iodine-131 macro aggregated albumin.

3. The *Xenon-133 study* was performed in sitting position, with four dorsal collimators directed towards the two upper and the two lower regions of the lungs.

a) For the *ventilatory* study, the patient was connected to a spirometer filled with a mixture of air and radio-active Xenongas. After equilibration with this mixture, the patient was told to take a deep breath and subsequently to expire as deep as possible.

The index of regional ventilation is calculated from the following formula:

$$\frac{V_1}{V_1 + V_2 + V_3 + V_4},$$

where the regional count rate change at the vital capacity manoeuvre is divided by the sum of the regional count rate changes of the 4 regions.

b) For the study of the regional *perfusion*, approximately 5 μCi of Xenon-133 in saline solution was injected as a bolus in an antecubital vein. The patient was asked to hold his breath after deep inspiration. The index of regional perfusion was again calculated by dividing the regional count rate change by the sum of the 4 regional count rate changes. The interpretation of the different techniques was made by different members of our group. The angiography and the MAA scanning were divided in 4 quadrants corresponding to the upper and lower regions of both lungs as it was done in the Xenon study. The quadrants were quoted on the following scale: Q_N (normal perfusion), Q_M (slightly diminished perfusion), Q_L (greatly diminished to absent perfusion). In order to obtain a semiquantitative comparison between the three techniques in the same patient a score system was established based on the difference in quoting for each technique. One point was attributed for a difference between Q_N–Q_M or Q_M–Q_L. A score of two points was attributed for a difference of Q_N–Q_L.

The results obtained in our series indicate that, in emphysema, there is a better correlation between the pulmonary angiography and the Xenon-technique, than between the angiography and the MAA scanning.

The most apparent reasons for this difference are:

1. The Xenon technique and the pulmonary angiography are two dynamic techniques, in contrast with the MAA scanning which is static.

2. The measurements of the regional count rate for Xenon were performed on the dorsal side of the patient in sitting position, while the MAA scanning was performed on the ventral side of the thorax of a patient in supine position.

Conclusion

In cases of localised pulmonary emphysema, there is a better correlation between the pulmonary angiography and the Xenon-133 study of the pulmonary perfusion than between the angiography and the MAA scanning.

In addition the Xenon study provides information about the regional ventilation.

Furthermore, in cases with severe alteration of the pulmonary perfusion, the Xenon study offers less. risk than the MAA scanning, which causes a temporary obstruction of a part of the already diminished pulmonary vascular bed. For these reasons we feel that the Xenon-133 technique should certainly be included in the study program of cases of pulmonary emphysema.

Selective Catheterization of the Bronchial Arteries and their Diagnostic and Therapeutic Use

S. Greco, F. Beritelli, C. Loreto, G.B. Cotroneo and G. Tafuri

According to recent anatomic studies, we have found that the bronchial arteries take origin from the initial segment of the descending aorta, at the level of the initial superior edge of the 6th thoracic vertebra, and less frequently slightly cephalad or caudally to the above level.

In the drawing of Fig. 1 are reported the relative percentage of the sites of origin, taken from our series.

The modality of origin of the bronchial arteries can be variable.

The bronchial arteries either right or left can take origin togheter from a "common trunk" or separately from the aorta.

The right bronchial arteries quite often take origin togheter with an intercostal artery ("Intercostal-bronchial trunk").

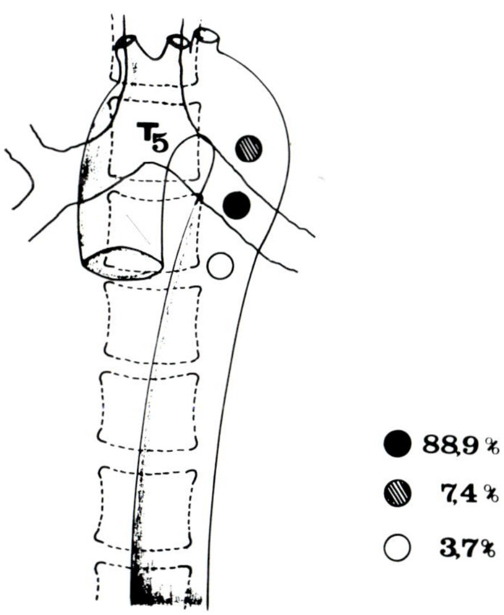

Fig. 1

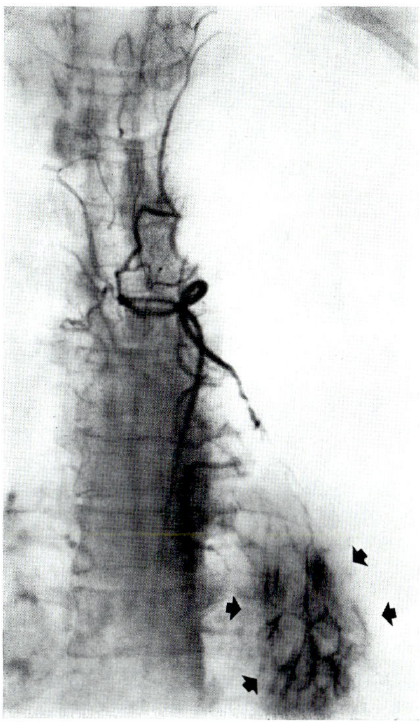

Fig. 2

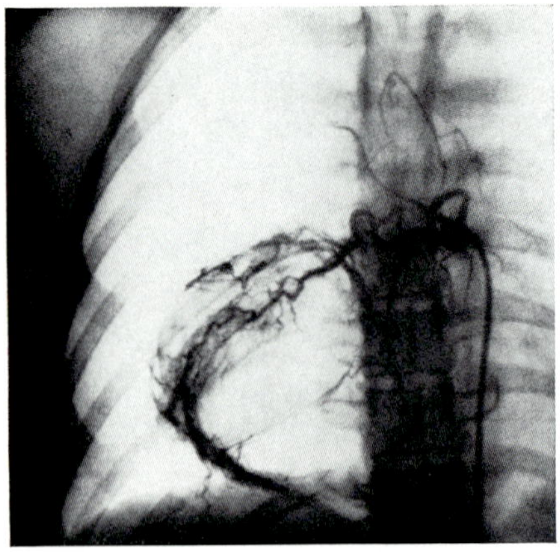

Fig. 3

For what is concerned with the various aspects of the selective angiography of the bronchial arteries, we will limit ourselves to discuss only those we think of more accurate diagnostic judgement in the study of the pulmonary pathology.

In the polycystic lung (Fig. 2) we have always noticed the presence of a rich vascularization which involves the arteries in their entire length with the result of characteristic images "multiple interferent circles".

In the pulmunary pathology due to bronchiectasis we have noticed constant hypervascularization, with vessels, with increased caliber and which describe a packed reticular pattern.

In the pulmonary echinococcosis as in cases of solitary air cyst (Fig. 3) the bronchial arteries maintain a normal morphology even though they show evidence of displacement of variable degree depending upon the dimension of the cysts.

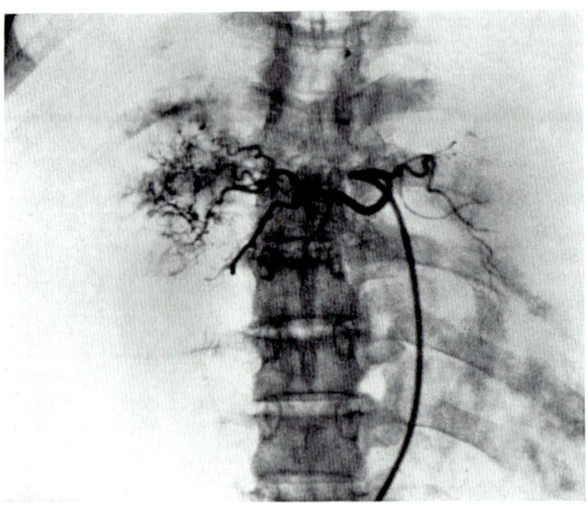

Fig. 4

Benign tumours show evidence of high vascularization around the tumour itself but the vessels never show the chaotic pattern, the tortuosity, the enlargement, the venous lakes and the disruption of the morphology typical of the malignant tumour.

In cases of primary broncho-pulmonary epithelial neoplasies we have almost always observed the existence of a characteristic neoplastic blood flow: ectasiae, fusiform pattern, "cork screw pattern", artero-venous fistulae, chaotic vascular entanglement (Figs. 4, 5a and b, 6a and b).

In some cases of peripheral tumour, "ball type tumuor" (Fig. 5a and b), we have noticed absence of vascularization in the neoplastic structure with a sharp cut off of the vessels at the periphery of the tumour.

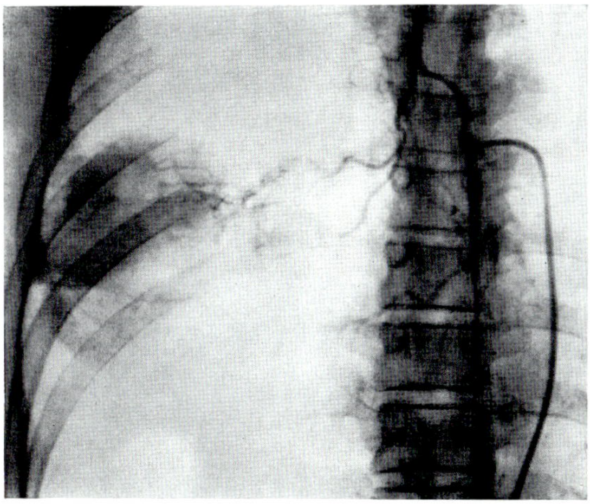

Fig. 5a

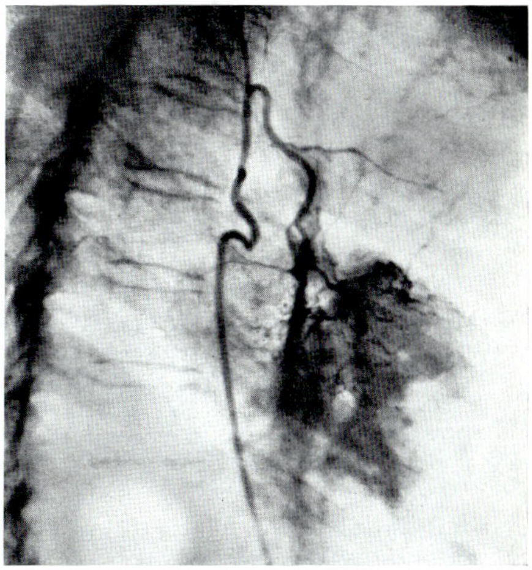

Fig. 5b

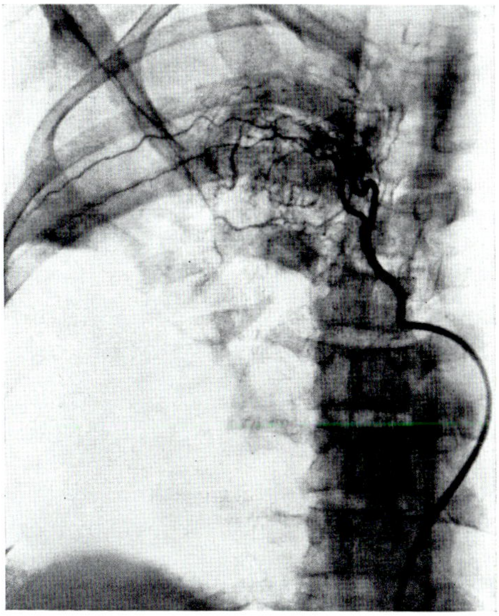

Fig. 6a

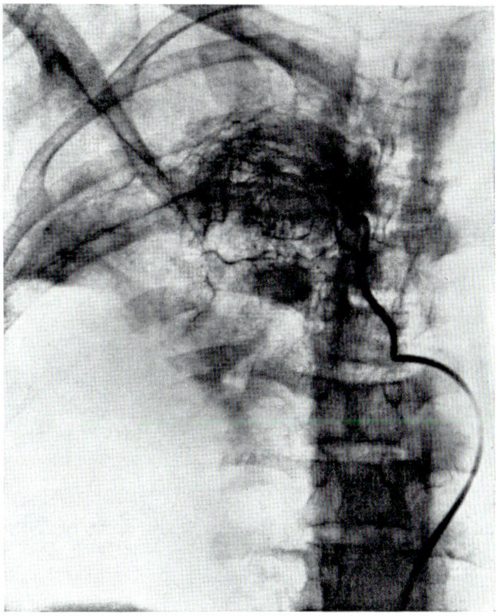

Fig. 6b

In the operative specimen, in such cases one could demonstrate large areas of necrosis.

In some other cases we have noticed a persistent tumour stain due to pooling of contrast material in the neoplastic structure (Fig. 6a and b).

In the pulmonary localization of Hodgkin's disease we have found that the angiographic pattern is not much different from that described for the primary malignancy of the lung (Fig. 7).

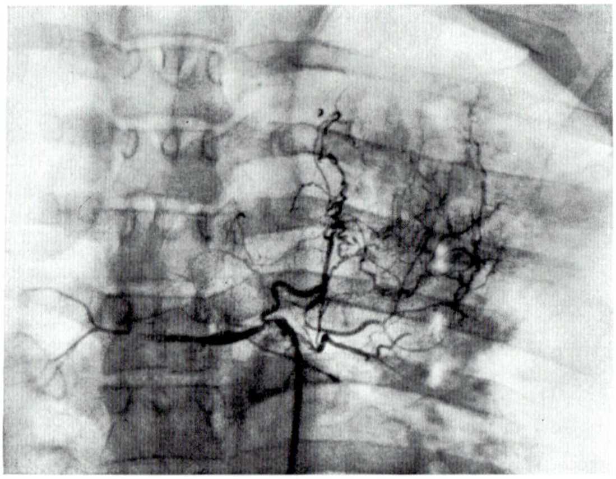

Fig. 7

In an attempt of obtaining useful informations about the conditions of the precapillary flow we have added to the angiography the "selective angioscintigraphy", which we have obtained by injecting a radioactive tracer in the bronchial artery.

We have found that the scintigraphic findings are generally not much different from the angiographic findings even though with the scintigram the tumour mass appeared to be usually larger.

We have also studied the tumour blood flow by injecting a radioactive tracer selectively in the bronchial artery.

The curves that we have obtained are important in the attempts of selective perfusion of vascular tumour with chemotherapeutics or with pre-irradiation compounds, to change the cellular radium sensitivity, actually being done in our Institute of Radiology at the University of Catania.

Summary

After brief notes of anatomy about the origin of the bronchial arteries we have briefly exposed the angiographic pattern formed in the study of the pulmonary pathology.

A brief discussion is also made about other diagnostic means ("selective angioscintigraphy", "Curves of the tumor blood flow" and therapeutic attempts by mean of selective perfusion.)

Evaluation of Pulmonary Function and Blood Flow Using Xenon-133 and a Scintillation (Anger) Camera

M. K. Loken

Xenon-133 and a Scintillation (Anger) Camera have been used extensively in our Nuclear Medicine Clinic during the past 4 years for the evaluation of pulmonary function and measurements of regional pulmonary blood flow. These studies are normally carried out with the patient in the upright position with the camera placed against the posterior thorax although a supine or prone position may also be used (Fig. 1). Details of the technique used for these studies have been considered elsewhere.

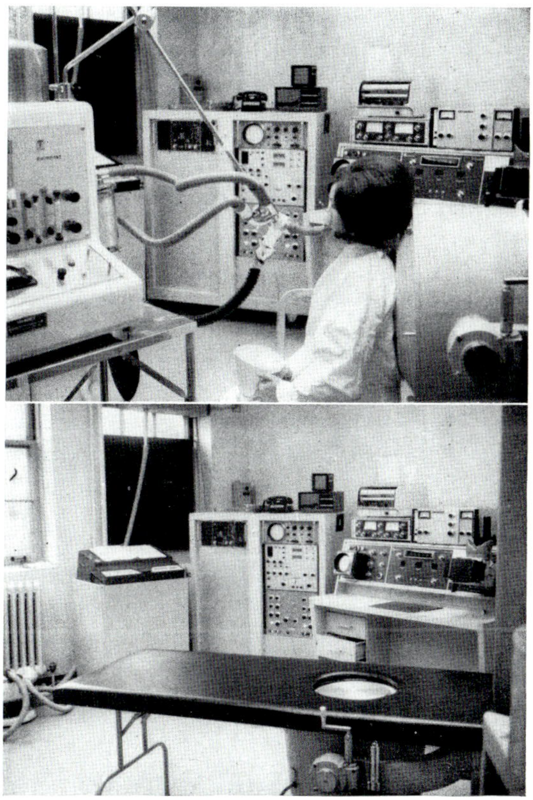

Fig. 1a and b

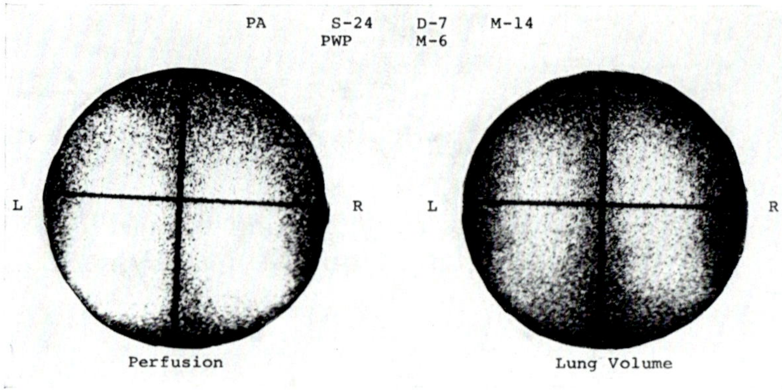

Fig. 2. Normal pulmonary hemodynamics

The distribution of Xenon administered as a saline solution intravenously into a patient studied erect with normal pulmonary hemodynamics is shown in Figure 2. Pressure measurements obtained with a catheter in the pulmonary artery bed are shown. A gradual decrease in blood flow from lung bases to apices is readily appreciated from the scintiphotograms. This gradient is more pronounced for blood flow than for ventilation as may be seen in the Calcomp plots from our computer of perfusion and ventilation indices (Fig. 3). This relationship causes the ventilation-perfusion ratio for the right lung of this normal subject to have a negative slope.

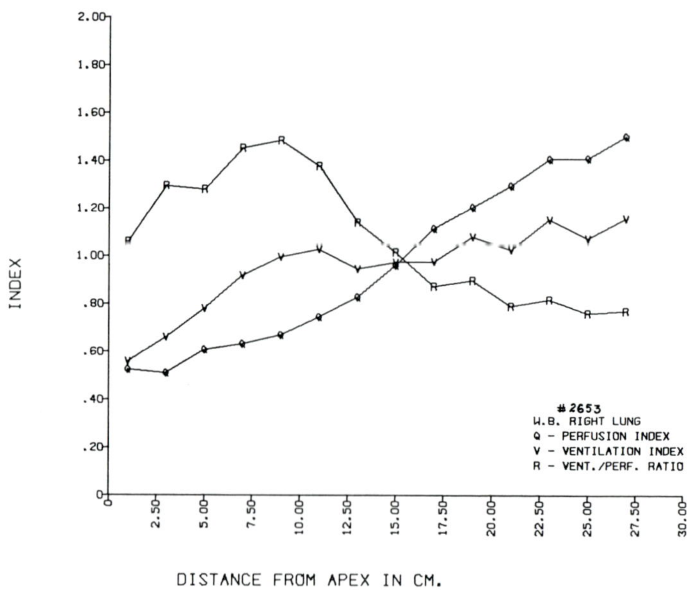

Fig. 3a

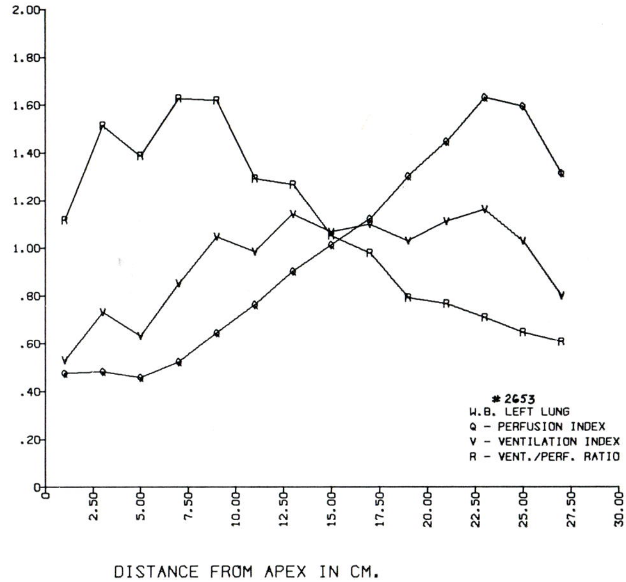

Fig. 3b

Pulmonary venous hypertension may cause a reversal of the perfusion and ventilation gradients. This may be seen in Figure 4 which shows scintiphotograms obtained during perfusion and ventilation studies in a patient with mitral stenosis. The elevation of pulmonary arterial pressures as measured during catheterization are also shown in this figure.

A chest radiograph and film from pulmonary angiogram of a patient with tetrology of Fallot are shown in Figure 5a. This patient had undergone a Blalock procedure with a subsequent occlusion of the right pulmonary artery. Figure 5b also

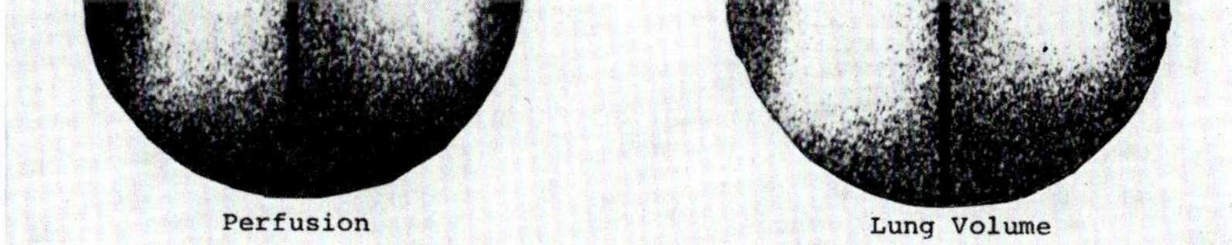

Fig. 4. Pulmonary venous hypertension

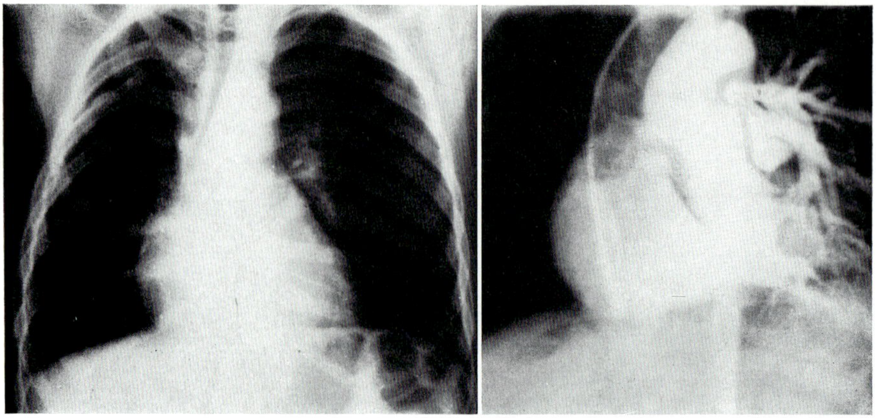

a

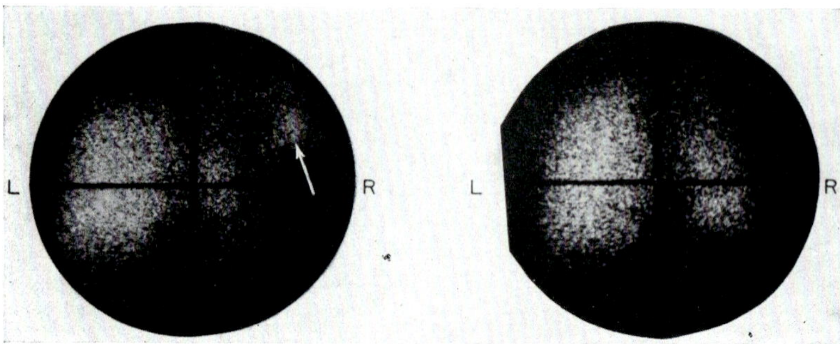

b

Fig. 5a and b. Right pulmonary artery occlusion a perfusion; b ventilation

shows two scintiphotograms obtained during perfusion and ventilation studies in this patient. The perfusion study shows the bolus passing through the right side of the heart into the left lung with essentially no perfusion of the right lung. Ventilation to the right lung is somewhat less than that on the left that is of sufficient magnitude to upset blood gases in this patient because of the "wasted ventilation" in the hemilung which is devoid of blood flow.

Two examples of pediatric patients with hyperlucency of the left lung are shown in Figure 6 and 7. In Figure 6 the pulmonary angiogram shows that there is a hypoplastic portion of the left pulmonary artery in a patient with a patent ductus arteriosis. The selected scintiphotograms also shown in this figure indicate a decrease in perfusion to the left lung because of the hypoplastic pulmonary artery but a uniform washout of the radioactive gas during ventilation. This should be contrasted with the findings in Figure 7 in a patient with congenital emphysema who shows very poor perfusion in the involved left lung, with this area retaining the radioactive xenon during the washout phase of the study.

An example of the use of Xenon-133 for the evaluation of a patient with pulmonary emboli is shown in Figure 8. The two scintiphotograms in the upper por-

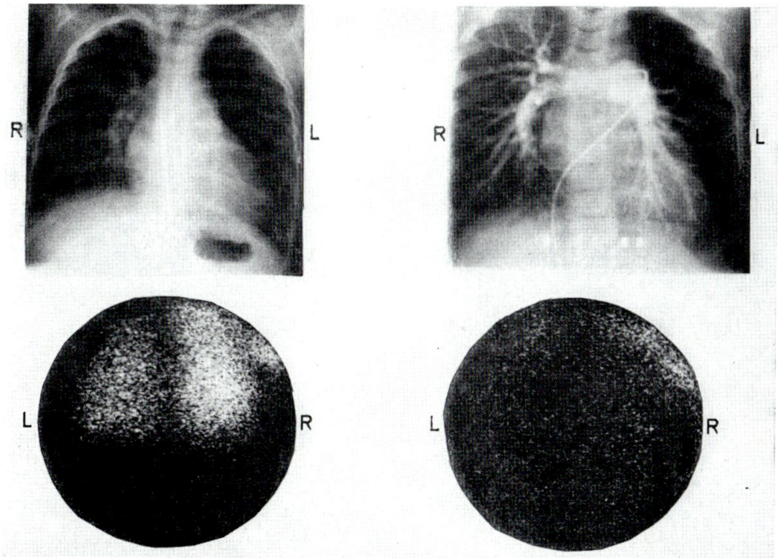

Fig. 6. Hyperlucency of left lung (A.E., 1077536, 3 yrs.) DX: Hypoplastic left pulmonary artery. Patent ductus arteriosus

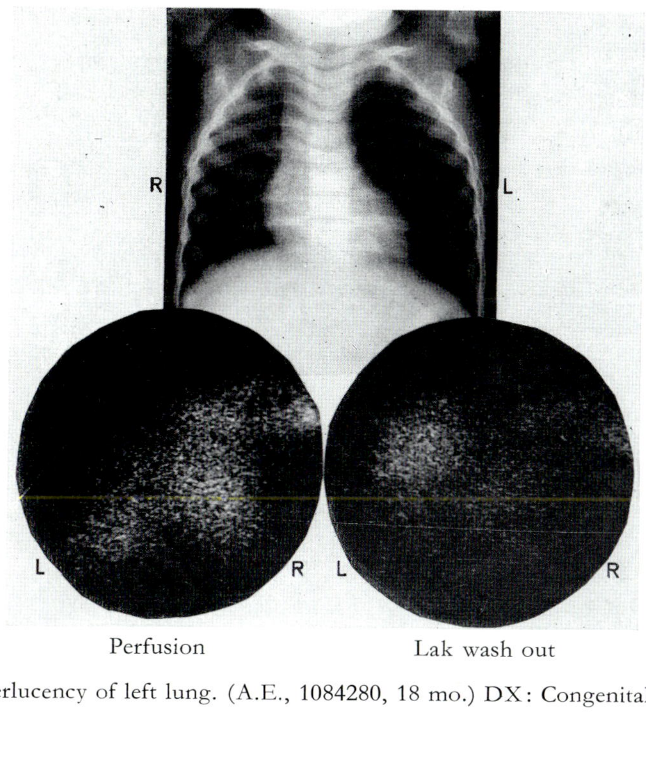

Perfusion Lak wash out

Fig. 7. Hyperlucency of left lung. (A.E., 1084280, 18 mo.) DX: Congenital emphysema

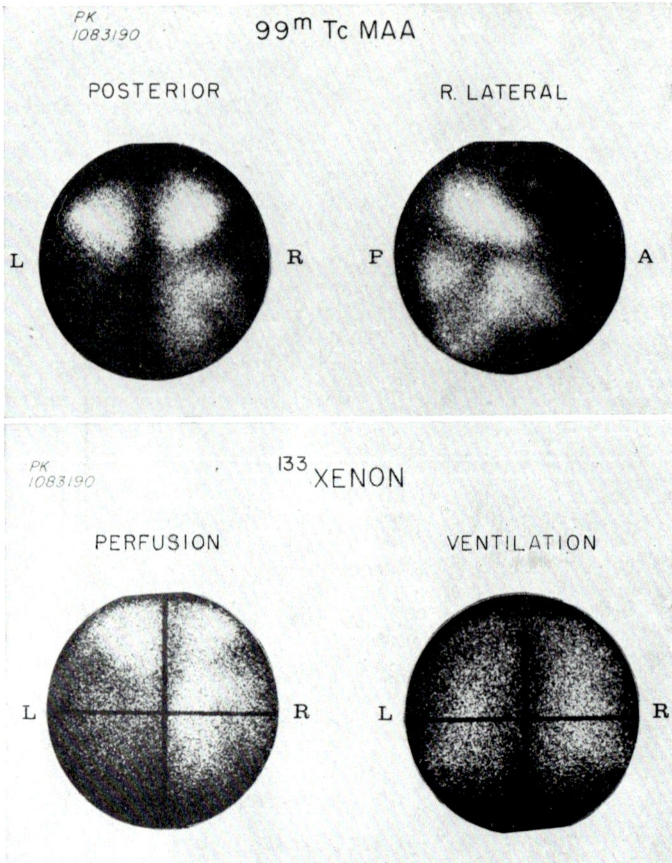

Fig. 8. Pulmonary Emboli

tion of this figure were obtained after the administration of 3 mCi of ^{99m}Tc macroaggregated albumin (MAA), show the typical wedge deformities associated with pulmonary emboli. The two lower scintiphotograms were taken during the Xenon portion of the study. The left-hand picture obtained after the intravenous administration of the Xenon-133-shows the wedge shaped perfusion defects. The picture on the right shows a pattern of normal ventilation which is typically found in patients with pulmonary emboli but without overlying obstructive lung disease.

Selected scintiphotograms of a patient with obstructive lung disease are shown in Figure 9. This patient was evaluated because of clinical symptoms thought compatible with multiple pulmonary emboli. The chest X-ray is unremarkable. A(MAA) macroaggregated albumin lung scan shows some irregularity in the perfusion pattern which was thought compatible with multiple small pulmonary emboli. This study was followed by a pulmonary angiogram, one film of which is also shown in this figure. There are multiple lucencies in the perfusion pattern which likewise were considered to represent multiple emboli. Three scintiphotograms from the xenon

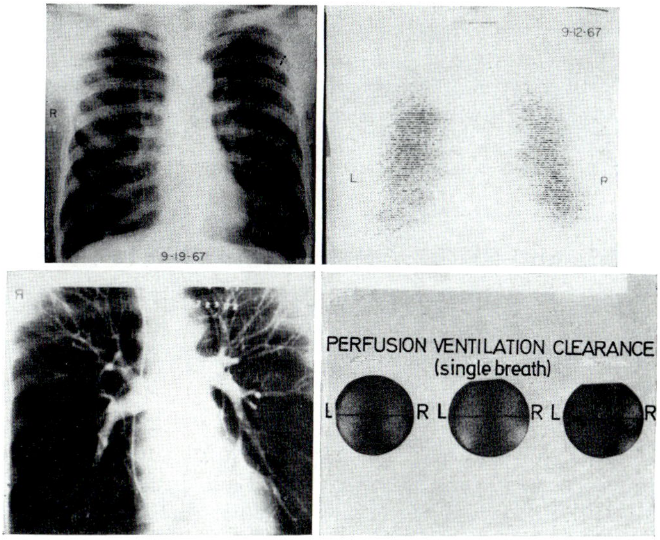

Fig. 9. Obstructive Lung Disease

study in this patient show irregularities in both perfusion and ventilation and an uneven pattern of Xenon clearance suggesting the appropriate diagnosis of chronic obstructive lung disease.

Conclusions

The preceding examples are shown as illustrations of the clinical value of Xenon-133 used together with a scintillation camera to evaluate pulmonary function and blood flow. We have found this technique to provide useful clinical data in more than 700 patients with a variety of pulmonary disorders. The addition of computer analysis, not discussed here, permits a quantitative approach to be made to regional pulmonary function which is particularly useful in the evaluation of medical and/or surgical intervention in patients with pulmonary disorders.

Diseases Pulmonary and Mediastinum

Angiographic and Scintigraphic Evaluation of the Circulation in Patients with Bronchial Cancer

V. JEŽEK, J. VANČOURA, VL. TEICHMANN, J. KOLÁŘ and J. ORT

An appropriate investigation of the lung ventilation and perfusion values may be of prime importance during the preoperative period in all patients with bronchial cancer. According to our experience it also enables some important predictions of the immediate functional results of a pulmonary resection in those patients.

In a group of 36 patients with microscopically proven bronchial cancers, functional, biochemical, angiographic and scintigraphic investigations have been performed and correlated during the preoperative period. Angiography has been performed by cathetrisation the right ventricle. 60–70 ml of 76% water soluble contrast medium have been injected within two three seconds by a pressure syringe and rapid seriography has been made in films 35 × 35 cm during the subsequent 6.5 sec with the AOT-Elema Schönander equipment. The blood analysis of samples collected via a catheter in a. femoralis has been made with a Van Styke equipment and a pH-meter (type Godard). At the same time the blood pressures have been measured with the Hellige tensometer. The heart minute volumes have been estimated according to FICKS and STEWARTS and HAMILTON. Scintigraphic investigations have been made after intravenous injections of 200 μCi ^{131}J-MAA with a PHO-DOT scanner (Nuclear Chicago) with a 19-hole focused collimator in patients in prone, supine and lateral positions.

According to the events the patients with bronchial cancer can be subdivided into the following three groups:

Group I. Patients with peripheric nodular cancers without hypoventilation, atelectasis or any influence on the blood circulation.

Group II. Central tumours with radiographic symptoms of hypoventilation, segmental or alar atelectasis, but without changes in the blood circulation in the lungs.

Group III. The main symptomatology of this group has been the same like in the second Group, but the blood circulation has been suppressed by tumorous invasion in the main vessels and sometimes by other additive complications, like by emphysema and similar.

In all patients some tendency for hyperventilation has been observed. The differences between the three main groups have not been statistically significant in this respect. The main values of blood saturation by oxygen in the Groups I and III have been about the same. In the second Group with perfunded atelectasis the saturation with oxygen is depressed. The main values of the CO_2-tension have been about the same in all 3 groups. The extent of the blood circulation in the lungs was different and varied in wide ranges. The Group III collected the most patients with tensions in a. pulmonalis above 20 Torr.

The angiographic as well as scintigraphic patterns in individual groups of patients have been of about the same value in reporting the state of perfusion of the atelectatic area. Thus, the scintigraphic evaluation brings less discomfort to the seriously ill patients.

The investigations have shown that the atelectasis influences in an important manner the interrelations between the ventilation and perfusion in the diseased area. From the physio-pathological point of view it is of prime importance whether there is any blood circulation in the atelectatic district at all, or at least in a lessened extent. In such cases less oxygen-saturated venous blood is added to the great circulation. For this reason the most depressed saturation of the arterial blood with oxygen has been found in the second Group of patients, suffering from heavy hypoxaemia (up to 67% of all cases investigated in this series). In the atelectasis with lessened perfusion, no mixture of this type could be stated.

The main conclusions drawn from these investigations are as follows: Some worsening of the lung function after resection of the lungs can be expected in the Group I, because here, a part of normally functioning lung district will be excluded. In the Group III, without any perfusion in the atelectasis, the diseased district does not substantially influence the circulation before the intervention and thus, the resection will cause only unimportant changes. But in the Group II the resection will abolish the venous mixture of hyposaturated blood to the circulation and the functional values in these patients can be improved by the resection of the atelectatic district.

Comparaison de l'angiographie et de la scintigraphie en pathologie pulmonaire

A. Bollaert, J. Schockert, J. C. Yernault, M. Payfa, Ph. De Costre, A. M. Ermans et A. de Coster

Nous avons étudié diverses pneumopathies par l'angiopneumographie I. V. et par la caméra à scintillation.

Nous nous sommes efforcés de localiser les lésions vasculaires et d'en apprécier le retentissement fonctionnel.

Technique

L'angiographie est réalisée par la voie I.V. La scintigraphie est réalisée au moyen de l'injection I.V. de 3 millicuries de macro-agregats d'hydroxyde ferrique marqué à l'Indium-113m (Davis, 1970) ou de microsphères techniticiées (5 millicuries de technetium (Biadine *et alii*, 1970) et de la caméra à scintillation «Pho-Gamma» Nuclear Chicago.

Les renseignements obtenus par les deux méthodes ont été systématiquement comparés.

La comparaison porte sur la localisation des troubles de la vascularisation et leur retentissement fonctionnel.

Dans un certain nombre de cas les résultates des deux examens ont été comparés à la consommation d'oxygène mesurée par bronchospirométrie séparée.

La localisation des lésions est un simple problème de lecture de clichés ou du scintigramme.

L'appréciation du retentissement fonctionnel des lésions pulmonaires à partir des angiographies est basée sur l'étude des diamètres vasculaires et des vitesses circulatoires intra-pulmonaires.

Nous établissons le profil du diamètre vasculaire moyen de l'artère aux veines d'un poumon selon une technique exposée dans des travaux précédents (A. Bollaert *et al.* 1961 et 1964) et nous en déduisons une appréciation quantitative du lit vasculaire pulmonaire exprimé en pourcentage. La comparaison des temps d'opacification du cœur droit et des poumons permet d'autre part d'apprécier la répartition du débit cardiaque droit dans chaque poumon.

En ce qui concerne la scintigraphie, l'adjonction d'un collimateur divergent permet d'explorer simultanément chacun des deux poumons. La caméra est reliée à une calculatrice électronique qui permet de chiffrer le degré de perfusion de chaque poumon (J. C. Yernault *et al.*, 1969; M. K. Loken *et al.*, 1970).

A l'état physiologique, le poumon droit assure 55% de la perfusion et le poumon gauche 45%.

Observations

Voici deux cas exemplatifs:

Observation No. 1 : Le premier patient, âgé de 59 ans, est atteint d'un cancer bronchique du lobe supérieur droit. L'angiographie montre une *amputation artérielle segmentaire apicale du lobe supérieur droit. Les artères segmentaires dorsale et ventrale sont abaissées*, et rétrécies. Elles donnent peu de collatérales qui ne se ramifient guère dans la périphérie du lobe (Fig. 1).

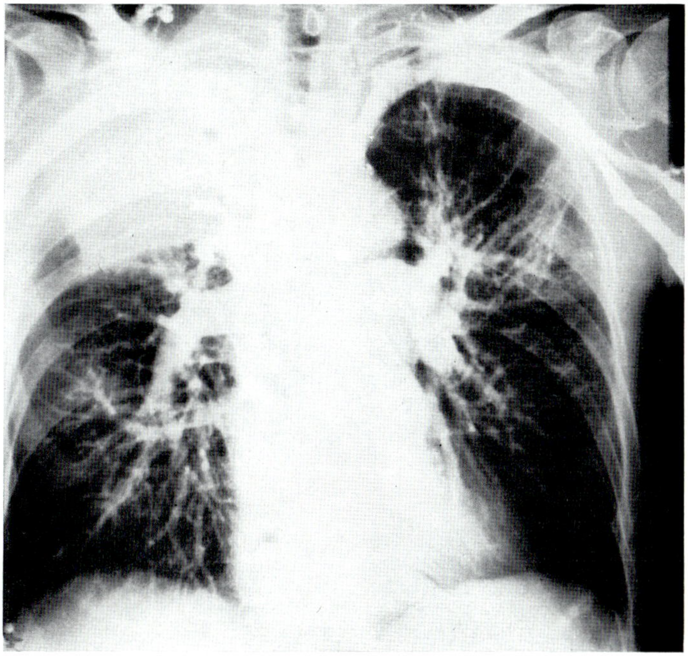

Fig. 1

Le diamètre de ces artères se réduit rapidement au delà des premières bifurcations et n'est plus mesurable.

Il existe une véritable stase de produit de contraste dans ces vaisseaux ce qui confirme la diminution extrême de la perfusion de ce lobe.

La capacité fonctionnelle est diminuée à 41 $^0/_0$ au niveau du poumon droit au lieu de 55% à l'état physiologique.

La scintigraphie confirme l'absence de perfusion dans les segments dorsal et apical du lobe supérieur droit et démontre que 38% seulement de la solution isotopique se retrouve au niveau du poumon droit (Fig. 2). Les évaluations topographiques et fonctionnelles de l'angiographie et de la scintigraphie sont donc très proches.

Observation No. 2 : Le 2e patient âgé de 61 ans, hypertendu, angoreux, a présenté à diverses reprises des hémoptysies et des épisodes d'insuffisance respiratoire dont l'étiologie n'a pas été établie par les examens traditionnels.

Une scintigraphie de routine révèle de multiples images d'hypoperfusion disséminées dans les deux champs pulmonaires. Elles sont particulièrement bien visibles

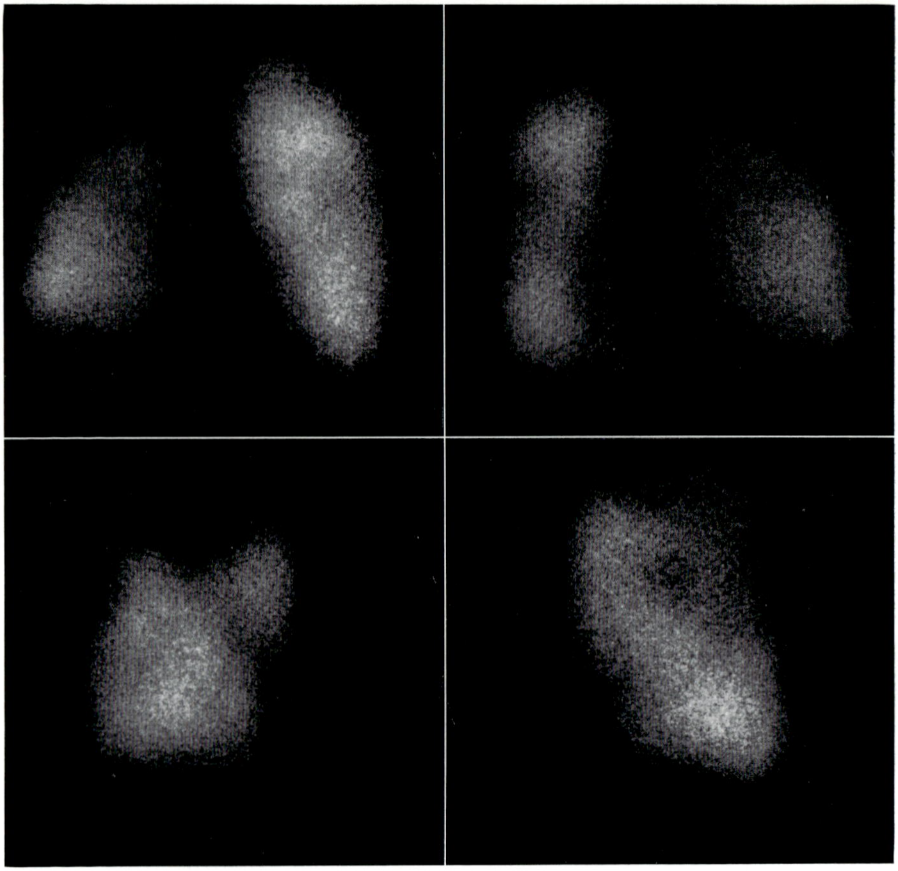

Fig. 2a–d

sur le cliché effectué en incidence postérieure au sommet droit et au niveau du tiers moyen du poumon gauche en incidence latérale gauche (Fig. 3).

L'angiographie montre des plages d'hypovascularisation dans la région sous-calviculaire droite. L'artère sous segmentaire axillaire droite est amputée à sa naissance. Tous les vaisseaux du lobe supérieur sont grêles, raccourcis et peu ramifiés.

A gauche, un thrombus s'observe dans l'artère lobaire inférieure avant la bifurcation segmentaire. Le tiers moyen du poumon gauche est peu vascularisé (Fig. 4).

L'angiogramme comme le scintigramme montrent des zones d'hypovascularisation bilatérale équivalentes dans les deux poumons, de sorte qu'il n'y a pas de variation significative de la perfusion dans chaque poumon.

Resultats et discussion

Trente pneumopathies ont été étudiées au moyen de ces deux techniques. Les résultats sont repris dans le tableau. En ce qui concerne la localisation des lésions, les résultats des deux méthodes concordent.

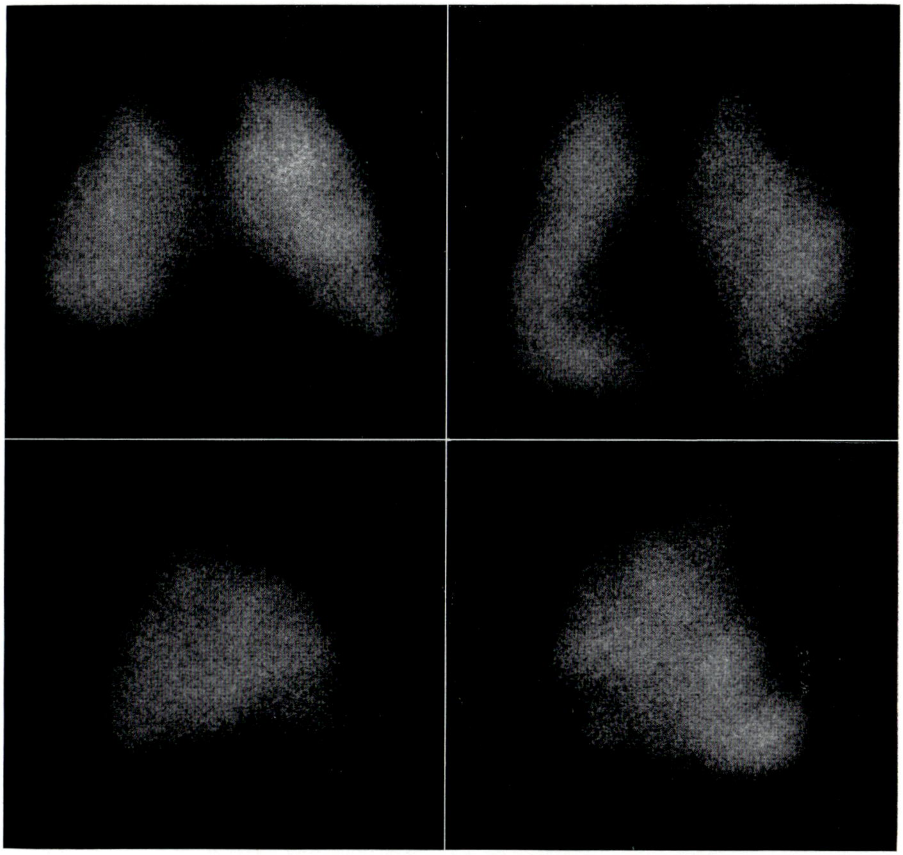

Fig. 3a–d

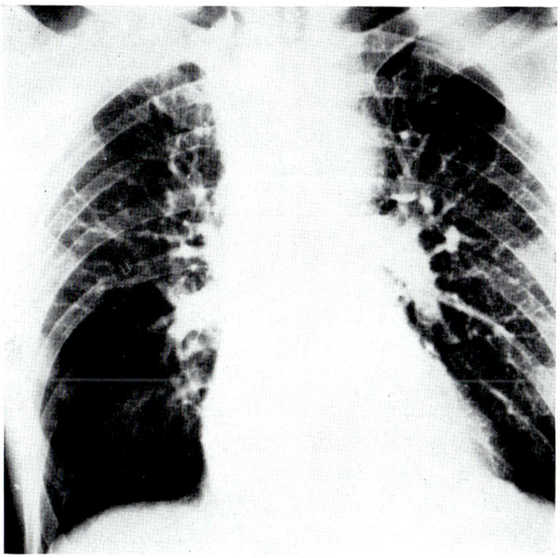

Fig. 4

Tableau. *Evaluation relative de la perfusion de chaque poumon*

		N. 55 % A droite *Evaluation par l'angiographie*		45 % A gauche *Evaluation par la scintigraphie*	
		Dr.	*G.*	*Dr.*	*G.*
1.	Néo bronchique	60	40	56	44
2.	idem	85	15	85	15
3.	idem	44	56	38	62
4.	idem	34	66	40	60
5.	idem	43	57	43	57
6.	idem	30	70	31	69
7.	idem	40	60	39	61
8.	idem	56	44	60	40
9.	idem	40	60	36	64
10.	idem	71	29	73	27
11.	idem	30	70	24	76
12.	idem	75	25	80	20
13.	idem	50	50	47	53
14.	idem	83	17	84	16
15.	idem	14	86	14	86
16.	idem	47	53	46	54
17.	Emboles pulmonaires	51	49	52	48
18.	idem	48	52	50	50
19.	idem	50	50	55	45
20.	idem	54	46	52	48
21.	idem	47	53	49	51
22.	idem	55	45	52	48
23.	idem	52	48	52	48
24.	idem	61	39	57	43
25.	idem	55	45	56	44
26.	Emphysème	68	32	70	30
27.	idem	68	32	63	37
28.	idem	15	85	20	80
29.	idem	54	46	44	56
30.	Malformation cong. vasculaire pulmonaire	48	52	52	48

Nous estimons néanmoins que l'angiographie apporte des renseignements morphologiques plus précis que la scintigraphie dans les néoplasies bronchiques. L'envahissement tumoral est mieux délimitable. La précision des informations obtenues sur le plan anatomique est supérieure à celle que fournit la scintigraphie.

En revanche, la scintigraphie sous incidences multiples est plus efficace dans la recherche des embolies pulmonaires. Elle excelle à révéler des zones d'hypovascularisation périphérique difficilement décelables à l'angiographie. Elle permet notamment une meilleure localisation dans le plan antéro-postérieur.

Les possibilités de l'angiographie nous semblent limitées dans les embolies pulmonaires. Il est rare qu'une angiographie soit effectuée en urgence pour cette affection. Nous pensons d'ailleurs que cet examen n'est pas sans danger en phase aiguë. L'angiographie est effectuée en général plus tardivement et il est exceptionnel qu'elle mette des images d'amputation en évidence au niveau des artères lobaires ou segmentaires. Dans la plupart des cas, il s'agit de lésions plus périphériques, moins bien délimitées.

Du point de vue fonctionnel, la concordance remarquable des résultats de l'angiographie et du scanning pulmonaire au moyen de la caméra est illustrée par le graphique ci-joint (Fig. 5).

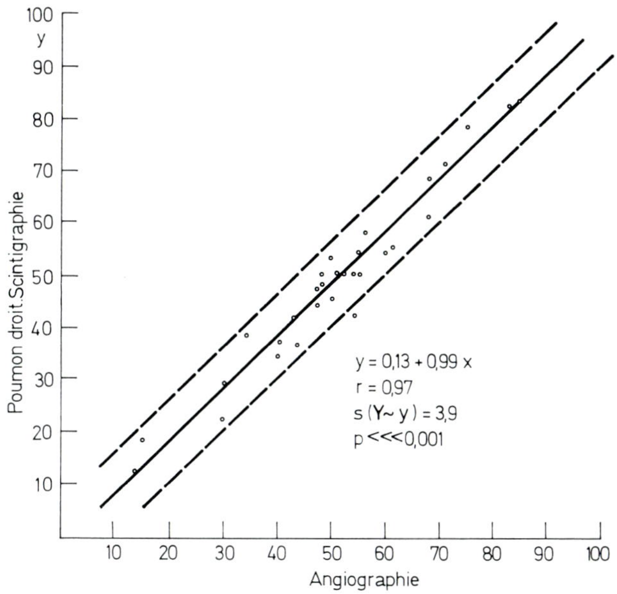

Fig. 5

Leurs résultats correspondent également avec les mesures de consommation d'oxygène, effectuées par bronchospirométrie séparée.

L'évaluation fonctionnelle par l'angiographie est inscrite en abcisse, et par le scintigraphie en ordonnée.

La corrélation que nous obtenons traduite par l'équation $Y = 0{,}13 + 0{,}99$ de X avec une valeur de $s = 3{,}9$ est très satisfaisante du point de vue statistique.

Un seul cas se situe en dehors des limites extrêmes de la relation, soit un coëfficient $p = 0{,}001$ qui ne remet pas la valeur de la correlation en cause. Ce point correspond à un emphysème. C'est dans cette affection que nous avons rencontré les plus grands écarts entre les valeurs fonctionnelles mesurées par l'angiographie et la scintigraphie. L'explication en réside probablement dans la différence de viscosité du produit de contraste et de la solution radioisotopique. Les molécules de celle-ci diffusent vraisemblablement moins rapidement et moins complètement à travers les vaisseaux arteriolo-capillaires rarefiés et rétrécis.

D'autre part la confrontation des données fonctionnelles obtenues par la scintigraphie et l'angiographie et les mesures de consommation d'oxygène par bronchospirométrie séparées permet de comprendre certaines discordances constatées précédemment entre les scintigrammes et la consommation d'oxygène de chaque poumon (Yernault *et al.*, 1968).

La scintigraphie montre parfois la persistance d'une perfusion dans des poumons atélectasiés alors qu'il n'y a aucune consommation d'oxygène décelable.

L'angiographie révèle que le produit de contraste pénètre dans les grosses artères de ces poumons, mais n'atteint pas les capillaires ni a fortiori les veines. La quantité de produit de contraste visible dans les grosses artères se traduit au scintigramme par une certaine activité radioisotopique mais celle-ci ne correspond pas à une perfusion efficace du point de vue de l'hématose. Le produit de contraste reflue des grosses artères vers l'artère pulmonaire contralatérale ou atteint les veines homolatérales en très faible quantité grâce à des shunts arterio-veineux non fonctionnels à l'état physiologique.

L'absence d'échanges gazeux dans les poumons pathologiques n'est donc pas surprenante.

Sur un plan plus pratique, l'appréciation fonctionnelle de la circulation pulmonaire par la scintigraphie sous incidences multiples est plus rapide, plus facile et plus précise que l'angiographie.

L'évaluation fonctionnelle d'un poumon d'après l'angiographie nécessite en effet des mesures nombreuses de diamètres vasculaires et de temps circulatoirs, parfois assez difficiles, toujours longues. Il faut signaler toutefois au bénéfice de l'angiographie que cette méthode permet des évaluations fonctionnelles séparées de chaque poumon, tandis que la scintigraphie et la bronchospirométrie ne peuvent donner que des appréciations relatives, d'un poumon par rapport à l'autre. Des réductions fonctionnelles bilatérales peuvent donc ne pas apparaitre quantitativement à la scintigraphie si le rapport de perfusion d'un poumon par rapport à l'autre n'est pas modifié, bien que dans la plupart des cas la scintigraphie révèle la présence de zones d'hypovascularisation.

Nous avons également comparé les résultats de l'angiographie au scintigramme pulmonaire classique avec scanner à balayage horizontal dans 15 cas de pneumopathies d'étiologies diverses. La comparaison n'est possible qu'en ce qui concerne la localisation des lésions, ce type de scintigraphie ne permettant pas une évaluation globale de la perfusion d'un poumon par rapport à l'autre dans notre expérience.

L'étude de ces dossiers révèle des discordances dans la localisation des lésions et dans l'appréciation de leur étendue entre les deux méthodes. L'angiographie est ici nettement plus précice.

Ce type de scintigraphie n'explore en effet pas l'entièreté d'un poumon mais préférentiellement un seul plan de l'organe, soit postérieur, soit antérieur. La durée de l'examen rend difficile l'étude des organes sous incidences multiples. Il en résulte que des lésions parenchymateuses localisées peuvent échapper à l'investigation.

Conclusion

La scintigraphie à caméra est certainement plus facile à mettre en œuvre que l'angiopneumographie. Elle donne d'excellentes évaluations fonctionnelles et devrait entrer dans le cadre des examens de routine. Par contre, l'angiographie donne des renseignements morphologiques plus précis et reste l'examen de choix dès qu'une thérapeutique chirurgicale est envisagée.

Summary

Angiography and scintigraphy have been performed in different pulmonary diseases: lung cancer, destroyed lung, emphysema and pulmonary embolism.

The morphologic and functionnal consequences of the parenchymatous lesions on the pulmonary circulation are studied.

The modification of the lung vascular pattern are studied, and quantified either by angiography and scintigraphy.

After comparison of the datas, some observations are made. The pulmonary angiography gives more detailed informations in lung cancer and destroyed lung than scintigraphy. This is most evident in appreciation of metastatic involvment of the mediastinum and hilus which is essential to determine the degree of operability.

Scintigraphy does not give such informations. On the contrary, scintigraphy gives immediately a very good and precise information in the research of pulmonary emboly, especially in the peripheral vessels.

Very often, scintigraphy reveals the abolition of pulmonary circulation in cases where traditional roentgen examination are negative.

A Radioisotopic Approach in the Diagnosis of Lung Cancer

M. Kaneko

It is very useful to have positive scientigraphy of tumor as a diagnostic tool. I talked in last International Congress of Radiology in Tokyo about the intra-arterial injection of radioisotope in the diagnosis of malignant tumor. I would like to introduce the method, expecially in the cases of lung cancer.

Method

Angioscanography was serially taken daily after intraarterial injection of radioiodinated macro-aggregated albumin (MAA) in a dose of 100 to 300 μCi into the bronchial artery in 14 cases of primary lung cancer, 2 cases of metastatic lung cancer and one case of lung abscess. After injection, in order to minimize the thyroid irradiation, Lugol solution was given to saturate the thyroid gland.

Rapid serial angioscintiphotography was taken by scinticamera immediately after injection of ^{99m}Tc pertechnetate or other radioisotopes such as ^{131}I-fibrinogen, ^{133}-Xe-solution and ^{67}Ga-citrate into the bronchial artery in 10 cases of primary lung cancer, 2 cases of metastatic lung cancer and each case of bronchial adenoma and lung abscess.

Results

In all 14 cases of lung cancer using regular MAA, angioscanography showed positive delineation of tumor. Five cases were apparantly positive immediately after injection. But other cases became positive several days later. When MAA less than 10μ was used in 2 cases, they were negative result, because the particle passed through the vascular bed of tumor.

It suggests that it is essential for the capillary bed of tumor to capture the particle and to retain them in the tumor in order to get the positive delineation.

Rapid serial angioscintiphotography showed longer remaining of ^{99m}Tc pertechnetate in the tumor and this phenomenon was accentuated by simultaneous injection of nor-adreanlin. ^{131}I-fibrinogen retained in the tumor fairly long time of 35 min, but ^{133}Xe showed negative result in 2 of 3 cases. ^{67}Ga-citrate showed good delineation of tumor even one day later, which suggests this substance has some affinity to the tumor.

Discussion

The positive scintigraphy is worthwhile to detect the tumor and to differentiate it from other condition, if the tumor can be positively scintigraphed in contrast to the negative background.

Serial angio-scanography and rapid serial angioscintiphotography are rather complicated techniques, because it is indispensable to inject the radioisotopes into the arterial branches including the vacular bed of tumor or region of interest.

In any case, the arteriography must be done first, so, it would be helpful to interpret the suspected tumor vessels in the arteriograms, when positive scintigraphy was obtained by serial angio-scanography or rapid serial angioscintiphotography.

The application of nor-adrenalin in these examinations was also studied. Normal arteries contract with nor-adrenalin, but tumor vessels contract poorly with nor-adrenalin, that makes tumor detection easier in these pharmacoangioscintiphotography.

Table

Case	Age	Sex	Diagnosis	Radiography	R.I.&Dose	Positive Scintigraphy	Time for positive Scintigraphy
1.	42	F	Primary Lung Cancer (Adenocarcinoma)	Main tumor	^{131}I-MAA 250 μCi	Main tumor	2 days
2.	54	M	Primary Lung Cancer (Sq. cell carcinoma)	Metastatic tumor	^{131}I-MAA 250 μCi	Metastatic tumor	1 day
3.	55	F	Primary Lung Cancer (Adenocarcinoma)	Main tumor & Lymph nodes	^{131}I-MAA 250 μCi	Main tumor & Lymph nodes	0 day
4.	56	F	Primary Lung Cancer (Atypical cells)	Main tumor	^{131}I-MAA 250 μCi	Main tumor	4 days
5.	67	M	Primary Lung Cancer (Tumor cells)	Main tumor & Lymph nodes	^{125}I-MAA 100 μCi	Main tumor & Lymph nodes	1 day
6.	52	M	Primary Lung Cancer (Adenocarcinoma)	Main tumor	^{125}I-MAA 250 μCi	Main tumor	0 day
7.	59	M	Primary Lung Cancer (Adenocarcinoma)	Main tumor	^{131}I-MAA 250 μCi	Main tumor	3 days
8.	52	M	Primary Lung Cancer (Adenocarcinoma)	Main tumor	^{131}I-MAA 250 μCi	Main tumor	0 day
9.	69	M	Primary Lung Cancer (Undifferentiated ca.)	Main tumor & Lymph nodes	^{131}I-MAA 250 μCi	Main tumor & Lymph nodes	2 days
10.	64	M	Primary Lung Cancer (Sq. cell carcinoma)	Main tumor	^{131}I-MAA 300 μCi	Main tumor	2 days
11.	60	M	Primary Lung Cancer (Sq. call carcinoma)	Main tumor	^{131}I-MAA 300 μCi	Main tumor	0 day
12.	56	M	Primary Lung Cancer (Sq. cell carcinoma)	Main tumor	^{131}I-MAA 300 μCi	Main tumor	2 days
13.	51	M	Metastatic Lung Cancer (Grawitz's tumor)	Metastatic tumor	^{131}I-MAA 250 μCi	Metastatic tumor	1 day
14.	60	M	Metastatic Lung Cancer (Gastric cancer)	Metastatic tumor	^{131}I-MAA 80 μCi	Metastatic tumor	0 day
15.	69	F	Primary Lung Cancer (Atypical cells)	Main tumor & Lymph nodes	^{131}I-MAA 80^{0} 5 m 250 μCi	(–) Liver	(–)

Table (continued)

Case	Age	Sex	Diagnosis	Radiography	R.I. & Dose	Positive Scintigraphy	Time for positive Scintigraphy
16.	43	M	Primary Lung Cancer (Adenocarcinoma)	Main tumor & Lymph nodes	^{131}I-MAA 90^{0} 10 m 250 μCi	(–) Liver	(–)
17.	59	M	Lung Abcess	Abcess	^{131}I-MAA 250 μCi	(–)	(–)
18.	35	M	Primary Lung Cancer (Undifferentiated ca.)	Main tumor & Lymph nodes	^{131}I-Fibrinog. 700 μCi	Main tumor	35 min
19.	64	M	Primary Lung Cancer (Sq. cell carcinoma)	Main tumor	^{67}Ga-citrate 2 mCi	Main tumor	3 days
20.	43	M	Primary Lung Cancer (Carcinoma simplex)	Main tumor & Lymph nodes	^{133}Xe-solution 4 mCi	(–)	(–)
21.	16	F	Metastatic Lung Cancer (Osteosarcoma)	Metastatic tumor	^{133}Xe-solution 1.7 mCi	(–)	(–)
22.	30	M	Metastatic Lung Cancer (Cystic adenoid ca.)	Metastatic tumor	^{133}Xe-solution 2.8 mCi	Metastatic tumor	4.5 min 30 sec
23.	53	M	Primary Lung Cancer (Adenocarcinoma)	Main tumor	^{99m}Tc O_4 1.0 mCi	Main tumor	0.5 min
24.	56	M	Primary Lung Cancer (Undifferentiated ca.)	Main tumor & Lymph nodes	$^{99m}TcO_4$ 10 mCi	Main tumor & Lymph nodes	1.5 min
25.	62	M	Primary Lung Cancer (Atypical cells)	Main tumor & Lymph nodes	$^{99m}TcO_4$ 5.0 mCi	Main tumor & Lymph nodes	1.5 min
26.	54	M	Primary Lung Cancer (Undifferentiated ca.)	Main tumor & Lymph nodes	$^{99m}TcO_4$ 1.8 mCi	Main tumor & Lymph nodes	4.0 min
27.	35	M	Primary Lung Cancer (Atypical cells)	Main tumor	$^{99m}TcO_4$ 5.4 mCi	Main tumor	4,5 min
28.	42	M	Primary Lung Cancer (Carcinoma simplex)	Main tumor	$^{99m}TcO_4$ 9.0 mCi	Main tumor	5.0 min
29.	72	M	Primary Lung Cancer (Sq. cell carcinoma)	Main tumor	$^{99m}TcO_4$ 10.5 mCi	Main tumor	10.0 min
30.	25	M	Bronchial adenoma	Main tumor	^{99} TcO_4 7.0 mCi	Main tumor	0.5 min
31.	36	M	Lung abscess	Abscess	$^{99m}TcO_4$ 11.0 mCi	Abscess lesion	1.0 min

Lungenszintigraphische Funktionskontrolle im Vergleich zu Röntgenuntersuchungen nach Thoraxtraumen

I. Staib, D. Maroske und H. Würdinger

Die Methodik, theoretischen Grundlagen und Risiken der Lungenszintigraphie darzustellen, erscheint vor diesem Auditorium nicht notwendig.

Durch eine Einzelbeobachtung nach einer Unterlappenresektion bei einem 9-jährigen Jungen stießen wir auf eine erhebliche Diskrepanz zwischen der konventionellen Röntgenuntersuchung und der Lungenszintigraphie.

Dadurch wurden wir zu einer prospektiven Studie an 28 Patienten mit Thoraxtraumen unterschiedlicher Genese angeregt. Wir stellen hier nur die Ergebnisse von 15 Patienten mit mindestens 4 oder mehr Rippenfrakturen einer Seite vor.

Untersuchungsschema

Die Erstuntersuchung erfolgte noch am Unfalltag, oder, wenn es der Zustand des Patienten nicht erlaubte, bis spätestens zum 5. Tag. Eine frühe Nachuntersuchung führten wir in der 1.–5. Woche nach Trauma, eine zweite Nachuntersuchung 12 bis 37 Wochen nach dem Trauma durch. Röntgenuntersuchung und Szintigramm wurden möglichst am gleichen Tag ausgeführt.

Befundbeurteilung

Pathologische Befunde wurden von 2 Untersuchern für beide Methoden in 4 Stufen eingeteilt (von gering bis sehr stark ausgeprägt).

Ergebnisse

Von 9 auswertbaren Erstuntersuchungen waren Röntgen und Szintigramm dreimal identisch, viermal zeigte das Szintigramm eine Stufe schwerere Veränderungen und einmal 2 Stufen stärkere pathologische Alteration.

Bei der ersten Nachuntersuchung waren von 13 auswertbaren Befunden 8 mal beide Methoden identisch, 3mal 1 Stufe und 2mal 2 Stufen das Szintigramm stärker pathologisch.

Von 4 Spätkontrollen war das Szintigramm einmal um eine Stufe stärker verändert.

Zusammenfassung und Folgerung

Das Szintigramm erwies sich in unseren Untersuchungen stets als empfindlichere Kontrollgröße. Da Durchblutung und Ventilationsgröße streng korreliert sind, kann das Szintigramm als wesentliche diagnostische Maßnahme zur Beurteilung der Lungenfunktion nach Thoraxtraumen herangezogen werden. Die Szintigraphie ist zu empfehlen, wenn der Röntgenbefund die Schwere des klinischen Bildes, insbesondere bei Anstrengung, nicht erklärt. Ferner als Verlaufskontrolle, besonders wenn blutgasanalytische oder spiroergometrische Messungen wegen ungenügender Kooperation des Patienten (Kind, Schädel-Hirntrauma etc.) nicht möglich sind.

Selective Arteriography of Tumours and First Experiences with Angioscintigraphy of the Mediastinum

H. RESCHKE

Selective arteriographic examination of the mediastinum with – electronic – substraction is able to demonstrate the vessels of even small tumours.

In cases where there remains doubt as to the presence of pathologic vascularization intraarterial injection of ^{131}JMAA is especially valuable.

With the exception of goiters and some tumours of the parathyreoid glands as well as the bony wall this region can not be examined by drugs specifically stored within organs.

On the other hand a ^{99m}Tc scanogram seldom will really impressively outline a tumour which is poorly defined by arteriography as was the case with this plasmocytoma of the sternum.

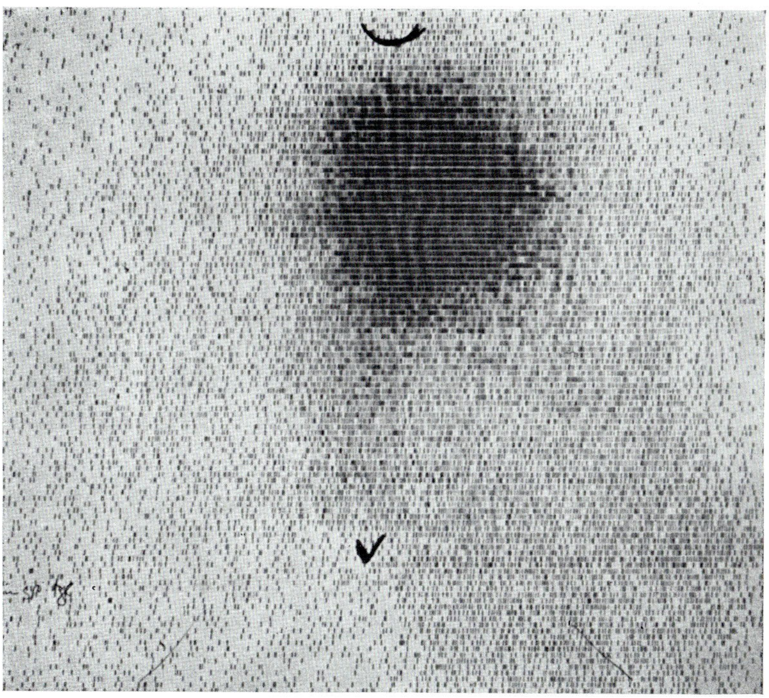

Fig. 1

In comparison of the arteriographic findings with the following scintigraphic studies it must be mentioned that the solution with 80–200μCi ^{131}JMAA – particles of 5–50 μ in size – has to be injected more slowly than the contrast medium. Reflux of the radiopharmaceutical in the aorta should be avoided.

The anterior mediastinum is perfused via the internal thoracic arteries.

Sometimes cervical arteries may atypically branch off from these vessels. Rarely the internal thoracic artery originates from an axillary artery. In about 10 % of cases the vessel bifurcates into two branches for the anterior and lateral aspects of the internal thoracic wall.

Occasionally arteriographic demonstration of the inferior anterior and the paracardial mediastinum can be accomplished via the inferior phrenic arteries.

The main branch of the internal thoracic artery, i.e. the pericardiacophrenic artery is visible in most arteriograms. If thymic or other small branches are visible within the anterior mediastinum in the adult patient, this unequivocally indicates pathologic lesions.

Even in tumours with only slight staining lesions from 20 mm diameter up can be outlined.

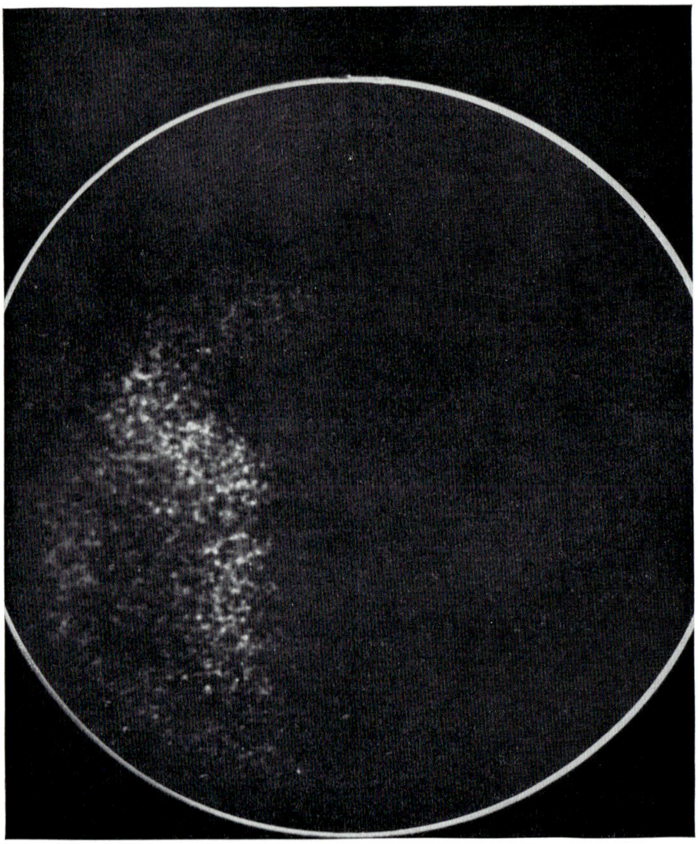

Fig. 2

This left mammary arteriogram shows a large (lymphogranulomatous) tumour by multiple extremely fine woven arteries and a partially better staining in the a.v. phase.

In the angioscintigram an intensive tumour staining is visible down to the hilum. The tumour being clearly outlined within the nearly homogeneous distribution of radioactivities in the left anterior thoracic wall (Fig. 1).

The only exception among 8 cases of tumour with positive angioscintigraphic findings was seen in a metastasis of a squamous cell-carcinoma which caused a defect in the upper right thoracic wall (Fig. 2). Arteriographically a deviation of arteries prevailed.

The medial portion of the mediastinum is supplied by the bronchial arteries as a link between the internal thoracic and the intercostal vessels. They may originate from the aorta with one to four branches.

Bronchial arteries often rise from the right third intercostal artery. Connexions with subclavian and thyroideal branches can be present. Such atypical vessels give rise to a variety of possible distribution of radioactivity.

Bronchial scanograms may resemble a lung scan. Different lobes can be visualized depending from the catheterized artery. The normal pattern of hilar and/or central mediastinal structures seems to be irregular and will outweigh the bronchial scan of the lung. The lower as well as the upper portion of the mediastinum appears scintigraphically almost empty.

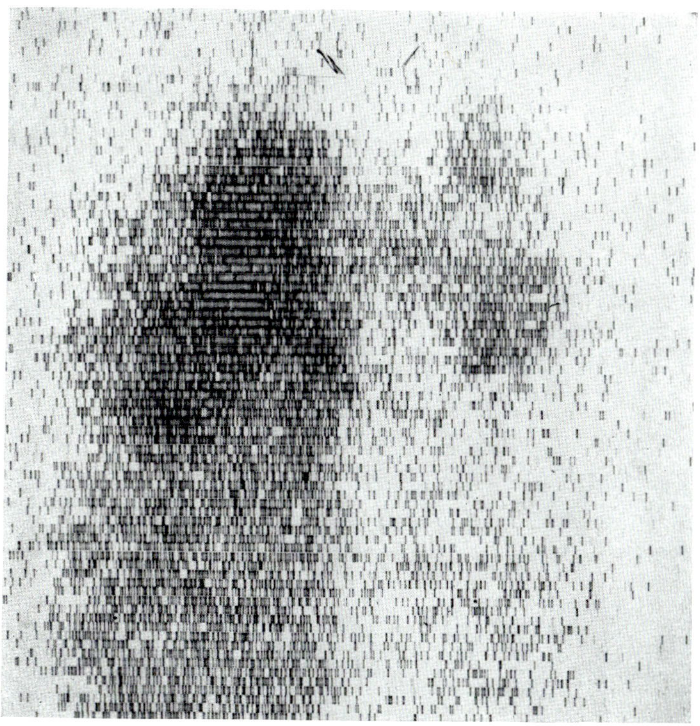

Fig. 3

Some tumours are supplied via the vasculature of the anterior as well as of the middle layers of the mediastinum (slide). The tumour-size seemed to be better demonstrated by the angioscintigram of this case of lyphogranulomatosis, which was injected via the right thoracic and left bronchial arteries. Radioactivity of the tumour as well as of the homogeneous distribution within the thoracic wall on the right are more intensive than that of the tumour and lung in the left bronchial scan (Fig. 3).

The posterior layer of the mediastinum and its wall must be examined via the intercostal arteries. They may have various unilateral anastomoses; however, controlateral anastomoses are rarlely seen. Size and shapes of angioscintigrams with their normally small-intercostal-areas of radioactivity vary depending on the anatomical conditions. Tumour scanning however is possible by accumulation as well as by filling-defects of the radioactivity presumably within the posterior wall of the thorax.

Summary

Arteriographically insignificant and/or uncertain demonstration of massiv tumours within the mediastinum can be ensured by injection of 80–200 μCi ^{131}JMAA. Most impressing are the as a rule positive findings in the scanograms of the anterior and middle mediastinal layers (Aa. thoracicae intt. and bronchiales).

Positive findings may also be seen in the retroesophageal space by filling of intercostal arteries.

Tumour infiltration of the thoracic wall occasionally will cause filling-defects.

Diseases of the Liver

Vergleichende vasographische und szintigraphische Untersuchungen zum Nachweis von Lebertumoren*

C. Winkler, A. Düx und E. Bücheler

Die Tumordiagnostik der Leber hat vor allem im Zusammenhang mit den Fortschritten der Leberchirurgie wesentliche Bedeutung erlangt. Leistungsfähige Methoden konnten röntgenologisch mit Hilfe vasographischer Verfahren und nuklearmedizinisch durch Anwendung der Szintigraphie entwickelt werden. Dabei ist es interessant festzustellen, wie sich die Untersuchungsmethoden in ihrer unterschiedlichen Aussagefähigkeit und klinischen Anwendbarkeit praktisch ergänzen.

Die *Splenoportographie* ist zur Lokalisation und Größenbestimmung pathologischer Leberveränderungen bevorzugt geeignet, weil die wandschwachen und sehr zahlreichen Portalgefäße raumfordernde Prozesse auch geringen Ausmaßes fast immer klar erkennen lassen. Eine Unterscheidung zwischen benignen und malignen Tumoren ist allerdings mit der Splenoportographie im allgemeinen nicht möglich. Demgegenüber kann eine solche Unterscheidung *mit der Arteriographie*, vor allem mit superselektiver Technik, erzielt werden, wenn es sich um Geschwülste mit gefäßreichem Stroma handelt und Tumorgefäße darstellbar sind. – Methodisch ergeben sich bei den vasographischen Verfahren heute kaum noch Probleme. Ein gewisser Aufwand – stationäre Durchführung der Untersuchung, Katheterisierung, evtl. Milzpunktion – muß in Kauf genommen werden. Kontrastmittelunverträglichkeit kommt in seltenen Fällen vor, ist aber als Komplikation im Rahmen der Problematik maligner Prozesse von untergeordneter Bedeutung.

Die *Szintigraphie* mit konventioneller Technik gibt Aufschluß über Parenchymdefekte, Form- und Lageveränderungen der Leber. Als Testpräparate kommen für die Tumordiagnostik in erster Linie kolloidale Substanzen, wie ^{99m}Technetium-Sulfurkolloid, ^{198}Goldkolloid etc. in Betracht. Auf die z.Zt. noch im Stadium des Experiments befindliche Positivdarstellung von Tumoren, etwa mit ^{67}Gallium oder ^{57}Cobalt-Bleomycin, soll im vorliegenden Zusammenhang nicht eingegangen werden. – Die Meßtechnik erfodert zwar auch bei Anwendung moderner, mit Einstellautomatik ausgerüsteter Szintigraphiegeräte ein gewisses Geschick und Erfahrung. Schwierigkeiten ergeben sich jedoch praktisch kaum noch, vor allem dann nicht, wenn mit einem geeigneten Speicherverfahren gearbeitet wird, das auch bei primär ungünstiger Wahl von Einstellparametern die Erzielung eines diagnostisch verwertbaren Szintigramms ermöglicht.

---

* Herrn Professor Dr. A. Gütgemann zm 65. Geburtstag gewidmet.

Außer den am meisten gebrauchten abtastenden Szintigraphen (Scannern) mit einem oder mehreren Detektoren werden in neuerer Zeit zunehmend auch Kamerasysteme mit einem stationären Detektor verwendet. Diese haben den Vorteil der schnelleren Bildgebung und können daher auch für kinetische Untersuchungen (Sequenzszintigraphie) eingesetzt werden. Weitere meßtechnische Unterschiede zwischen Scan-

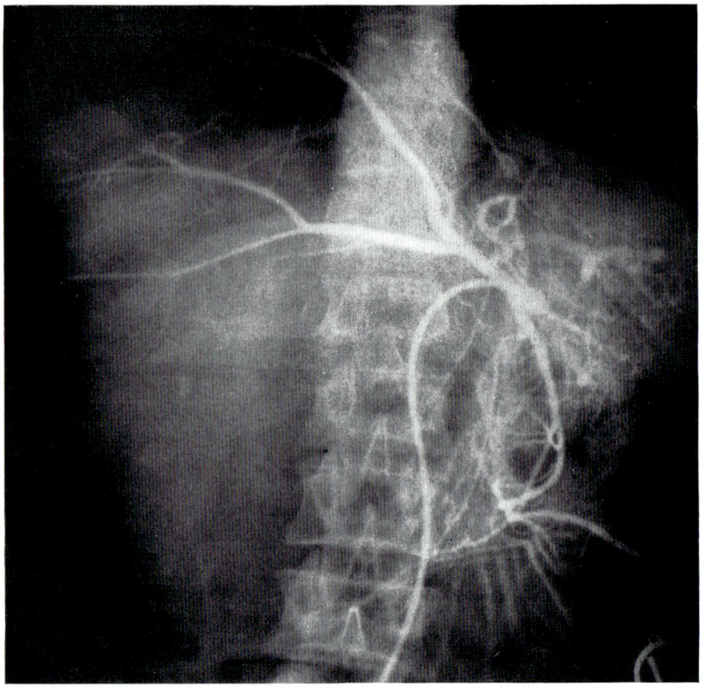

a

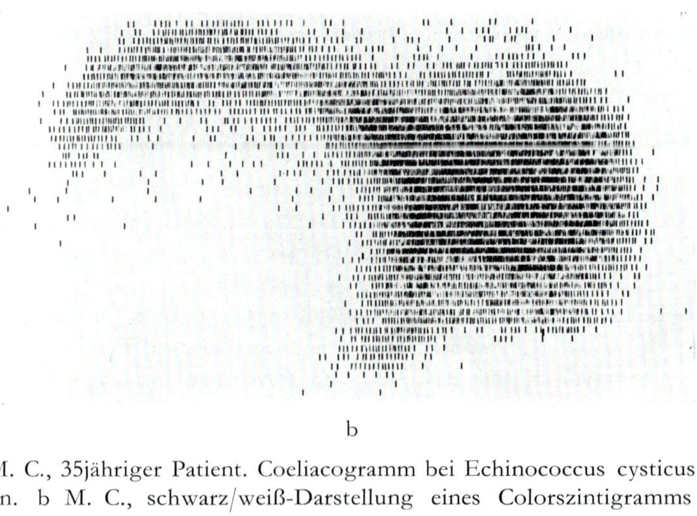

b

Abb. 1a. M. C., 35jähriger Patient. Coeliacogramm bei Echinococcus cysticus im rechten Leberlappen. b M. C., schwarz/weiß-Darstellung eines Colorszintigramms der Leber. Große Echinococcus-Solitärcyste ner und Szintikamera (bezüglich der Auflösung etc.) sind im übrigen hier nicht zu erörtern. Erwähnt sei lediglich, daß sowohl Szintigraphen mit mobilem wie auch mit stationärem Detektor in Verbindung mit einem Computer betrieben werden können und daß diese Technik vor allem für die Kameraszintigraphie entscheidende Fortschritte erbracht hat. An einem speziellen Beispiel soll dies unten erläutert werden. Zunächst wollen wir uns auf den Tumornachweis mittels der allgemein gebräuchlichen konventionellen Szintigraphie beschränken und deren Ergebnisse anhand von typischen Fällen mit denen der Angiographie vergleichen.

Abb. 1a zeigt das Coeliacogramm einer Leber, in deren rechtem Lappen sich eine riesige Echinococcuscyste entwickelt hat. Man erkennt die Distension und Verlagerung der Segmentarterien sowie die große Gefäßaussparung im gesamten Bereich des raumfordernden Prozesses.

Abb. 1b stellt das zugehörige Szintigramm dar. Der Parenchymdefekt im rechten Lappen ist nach Form und Ausdehnung klar erkennbar. Die glatte Randbegrenzung der annähernd kreisförmigen Projektion des Bereiches fehlender Kolloidspeicherung deutet in Verbindung mit der Größe des Defektes auf das Vorliegen einer Cyste hin. Der linke Leberlappen erscheint relativ groß. Er speichert vermehrt Kolloid, ist nach links verdrängt und überlagert die Milz.

Im Coeliacogramm der Abb. 2a haben sich Metastasen eines Nebennierencarcinoms in unterschiedlicher Weise dargestellt. Cranial im rechten Lappen finden sich typische Tumorgefäße und multiple Geschwulstanfärbungen, darunter Bezirke mit

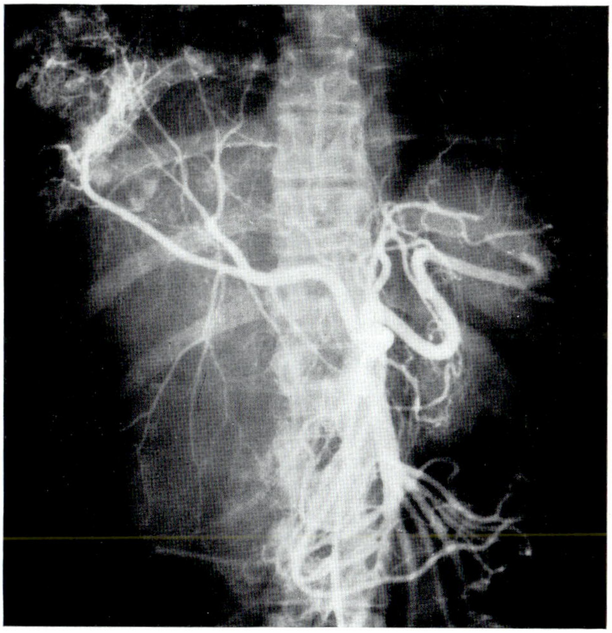

a

Abb. 2a. E. K., 21jährige Patientin. Coeliacogramm. Metastasen eines Nebennierencarcinoms mit unterschiedlicher Vascularisation

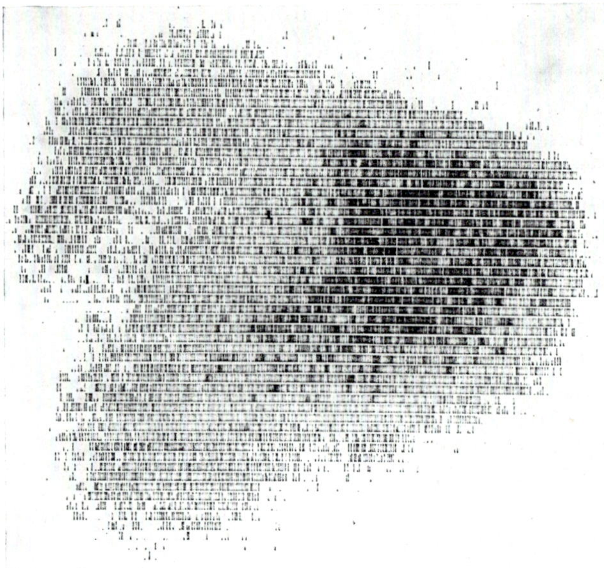

b

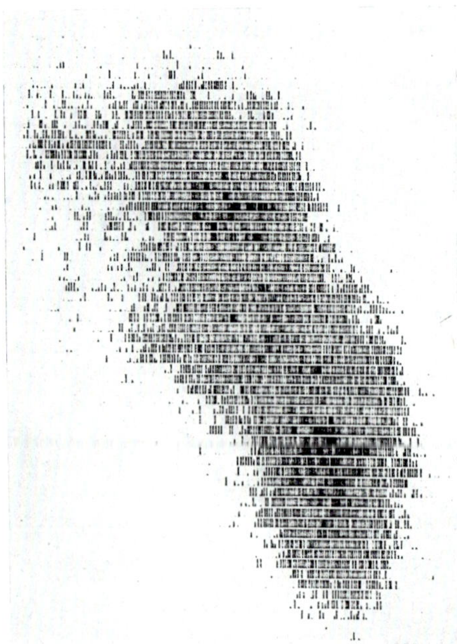

c

Abb. 2b. E. K., schwarz-weiß-Darstellung eines Colorszintigramms der Leber. Weitgehende Destruktion des rechten Lappens durch den metastatischen Tumorprozeß. c E. K., rechtsseitliche Aufnahme des Leberszintigramms. Bei weitgehender Destruktion des rechten Lappens durch den vorwiegend dorsal entwickelten Tumorprozeß Ventralverdrängung des Restparenchyms

Verdrängung und weitgehender Rarefizierung der Arterien. – Wenngleich im vorliegenden Fall die Diagnose eindeutig gestellt werden konnte, deutet der Befund generell auf die Problematik der Artdiagnostik bei metastatischen Tumoren hin, die häufig gering vascularisiert sind und deren Malignität in solchen Fällen auch arteriographisch nicht ohne weiteres definierbar ist. – Im Szintigramm der Abb. 2b finden sich im gesamten Areal des rechten Lappens unterschiedlich starke Speicherausfälle, die auf weitgehende Destruktion dieses Leberbereichs schließen lassen. Der relativ große linke Lappen zeigt eine unregelmäßig konturierte Abgrenzung und ist nach links bis über die Milzregion verdrängt. In der rechts-seitlichen Aufnahme der Abb. 2c erkennt man die durch dorsale Entwicklung des raumfordernden Prozesses zur vorderen Bauchwand verdrängten Anteile des noch intakten Parenchyms, vorwiegend des linken Lappens. Der cranio-dorsal gelegene rundliche Bezirk aufgelockerter Aktivitätsakkumulation stellt angedeutet die nicht vergrößerte, normal Kolloid speichernde Milz dar.

Im Coeliacogramm der Abb. 3a, das nach positivem, auf Echinococcus hydatidosus hinweisenden Ausfall des Cosonitests aufgenommen wurde, findet sich eine weitgehend unauffällige Darstellung der intrahepatischen Arterien – bis auf eine geringgradige, bogenförmige Verlagerung einzelner Segmentarterien im craniolateralen Abschnitt des rechten Lappens. – Auch die in Abb. 3b dargestellte Frontalaufnahme des Leberszintigramms ergibt, wenn überhaupt (im farbigen Original), nur einen diskreten Hinweis auf eine Veränderung des Speichermusters rechts cranial. Dagegen zeigt die rechtsseitliche Aufnahme der Abb. 3c deutlich einen rundlichen Speicherausfall

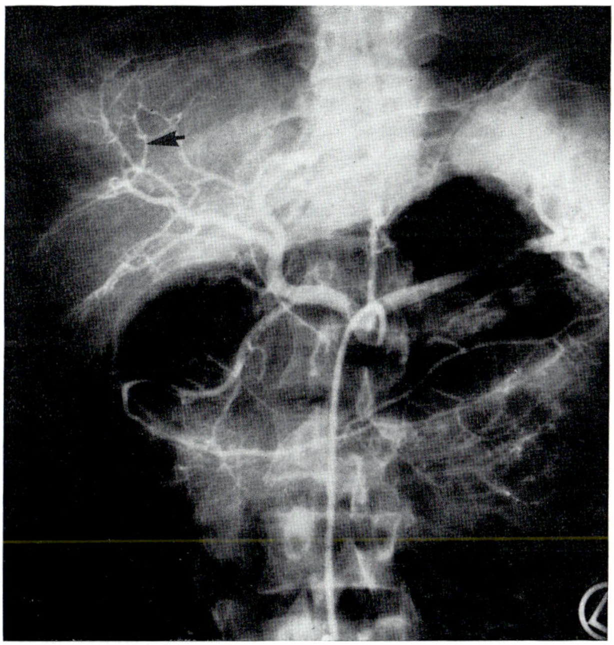

a

Abb. 3a. G. M., 24jähriger Patient. Coeliacogramm bei Echinococcus cysticus im rechten Lappen. Geringgradige Verlagerung einzelner Segmentarterien (Pfeil)

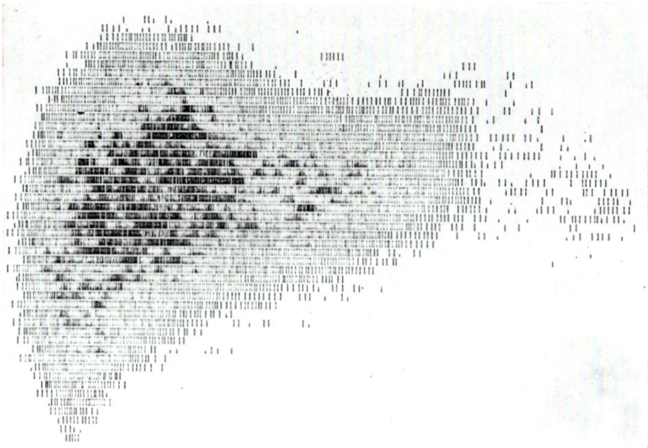

b

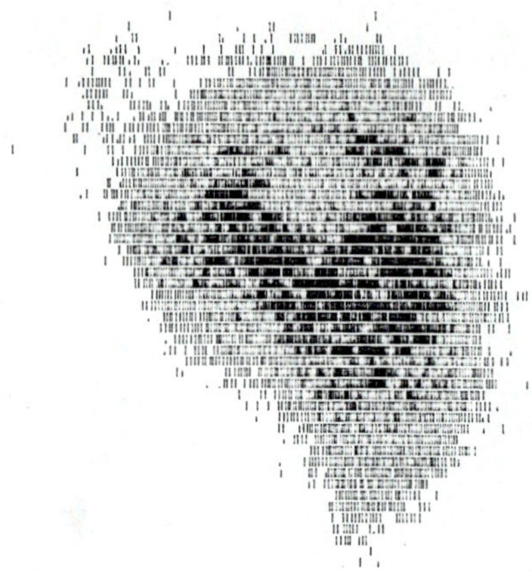

c

Abb. 3b G. M., schwarz-weiß-Darstellung eines Colorszintigramms der Leber (Frontalebene). *Im farbigen Original* erkennt man eine geringfügige Normabweichung des Speichermusters im Cranialbereich des rechten Lappens. c G. M., rechts-seitliche Aufnahme des Szintigramms. Deutliche Darstellung eines Parenchymdefektes im cranialen Abschnitt der Leber

in der im übrigen normal erscheinenden Seitenprojektion der Leber. Bei dem Parenchymdefekt handelte es sich nach dem Operationsbericht um eine etwa taubeneigroße, uniloculäre Echinococcuscyste.

In den vorbeschriebenen Befundvergleichen wurden in nuklearmedizinischer Hinsicht ausschließlich Aufnahmen der konventionellen Szintigraphie angeführt. Anhand eines weiteren Falles sei auch auf eine der neuen Möglichkeiten der szintigraphischen Diagnostik hingewiesen, die sich durch die Entwicklung der Computerszintigraphie ergeben haben. Das Leberszintigramm der Abb. 4a wurde bei einer Patientin aufgenommen, bei der 6 Jahre zuvor wegen einer Lebercirrhose mit Varizenblutung eine

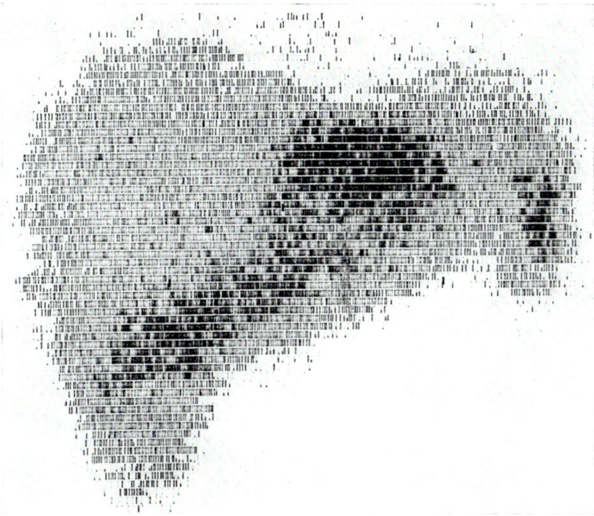

a

Abb. 4a. A. P., 61jährige Patientin. Schwarz-weiß-Darstellung eines Leberszintigramms, das 6 Jahre nach portocavaler Anastomose bei Lebercirrhose aufgenommen wurde. Großer, umschriebener Speicherdefekt im rechten Lappen. Klinisch Verdacht auf Carcinom

portocavale Anastomose angelegt worden war. Nach dem klinischen Befund hatte sich jetzt der Verdacht auf die Entwicklung eines Lebercarcinoms ergeben. In der konventionellen Aufnahme findet sich ein erheblich von der Norm abweichendes Speichermuster mit bevorzugt im rechten Lappen umschrieben reduzierter Kolloidakkumulation. Das Projektionsbild der mäßig vergrößerten, vermehrt Kolloid speichernden Milz läßt sich nur undeutlich von dem des linken Leberlappens abgrenzen.

Zur Klärung der Frage, ob der Speicherdefekt im rechten Lappen durch einen vascularisierten Tumor im Sinne eines hepatocellulären Carcinoms verursacht worden war, wurde eine Computer-Sequenzszintigraphie mit der Szintillationskamera durchgeführt. Dabei werden nach i.v.-Applikation des Testkolloids in Intervallen von 5 sec Szintigramme aufgenommen und die Verteilungsmatrizen zunächst auf einen Magnetplattenspeicher übertragen. Nach anschließender Ausgabe eines Summationsbildes auf Analogsichtgerät oder per Schnelldrucker werden, wie in Abb. 4b dargestellt, zwei Areale definiert, von denen eins dem tumorverdächtigen Bereich und das zweite einem Vergleichbereich im normal speichernden Leberanteil zugeordnet ist. Über diesen interessierenden Regionen werden vom Rechner aus der Szintigrammsequenz anhand eines entsprechenden Programms die Zeitaktivitätsverläufe ermittelt und als Kurven ausgegeben. In Abb. 4d sehen wir einen normalen, dem Vergleichsbereich zugehörigen Akkumulationsverlauf mit einer langsam bis zum Ende der Untersuchung ansteigenden Kurve. Demgegenüber ist es bei Abb. 4c zu einem sehr raschen Anstieg der Kurve bereits in den ersten Sekunden gekommen, entsprechend einem schnellen Einschuß der Radioaktivität mit dem Blutstrom in den betr. Gewebsbereich. Danach zeigt sich ein fast plateauartiger Verlauf, dessen Niveau bei Beendigung der Meßreihe deutlich unter der im Vergleichsbereich erreichten Aktivitätsak-

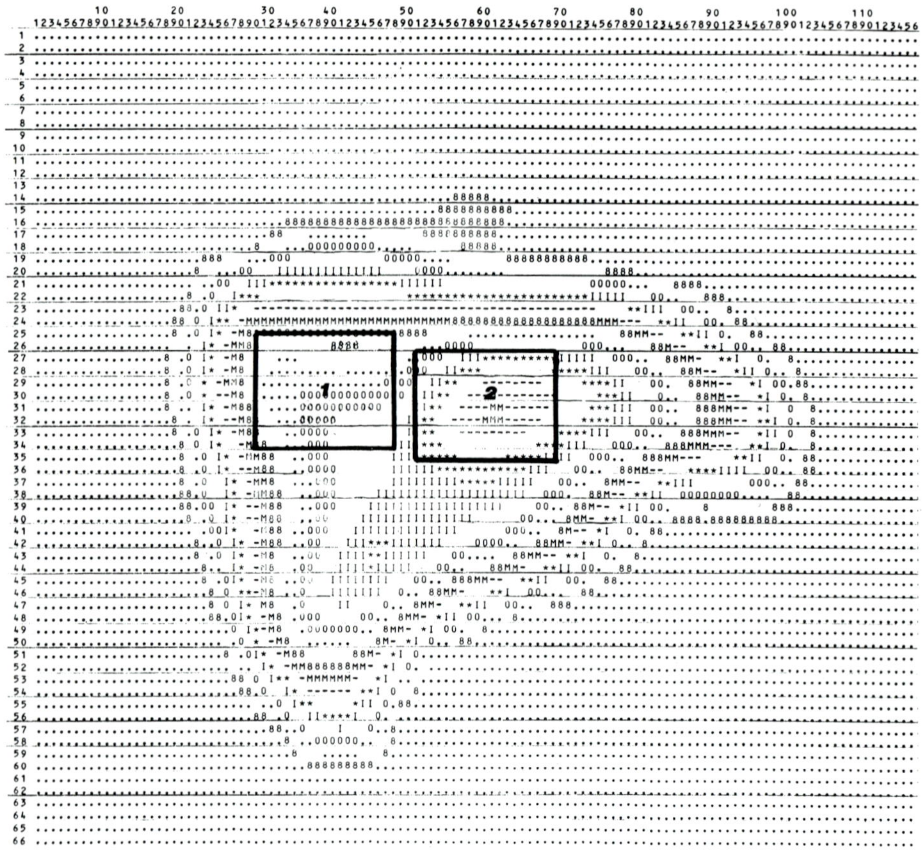

b

Abb. 4b. A. P., Schnelldruckerausgabe eines Computerszintigramms der Leber. Isointensitäts-Zonendarstellung. 1 = Region des Tumor-verdächtigen Bereichs, 2 = Vergleichsbereich (s. zugehörige Kurven Abb. 4c und d)

kumulation liegt. Nach diesem Auswertungsergebnis wurde auf das Vorliegen eines stark vaskularisierten Tumors im rechten Lappen der cirrhotischen Leber geschlossen. Das superselektive Hepaticogramm der Abb. 4e bestätigt diese Diagnose. Man erkennt das ausgeprägte Tumorgefäßkonvolut im oberen Abschnitt des rechten Leberlappens, das dem tatsächlich vorliegenden Cirrhose-Carcinom entsprach.

Abschließend sei noch ein Beispiel für eine neuartige Aufgabenstellung der radiologischen Leberdiagnostik angeführt, die sich im Rahmen der Transplantationschirurgie ergeben hat. Die Untersuchungen beschränken sich hier nicht auf die praeoperative Lokalisation und Differenzierung des Tumorprozesses, sie erstrecken sich vielmehr auch auf postoperative Kontrollen des Lebertransplantates.

Abb. 5a zeigt das Splenoportogramm eines 30jähr. Patienten, bei dem ein ausgedehntes Lebercarcinom vorlag. Man sieht, daß der Tumor nicht nur zu einem völligen Verschluß des rechten Pfortaderhauptastes, sondern auch bereits zu einer hochgradigen Stenosierung des linken Portalastes geführt hatte. Im Arteriogramm fanden

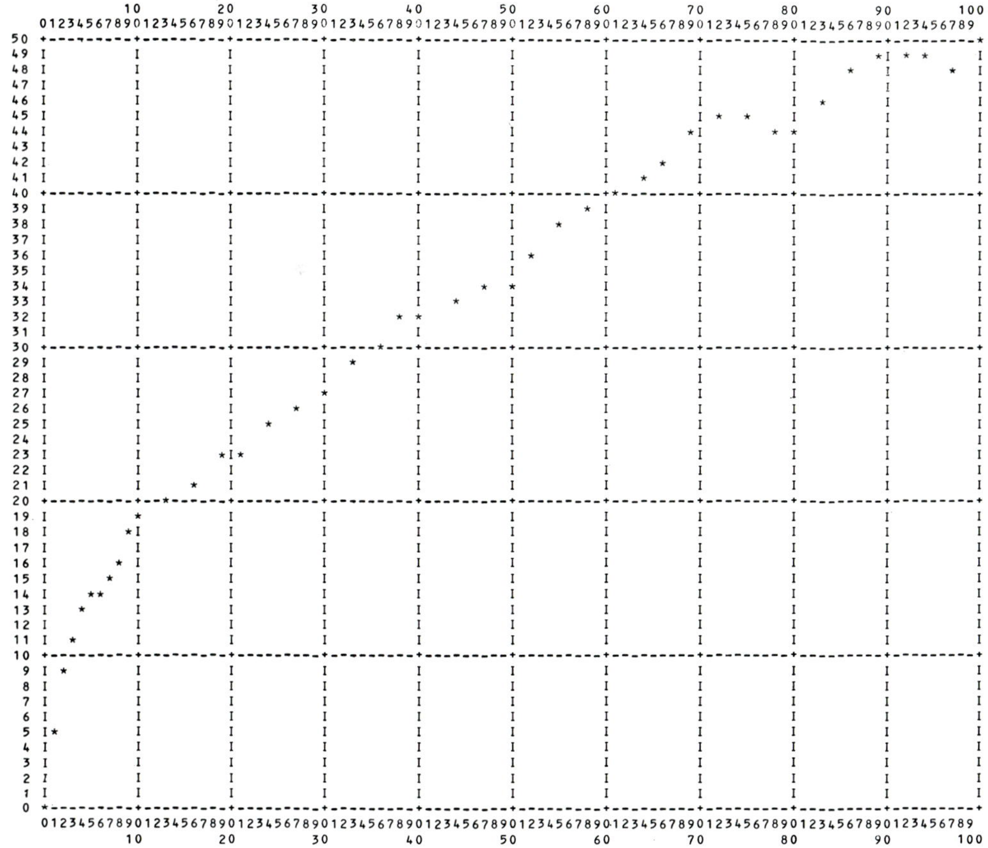

c

Abb. 4c und d A. P., Computerausgaben der Zeit-Aktivitätsverläufe in den interessierenden Regionen (nach i. v.-Applikation von Tc^{99m}-Kolloid): c (oben) im Tumorbereich, d im normal akkumulierenden Vergleichsbereich. d A. P., superselektives Hepaticogramm. Ausgedehntes Tumorgefäßkonvolut im Cranialabschnitt des rechten Lappens bei hepatocellulärem Carcinom in der cirrhotischen Leber

sich massenhaft Tumorgefäße im Bereich des rechten Lappens. Das Szintigramm der Abb. 5b läßt die weitgehende Destruktion der Leber erkennen, die durch Ausbreitung des raumfordernden Prozesses im gesamten Organ stark vergrößert erscheint und die nach cranial verdrängte Milz z.T. überlagert.

1969 wurde von Gütgemann in der Bonner Chirurgischen Universitätsklinik das tumorbefallene Organ entfernt und eine Lebertransplantation durchgeführt. Nach der erfolgreichen Operation konnte der Einheilungsprozeß des Transplantates szintigraphisch verfolgt werden, wobei sich Rejektionsreaktionen z.T. bereits vor der Beobachtung anderer Symptome im Szintigramm zeigten. Die sich anbahnenden Reaktionen kamen – offenbar infolge einer Alteration der Organperfusion – in quantitativ nachweisbaren Verminderungen der Kolloidspeicherung im hepatischen RES

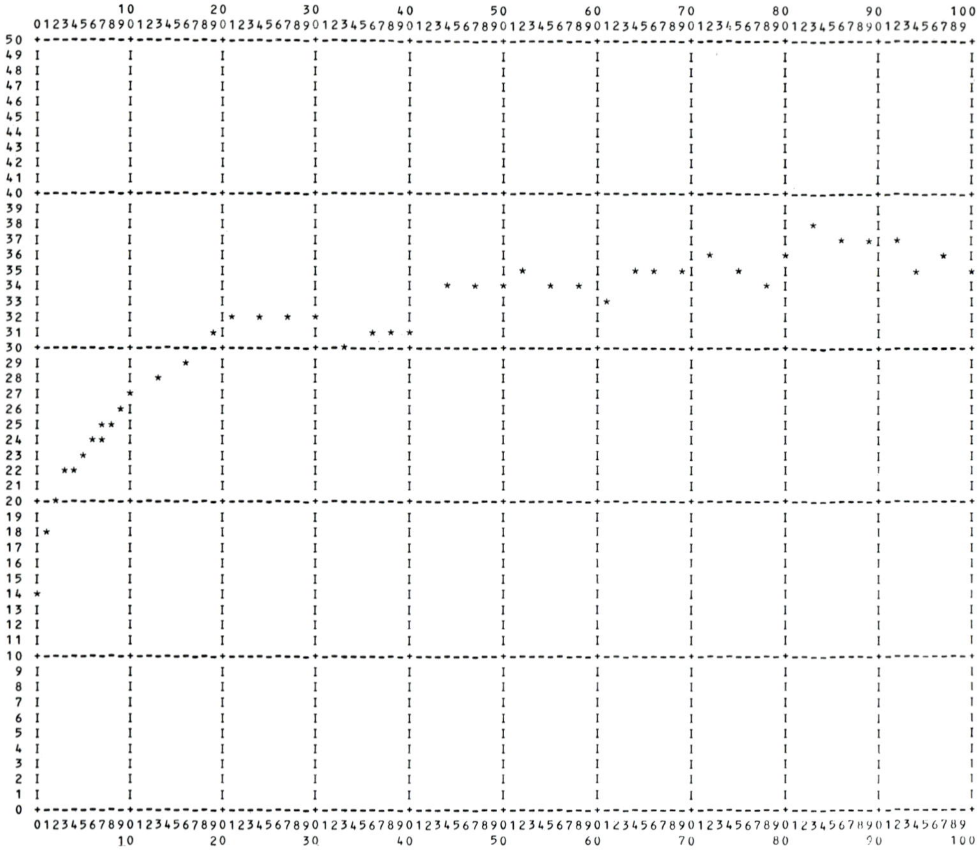

d

bei gleichzeitig vermehrter Aktivitäts-Akkumulation in der Milz zum Ausdruck. Aus der szintigraphischen Untersuchungsserie kann hier nur das kurz vor Entlassung des Patienten aus der stationären Behandlung konventionell aufgenommene Szintigramm dargestellt werden. Abb. 6 zeigt die Aufnahme des transplantierten Organs, das nach Form und Größe weitgehend normal erscheint. Auch das Aktivitätsverteilungsmuster weicht nur in geringem Maße von der Norm ab; im Bereich des Leberhilus findet sich etwas herabgesetzte Kolloidspeicherung, offenbar infolge einer gewissen Beeinträchtigung des Parenchyms durch die Operationsmaßnahmen. Die Milz ist klar vom linken Leberrand abgegrenzt. Sie erscheint nur leicht vergrößert und zeigt eine kaum über das normale Maß hinausgehende Kolloidspeicherung. – Wenn auch eine ausführlichere Darstellung des Falles im vorliegenden Rahmen nicht möglich ist, so mag das Beispiel doch prinzipiell auf die Vorteile der Szintigraphie für Verlaufskontrollen nach Lebertransplantationen hinweisen: die beliebig häufige Wiederholbarkeit der Untersuchung und die damit erzielbaren Aufschlüsse über Organdurchblutung, Rejektionsreaktionen, evtl. Abszeßbildungen oder partielle Nekrotisierungen, Dislokalisation z.B. durch subphrenische Prozesse etc. –

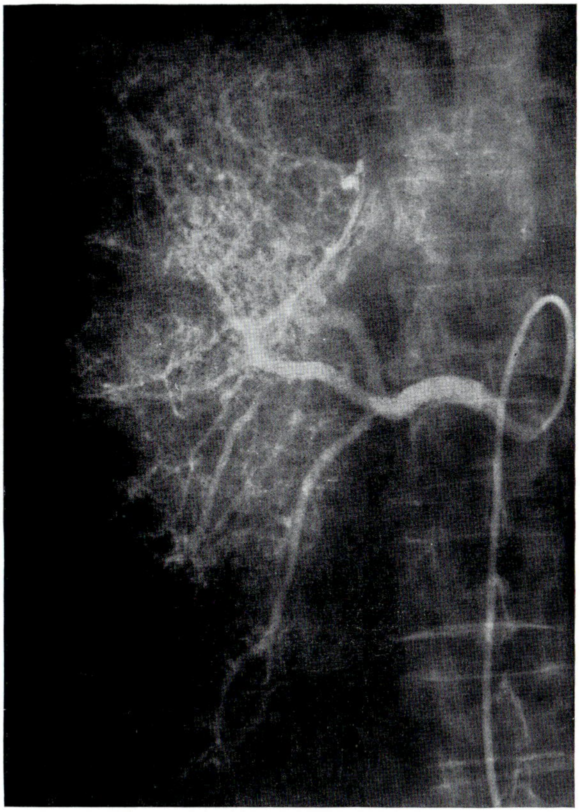

e

Abb. 4e. A.P., superselektives Hepaticogramm. Ausgedehntes Tumorgefäßkonvolut im Cranialabschnitt des rechten Lappens bei hepatocellulärem Carcinom in der cirrhotischen Leber

In den Betrachtungen des vorliegenden Referates über den Einsatz von Angiographie und Szintigraphie im Rahmen der Leberdiagnostik bei Tumorprozessen sollte versucht werden, die heute radiologisch gegebenen Möglichkeiten vergleichend zu skizzieren. Bei der notwendigen Beschränkung auf wenige Beispiele konnten dabei nur einige der wesentlichsten Aspekte exemplarisch aufgezeigt werden.

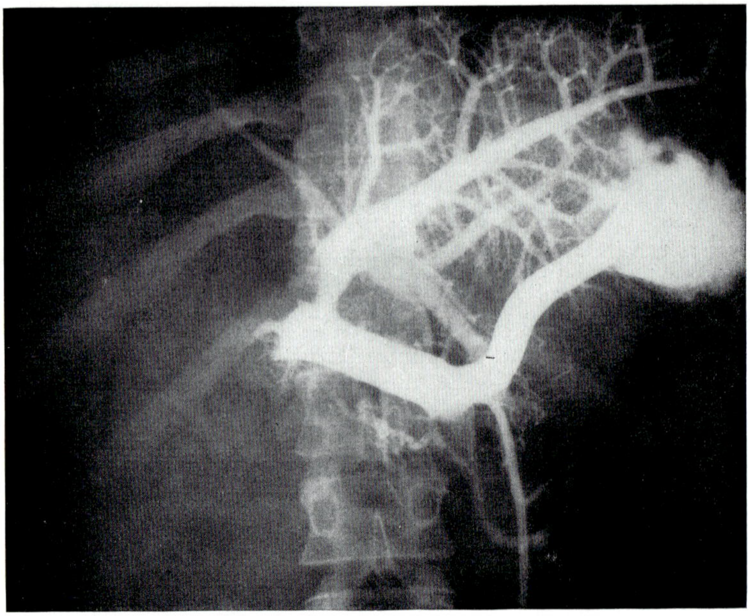

a

b

Abb. 5a. V. G. 30jähriger Patient. Splenoportogramm bei Hepatozellulärem Carcinom. Verschluß des rechten Pfortaderhauptastes, Stenosierung des linken Portalastes. b V. G. Schwarz-weiß-Darstellung des Colorszintigramms der Leber bei ausgedehnten, multiplen Parenchymdefekten im gesamten Leberbereich. Partielle Überlagerung der mäßig vergrößerten Milz

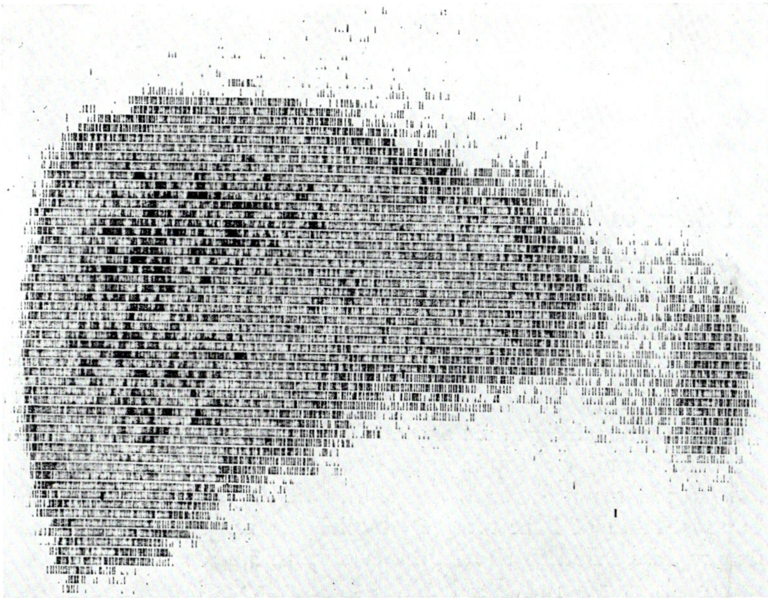

Abb. 6. V. G. Schwarz-weiß-Darstellung des Colorszintigramms der transplantierten Leber. Normale Form und Größe des Organs. Weitgehend normales Verteilungsmuster des Testkolloids, nur gering verminderte Kolloidspeicherung im Hilusbereich (s. Text)

Zusammenfassend läßt sich sagen, daß nach den vorliegenden Erfahrungen die röntgenologischen und nuklearmedizinischen Methoden etwa gleichermaßen diagnostisch von Interesse sind und sich in ihren verschiedenen Prinzipien bzw. Anwendungsmöglichkeiten in wertvoller Weise ergänzen. Bevorzugt geeignet zur Größenbestimmung von Tumoren ist das Splenoportogramm, zur Artdiagnostik das Arteriogramm und zur Vorfelddiagnostik bzw. für Verlaufskontrollen das Szintigramm. In Form der Computerszintigraphie scheint sich zudem eine methodische Entwicklung anzubahnen, die eine nicht unbeträchtliche Erweiterung der bisherigen Möglichkeiten erwarten läßt.

A Comparison of Angiographic and Scintigraphic Examinations of the Liver and the Results of Histology

E. Raschke

From 1965 until 1970 96 patients were treated in the Chirurgische Universitätsklinik Bonn in whom scintigraphic and angiographic examinations were compared with intraoperative and/or autoptic intrahepatic findings. The comparison of these diagnostical procedures prooved a superiority of angiographs over radionuclear tests in demonstration of liver tumors expecially in respect to their classification. Splenoportographies failed to show tumors only in 3,6% in cases of complete or partial thrombosis of the portal vein. The arteriographs had a failure of 5% and scintigraphic tests such of 6,5%. The combined analysis of all 3 methods left only one carcinoma unrecognised which was growing diffusely in a cirrhotic liver. The size of the single nodes did not exceed 1.5 to 2 cm in diameter. In simultaneously existing diffuse damages of the liver a false-positive tumor interpretation amounted on arteriographic studies to approximately 7,5%, in splenoportograms to almost 10,7% and in scintigraphic examinations to 12,9%. A method demonstrating the vascular system – primarily the hepatic arteriography – has the distinct advantage of differentiation of benigne and malignant intrahepatic tumors. According to Prof. Winklers studies there seem to develop new possibilities with radionuclear methods.

An exact diagnosis of different malignant growths is, however, only feasable by microscopic examination. The exploratory laporatomy requires more than any other diagnostic procedure a clear-cut indication and should, therefore, be considered at the very end of all methods.

Scintigrapic studies of intrahepatic tumors gain importance for the same reason because with experienced technique they can be performed without endangering the patient with a high degree of diagnostical certainty. In regard to the required surgical procedure the angiogram i.e. arteriogram and splenoportogram is still a must in diseases of the liver. Sometimes after removal of the primary tumor in selected patients partial resections of the liver to excise solitary metastases are successful. In dubious cases the exploratory laporatomy should be reserved for patients in whom during this operation a radical procedure can be done if the tumor is anatomically operable.

Diagnose primärer und sekundärer Lebertumoren

A. Bischof-Delaloye und B. Delaloye

Leider steht uns heute noch keine Substanz zur Verfügung, die sich selektiv im tumoralen Gewebe anreichert und so einen genauen Nachweis von Neoplasmen erlaubt. Wir müssen uns daher mit dem Nachweis kalter Zonen begnügen, also mitten in funktionellem Gewebe die Bereiche darstellen, die die radioaktive Substanz nicht zu konzentrieren vermögen.

Zur Lösung dieser Aufgabe stehen uns heute eine Vielzahl von Substanzen, Radioisotopen und Detektoren zur Verfügung, von denen wir nur die besprechen wollen, die wir zum jetzigen Zeitpunkt für die geeignetsten halten.

Unsere Erfahrung beruht auf der Auswertung von 6830 Szintigrammen, aufgezeichnet nach Radiogoldkolloid-Injektion und von 1200 Dokumenten der Gammakamera nach i.v. Injektion von Technetium-99m-Schwefelkolloid. Wir haben festgestellt, daß beim Verdacht einer Invasion der Leber durch neoplastisches Gewebe,

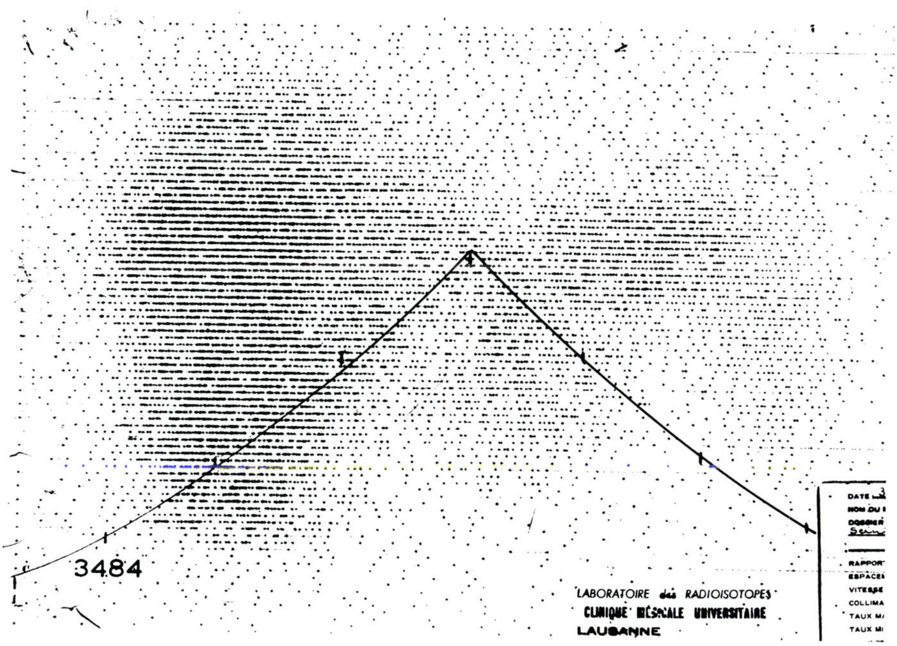

Abb. 1

besonders wenn es sich um die Aufdeckung kleiner Bezirke handelt, die letztere Methode erfolgreicher ist.

10–15-min nach der Injektion von 2 mCi Technetium-99^{m}-Schwefelkolloid beginnen wir mit der Aufzeichnung. Die geringe Energie des Technetiums erlaubt uns, eine Beeinflussung durch tieferliegende Schichten weitgehend auszuschalten

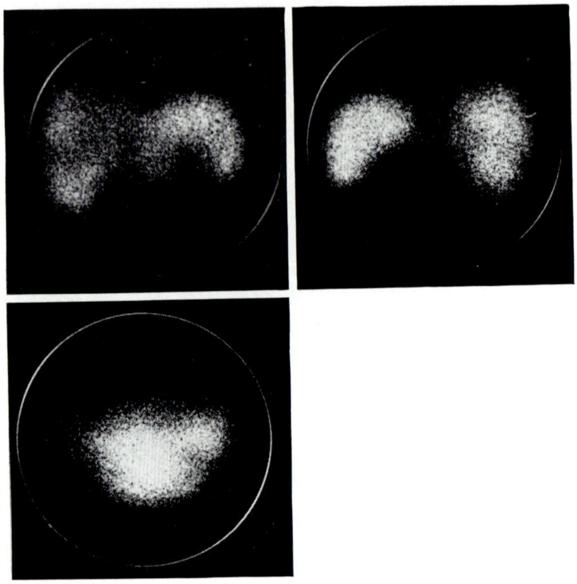

1130

Abb. 2a–c

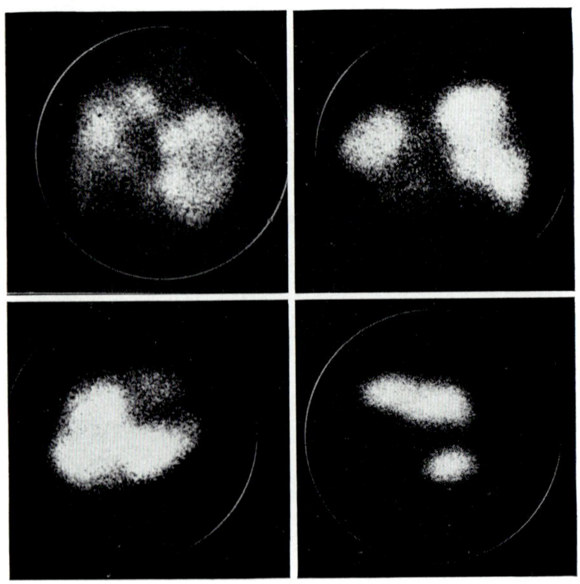

3196

Abb. 3a–d

und so die Leber von drei verschiedenen Seiten aus (ventral, dorsal und rechtslateral) bis jeweils in eine Tiefe von 4–5 cm, d. h. also den größten Teil ihres Parenchyms zu untersuchen.

Zur Aufzeichnung verwenden wir die Szintillationskamera nach Anger (Pho Gamma III, Nuclear Chicago). Der Szintigraph arbeitet zu langsam und ist besonders bei der Suche nach kleinen Defekten zu wenig genau.

Um wirklich verläßliche Aussagen machen zu können, schien es uns notwendig, unsere Ergebnisse quantitativ auszuwerten. Deshalb haben wir unsere Kamera an ein Datenverarbeitungssystem angeschlossen. Als digitalen Speicher benützen wir einen zweidimensionalen 1600-Kanal-Analysator. Dieser ist über ein Interface direkt an einen Computer PDP8 angeschlossen. Der Rechner ist mit einem 8000-Wort-Speicher versehen und hat als Zusatzgeräte einen Teletype ASR33 der zum Dialog dient, zwei Magnetbandspeicher und einen "Incremental Plotter" zur Aufzeichnung der Isoaktivitätslinien.

Zur Demonstration möchten wir einige Dokumente zeigen.

Nach intravenöser Injektion von 300 μCi Radiogoldkolloid haben wir dieses Szintigramm (Abb. 1) bei einer Patientin mit einem Mamma-Carcinom aufgezeichnet, das auf den ersten Blick eine vergrößerte Leber erkennen läßt, die besonders in ihrem

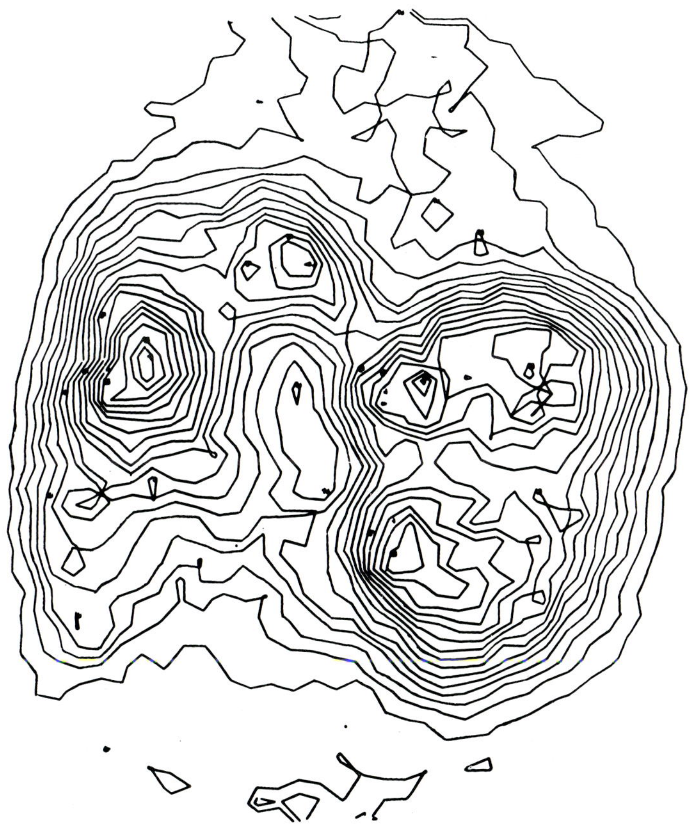

Abb. 4

linken Lappen heterogen ist. Daneben stellen wir eine Hilusvergrößerung und eine Betonung der Cava-Furche fest. Außerdem besteht eine bedeutende extrahepatische Speicherung des Kolloids, die Milz ist gut dargestellt.

Auf der Aufnahme der Szintillationskamera nach intravenöser Injektion von 2 mCi Technetium-99m-Schwefelkolloid (Abb. 2) bemerken wir in ventraler Projektion (a) einen Defekt im rechten unteren Leberlappen, von dorsal etwas weniger sichtbar (b), da er hier weniger ausgedehnt ist, wie auch die rechtslaterale Projektion (c) bestätigt.

Auf den analogen Dokumenten (Abb. 3), die unter den gleichen technischen Bedingungen wie Abbildung 2 bei einer anderen Patientin erzielt wurden, fallen uns in ventraler Ebene eine Lebervergrößerung und mehrere Aussparungen in beiden Leberlappen auf. Von dorsal ist nur eine Aussparung rechts-marginal sichtbar, auf der rechtslateralen Projektion hingegen sind die Defekte des rechten cranialen Leberlappens deutlich sichtbar. Auf der linkslateralen Projektion bemerkt man nur eine kleine Aussparung.

Wenn wir dieses Ergebnis mit Hilfe unseres Rechners quantitativ auswerten, erhalten wir eine Darstellung der Isoaktivitätslinien (Abb. 4). Die funktionellen Bereiche treten dabei noch besser hervor als auf dem analogen Bild. Vor allem aber kann ihr funktioneller Wert quantitativ erfaßt werden. So sehen wir, daß zwischen den noch gesunden und den erkrankten Bezirken ein Aktivitätsabfall von bis zu 80% besteht.

Scintigraphie et angiographie dans le diagnostic – du kyste hydatique du foie

DJ. RAHMOUNI

En terre d'endémie hydatique le pronostic est encore mauvais et cela principalement du fait des complications infectieuses et hémodynamiques.

La scintigraphie montre le défect et l'hypertrophie compensatrice du lobe hépatique sain.

L'angiographie du tronc coeliaque, de l'artère mesentérique supérieure et de la veine cave inférieure:

1. Précise la nature avasculaire du défect isotopique.
2. Montre un liseré en cas d'infection.
3. Délimite la vésicule biliaire et permet de poser le diagnostic de cholecystite.
4. Précise les rapports avec les vaisseaux.
5. Soulève l'hypothèse de cirrhose biliaire.
6. Enfin pose le diagnostic d'hypertention portale et de Budd-Chiari.

Dans de nombreux cas, quand le kyste a une extention extra-parenchymateuse, seule l'angiographie permet le diagnostic positif et différenciel.

Les deux méthodes sont complémentaires et doivent éliminer la splénoportographie qui peut être dangereuse dans certains cas.

Comparative study of Angiography and Scanning in Diseases of the Liver

P. Rossi and H. R. Gould

The study comprises review of approximately 1500 liver scans and 500 celiac anteriograms performed in the last few years at St. Vincent's Hospital in New York City. Over 100 patients were examined by both techniques (liver scan and celiac arteriography). Of these cases studied by combined approach, the cases selected also had confirmation of findings either by liver biopsy or by surgical or post-mortem studies. The various angiographic signs for each disease were tabulated and classified. The accuracy, relative value, advantages of each method will be presented.

Angiographische und szintigraphische Untersuchungen der Abdominalorgane

R. Höfer

Die angiographische Darstellung der Gefäße der Abdominalorgane vor allem nach selektiver Katheterisierung der Hauptstämme wie der A. coeliaca und der A. mesenterica cranialis hat seit den Publikationen von Ödmann im Jahre 1958 weite Verbreitung gefunden. Nachdem Taplin und Wagner zeigen konnten, daß sich das Capillarbett der Pulmonalarterie mit radioaktiv markierten Albuminpartikeln einer Größe von 5–50 micron szintigraphisch sehr gut darstellen ließ und nachdem sich in einer großen Anzahl von Untersuchungen gezeigt hatte, daß diese Mikroembolien keinerlei Funktionsstörung verursachen, war es naheliegend, auch andere Gefäßgebiete auf diese Weise zu untersuchen. Der intraarteriellen Applikation der Albuminpartikel in leicht zugängige Arterien, wie etwa der A. brachialis oder der A. carotis folgte bald die Applikation durch einen Katheter in die Gefäße der abdominellen Aorta. Der große Aufschwung ,den szintigraphische Techniken in den letzten 10 Jahren genommen hatten, begünstigte diese Entwicklung, obwohl von vornherein anzunehmen war, daß die Angioszintigraphie hinsichtlich der Organdarstellung nur bedingt mit der röntgenologischen Angiographie in Konkurrenz treten könnte. Allerdings ergeben sich aus der angioszintigraphischen Technik andere diagnostische Informationen als die reinen Organabbildungen ,durch die die Angioszintigraphie zu zusätzlicher Bedeutung gelangt.

Grundsätzlich liefert die angioszintigraphische Untersuchung eines Gefäßbezirkes 3 Informationsqualitäten, wie es Ueda instruktiv dargestellt hat.

1. Die direkte Information nach Injektion der Albuminpartikel in ein arterielles Gefäß ist die Darstellung des gesamten von diesem Gefäß versorgten Capillarbettes, das sog. Perfusionsszintigramm.

2. Bestehen Verbindungen zwischen dem Gefäß, in das die Partikel injiziert werden und dem venösen Schenkel des Versorgungsgebietes, so wird ein Teil der Partikel das dem Gefäß zugeordnete Capillarbett umgehen und im ersten nachgeschalteten Kapillarfilter (meist ist dies die Lunge) steckenbleiben und dort szintigraphisch nachzuweisen sein. Wir haben auf diese Weise die Möglichkeit, arteriovenöse Shunts zu diagnostizieren.

3. Werden von dem Gefäß, in das die Partikel injiziert werden, mehrere diskrete Capillargebiete versorgt, so ist es möglich, aus der in jedem der beiden Capillarfilter enthaltenen Aktivität darauf zu schließen, welcher Anteil des Blutstromes im Hauptgefäß jedem der Capillargebiete zuströmt.

Für alle diese drei Möglichkeiten der Anwendung der Angioszintigraphie liegen für die Gefäße der Bauchaorta Untersuchungen vor.

1. Die Darstellung von Abdominalorganen mit Hilfe der Perfusionsszintigraphie stößt durch die Anatomie der Gefäßversorgung auf große Schwierigkeiten, da es praktisch unmöglich ist, den Katheter, durch den die Partikel injiziert werden, so selektiv einzuführen, daß ein *nur das interessierende Organ* versorgendes Gefäß erreicht wird. Selbst bei ausgefeiltester Technik der selektiven Katheterisierung, wird man sich mit Katheterpositionen zufrieden geben müssen, die eine gleichzeitige perfusionsszintigraphische Darstellung verschiedener Organe mit verschiedener Intensität ergeben, was die Interpretation der gewonnenen Bilder schwierig macht und die diagnostische Aussagekraft im Vergleich mit der röntgenologischen Angiographie einschränkt. Der Vorteil im Vergleich mit der röntgenologischen Angiographie bleibt hier, daß das Perfusionsszintigramm eine Fixierung der Parenchymphase darstellt.

Praktisch wurde diese Methode von uns (OGRIS) bisher in erster Linie zur Darstellung des Pankreas verwendet, wobei versucht wird, die Katheterspitze möglichst weit in die A. hepatica communis vorzuschieben. Es kommt dabei zu einer sich überlagernden Darstellung, insbesondere von Leber und Pankreaskopf, sowie einer Aktivität im Magen aus der A. gastrica dextra. Während es nicht möglich ist, die gastrische Aktivität zu korrigieren, läßt sich durch jede gangbare Subtraktionsmethode – wir verwendeten die fotographische Subtraktion nach Injektion von Goldkolloid – die Leberaktivität vom Perfusionsszintigramm der A. hepatica communis subtrahieren, wodurch Darstellungen des Pankreas bzw. von Pankreastumoren von zufriedenstellender Qualität gewonnen werden können. Es muß jedoch zugegeben werden, daß die Kombination von röntgenologischer Angiographie mit technisch ausgefeilter Pankreasszintigraphie mit Selen-Methionin hier bessere Resultate bringt. Auch bei der reinen Abbildung von Leber und Milz hat sich die Angioszintigraphie bisher nicht durchgesetzt, obwohl für die Darstellung z. B. von Infarkten in diesen Organen die Angioszintigraphie die Technik der Wahl sein sollte.

Gelegentlich kann der Nachweis, ob ein abdomineller Tumor aus der Mesenterica superior versorgt wird, oder nicht, Aufschlüsse über einen Tumor bringen, wie etwa bei einem beobachteten Ovarialcystom, doch kann natürlich die gleiche Information durch die röntgenologische Angiographie geliefert werden.

Ein weiteres Anwendungsgebiet der Perfusionsszintigraphie der Abdominalorgane ist die Darstellung der Nieren und vor allem der Nebennieren, die durch Injektion des Kontrastmittels in die Bauchaorta im Bereich des Abganges der Aa. renales bzw. der Aa. suprarenales oder aber, wie HAAS zeigen konnte, nach selektiver Katheterisation der rechten oder linken A. phrenica möglich ist.

2. Während die perfusionsszintigraphische Darstellung der Abdominalorgane bisher keine entscheidenden Fortschritte gebracht hat, verspricht die Shuntbestimmung eine Bereicherung unserer diagnostischen Möglichkeiten zu sein. Der einfachste Zugang zu dem interessierenden Gefäß, der Vena portae, ist in diesem Fall die Punktion der Milz und die intralineale Injektion des Indikators, wie bei der Splenoportographie. Normalerweise werden die mit der Vena lienalis abtransportierten Albuminpartikel in die Vena portae transportiert und bleiben in den Capillaren bzw. Präcapillaren der Leber stecken. Szintigraphisch findet sich Aktivität im Milzdepot und in der Leber. Bestehen portosystemische Kurzschlüsse, so wird ein Teil der Partikel direkt in den venösen Kreislauf geshuntet und kann dann in den Lungencapillaren wiedergefunden werden: szintigraphisch stellen sich nunmehr Milzdepot,

Leber und Lunge dar. Diese Methode erwies sich bei unseren Untersuchungen als sehr empfindlich.

Neben dem qualitativen Nachweis von Shunts ist mit dieser Methode auch ohne weiteres eine Quantifizierung möglich, sei es nach der Methode von Mostbeck, sei es unter Verwendung einer Kamera mit Vielkanal, wie wir es bei cerebralen Shunts praktizieren.

3. Zirkulationsgrößen in den Abdominalorganen bei Veränderungen des portalen Druckes sind für den Kliniker von großem Interesse und jede neue Methode, die grundsätzlich Information zu dieser Problematik bringt, bedeutet eine wertvolle Bereicherung unserer diagnostischen Möglichkeiten.

Die einleitend angeführte dritte Anwendungsart der Angioszintigraphie, nämlich die Bestimmung des relativen Blutangebotes an verschiedene Kapillargebiete aus einem Stammgefäß, wurde von Ueda zur Schätzung der relativen Durchblutung von Leber und Milz verwendet.

Nach besonders sorgfältiger Positionierung der Katheterspitze in der Arteria coeliaca möglichst weit proximal vom Abgang der Arteria hepatica und der Arteria lienalis wird unter konstantem Druck makroaggregiertes Albumin injiziert und daraufhin die Aktivität über Leber und Milz szintigraphisch registriert. Normalerweise ist das arterielle Blutangebot an Leber und Milz annähernd gleich groß, bei der Cirrhose kommt es zu einer wesentlichen Bevorzugung der Leber, während bei der idiopathischen portalen Hypertension etwa die Milz den Großteil des arteriellen Blutes erhält.

Zusammenfassend ist die Angioszintigraphie der Abdominalorgane, soweit es die Organdarstellung durch eine fixierte Parenchymphase betrifft, durch die Schwierigkeit der selektiven Katheterisierung und die sich daraus ergebenden Überlagerungen sich abbildender Organe kompliziert. Wieweit angioszintigraphische Untersuchungen mit der röntgenologischen Angiographie konkurrieren bzw. diese ergänzen können, muß erst durch größere Untersuchungsserien gezeigt werden. In der Shuntdiagnostik aber und der Schätzung der Verteilung des Blutangebotes aus einem arteriellen Stammgefäß hat die angioszintigraphische Technik jedenfalls neue Möglichkeiten eröffnet.

Combined Angiographic and Scintigraphic Investigations of the Liver

L. M. Freeman

In the past decade, liver scanning has contributed greatly to the diagnosis and understanding of a number of hepatic disorders such as benign and malignant neoplastic processes (primary and secondary), inflammatory disease, diffuse parenchymal diseases such as cirrhosis and traumatic lesions.

However, the findings as seen on scan are relatively nonspecific. Benign hepatic cysts, abscesses and metastatic disease would all present as single or multiple filling defects. Pseudomasses in cirrhosis could not accurately be differentiated from a superimposed hepatoma on the basis of scan alone. The end result of a traumatic lesion may be seen on the scan as a filling defect which usually represents a hepatoma. However, the underlying damage causing the bleeding would remain a mystery without further investigation.

Celiac angiography has offered a definitive solution to most of these aforementioned problems and has in this fashion complemented and clarified the findings seen on the hepatic scan. The better resolution of the radiographic study has on occasion given clearer delineation of lesions that may have been suspected or even entirely missed on the scan. The extent of a disease process is often better appreciated when the results of both the scan and angiogram are available.

Recent advances in hepatic surgery have also created a need for precise anatomic delineation of the vascular supply to the liver. Celiac angiography affords one the opportunity to obtain this extremely valuable and necessary information.

Hepatic scanning is an easily performed innocuous procedure that may be used even in seriously ill patients. Stationary camera devices have significantly decreased the time required to perform the study. Celiac angiography requires skill and more specialized equipment to perform. It has often clarified problems that have existed on the scan and therefore, when used in specific selected situation has helpfully complemented the radioisotope procedure.

Zur Angiographie-Szintigraphie im Abdominalraum

H. G. Claus und J. P. Haas

Die günstigen Erfahrungen mit der Angioszintigraphie der Nieren waren für uns Anlaß, diese Methode auch auf die Leber, Milz und den Darm auszudehnen.

Bei der Angioszintigraphie der Leber ist die oft doppelte, aus dem Stromgebiet der A. coeliaca und der A. mesenterica cranialis stammende Blutversorgung zu berücksichtigen. Als Beispiel hier das Angioszintigramm eines Patienten, bei dem wir uns wegen einer zweizeitigen Milzruptur mit großem perilienalem Hämatom auf die selektive Untersuchung der A. coeliaca beschränkten. Dadurch ist es zu einer starken Anreicherung im linken Leberlappen gekommen; die rechte Leberarterie entspringt aus der A. mesenterica cranialis. Die auffallend geringe Aktivitätsanreicherung der Milz ist sehr wahrscheinlich die Folge einer starken Minderdurchblutung nach Ruptur. Normalerweise wird die in die A. coeliaca injizierte Aktivität überwiegend von der Milz akkumuliert.

Bei diesem Patienten mit Zustand nach Cholecystektomie war offenbar unter der Operation ein größerer Ast der Leberarterie unterbunden worden, die arterielle Gefäßversorgung der Leber erfolgt z. T. über Kollateralen. Die arterielle Minder-

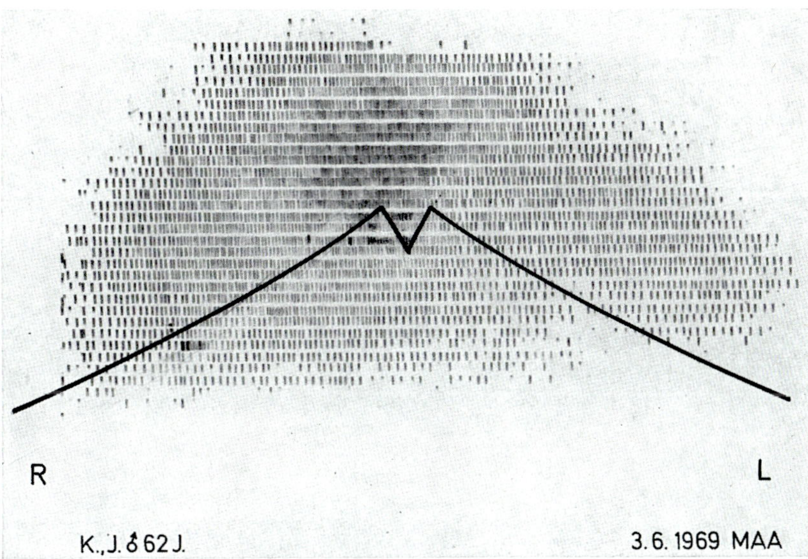

Abb. 1

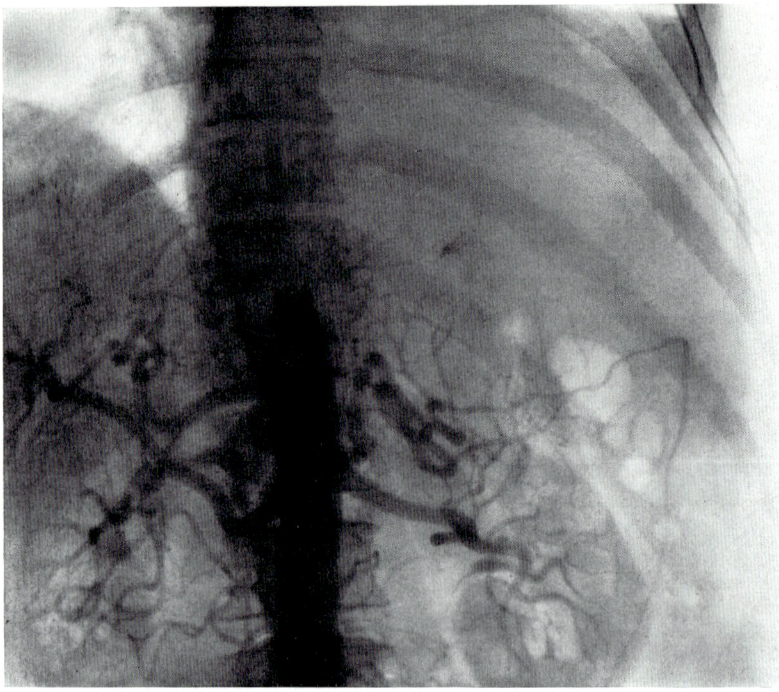

Abb. 2

durchblutung und die Größe des hiervon betroffenen Leberbezirkes gehen wesentlich besser aus dem Angioszintigramm als aus dem Technetium-99-m-Schwefel-Kolloid-Szintigramm hervor.

Ähnlich war dies auch bei raumfordernden Leberprozessen, wie Cysten und Metastasen.

Bei dieser Patientin mit zweimal operierten Echinokokkuscysten läßt das Angioszintigramm wesentlich besser als das Technetium-99m-Schwefel-Kolloid-Szintigramm die cystenbedingten Aktivitätsaussparungen erkennen. Ja, es zeigt sogar besser als das Angiogramm die Ausdehnung, Lage und Größe der Echinokokkuscysten.

Was unserer Auffassung schon von sich aus für die Angioszintigraphie der Leber spricht, ist die Größe dieses parenchymatösen Organes sowie sein Volumen. Durch die vielen intrahepatischen Gefäßvariationen, Gefäßüberkreuzungen und Überlagerungen ist die angiographische Orientierung oft erschwert. Nicht selten werden kleinere raumfordernde Prozesse, Kontrastmittel anreichernde oder aussparende, durch die beträchtliche Parenchymdicke dieses Organes überlagert oder verdeckt. Bei solch unklaren Prozessen stellt das Angioszintigramm nicht nur eine gute Ergänzung dar, sondern es besitzt den Vorzug der leichten Darstellungsmöglichkeit in der 2. Ebene.

Am Darm nahmen wir angioszintigraphische Untersuchungen bei Entzündungen und Tumoren vor. Dies ist das Angioszintigramm eines durch Laparatomie bestätigten, inoperablen Rezidivs eines Mesenterialfibroms, das zu einer erheblichen

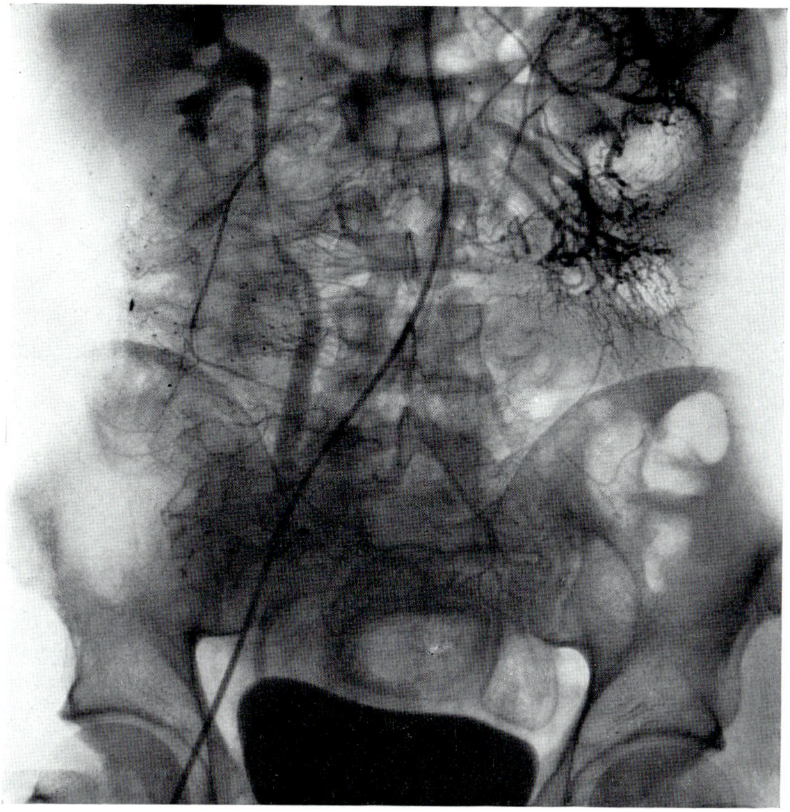

Abb. 3

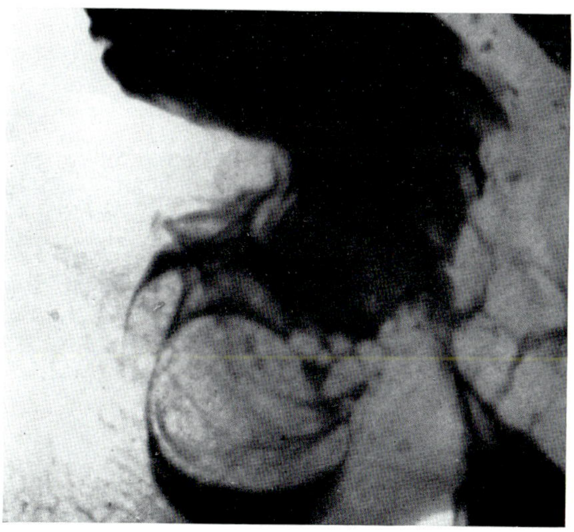

Abb. 4

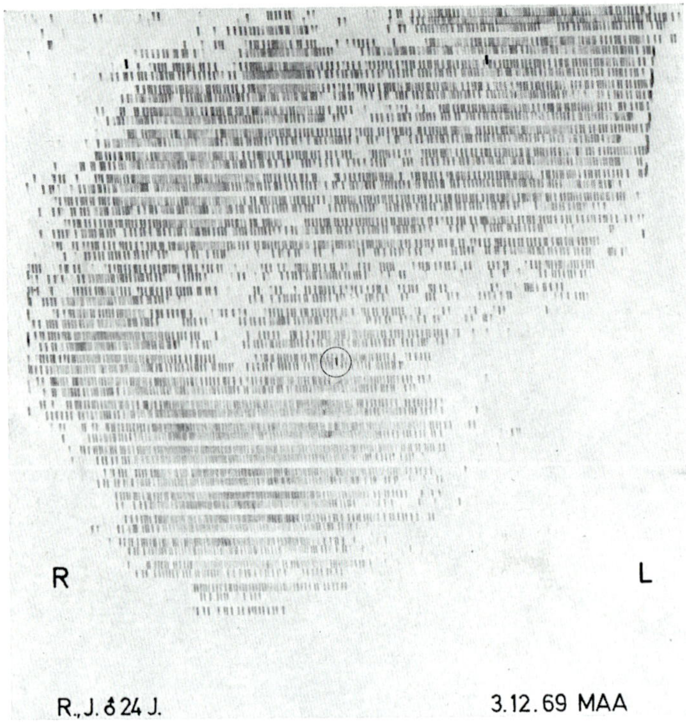

Abb. 5

Verdrängung der Darmgefäße geführt hat. Möglicherweise könnte man mit zunehmender Erfahrung in der Lage sein, aufgrund des angioszintigraphischen Bildes Aussagen über die *Benignität* und *Malignität* eines Tumors zu machen.

Auch bei den entzündlichen Darmerkrankungen konnten wir in der Ausdehnung und Lokalisation eines Prozesses eine gute angiographische und angioszintigraphische Übereinstimmung feststellen. Hier das angiographische Bild eines bei der Magen-Darm-Passage festgestellten Morbus Crohn, hier die Aktivitätsanreicherung im Bereich des erkrankten ileo-kolischen Darmabschnittes. Weitere Untersuchungen werden noch klären müssen, ob die angioszintigraphische Darstellbarkeit solcher Darmprozesse von der jeweiligen Verlaufsform und -phase der Entzündung abhängt.

Zusammenfassend kann gesagt werden, daß unsere ersten angioszintigraphischen Ergebnisse an Leber, Milz und Darm ermutigend sind. Die einzelnen Indikationen müssen aber noch genauer herausgearbeitet werden.

Comparative Studies on the Informational Value of Angiography, Scintigraphy and Ultrasonic Scanning in Hepatic Disorders

H. Imhof, Ch. Jantsch, A. Kratochwil, H. Pokieser and H. Umek

Using a total case material of 20 patients with various hepatic disorders – verified by biopsy or autopsy – the value of the information provided by the diagnostic techniques listed below was compared:

1. Angiography carried out as selective celiacography, using the standard method.
2. Scintigraphy – with an Anger camera[1] under conditions of respiratory arrest, following intravenous injection of TcS colloid; with a linear scanner following administration of Au-colloid.
3. Ultrasonic scanning – using a combined "A" and "B" scanner (Kretz).

Results

Out of 20 cases (Table) had carcinoma of the liver and 6 hepatic metastases. In all instances the tumorous formations were larger than 2 cm in diameter. Scintigraphy revealed the blastomas in all cases. Angiography of the celiac artery and ultrasonic techniques failed to discover a peripheral metastasis with the size of a tangerine which was located in the right hepatic 6 patients suffered from cirrhosis of the liver; in three of those no verification was possible by either of the three techniques.

The third group included cholestases of extrahepatic origin, one case of steatosis and one of chronic hepatitis. Examination of these patients was carried out in order to find evidence of a blastomatous process. Ultrasound and angiography both furnished a false positive diagnosis in case of a pancreas carcinoma with cholestasis and cholangitis. Echogram (ultrasound) and scintigram visualized structures highly suspicious of metastases in a case involving steatosis with giant hepatomegaly; however, neither angiography nor autopsy confirmed the echographic findings. All three techniques wrongly interpreted a large space-occupying process on the hepatic hilus as a metastatic growth of a gastric carcinoma that had been surgically removed three years before. Autopsy, however, revealed a choledochus carcinoma with regional lymph node metastases as the primary source – the liver as such being free from metastases.

---

1 We are grateful to the Clinic for Psychiatry and Neurology of the University of Vienna (Acting Head Dr. P. Berner) for putting their equipment at our disposal.

Table

	Scintigraphy	Angiography	Ultrasound
Tumors (primary and secondary): $n = 8$			
♂ B. L. N. hep.	+	+	+
♂ E. A. N. hep.	+	+	+
♂ Sch. L. Metastases in N. ventr.	+	+	+
♂ B. A. Metast. in N. duct. chol.	+	—	—
♂ M. R. Met. in N. coli	+	+	+
♂ H. H. Met. in hypernephroma	+	+	+
♀ F. J. Met. in N. pancr.	+	+	+
♀ P. G. Met. in N. pancr.	+	+	
Wrong Diagnoses:	0	1	1
Cirrhoses: $n = 6$			
♂ B. A. Cirr. hep. and N. pancr.	+	+	+
♂ K. H. Cirrh. hep.	+	+	—
♀ H. J. Cirrh. hep.	+	—	+
♂ G. E. Cirrh. hep.	+		+
♂ St. H. Cirrh. hep. and N. pancr.	—	+	+
♂ B. O. Cirrh. hep. and N. pancr.	+	+	+
Wrong Diagnoses:	1	1	1
Miscellaneous: $n = 6$			
♀ H. H. persisting hepatitis	—	—	—
♂ D. L. Cholestase	—	—	—
♂ S. K. N. duct. chol., meta ad portam hep.	+	+	+
♂ K. H. Cholestase in N. pancr., Cholangit.	—	+	+
♂ D. A. Steatosis, hypernephroma	+	—	+
♂ W. O. Cholestase in N. pancr.		—	—
Wrong Diagnoses:	2	2	3

Discussion

In 68 83% of the cases scintigraphy according to McAffee et al. successfully visualizes secondary blastomas; the same holds true of the scintigram according to Nagler, Bender, and Blau. Angiography in addition serves to locate centrally positioned tumors or small, richly vascularized tumorous structures of rare types (carcinoid growths, tumors of the islets of Langerhans, melanomas, tumors of the adrenal cortex).

In livers restructured due to cirrhosis, all three techniques were subject to errors because of the difficulty of differentiating regenerated areas of varying sizes from neoplastic processes. In cases where cholestasis is difficult to diagnose, angiography and the use of ultrasound scanning may furnish information on the primary process by visualizing adjacent organs.

Of the three techniques discussed, angiography alone allows a diagnosis of the type of tumor by direct visualization of the tumorous vessels.

Judging from the experience we have incurred, the diagnostic usefulness of the three techniques – scintigraphy, angiography and ultrasound – is about the same. However, the sources of error are different in each and therefore combined application results in a higher degree of diagnostic certainty.

In the future computer scintigraphy, super-selective angiography, pharmaco-angiography as well as more sophisticated techniques of applying ultrasound will improve the results still not satisfactory.

Pharmacoangiography by Intra-Arterial Injection of Nor-Adrenalin

M. Kaneko

Introduction

In 1966, 0.2 mg of nor-adrenalin was introduced into the celiac artery and marked contraction of the artery was observed. Thereafter, the dose was reduced to 0.1 mg or less to find out the minimum dose for the better pharmaco-angiography. The timing of injection was also investigated. The purposes of this paper are

1. to decide the dose of nor-adrenalin, and
2. to decide the timing of injection.

Method

Nor-adrenalin solution 1 mg/cc was diluted 5 to 10 times by saline for arterial injection. The patient for pharmaco-angiography was selected in the catergory of lower blood pressure than 150 in systolic and 100 in diastolic pressure and no abnormality of ECG. Blood pressure changes were measured, immediately after intra-arterial injection of noradrenalin, until they returned to normal. In the first series of 80 cases, the angiography was started after blood pressure elevation was observed. The doses of nor-adrenalin were 0.1, 0.08, 0.06, 0.04 and 0.02 mg. The arteries examined were mostly celiac artery and beside this, sup. mesenteric, renal, bronchial

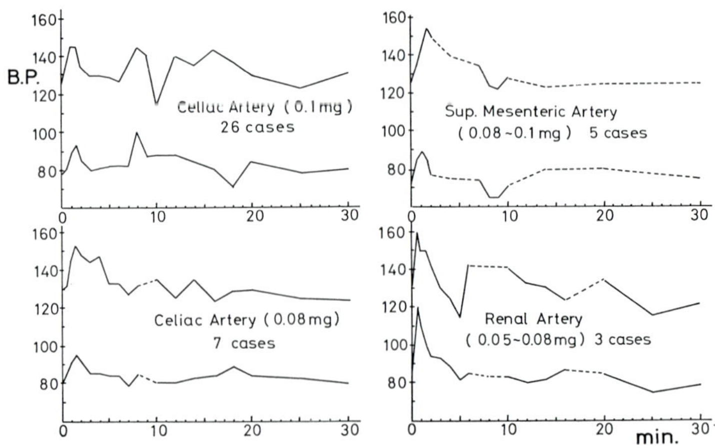

Fig. 1. Blood pressure changes by intra-arterial nor-adrenalin injection

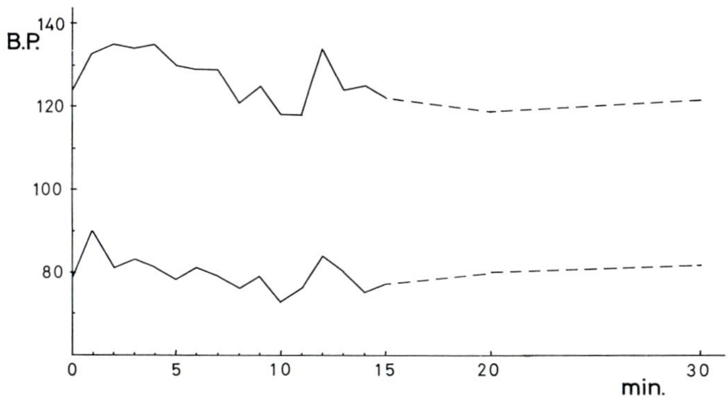

Fig. 2. Blood pressure changes by simultaneous intra-arterial injection of nor-adrenalin and contrast media. Celiac artery (nor-adrenalin 0.02 mg); 20 cases

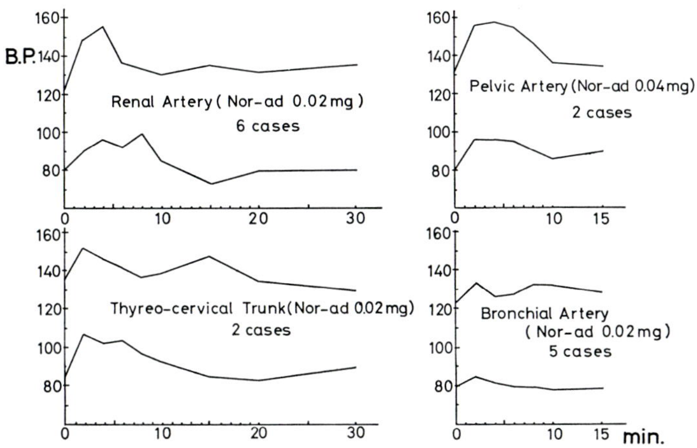

Fig. 3. Blood pressure changes by simultaneous intra-arterial injection of nor-adrenalin and contrast media. Celiac and sup. mesenteric arteries (nor-ad. 0.04 mg); 65 cases

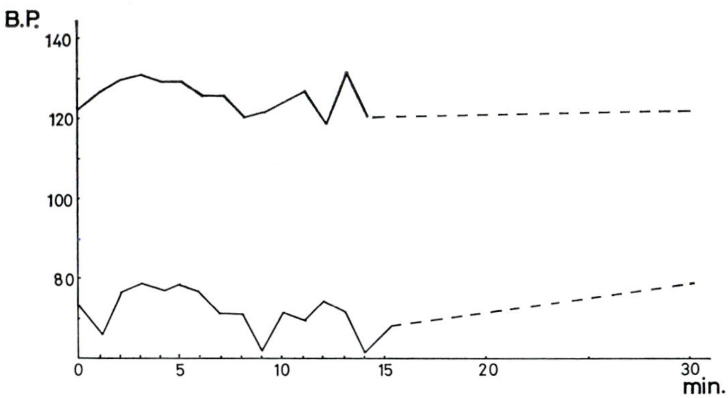

Fig. 4. Blood pressure changes by simultaneous intra-arterial injection of nor-adrenalin and contrast media

and pelvic arteries were injected. The dose of contrast medium and the pressure of injection were reduced to slightly less than normal angiography, to prevent the overflow from the catheter.

For the 2nd series of cases, simultaneous injection of nor-adrenalin and contrast medium was done. Celiac arteries were mostly examined for the malignant disease of liver, gall bladder and pancreas etc. The dose for celiac, sup. mesenteric and pelvic arteries was 0.04 mg and for renal, bronchial and thyreocervical was 0.02 mg. In the last series of 20 cases, 0.02 mg of nor-adrenalin was simultaneously injected with contrast medium to celiac artery. In these simultaneous injection, the dose of contrast medium and the pressure of injection were the same as conventional method. Blood pressure was measured before and after angiography until the pressure returned to normal state.

Results

In the first series, 63 celiac, 7 sup. mesenteric, 5 renal, 3 pelvic and 2 bronchial arteries were examined in total number of 80 cases. The elevation of blood pressure raised upto maximum in 2 to 3 min and returned to normal within 10 min in most of the cases with celiac artery injection. For renal arteries, it took more time to return to normal state. In some cases, lower blood pressure was recorded before it returned to normal.

The results of angiography were classified into 4 groups. Group I: Contraction of the artery was more than $^1/_2$ and other unnecessary arteries were also visualized due to the overflow of contrast medium.

Group II: Contraction was between 1 and $^1/_2$, but the same vascular demonstration as Group I.

Group III: Contraction was between 1 and $^1/_2$, and ideal demonstration of vasculature without overflow of the contrast medium. Group IV: Almost no visible contraction of the artery without any effect.

As in the cases of celiac artery, the results were summarized in the table and the dose of 0.04 mg showed appropriate to have most in group III.

In macro-roentgenography of renal artery, glomerulography is possible and it is further advantageous to inject noradrenalin after contrast medium injection, which arrested the renal blood flow for a while and oppacified the glomeruli more distinctly.

In the 2nd series, simultaneous injection was done by filling the nor-adrenalin in the catheter and by injecting the contrast medium at the same time into the artery. The cases were 80 in total, including 63 celiac, 2 sup. mesenteric, 6 renal, 2 pelvic, 5 bronchial and 2 thyreo-cervial. 0.04 mg was introduced into the celiac artery, and the mean elevation of blood pressure was 21 in systolic and 12 in diastolic. The duration was also within 10 min.

In this series, no contraction was observed in the main branches of the artery, but in the periphery. Proximal branches were also well demonstrated to the periphery and most favorably the tumor vessels were more clear and the tumor stain was more contrasted with the contraction of normal arteries. It was surprising to demonstrate the lymph node invaded by malignancy with this simultaneous injection of nor-adrenalin and contrast medium. It was obvious that all the contrast medium had been injected into the artery before the artery began to contract in about 3 sec later,

Table. *Effects of intra-arterial injection of Nor-Adrenalin*

Group			I	II	III	IV	
Arterial Contraction (++: 0–1/2; +: 1/2–1; –: 1)			++	+	+	–	
Demonstration of Tumor Vessels and/or Proximal Branches			+	+	+	–	
Demonstration of other Vessels			+	+	–	–	
Injected Arteries	Dose	Mean Blood Pressure Elevation (max/min)					Total
Ceriac A.	0.1 mg	27/15	10	5	9	2	26
Ceriac A.	0.08 mg	20/14	1	2	5	0	8
Ceriac A.	0.06 mg	29/14	5	5	4	0	14
Ceriac A.	0.04 mg	26/11	3	1	9	2	15
Sup mesent A.	0.1 mg	27/22	3	1	3	0	7
Renal A.	0.08 mg	32/25	1	0	0	0	1
Renal A.	0.06 mg	10/10	0	0	1	0	1
Renal A.	0.04 mg	37/23	0	1	1	0	2
Renal A.	0.02 mg	30/30	0	0	0	1	1
Pelvic A.	0.1 mg	70/20	0	0	1	0	1
Pelvic A.	0.04 mg	36/22	0	1	1	0	2
Bronchial A.	0.02 mg	20/23	1	0	1	0	2
Total			24	16	35	5	80

therefore, no overflow of the contrast medium and rejection of the catheter had been rarely observed.

In last series of 20 cases, the simultaneous injection of nor-adrenalin in the dose of 0.02 mg into the celiac artery revealed the effectiveness of nor-adrenalin on the artery and good demonstration of tumor vessels and tumor stain. But in 5 of 20 cases, no effect of nor-adrenalin was obtained. The mean elevation of blood pressure was 12 in systolic and 6 in diastolic. But in most of cases the blood pressure change was very slight or nothing, and in some cases, the blood pressure was lowered without initial elevation. Therefore, 0.04 mg was apperantly more consistent in the effect of nor-adrenalin than 0.02 mg.

Discussion

Pharmaco-angiography was first applied by Abrams, H. L. in 1962 to renal artery and it has been given a good attention as an interesting method of angiography to demonstrate the tumor vessels since 1964. But the method is not yet completely established for the kind of drug, the dose and the timing of administration, suitable for the pharmaco-angiography. Noradrenalin seemed suitable for the aged patients, because of less influence on the heart and greater effect on the peripheral vessels. The dose was sufficient enough with 0.04 mg for celiac artery, and it seemed the less, the safer for the risk. But 0.02 mg is still effective on the artery, therefore, the dose must be investigated further for the appropriate dose. The timing of injection is most important for demonstrating the tumor vessels and stain.

Simultaneous inection is one of the excellent ways to do so. But, KAHN, in Harvard Univ., had given warning of increasing toxicity, when simultaneous injection of contrast media and nor-adrenalin was made in animal experiment. But in our cases, no side effect of contrast medium has been experienced with simultaneous injection so far.

One shot therapy, that is injecting chemotherapy drug into the artery with one procedure, or radioisotope injection was also carried out, combined with nor-adrenalin, and it was learned useful for tumor selectivity and long retaining in the tumor.

Conclusion

As a pharmaco-angiography, when nor-adrenalin was applied for intra-arterial injection, the elevation of blood pressure was minimal and transient in a dose of 0.04 mg. Simultaneous injection of nor-adrenalin and contrast medium was useful for demonstrating tumor vessels, stain, and lymph node invaded by malignancy, as well, which made this technique more valuable.

Comparative Study of Angiography and Scintigraphy in the Diagnosis of Liver Disease

T. SASAKI

It has been developed the various diagnostic tools in the examination of liver disease. Particularly in the radiology field there has been developed the selective hepatic angiography (Seldinger technique), liver scanning (Scintiscanner) and liver scintiphotography (Scinticamera).

In order to evaluate the diagnostic values of these three radiological examining methods, the radiological informations obtained from these methods are comparatively studied.

Methods and Materials

The liver scanning is taken with Shimadzu 30-type 3 in. scanner, in the antero-posterior view in the supine position following the injection of 150 μCi of ^{198}Au-colloid.

The liver scintiphotography is performed with Nuclear Chicago Pho/Gamma Scinticamera in a several exposures such as AP, oblique and lateral views in the supine position following the injection of ^{198}Au-colloid and/or ^{99m}Tc-S-colloid.

The selective hepatic angiography is performed with a Seldinger technique using Ödman green catheter. The contrast medium Angiografin 30 ml is injected automatically under the pressure of 2 kg/cm^2. The exposure factors are 85 kVp, 300 mA and 0.08 sec. The films are taken one per second for a period of 15 sec.

The cases subjected to study are as follows: Primary hepatic cancer 16, metastatic hepatic cancer 65 (gastric cancer 27, gastric sarcoma 1, pancreatic cancer 10, renal cancer 2, ureteric cancer 1, colonic cancer 11, papilla cancer 2, ovarial cancer 1, lung cancer 5, biliary cancer 1, duodenal cancer 1, esophageal cancer 1, pharyngeal cancer 1, melanoma 1).

In the casuistics review 6 cases of primary hepatic cancer and 7 of liver metastasis were demonstrated.

Results

In order to evaluate the diagnostic value for three methods such as liver scanning, liver scintiphotography and hepatic arteriography, the grades of diagnostic ability are divided into 4 categories such as impossible to diagnose, possible to diagnose, easily possible to diagnose and measurablly possible to diagnose.

The diagnostic abilities are evaluated to 87.5, 87.5 and 100% in primary liver cancer respectively and 75.4, 92.3 and 100% in metastatic liver cancer respectively in scanning, scintiphotography and hepatic arteriography.

The degree of diagnostic ability is improved in the order of scanning and scintiphotography and then arteriography.

On the other hand the cases examined with ^{198}Au-colloid and ^{99m}Tc-S-colloid are compared with hepatic arteriography. ^{99m}Tc-S-colloid liver scintiphotography can be taken within the exposure time of 20 sec with the patient's breath-hold. This makes the scintigram much clear when compared to that of ^{198}Au-colloid scintiphotography.

Discussion and Conclusion

Liver scanning and liver scintiphotography indirectly demonstrate the lesions as a negative defect. On the other hand the hepatic arteriography directly demonstrates the lesions as vascular increase and tumor stain.

In the scanning and scintiphotography of the liver, ^{198}Au-colloid is up-taken into the normal liver tissues. Therefore the lesions are presented as a negative defect which is rather difficult to recognize as a lesion for us.

When compared to liver scanning, the liver scintiphotography by scinticamera is superior in view of resolving power. That is, the resolving power is 20×20 mm in scanning and that is 10×10 mm in scinticamera. In scintiphotography the exposure time is much shorter than that of scanning. This makes possible to take the liver scintiphotography in a various directions.

And recently ^{99m}Tc-S-colloid liver scintiphotography come into practice. It makes possible to take the scintigram with breath-hold. The image quality of liver scintigraphy is improved because of less motion secondary to respiration.

Hepatic arteriography can be shown the lesion with detail vascular architecture, as a possitive shadow such as tumor stain and vascular increase. The diagnostic ability is superior than that of scanning and scintiphotography.

Liver scintiphotography is improved in diagnostic ability when compared to liver scanning, and is nearly closer to that of hepatic arteriography.

Angiography and Comparative Scintigraphic Findings in Space-occupying Lesions of the Liver

R. Steckenmesser, S. Bayindir, N. Heger and S. F. Grebe

Space-occupying lesions of the liver can be detected scintigraphically when they reach a dimension of 3–4 cm in diameter. Non-vascularised processes can be displayed at a sice of between 2–3 cm in diameter by the use of selective arteriography, vascularised processes even at a sice of less than 1 cm. Marginal and diffuse expansion

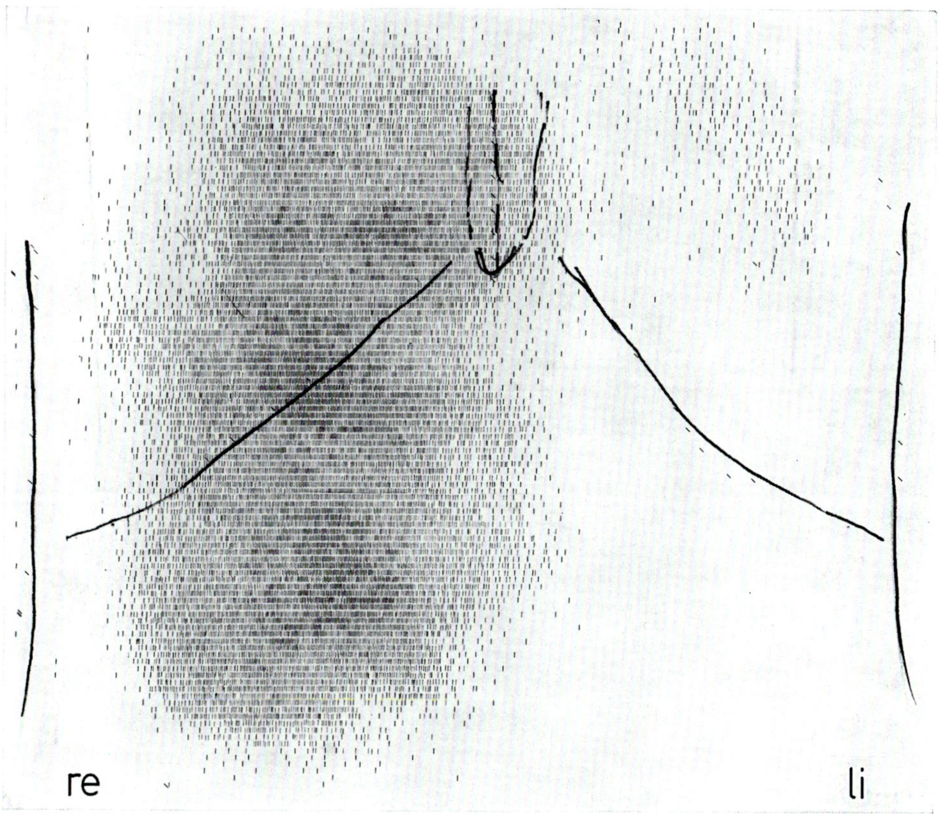

Fig. 1. The liver scanning of a 50-year-old patient in whom bilateral cystic kidneys were found 17 years ago, shows a caudal enlargement of the liver with marginal polycycloidally limited accumulation defects and reduced accumulation within the liver

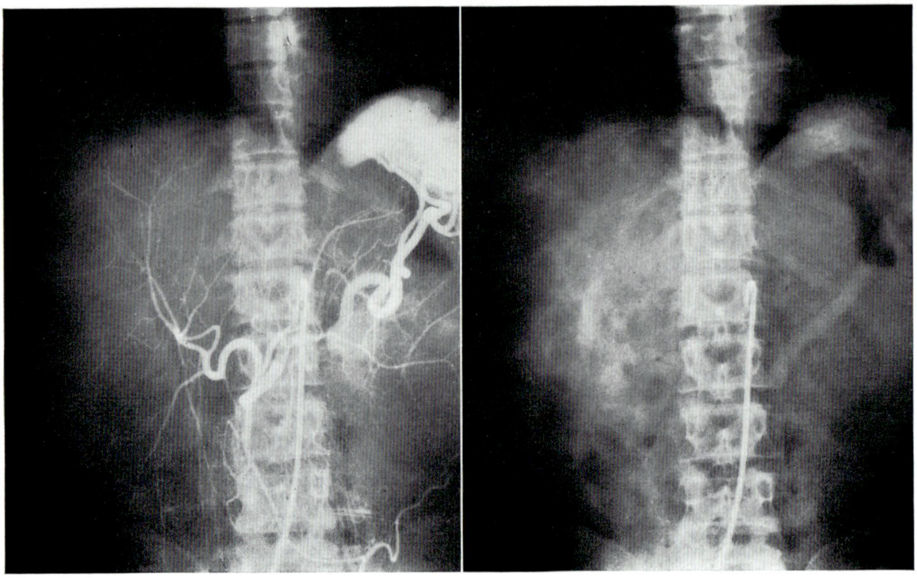

a b

Fig. 2. a In the arterial phase the coeliacography in the same patient shows an enlargement of the liver with arch-like stretched vessels and poorly vascularised areas in – between. The arteries are remarkably frail compared to the large liver. The diagnosis read cystic liver.
b The same patient, parenchymal phase (proof by autopsy)

facilitates the detection by scintigraphy and arteriography. As the performance of scintigraphy is not at all complicated it becomes – to an increaring extent – the primary screening test when a space-occupying process of the liver is suspected.

While the scanning allows only to detect a space-occupying process of the liver, the arteriography of the liver can often – because of the alterated vascular structure – indicate the type of a tumour and allow decision whether it is benign or malignant.

The selective arteriography of the liver is indicted:

1. in all scanning defects that cannot be related to a certain disease,

2. in scintigraphically detected processes of the liver before the surgical intervention,

3. in all dubious scintigraphic findings.

The following angiograms and scintigrams are supposed to demonstrate the potentials and limits of the both methods.

Hepatic Scintigraphy and Venography in the Budd-Chiari Syndrome

E. J. Wood, A. S. Tavill and L. Kreel

At the Royal Free Hospital in London, a diagnosis of the Budd-Chiari Syndrome (hepatic vein outflow block) has been made in 14 patients. In this condition both the liver scans and venograms display characteristic appearances.

The liver scans were carried out using radioactive colloids of ^{198}Au, ^{99m}Tc and ^{113m}In. In all but one of the patients, the anterior-posterior scan showed predominant uptake of colloid in a region near the mid-line (Fig. 1). The right lateral scan (Fig. 2) – here in a different patient – may indicate this predominant uptake to originate from the posterior part of the liver.

The liver at post-mortem of one of our patients – in horizontal section – (Fig. 3) showed intense congestion of the right lobe and a lesser degree of congestion of the left lobe. However, the enlarged caudate lobe appeared to be comprised almost wholly of yellow-brown nodular regenerating liver tissue. Both right and left hepatic veins were occluded by thrombi. On further examination, the venous drainage of the caudate directly into the inferior vena cava appeared to be intact. This can be seen more clearly in close-up (Fig. 4): this also demonstrates collateral vessels in the bridge

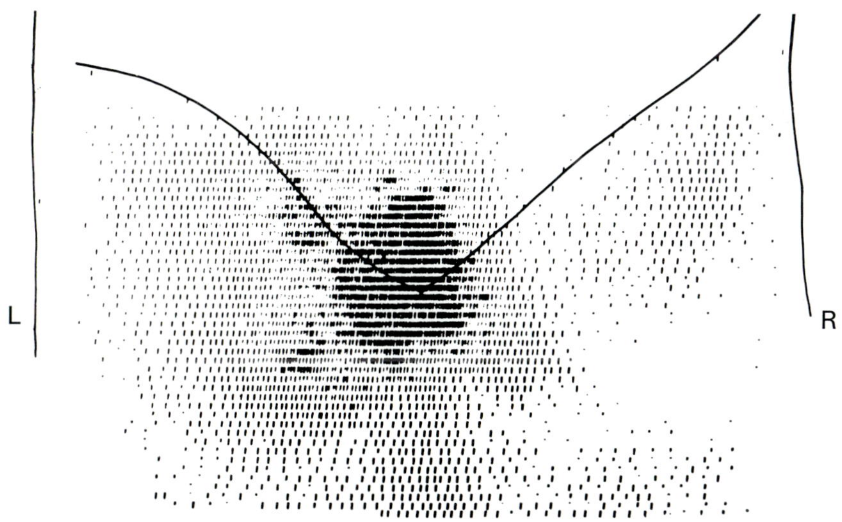

Fig. 1

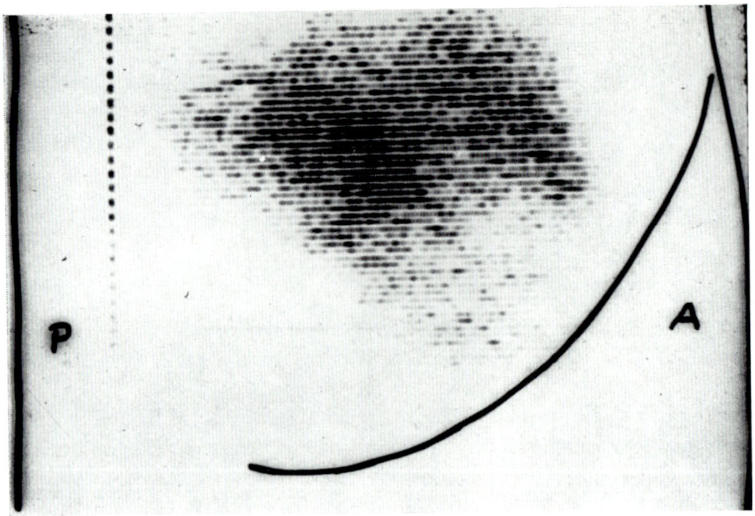

Fig. 2

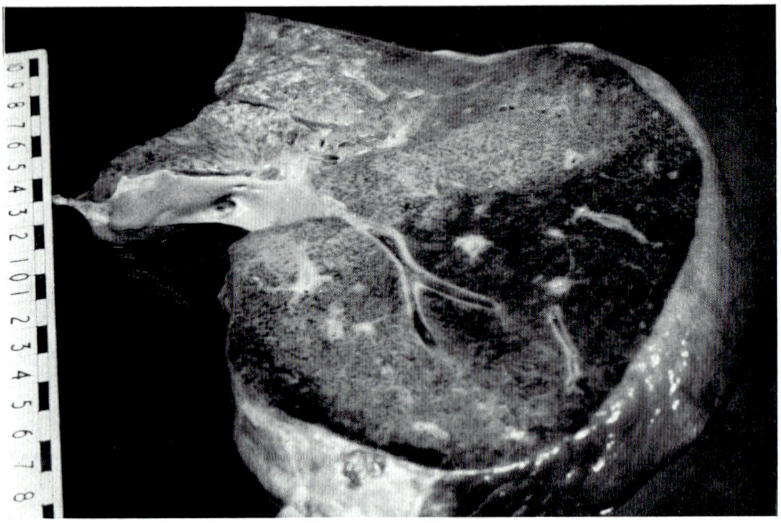

Fig. 3

of tissue between the left and caudate lobes. My colleagues Dr. TAVILL and Dr. KREEL carried out post-mortem injection of contrast medium into the inferior vena cava (Fig. 5). Free reflux of contrast medium into the hepatic venous system draining the caudate lobe can be seen. The scan appearances in Budd-Chiari Syndrome appear to be caused by selective uptake of radioactive colloid into the swollen caudate lobe, which retains its separate venous drainage. It is only possible to speculate why this occurs; it may perhaps be concerned with the sparing of Kupffer cell function in the caudate lobe. Alternatively it may be due to the failure of the Kupffer cells in the

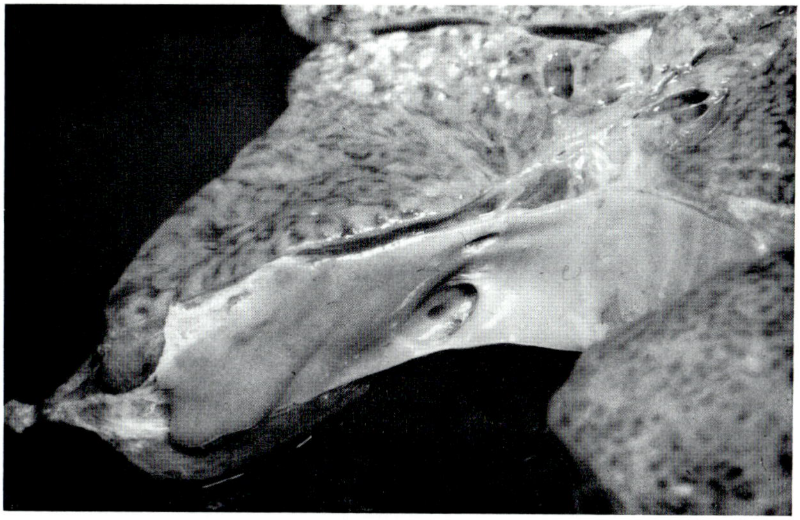

Fig. 4

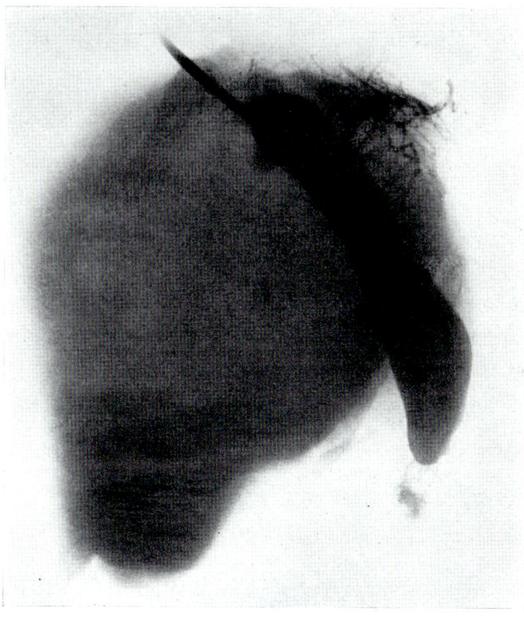

Fig. 5

right and left lobes of the liver to take up the colloid because of stagnation or shunting of blood flow in these regions of hepatic vein block.

A characteristic pattern seen on the hepatic venogram when the catheter can be *wedged* within a blocked hepatic vein, is a "spider-web" network of contrast medium (Fig. 6). This is caused by penetration of the contrast medium from the tip of the catheter into the finest venous radicles which in this situation are dilated. Any patent

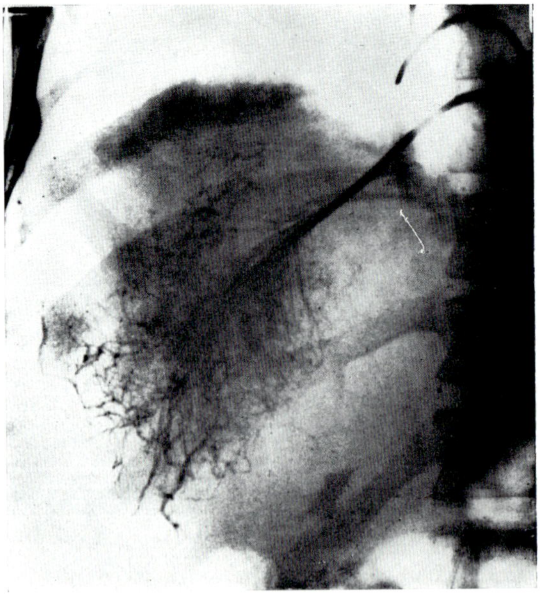

Fig. 6

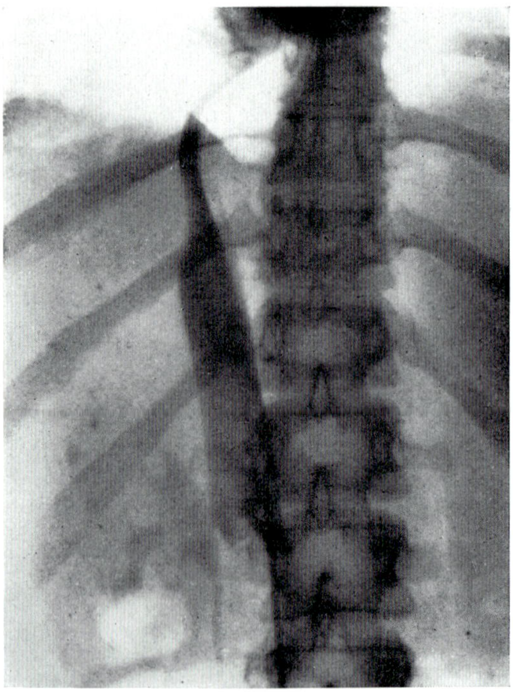

Fig. 7

collateral veins present may also be filled and displayed as a coarse network which may also be seen where occlusion of the hepatic veins is incomplete. This appearance is quite unique (the strands of the contrast medium are particularly well defined), and quite unlike the fine sinusoidal pattern of the normal venogram, or the coarse sinusoidal pattern seen in cirrhosis. This "spiders-web" network pattern, *as well as* the demonstration of the actual partial or total occlusion of a hepatic vein, is considered to be pathognomic of the Budd-Chiari Syndrome.

The inferior vena cavagrams are also of interest (Fig. 7). Here a distinct *side-to-side* narrowing of the upper part of the inferior vena cava can be seen, caused by extrinsic pressure from the hypertrophied caudate lobe of the liver. By comparison, *anterior-posterior* compression of the inferior vena cava is small. The reason for this is illustrated in Fig. 8, which shows a posterior view of a liver at post-mortem. This inferior

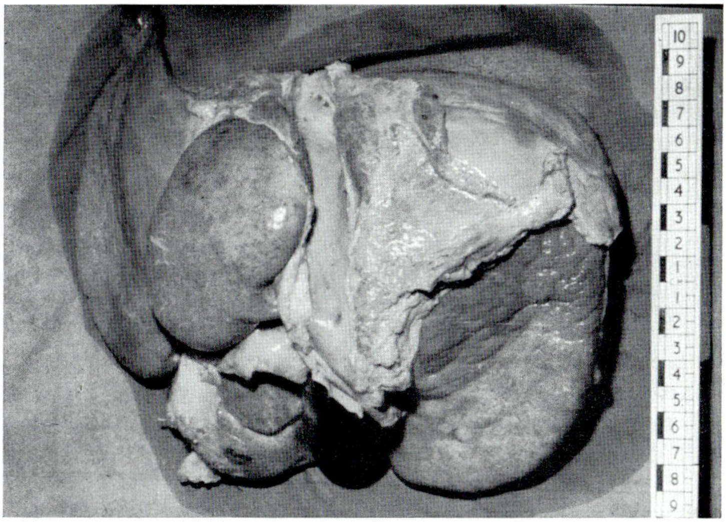

Fig. 8

vena cavagram pattern is probably diagnostic, and also helpful in the understanding and interpretation of the underlying pathology. In 4 cases, actual complete obstruction of the inferior vena cava was observed.

The liver scan is best used as an initial simple screening test in the diagnosis of the Budd-Chiari Syndrome (Table): the appearances described may be useful as an indication for further detailed investigation of the patient by the more complicated techniques of vascular radiology.

Table

Budd-Chiari-Syndrome: –	
	Summary
14 patients:	
Liver-Scan: –	simple inital screening test. caudate lobe uptake of radiocolloid.
Vascular Radiology: –	detailed investigation by hepatic venogram ("spider-web" pattern)/inferior vena cavagram (side-side narrowing).

Vergleichende angio- und szintigraphische Untersuchungen beim experimentellen Verschlußikterus

D. Beduhn und H. Kampmann

Die Differentialdiagnose des Ikterus bereitet trotz Einsatz aller modernen klinischen und blutchemischen Untersuchungsmethoden Schwierigkeiten. In 10–20% ist eine Differenzierung zwischen intra- und extrahepatischem Verschlußikterus nicht möglich. Im Tierexperiment wurden am Hund angiographische und szintigraphische Untersuchungen vorgenommen, um folgende Fragen zu klären:

1. Welche Gefäßsysteme der Leber sind neben den Gallenwegen beim Verschlußikterus beteiligt?
2. Sind die Gefäßveränderungen angio- und szintigraphisch zu verifizieren?
3. Können die erhobenen Befunde zur Diagnostik des Verschlußikterus in der Medizin herangezogen werden?

An 20 Hunden wurden nach Unterbindung des Choledochus 130 angio- und szintigraphische Untersuchungen der arteriellen Lebergefäße, des Pfortadersystems und der ableitenden Gallenwege durchgeführt (Tabelle).

Tabelle. *130 experimentelle angio- und szintigraphische Untersuchungen*

Art der Untersuchung	Zahl der Untersuchungen 1 Ebene	2 Ebenen
Coeliacographie	31	18
Portographie	25	7
Cholangiographie	22	7
Szintigraphie	20	—

Gallenwege

Die ersten Veränderungen treten erwartungsgemäß am Gallengangsystem auf. 3 Tage nach Choledochusverschluß kann bereits eine Erweiterung der zentralen Gallengänge festgestellt werden, während die peripheren Äste noch unverändert enggestellt sind. Nach weiteren 5 Tagen sind auch die intrahepatischen Gallengänge erweitert. 14 Tage nach Ligatur des Choledochus ist das gesamte Gallengangsystem exzessiv aufgetrieben. Zu diesem Zeitpunkt besteht eine erhebliche Erhöhung des Bilirubinspiegels im Serum von durchschnittlich 10,2 mg% (Abb. 1).

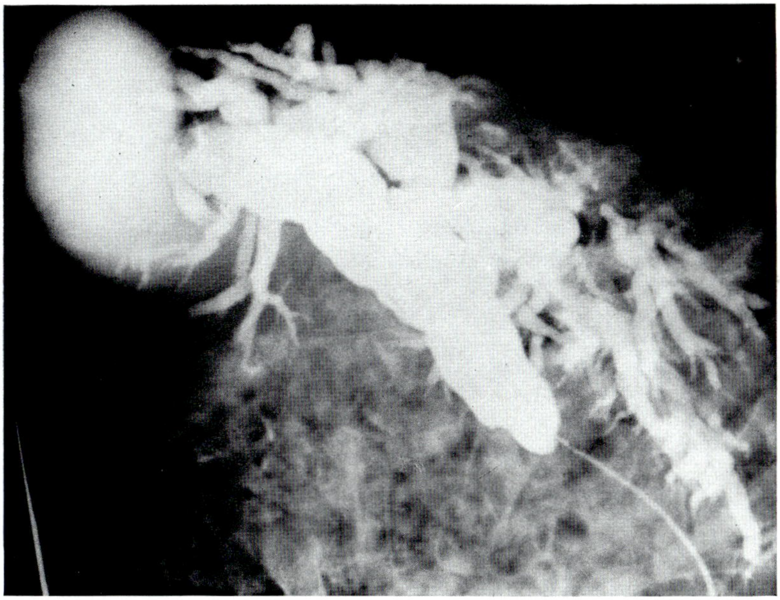

Abb. 1. Cholangiographie. Excessive Dilatation des zentralen und peripheren Gallengangssystems mit unregelmäßiger Begrenzung bei einem Serumbilirubinspiegel von 9,8 mg % und einem Druck von 38 cm H_2O im Gallengangssystem

Der manometrisch gemessene Druck im Gallengangsystem steigt von den Normalwerten mit 9 cm Wassersäule am 1. Tag bis zu Meßwerten zwischen 26–28 cm H_2O in der Zeit zwischen dem 12. und 20. postoperativen Tag an.

Funktionsszintigraphie

Der komplette Gallengangsverschluß ist szintigraphisch mit ^{131}J-Bengalrosa leicht zu verifizieren. In den ersten Tagen nach Gallengangsverschluß ist eine zeitgerechte Verlagerung der Radioaktivität von der Leberperipherie in die zentralen Leberanteile, d. h. in die Gallenblase und extrahepatischen Gallenwege zu beobachten. Es erfolgt kein Übertritt der Radioaktivität ins Intestinum. Die Zeit-Aktivitätskurven des Herzens und des rechten Leberbereiches zeigen einen regelrechten Verlauf. Die ermittelten Halbwertzeiten liegen im Normbereich. Die Kurve des zentralen Leberanteiles nimmt einen konstant steilen Anstieg, als Zeichen eines Aktivitätsaufstaues in den extrahepatischen Gallengängen und der Gallenblase. Besteht der Verschluß länger als 5 Tage, läßt sich szintigraphisch keine Aktivitätsanhäufung im Gallenblasen- und Leberpfortaderbereich mehr nachweisen (Abb. 2).

Ein über 3 Wochen hinaus bestehender Verschlußikterus führt infolge der Gallenstauung zu einer sekundären Leberparenchymschädigung, die sich funktionsszintigraphisch in einer deutlich verzögerten Aktivitätsaufnahme des Leberparenchyms, einer signifikanten Aktivitätsaussparung in jenem Leberbereich, der in der frühen Stauungsphase durch eine erhöhte Aktivitätskonzentration gekennzeichnet

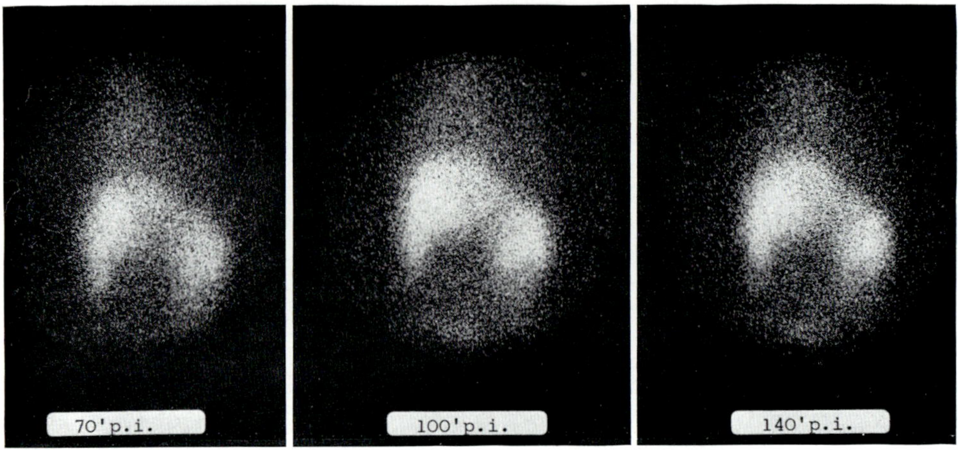

a

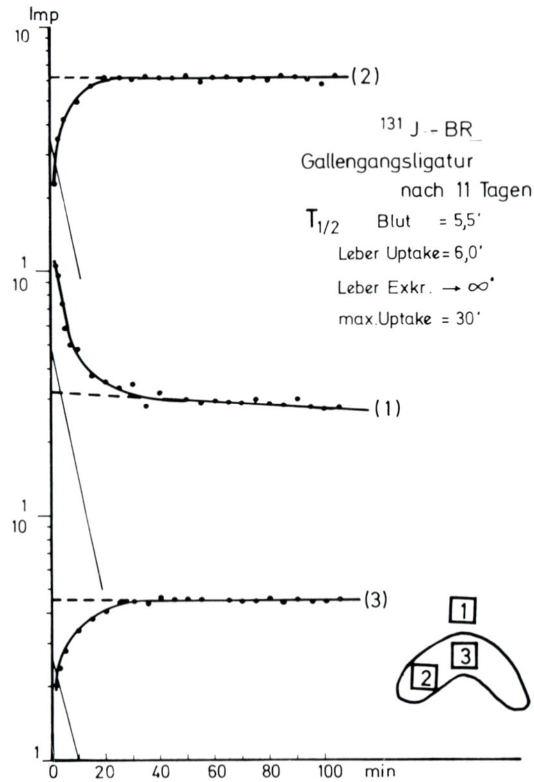

b

Abb. 2a und b. Leberfunktionsszintigraphie. a Kameraszintigraphie, b Zeitaktivitätskurven. Die Aktivitätsaufnahme in der Leber ist zeitlich verzögert (Kurve 1, Abb. 2b). Da kein meßbarer intrahepatischer Aktivitätstransport stattfindet, zeigt die Kurve nach Erreichen eines Maximums einen gradlinigen Verlauf, gleicher Verlauf der Kurve 3, da kein extrahepatischer Aktivitätsaufstau. Blutclearencezeit (Kurve 1) entsprechend verlängert ist, einer kompensatorischen Ausscheidung über die Niere und einem erhöhten Aktivitätsuntergrund äußert.

Coeliacographie

In der Leber kommt es parallel zu den entzündlichen Umbauvorgängen beim Verschlußikterus zu einer Weitstellung der Leberarterien. Beim Vergleich einer Coeliacographie vor und nach Choledochusverschluß, ist eine deutliche Kaliberzunahme der zentralen und peripheren Leberarterien zu beobachten. Gleichzeitig ist eine vermehrte Vaskularisation in den peripheren Leberabschnitten zu erkennen.

Im Rahmen des Verschlußikterus kommt es mit der Stauung im Gallengangsystem zu erheblichen entzündlichen Umbauvorgängen, die vom Pathologen als pericholangiolaere, chronisch-entzündliche oder leukocytaere Infiltrationen beschrieben werden (Rössle,1930; Kaufmann, 1960). Diese feinmikroskopischen Umbauvorgänge gehen mit einer erheblichen Vermehrung des Gefäßnetzes einher und erzeugen damit im Angiogramm das Bild der Hypervaskularisation. Im Spätstadium sind die Schlängelungen der weitgestellten Gefäßareale ebenso im Sinne der entzündlichen Alteration zu deuten wie Kalibersprünge und Wandunregelmäßigkeiten der Leberarterien (Abb. 3).

Portographie

Die Veränderungen am Pfortadersystem manifestieren sich meist zwischen der 2. und 3. postoperativen Woche in Form mäßiger Erweiterung der zentralen und peripheren Pfortaderäste. Während sich bei den präoperativen Portographien die

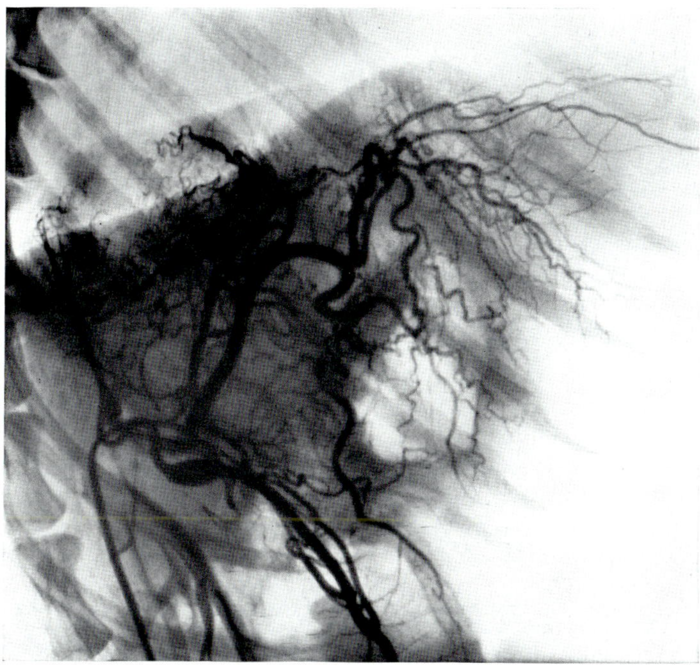

Abb. 3. Seitliche Coeliacographie. Weitstellung des gesamten arteriellen Gefäßnetzes, besonders in den peripheren Abschnitten mit Kaliberschwankungen

Leber vollständig homogen anfärbt, finden sich beim Verschlußikterus im Portogramm Aussparungen in der Leberopazität, die durch Umbauvorgänge in der Leber mit Stauung in den sinusoiden Kapillaren und den kleinen Venen hervorgerufen werden. Im weiteren Verlauf zeichnet sich eine Rarefizierung der peripheren Pfortaderäste ab. Bei Kontrolluntersuchungen 5–7 Wochen nach Verschluß des Choledochus findet siche eine Pfortaderthrombose mit ausgedehntem Kollateralkreislauf über umbilikale und paravertebrale Venen. Als weiteres Zeichen der Thrombose ist bei diesen Tieren Aszites festzustellen (Abb. 4).

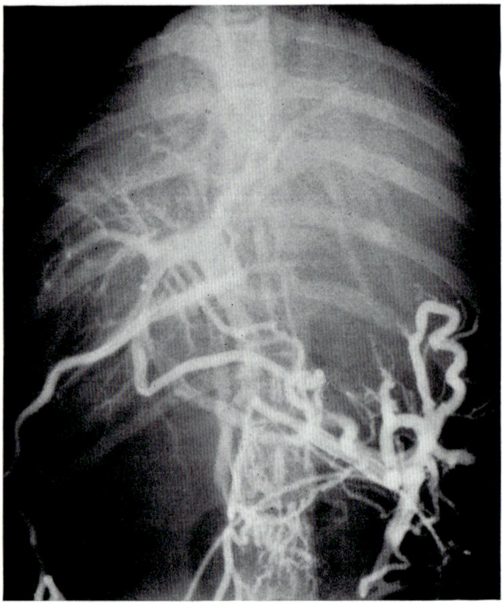

Abb. 4. Portographie. Pfortaderthrombose mit ausgedehntem Kollateralkreislauf über Mesenterial-, Umbilical- und Bauchwandvenen mit Wiederauffüllung der intrahepatischen Pfortaderäste

Diskussion und Zusammenfassung

In der 1. Woche des Verschlußikterus sind – neben röntgenologisch erfaßbaren Veränderungen am Gallengangsystem mit Druckerhöhung – besonders mit der Funktionsszintigraphie Aussagen über die Art des Verschlusses möglich. In der 2. Woche manifestieren sich die Folgen der Gallestauung in Form einer vermehrten arteriellen Vaskularisation der Leber mit Weitstellung der Gefäße, Kaliberschwankungen und Wandunregelmäßigkeiten. Umbauvorgänge in der Leber werden beim Verschlußikterus auch im Portogramm erkennbar. Wenn sich auch die Druckverhältnisse im Pfortadersystem des Hundes nicht wesentlich ändern, so bedeutet doch die Deviation und Infiltration mit teilweiser oder vollständiger Thrombose der V. portae ein sehr entscheidendes Kriterium in der Diagnostik des Verschlußikterus.

Neben der perkutanen transhepatischen Cholangiographie sollte bei der Diagnostik der Verschlußikterus auch der Arteriographie und der Portographie mehr Aufmerksamkeit gewidmet werden, wie die experimentellen Untersuchungen gezeigt haben.

A Comparison of Isotope Scanning and Angiography in the Diagnosis of Liver Disease

R. J. ALFIDI and A. RODRIGUEZ-ANTUNEZ

Over the past 4 years, approximately 750 isotope scans of the liver and 550 celiac angiograms have been performed at the Cleveland Clinic. These two procedures were found to be coincident in 120 cases. These cases were reviewed to compare the diagnostic accuracy of these two procedures and further to determine in which disease process one or the other was more useful. Due to the lack of time, methods will not be discussed.

The pathologic state of the liver was determined in most cases by an autopsy or biopsy, either needle or surgical. In the living patients where these are not available, the clinicians final diagnosis based on clinical, laboratory, and sufficient follow-up evidence was used. Of the 120 cases there was insufficient follow-up information in twenty. This left us with 100 cases.

The 100 cases are subdivided into those that are normal, and into the various disease entities found. There were 31 normal patients. The scan was read as abnormal in 15 for a false-positive rate of 48%. The arteriograms read as abnormal in 10 for a false-positive of 32%.

Of the 44 patients with primary or secondary carcinoma, only two of the scans were read as normal for an accuracy of 95%. Arteriography showed 30 abnormal for an accuracy of 68%. In the 19 cases of cirrhosis the scan showed 17 abnormals for a 90% accuracy. By arteriography half were normal and half were considered abnormal. In the three cases of liver cysts, both the scan and the arteriogram showed the abnormality in all cases. The one case of hepatitis showed abnormalities on the scan, but the arteriogram was normal. On the other hand, the single case of hemangioma did not show any changes on the scan but was diagnosed by arteriography. Both the scan and the arteriogram showed abnormalities in the one case of vascular hamartoma.

Overall accuracy shows the scan wrong in 20% and correct in 80% of the cases. By angiography, there was an overall accuracy of 35% wrong and 65% correct diagnosis. Very high accuracy of scans has been reported in early years. More recently, after careful correlation of the scan with the complete pathological findings, the accuracy rate has come down somewhat. The 48% false-positive rate reported here is the highest found in a review of the literature, however, on the other hand the incidence of false-negatives in this serie of 9% is one of the lowest reported.

The angiographic findings of hepatoma are stretching of the larger intra-hepatic vessels and neovascularity. Also common to hepatoma is an hypertrophied hepatic artery, secondary to the increased blood flow through the tumor.

In the latter phases of the arteriogram the delayed flow and slow emptying of these abnormal vascular structures in the tumor are demonstrated.

On the scan, the primary carcinoma shows up as large "cold spots" with the isotope being taken up only by the normal tissue.

Metastases to the liver can be divided into the vascular and avascular types. The vascular types are relatively easy to recognize on the angiogram because of the neovascularity or tumor vessels. Also often present, are the signs of mass with stretching and displacement of the larger intra-hepatic vessels. Unfortunately, the vascular metastases are much less common than the avascular type.

The late hepatogram phase showing tumor staining in the very mottled hepatogram.

The scans show the very irregular uptake with many areas of decreased or no radioactivity. These areas represent metastatic tumor masses.

Two areas of neovascularity are demonstrated. First of all the bizarre vessels seen throughout the right lobe of the liver and then the tumor vessels seen on the left side of the abdomen. This is an example of leiomyosarcoma which is primary in the stomach with metastases to the liver.

The scan again demonstrated the numerous areas of decreased or absent uptake particularly in the right upper portion of the liver.

In chronic cirrhosis, the liver is usually small and the vessels are shortened and may show a cork-screwing effect. Reports by ALFIDI et al. and POLLARD showed that these vessel changes are non-specific for cirrhosis and that the diagnosis by angiography is limited at best.

The hepatogram phase of the arteriogram showed mottling throughout the liver secondary to the differential amounts of contrast in various parts of the diseased liver.

The liver scan in cirrhosis may show the liver to be either enlarged or small. The main changes are those of the mottled uptake of radioactivity. Splenomegaly and increased isotope uptake in the spleen are often present in cirrhosis.

Cystic disease may be simple, polycystic or pericytic in type. The only evidence of abnormality on the early arterial phase is a slight absence of vessels and some stretching around that slightly hypovascular area.

A large cyst within the liver was very well demonstrated by decreased contrast material in the area of the cyst. There was a slight increase in density of the hepatogram immediately around the cyst.

The scan faintly showed a 6 to 8 cm area of decreased uptake in the area of the porta hepatis.

Conclusion

We have reviewed 100 cases where the liver was studied both by angiography and by isotope scanning. A large number of false-positives was found with scanning. False-negatives were very low. The abnormal findings of scans were non-specific and correlation with any particular diagnosis was poor. The overall accuracy was 80%. With angiography, the percent of false-positives and false-negatives were approximately equal. The findings of the various diseases were quite specific and showed good correlation with the pathologic reports. Overall accuracy was only 65%.

Hepatic Scan and Arteriogram in the Preoperative Diagnosis of Circumscribed Liver Diseases

K. HUPE, D. MAROSKE, H. DOMBROWSKI and K. JOSEPH

With the exception of multiocalized liver metastases the circumscribed liver diseases have an operative indication. Of preoperative interest is:

1. Localisation of the disease.
2. Extent and operability of the process.
3. Character of the disease.
4. Information over the operative technique.

In the *scan* the pathological area displays a space-occupying defect located in the liver, and the size of the process can be estimated.

The *angiogram* gives the surgeon a diagram so that precise information over the localisation and extension is known. From this diagramatical information the character of the process can be obtained. The knowledge from the angiogram eases the decision for operation and the choice of operative technique.

Four Examples

1. The scan of a 52 year old patient with an unspecific liver abscess containing 6000 ml shows the space-occupying defect on the right lobe of the liver, but not in the upper area of the abscess. The angiogram shows the expansion of the liver abscess and the elevation of the surface tissue of the liver towards the clavicle.

2. The scan of a 40 year old patient with an amebic abscess shows a space-occupying defect of the size of a fist in the lateral part of the right liver lobe. The angiogram shows an avascular intrahepatic process.

3. In a 49 year old patient, were a pancreatic-cyst was suspected by clinical and scanning observation, the liver angiogram indicated a hypervascular intrahepatic process in the left liver lobe. Due to the pathological formation of blood vessels it was thought a malignant growth, which was confirmed histologically as a solid carcinoma.

4. By a 20 year old patient with 3 large echinococcuscysts, the scan shows almost a complete space-occupying defect in the left liver lobe, and in the right caudal part a space-occupying defect of the size of two fists. The angiogram shows left two and right one avascular space-occupying process. In a two-stage-operation the two cysts of the left lobe were removed first and four weeks later the cyst of the right lobe.

Postoperative the liver regeneration of the right lobe was complete, whereas the regeneration of the left lobe was absent. This was well indicated by the scan.

In conclusion we can say, that for the surgical intervention the angiogram gives the most precise anatomical information.

Value and advantage of the scan is: it is a simple method, less strainious for the patient,

it can often be repeated,

can be used for diagnoses of space-occupying defects and for control of liver regeneration in the postoperative period.

Diagnostische Wertigkeit der abdominalen Arteriographie

W. Wenz und J. Wawersik

Die Bedeutung der abdominalen Arteriographie im Einzelfall ist unbestritten. Welches Gewicht kommt diesem Spezialverfahren im Rahmen der Gesamtzahl diagnostischer Maßnahmen eines gemischten chirurgischen Krankengutes zu und wie groß ist die Wahrscheinlichkeit, dadurch eine richtige Diagnose zu finden?

In dieser Analyse von 2771 konsekutiven stationären Patienten der Chirurg. Univ.-Klinik Heidelberg sind 66% aller Kranken in irgendeiner Form einer Röntgenuntersuchung zugeführt worden. Dabei dominieren die konventionellen Röntgenverfahren. Angiographien wurden in 14% dieser Stichprobe durchgeführt, darunter 51 abdominelle Arteriographien. Diese Untersuchung wird demnach im Vergleich zu konventionellen Röntgenmethoden bei Abdominalerkrankungen relativ selten angewandt (Abb. 1).

Die im Rahmen unserer Erhebung durchgeführten abdominellen Arteriographien betreffen ein gemischtes Kollektiv (Tumoren, Entzündungen, Gefäßverschlüsse) und führten 30mal zu einer richtig positiven, 8mal zu einer richtig negativen Diagnose (Tabelle). In 7 Fällen war die angiographische Diagnose fraglich; bei positiver

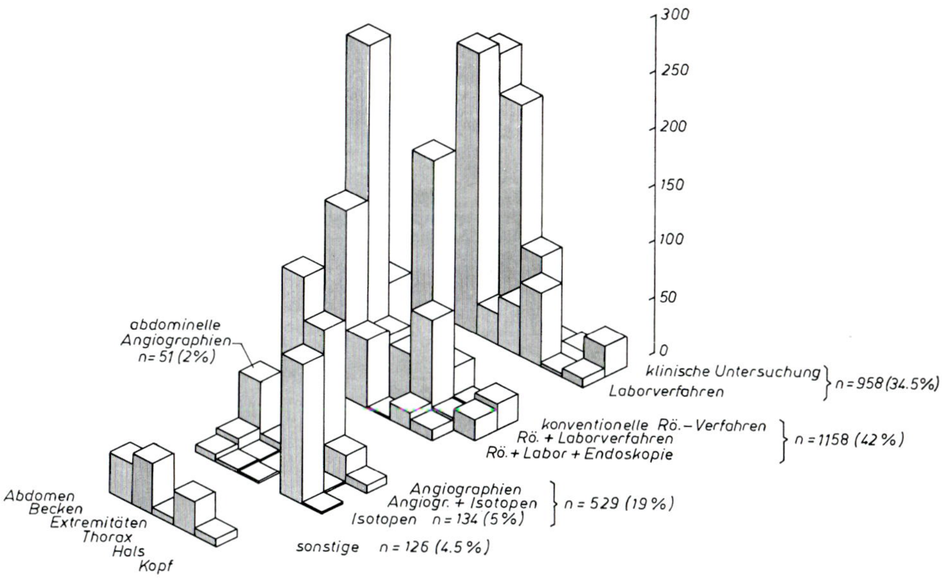

Abb. 1. Häufigkeitsverteilung diagnostischer Maßnahmen

Tabelle. *Beziehung zwischen angiographischem Befund und Krankheit in einem gemischten Kollektiv*

Fragliche Befunde – in Klammern – pos. interpretiert			
angiographischer Befund	Krankheit pos.	Krankheit neg.	Summe
pos.	35 (5)	4 (2)	39
neg.	4	8	12
Summe	39 (5)	12 (2)	51 (7)

Spezifität: 0,67; Sensibilität: 0,90; Fehler I: 0,10; Fehler II: 0,33

Beziehung bei abdominellen Tumoren			
angiographischer Befund	Krankheit pos.	Krankheit neg.	Summe
pos.	186 (26)	20 (10)	206
neg.	30	27	57
Summe	216 (26)	47 (10)	263 (36)

Spezifität: 0.57; Sensibilität: 0,86; Fehler I: 0,14; Fehler II: 0,43

Interpretation wären 2 Befunde falsch positiv gewesen. Daraus resultiert eine Sensibilität von 90%. Die Wahrscheinlichkeit, einen tatsächlich Kranken als solchen zu entdecken, ist also relativ hoch.

Diesem Ergebnis sei die Analyse von 263 Fällen mit einem abdominellen Tumor gegenübergestellt. Die Sensibilität, d. h. die Wahrscheinlichkeit eines richtig positiven Befundes liegt in der gleichen Größenordnung wie in dem gemischten Kollektiv, sofern auch hier die fraglichen Befunde positiv gedeutet werden. Unter dieser Voraussetzung ist aber die Spezifität, d. h. die Sicherheit für den Ausschluß der tatsächlich nicht Kranken (Fehler II = 0,43) gering. Selbst wenn fragliche Befunde grundsätzlich negativ interpretiert würden, beträgt das Risiko eines falsch positiven Befundes bei abdominalen Tumoren 21%.

Daraus ergibt sich, daß die viszerale Arteriographie besser geeignet ist, bei hinreichendem Krankheitsverdacht einen Tumor nachzuweisen. Sie ist aber weniger wirksam, wenn es bei unsicheren klinischen Verdachtsmomenten darauf ankommt, die tatsächlich nicht Kranken auszuschließen oder anders ausgedrückt: es besteht die Tendenz angiographischen Symptomen im Bauchraum eine übertrieben starke pathomorphologische Bedeutung zuzuordnen.

Diseases of the Spleen

Szintigraphische und angiographische Milzdiagnostik – ein Vergleich bei Hämoblastosen

K. Hennig, W.-G. Franke und H. Platzbecker

Die Arteriographie und die Szintigraphie der Milz haben in den letzten Jahren eine zunehmende Verbreitung erlangt. Es liegen Erfahrungen an größeren Patientenzahlen vor, und Indikationen für beide Untersuchungsverfahren wurden abgesteckt. Für die Milzarteriographie werden heute folgende Indikationen angegeben:

a) Bestimmung von Lage, Größe und Form des Organs,
b) zum Nachweis von Gefäßprozessen,
c) bei einer Splenomegalie,
d) zur Ausschluß- und Identifikationsdiagnostik linksseitiger Oberbauchtumoren,
e) bei entzündlich-infiltrativen oder tumorösen Milzparehcnymprozessen,
f) anstelle der Splenoportographie, wenn diese mit erhöhtem Risiko verbunden ist,
g) bei entzündlichem und tumorösem Befall von Pankreaskörper und -schwanz.

Für die Milzszintigraphie lassen sich – nach Fischer bzw. Feine und zum Winkel – folgende Indikationen stellen:

a) Bestimmung von Lage, Größe und Form des Organs,
b) Differentialdiagnose von Tumoren im linken Oberbauch,
c) Feststellung von Parenchymläsionen der Milz bei Tumoren, Infarkten, Zysten usw.,
d) Nachweis von Nebenmilzen,
e) Verlaufskontrollen, insbesondere unter der Therapie.

Man erkennt, daß in einigen Fällen beide Verfahren hinsichtlich ihrer Indikationen miteinander konkurrieren. Es bedarf daher einer sorgfältigen Abwägung der Vor- und Nachteile beider Verfahren, um zu entscheiden, wann das eine oder das andere oder eine Kombination beider Verfahren am vorteilhaftesten ist.

Bei uns kommen verhältnismäßig viele Patienten mit Hämoblastosen zur Untersuchung und Behandlung. Der Nachweis einer Mitbeteiligung der Milz ist von wesentlicher Bedeutung für Diagnose und Prognostik und beeinflußt das therapeutische Vorgehen. Es blieb durch den Überweisungsweg mehr oder weniger dem Zufall überlassen, ob eine röntgenologische oder nuklearmedizinische Milzdiagnostik erfolgte. Aufgrund der bisher vorliegenden Ergebnisse von über 400 szintigraphischen und etwa 60 arteriographischen Untersuchungen bei Hämoblastosen entschlossen wir uns, den Wert dieser Methoden an 50 Patienten dieser Krankheitsgruppe zu überprüfen, bei denen beide Verfahren zur Anwendung kommen sollten.

Die Tabelle gibt einen Überblick über die Zusammensetzung des Patientengutes.

Szintigraphisch wurden alle Patienten untersucht, die Arteriographie konnte 8mal nicht durchgeführt werden: 4mal wegen Gefäßsklerose, 1mal wegen hämorrhagischer Diathese, 2mal wegen schlechten Allgemeinzustandes und 1mal wegen Ablehnung durch den Patienten.

Tabelle

Polyzythaemia vera	7
Lymphogranulomatose	12
Retikulosarkomatose	13
Lymphosarkomatose	5
Lymphatische Leukämie	8
Myeloische Leukämie	3
Morbus Brill-Symmers	2

Für die Milzarteriographie wurde eine Katheterisierung des Truncus coeliacus vorgenommen, wobei versucht wurde, die Katheterspitze so zu legen, daß der größte Teil des Kontrastmittels in die A. lienalis abfloß; bei einem geringen Teil der Fälle gelang eine superselektive Milzarteriographie ohne weitere Manipulationen. Hinzu kommen die Fälle, bei denen die A. linealis direkt aus der Aorta entsprang. Je nach Größe der Milz injizierten wir 20–70 ml Visotrast 290 mittels Druckspritze, wobei möglichst ein Fluß von 10 ml/sec eingehalten wurde. In der Regel jedoch verzichteten wir auf die superselektive Milzarteriographie, weil es sich einerseits um überwiegend ältere Patienten handelte, bei denen die Sondierung der Milzarterie schwierig, bisweilen unmöglich ist, und andererseits, weil gerade bei der superselektiven Angiographie häufiger Komplikationen auftreten. Die Aufnahmen erfolgten mit dem Blattfilmwechsler der Firma Elema-Schönander, wobei in einigen Fällen Aufnahmen alternierend in zwei Ebenen angefertigt wurden. Komplikationen traten in dieser Patientengruppe nicht auf.

Zur Milzszintigraphie verwenden wir seit einiger Zeit fast ausschließlich Technetium-markierte Erythrocyten. Unser Markierungsverfahren wurde gemeinsam mit dem Zentralinstitut für Kernforschung Rossendorf entwickelt, das auch die Technetium-Generatoren liefert (Bezug über Isocommerz GmbH Berlin-Buch, Lindenberger Weg). Es enthält als wesentlichen Bestandteil eine Erhöhung der Reduktionskapazität des Hämoglobins durch Zusatz von Zinn-Ionen zur Erythrocytensuspension vor der Markierung. Die einzelnen Arbeitsgänge wurden von uns bereits ausführlich beschrieben. Die so erzielte Markierung zeichnet sich durch strenge Reproduzierbarkeit, hohe Markierungsausbeute von 85–95% und große Stabilität in vitro und in vivo aus. Die Erythrocyten werden anschließend in bekannter Weise thermisch alteriert. Die Qualität der Szintigramme übertrifft wegen der bei Technetium erreichbaren höheren Impulsrate diejenige der mit ^{51}Cr geschriebenen. Die Szintigramme wurden in mehreren Lagen des Patienten mit dem Magnascanner 500 bzw. mit einem von uns modifizierten Siemens-Nucleographen angefertigt.

Bei den Patienten mit Hämoblastosen stehen im Rahmen der Milzdiagnostik die Beurteilung des Organs hinsichtlich Lage, Form und besonders der Größe sowie der Nachweis maligner Veränderungen bzw. von Infarkten im Vordergrund.

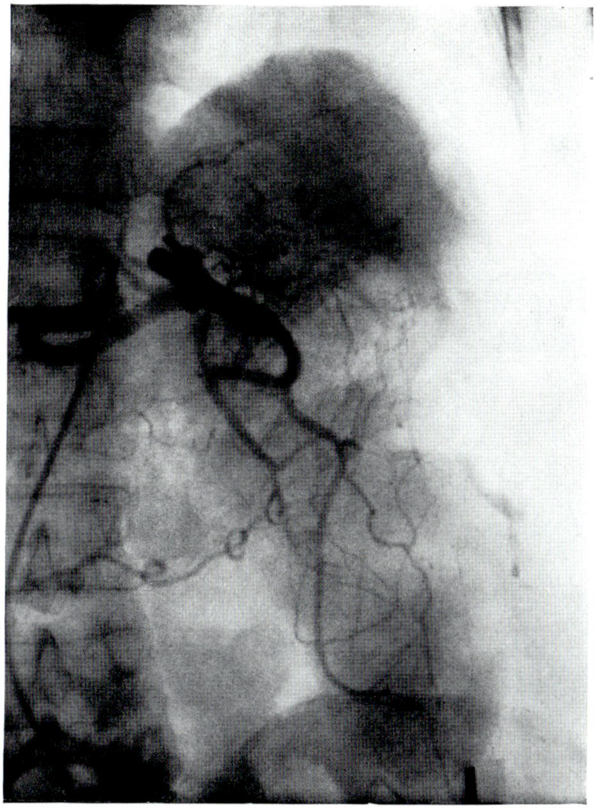

Abb. 1. Milzarteriogramm bei Polyzythaemia vera. Annehmbar Durchblutungsstörungen im Bereich des oberen Milzpoles

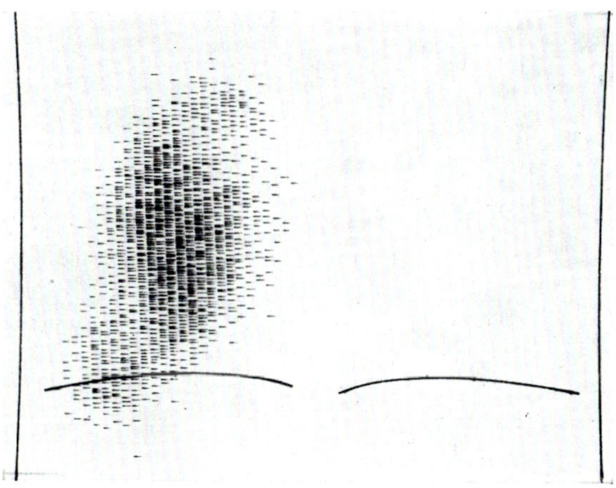

Abb. 2. Rückenlage-Szintigramm zu Abb. 1. Infarkt dicht am oberen Milzpol

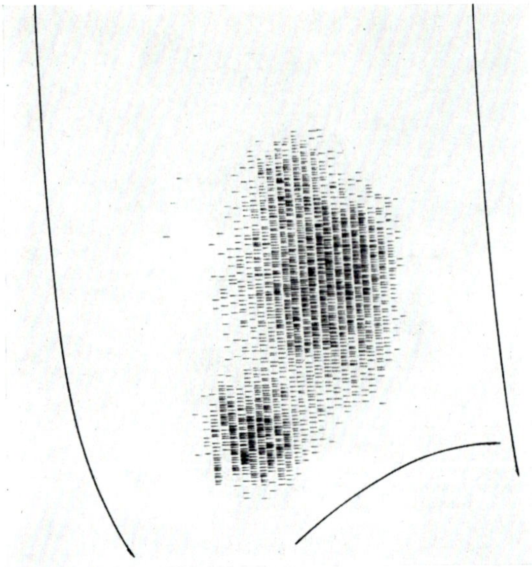

Abb. 3. Seitenlage-Szintigramm zu Abb. 1. Speicherungsstörungen im unteren Milzbereich

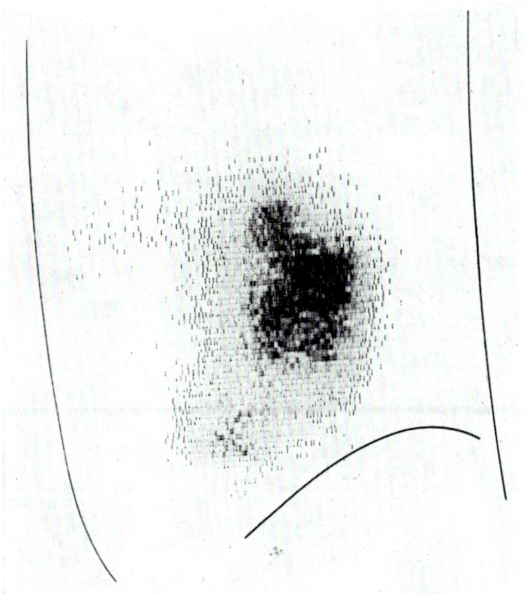

Abb. 4. Seitenlage-Szintigramm zu Abb. 1. Schwarz-Weiß-Wiedergabe eines Colorszintigrammes. Rückbildung der Durchblutungsstörungen nach Radiophosphor-Therapie

Die Darstellung der Milz und damit ihre Beurteilung hinsichtlich Lage, Größe und Form gelingt bekannterweise mit beiden Methoden. Beim überwiegenden Teil der Patienten war die Milz vergrößert. Die Szintigraphie ist für den Nachweis einer Milzvergrößerung wegen des Fehlens jeglicher Komplikationen, wegen der geringen Belastung des Patienten und wegen der nahezu beliebigen Wiederholbarkeit eindeutig im Vorteil.

Raumfordernde Prozesse bzw. Infarkte manifestieren sich im Milzszintigramm als Speicherungsstörungen. Bei unserem gesamten Patientengut an Hämoblastosen konnten wir Speicherungsstörungen bei rund einem Viertel aller Patienten beobachten; bei der diesem Vergleich zugrundeliegenden Patientengruppe war dieser Anteil zufällig höher. In 7 Fällen konnte bei Speicherungsstörungen im Milzszintigramm bei der Autopsie die Milz histologisch untersucht werden; dabei wurde in jedem Falle ein dem Krankheitsbild entsprechendes pathologisch-anatomisches Korrelat zu den Speicherungsdefekten nachgewiesen. Es handelte sich 3mal um eine Lymphadenose, 2mal um eine Lymphosarkomatose und je 1mal um ein Retothelsarkom und eine Lymphogranulomatose.

Bei den Patienten mit Speicherungsstörungen im Szintigramm kamen im Milzarteriogramm enggestellte arterielle Gefäße mit teilweise gestrecktem Verlauf sowie insgesamt eine rarefizierte Gefäßarchitektur vor. Die im Vergleich zur Milzgröße in diesen Fällen oft relativ schmale A. lienalis und die homogene, oft nur flaue Anfärbung der Milz in der Parenchymphase, ließen uns diese Veränderungen als Fibrosefolgen deuten. Nur in 2 Fällen war wegen auffallend bogig verlaufender arterieller Äste und einer inhomogenen Parenchymanfärbung an eine echte Raumforderung zu denken. Pathologische Gefäße als sichere Zeichen des malignen Wachstums haben wir intralienal nicht nachweisen können.

Besonders die große, fibrosierte Milz bietet angiographisch bei der Abgrenzung zwischen entzündlichen, stauungsbedingten und durch tumoröse Infiltrationen verursachten Organvergrößerungen erhebliche Schwierigkeiten. Es ließ sich jedoch bei allen Fällen mit Speicherungsstörungen im Szintigramm auch ein mehr oder weniger ausgeprägtes angiographisches Korrelat beobachten. Auffallend war dabei, daß sich in der Regel der Befund szintigraphisch scharf abgrenzen ließ, während dies im Angiogramm nicht der Fall war. Waren im Szintigramm keine Speicherungsstörungen zu erkennen, so konnte in jedem Falle auch das Gefäßbild nicht beanstandet werden.

Als Beispiel läßt das Arteriogramm (Abb. 1) einer 68jährigen Patientin mit einer Polyzythaemia vera Durchblutungsstörungen im Bereich des oberen Milzpoles annehmen. Nach dem Szintigramm (Abb. 2) mit einer deutlichen, annähernd dreieckigen Aussparung etwas unterhalb des oberen Milzpoles ist in Verbindung mit dem Grundleiden am ehesten an einen durchgemachten Infarkt zu denken. Die gleichzeitig vorhandene Speicherungsstörung im unteren Milzbereich fällt besonders im Seitenlagenszintigramm (Abb. 3) auf. 4 Monate nach der angeschlossenen Radiophosphor-Therapie hatten sich die Durchblutungsstörungen deutlich zurückgebildet (Abb. 4).

Bei einem 38jährigen Patienten mit einer Retikulosarkomatose fielen im Milzarteriogramm (Abb. 5) die deutlich rarefizierte intralienale Gefäßaufteilung und die teilweise etwas bogig verlaufenden Gefäße auf. Die V. lienalis und die Pfortader stellten sich nicht dar. Das Milzszintigramm (Abb. 6. u. 7) imponiert durch ausgedehnte, hochgradige Speicherungsstörungen, nahezu über die ganze Milz ver-

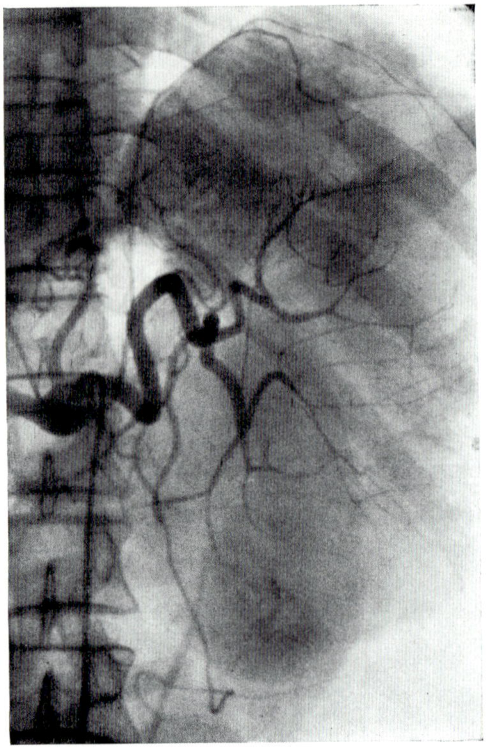

Abb. 5. Milzarteriogramm bei Retikulosarkomatose. Rarefizierte intralienale Gefäßaufteilungen, teilweise etwas bogig verlaufende Gefäße

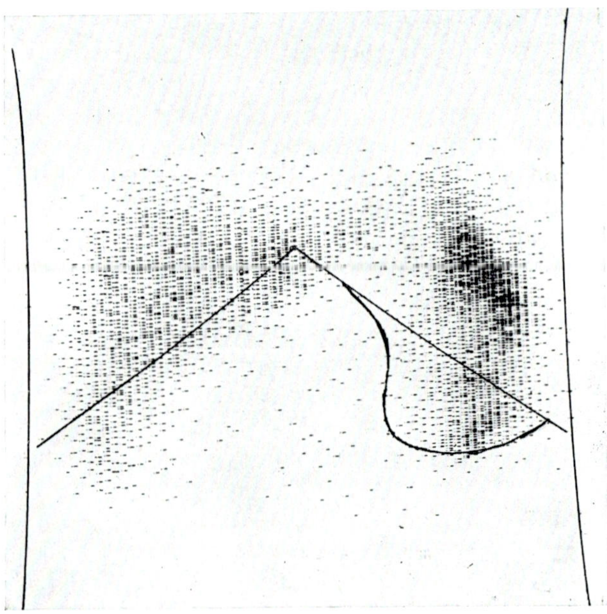

Abb. 6. Rückenlage-Szintigramm zu Abb. 5. Ausgedehnte, hochgradige Speicherungsstörungen bei Splenomegalie

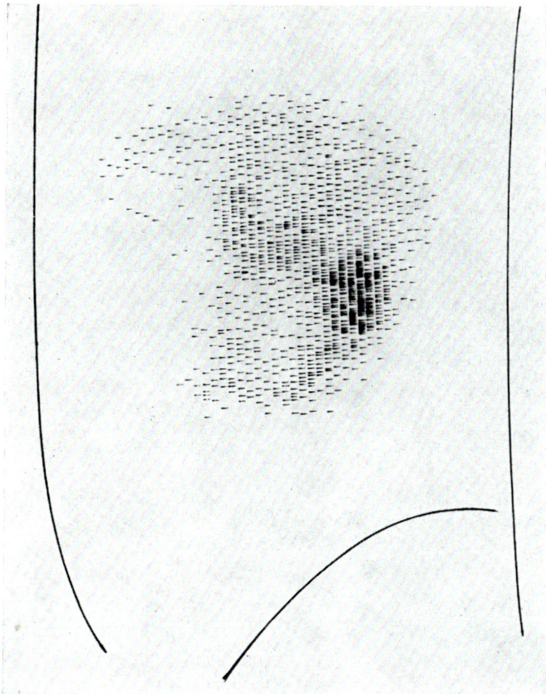

Abb. 7. Seitenlage-Szintigramm zu Abb. 6

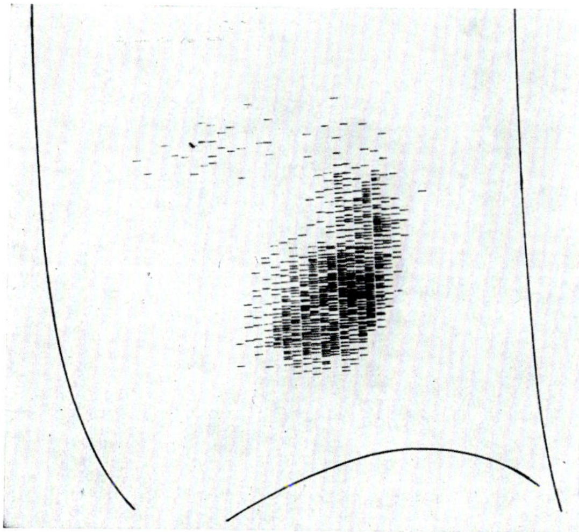

Abb. 8. Kontroll-Szintigramm zu Abb. 7 nach Röntgen- und Chemotherapie. Rückbildung der Milz auf normale Größe

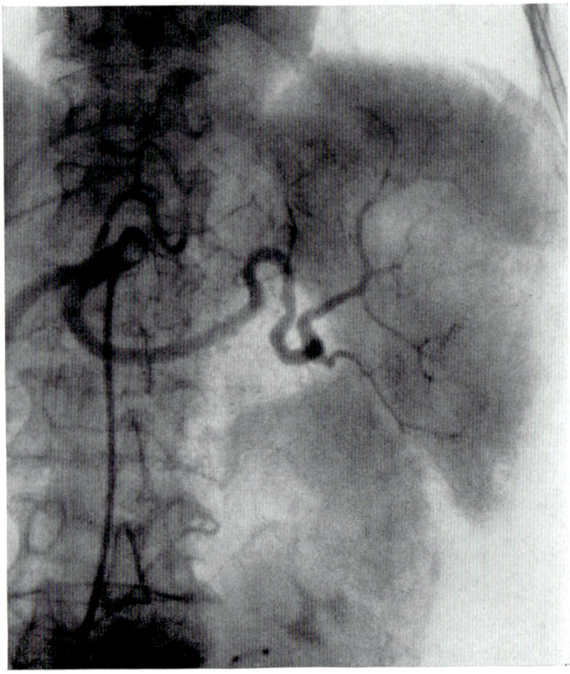

Abb. 9. Milzarteriogramm bei Retikulosarkomatose. Verengung der A. lienalis und der intralienalen Gefäße

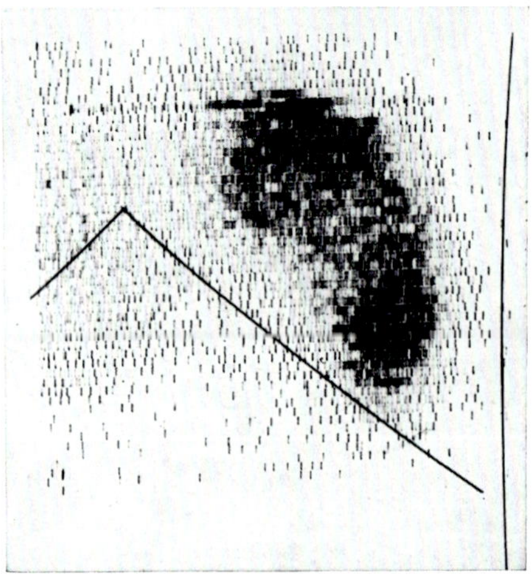

Abb. 10. Rückenlage-Szintigramm zu Abb. 9 (Colorszintigramm). Zentrale Speicherungsverminderung

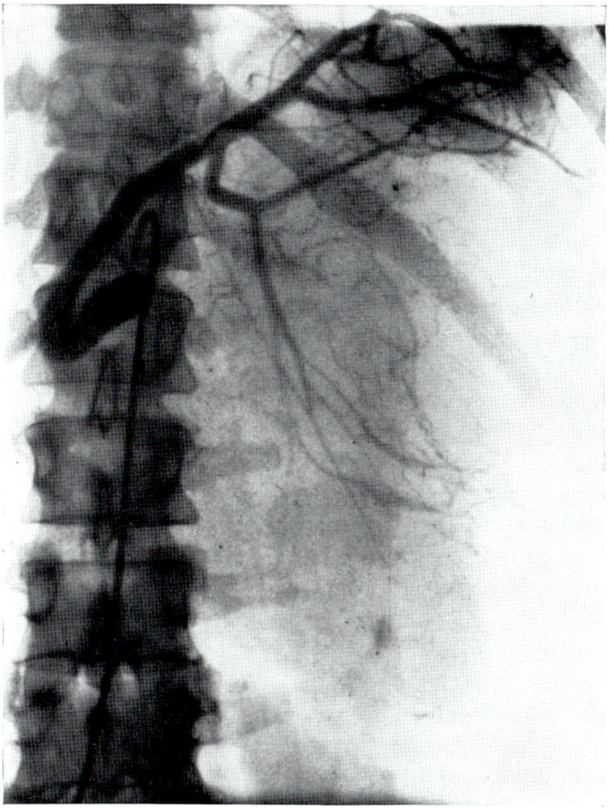

Abb. 11. Behandeltes Retothelsarkom und unklarer großer Oberbauchtumor. Milzarteriogramm: Pankreasschwanztumor

teilt. Reichlich ein Jahr später hatte sich nach erfolgter Chemotherapie die Milz auf normale Größe zurückgebildet (Abb. 8). Speicherungsstörungen lassen sich nur noch im oberen Anteil der Milz nachweisen.

Im Arteriogramm (Abb. 9) einer 69 Jahre alten Patientin mit einer Retikulosarkomatose sind die Gefäßveränderungen besonders deutlich. Es ist eine Verengung der A. lienalis sowie der intralienalen Gefäße zu verzeichnen. Szintigraphisch (Abb. 10) fällt eine zentrale Speicherungsverminderung auf. Die kräftige Mitdarstellung der Leber läßt auf eine erhebliche globale Drosselung der Durchblutung schließen. In Verbindung mit dem Grundleiden sind auch hier am ehesten destruktive Veränderungen anzunehmen.

Beim letzten Beispiel liegt ein behandeltes Retothelsarkom vor. Ein zu tastender großer Oberbauchtumor konnte nach dem Milzarteriogramm (Abb. 11) als Pankreasschwanztumor identifiziert werden. Dieser Befund wurde operativ bestätigt, histologisch wurde er als ein neurogenes Sarkom ohne Zusammenhang mit der ursprünglichen Geschwulsterkrankung angesehen. Szintigraphisch (Abb. 12 u. 13) mußte bei der klinisch als Milztumor imponierenden Oberbauchgeschwulst ein Zusammenhang mit der Milz negiert werden. Eine weitere nuklearmedizinische Abklärung konnte

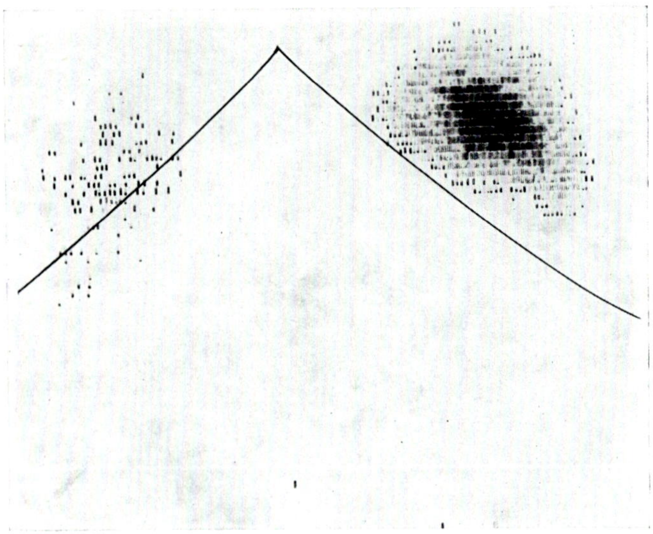

Abb. 12. Rückenlage-Szintigramm zu Abb. 11 (Colorszintigramm). Kein Zusammenhang des Oberbauchtumors mit der Milz

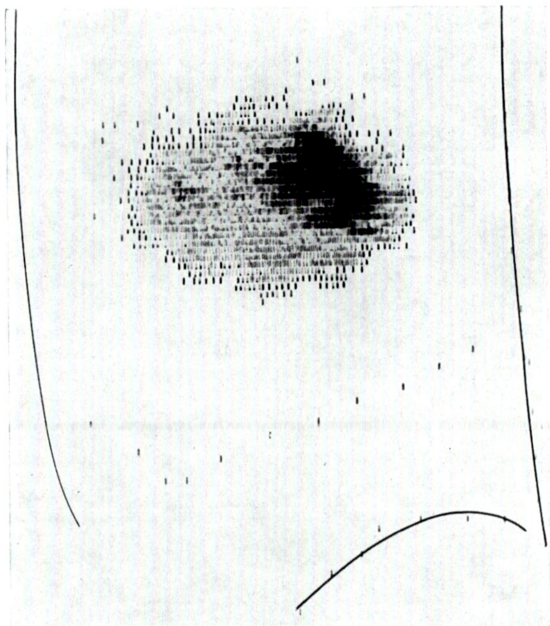

Abb. 13. Seitenlage-Szintigramm zu Abb. 12 (Colorszintigramm)

wegen der inzwischen vorliegenden arteriographischen Untersuchungsergebnisse unterbleiben. Den Nachweis des Pankreasschwanztumors hätte erst die Pankreasszintigraphie erbracht.

Wie auch die Beispiele zeigen, ist die Arteriographie zur Beurteilung der Milz bei Hämoblastosen keineswegs aufschlußreicher als die Szintigraphie. Die arteriographisch zu beobachtenden Veränderungen der Gefäßarchitektur waren häufig nur minimal und schwierig zu interpretieren. Auch in den Fällen, in denen bioptisch oder bei der Sektion eindeutiges Tumorgewebe in der Milz nachgewiesen werden konnte, kamen nicht alle Kriterien des malignen Tumorwachstums vor.

Die Überlegenheit der Arteriographie in differential-diagnostischer Hinsicht kommt hier nicht zur Geltung, da eine Hämoblastose als vorliegende Krankheit bekannt ist. Jedoch bietet die Arteriographie die Möglichkeit der gleichzeitigen perilienalen Diagnostik, die bei der nuklearmedizinischen Diagnostik weitere Untersuchungen erforderlich macht.

Die Bedeutung der arteriellen Gefäßdarstellung zur Erfassung des sogenannten Rückflußportogramms bleibt vorwiegend auf Lebererkrankungen beschränkt. Aufgrund unserer Untersuchungsergebnisse und in Anbetracht der Komplikationsmöglichkeiten bei der Arteriographie sowie der Belastung für den Patienten, erachten wir bei Hämoblastosen zur Beurteilung der Milz die Szintigraphie als ausreichend. Zur Ergänzung halten wir die Arteriographie nur in besonders gelagerten Fällen für erforderlich.

Zusammenfassung

Der Nachweis einer Mitbeteiligung der Milz bei Hämoblastosen ist von wesentlicher Bedeutung für Diagnostik und Prognostik und beeinflußt das therapeutische Vorgehen. Die klinische Feststellung der Milzgröße gelingt häufig nicht und ist mit einer relativ großen Unsicherheit behaftet.

Als diagnostisches Verfahren kommen neben indirekten röntgenologischen Methoden die selektive Milzangiographie und die Milzszintigraphie in Betracht.

Nur die Gefäßdarstellung und die Szintigraphie gewähren auch Einblick in strukturelle Veränderungen. Mit vorliegender Arbeit werden die Ergebnisse bei Patienten, die sowohl mit der selektiven Katheterangiographie nach Seldinger, als auch mit der Milzszintigraphie untersucht wurden, mitgeteilt.

Die Milzgröße ist mit beiden Verfahren zu ermitteln. Bei allen Fällen mit Speicherungsstörungen im Szintigramm war ein mehr oder weniger ausgeprägtes arteriographisches Korrelat zu beobachten; die Veränderungen der Gefäßarchitektur waren jedoch häufig nur minimal und schwierig zu interpretieren. Fehlten im Szintigramm Speicherungsstörungen, so konnte auch das Gefäßbild nicht beanstandet werden.

Die Ergebnisse lassen die Schlußfolgerung zu, daß für die klinischen Belange die einfache und risikolose Milzszintigraphie allein sich im allgemeinen als ausreichend erweist.

Möglichkeiten und Grenzen der Milzszintigraphie

J. Fischer

Im Vergleich zur Szintigraphie anderer Organe hat sich die Milzszintigraphie in den vergangenen 10 Jahren nur zögernd durchgesetzt. *Ein* Grund dafür ist die häufig anzutreffende Überzeugung, daß eine Milz, die nennenswert vergrößert ist, von dem Erfahrenen stets auch getastet werden kann. Ein *anderer* Grund ist der, daß man die Milz entfernen kann, anscheinend, ohne nachhaltige Auswirkungen für den Organismus. Hierbei wird allerdings übersehen, daß die Milz die stärkste räumliche Konzentration an retikuloendothelialem Gewebe darstellt, und daß Veränderungen in der Milz in einem bestimmten Umfange Rückschlüsse auf das gesamte Retikulohistiocytäre System zulassen.

Schließlich müssen wir bekennen, daß wir nur vage Kenntnisse darüber besitzen, warum eine Milzvergrößerung bei einzelnen Erkrankungen überhaupt auftritt. Wie falsch darüber hinaus unsere bisherigen Vorstellungen in der klinischen Medizin über Häufigkeit und Umfang von Milzvergrößerungen waren, soll im ersten Teil meiner Ausführungen gezeigt werden.

Die Milzszintigraphie

Eine Verbindung, die sich spezifisch in der Milz anreichert, ist noch nicht bekannt.

Die Milzszintigraphie erfolgt deshalb auch heute noch auf einem Umwege mit Hilfe von Erythrocyten, die durch physikalische oder chemische Einwirkungen künstlich geschädigt worden sind. Durch die künstliche Alteration verliert der Erythrocyt mit seiner normalen Form auch seine normale Flexibilität oder Fluidität. Er wird sphärisch und starr und kann sich nicht mehr verformen. Nach der Injektion in die Blutbahn werden solche künstlich geschädigten Erythrocyten obligat und definitiv im retikulären Maschenwerk der Milz festgehalten.

Zur Markierung der Erytrocyten wird radioaktives Chrom, radioaktives Quecksilber oder radioaktives Technetium, neuerdings auch radioaktives Rubidium verwendet.

In der Zukunft dürfte der Markierung mit ^{99m}Tc wegen der günstigen physikalischen Charakteristica dieses Isotops, eine besondere Bedeutung zukommen.

Nachdem wir 1966 zusammen mit Wolf und Leon auf die prinzipielle Möglichkeit der Erythrocytenmarkierung mit Pertechnetat hingewiesen und die ersten Milzszintigraphien mit Hilfe von ^{99m}Tc markierten, wärmealterierten Erythrocyten durchgeführt haben, wurde die Präparationsmethodik in den letzten Jahren weiter ausgebaut.

Unabhängig voneinander zeigten Berger und Johannson aus Rostock und Nouel und Brunell aus Rouen, daß durch die *Vorbehandlung* der Erythrocyten mit Zinnchlorid die *Inkubationsausbeute* und die *Stabilität* der Markierung wesentlich verbessert werden. Eigene Untersuchungen konnten diese Erfahrungen bestätigen.

In einem optimalen Bereich des Sn-Ionen-Gehaltes können 80–90% des angebotenen ^{99m}Tc fest an die Erythrocyten gebunden werden. Zur Markierung wird 1 mCi^{99m}Tc eingesetzt.

Die quantitative Abschätzung der Milzgröße

Führt man die Szintigraphie der Milz unter Standardbedingungen aus, so kann durch planimetrische Bestimmung des Flächeninhalts des Szintigramms ein quantitatives Maß für die Größe der Milz gewonnen werden. Zwischen dem Querschnitt des Organs, der sich im Seitenlagenszintigramm manifestiert, und dem Volumen der Milz bestehen ersichtliche Zusammenhänge:

Der Proportionalitätsfaktor wurde von uns aufgrund von Splenektomien und Autopsien ermittelt und hat einen Zahlenwert von 0,3. Mit einer Formel läßt sich aus dem Milzszintigramm das Milzgewicht in vivo bestimmen. Die Überprüfung der Korrelation zwischen dem szintigraphisch ermittelten und dem tatsächlichen Milzgewicht bei über 70 splenektomierten Patienten ergab eine gute Übereinstimmung auch bei sehr großen Milzen.

Die quantitative Bestimmung der Milzgröße hat eine praktische Bedeutung. Mit Hilfe der Milzszintigraphie war es erstmalig möglich, objektiv festzustellen, in welchem Umfange mit der Palpation eine Vergrößerung der Milz überhaupt aufgedeckt werden kann.

Das Ergebnis einer systematischen Studie, die wir zusammen mit Wolf seit 7 Jahren durchführen, kann in zwei Sätzen zusammengefaßt werden.

Milzszintigraphien in über 4000 Fällen zeigen, daß nur ein Drittel der vergrößerten Milzen klinisch aufgedeckt werden. Rund 70% können klinisch nicht festgestellt werden.

50% der Milzen mit einem Gewicht zwischen 600–750 g und immerhin noch 20% der Milzen mit einem Gewicht zwischen 900 und 1600 g werden nicht getastet.

Daraus ergibt sich eine Folgerung zwangsläufig: Wenn die Milz als ein relevanter Parameter registriert werden soll, kann man auf die szintigraphische Größenbestimmung nicht verzichten. Tut man es dennoch, so muß man wissen, daß man auf eine wesentliche klinische Information bewußt verzichtet.

Die Funktionsanalyse

Wärmegeschädigte Erythrocyten sind obligat eliminationspflichtig.

Die Geschwindigkeit der Extraktion aus dem Blut und der Umfang der Anreicherung in der Milz hängen von der Durchblutung der Milz und von der Beschaffenheit der *Filtrationsräume* ab. Unter letzteren versteht man die Gesamtheit des retikulären Maschenwerkes der roten Pulpa.

Histologische Umbauprozesse, wie sie z. B. in ausgeprägter Weise bei Systemerkrankungen, aber auch bei vielen anderen Erkrankungen auftreten, können diese Räume so modifizieren oder reduzieren, daß ihre Filterfunktion eingeschränkt wird. Dies führt zu einer Verzögerung der Extraktion der wärmealterierten Erythrocyten aus dem Blut und zu einer verminderten Anreicherung in der Milz.

Umgekehrt kann man immer dann, wenn die Clearance der wärmegeschädigten Erythrocyten aus dem Blut verzögert erfolgt, annehmen, daß die Mikroarchitektur der Milz gestört ist. Der Grad der Verzögerung der Clearance ist ein Maß für die Umbauprozesse in der Milz.

Es kann somit festgehalten werden: Die normale Milz kann ein akutes Angebot von 3–5 ml wärmealterierter Erythrocyten schnell aus dem Blut extrahieren und sequestrieren. Die krankhaft veränderte Milz dagegen kann, auch wenn sie stark vergrößert ist, diese Funktion nur noch partiell erfüllen.

Mißt man nach der Injektion in geeigneter Weise den zeitlichen Verlauf der Konzentration der Radioaktivität im Blut, so zeigt sich folgendes:

Beim Gesunden erfolgt ein rascher Abfall der Radioaktivität; schon nach 5–10 min werden 50% des Ausgangswertes erreicht. Beim Auftragen der Meßergebnisse in halblogarithmischen Maßstab ergibt sich eine biphasische Kurve, die aus zwei Exponentialfunktionen zusammengesetzt ist. Etwa 70% der injizierten Aktivität werden mit einer kurzen Halbwertzeit von etwa 3–5 min aus dem Blut extrahiert und mit gleicher Halbwertzeit in der Milz angereichert. Die übrigen 30% werden sehr viel langsamer aus dem Blut entfernt.

Das Funktionsbild der Milz hinsichtlich der Elimination von künstlich geschädigten Erythrocyten kann somit durch drei Zahlenwerte charakterisiert werden:

1. Die Halbwertzeit der Elimination der Radioaktivität und damit der wärmealterierten Erythrocyten aus dem Blut – ohne Zerlegung der Eliminationskurve in ihre Komponenten. Normalerweise beträgt diese Halbwertzeit *6–10 min*. In ihr widerspiegelt sich sowohl der Eliminationsfaktor Milz als auch der Eliminationsfaktor des extralienalen retikuloendothelialen Systems.

2. Die Halbwertzeit der Elimination der milzspezifischen Komponente; normalerweise beträgt sie *3,5–5,5min*

3. Der Anteil (in Prozent der injizierten Aktivität), der mit der kurzen Halbwertzeit aus dem Blut extrahiert wird. Er beträgt normalerweise *60–75%*.

Während der akuten Phase der Erkrankung, etwa einer akuten Leukose, können die Funktionsparameter hochgradig gestört sein.

Nach der Behandlung und nach weitgehender Rückbildung der Milzgröße und Normalisierung des histologischen Aufbaus erfolgt die Clearance wieder normal.

Dieses Beispiel soll den grundsätzlichen Informationsgewinn aufzeigen, der sich aus der Clearance-Untersuchung mit wärmealterierten Erythrocyten ergibt.

Abschließend möchte ich noch zeigen, wie häufig Veränderungen der Milzgröße und des Funktionsbildes vorkommen und wie hochgradig bei einzelnen Erkrankungen die Abweichungen von der Norm sein können.

Ergebnisse der Funktionsprüfung und Szintigraphie der Milz von insgesamt 344 Patienten mit hämatologischen und onkologischen Erkrankungen:

Mit Ausnahme der Myelofibrose ist bei allen anderen Krankheitsgruppen der Sequestrationsindex stark herabgesetzt, selbst bei sehr großen Milzen, z. B. bei der chronisch myeloischen Leukämie ist die Aufnahme der wärmealterierten Erythrocyten hochgradig eingeschränkt.

Auch bei Hepatopathien finden wir ausgeprägte Störungen des Funktionsbildes, wobei sich der Sequestrationsindex beim Übergang einer Hepatitis in eine Cirrhose verschlechtert.

Comparative Study of Angiography and Scanning in Diseases of the Spleen

H. R. Gould and P. Rossi

With the advent of selective catheterization techniques, angiography has been expanded to study specific organs in the body. We have attempted to compare the accuracy and relative value of both scanning and angiography in the study of various diseases of the spleen.

The spleen scans were performed as part of routine liver scans, using 2 mCi of Technetium-99m Sulphur Colloid. Approximately 5–10 % of the injected dose is taken up by the reticulo endothelial system of the spleen, and adequate spleen scans are usually obtained on routine four-view scans of the liver.

The angiograms were performed after selective celiac or splenic artery catheterizations using 50–60 cc of Renografin 76% injected at a flow rate of 6–15 cc per sec Filming is obtained at 1 film per sec for 10 sec and 1 every 3 sec fir an additional 15 sec.

The most common neoplasms which involve the spleen are the lymphomas. Discrete nodular tumor masses occur in reticulum cell sarcoma and Hodgkins Disease, but not in lymphocytic or lymphoblastic lymphoma.

The first case was a 23 year old male, admitted with a 5 month history of low back pain and generalized muscle aches. Radiographic examination revealed multiple vertebral lesions, right hilar enlargement, mediastinal and paravertebral soft tissue masses, and splenomegaly. A Technetium-99m Sulphur Colloid scan revealed hepatosplenomegaly with multiple defects in both the liver and spleen. A selective splenic arteriogram showed stretched vessels in the arterial phase, with sharply demarcated radiolucent lesions in the capillary phase. Bone marrow aspiration revealed a homogeneous population of very primitive cells, consistent with reticulum cell sarcoma.

Metastases from other tumors are rare, and usually occur with generalized carcinomatosis. An exception of this generalization is widely disseminated melanoma where the spleen is involved in about one-half of the cases. We have had three cases with metastatic melanoma of the spleen.

The first of these was a 22 year old male who had a previous excision of a melanoma in the left neck. 1 year later, a small lung nodule was seen on routine X-ray. A Technetium-99m Sulphur Colloid scan revealed a normal liver but the spleen was slightly enlarged with defects in both the upper and lower poles. A celiac arteriogram revealed marked displacement of the superior and inferior branches of the splenic artery, and an abnormal vascularity with a mottled appearance in the early capillary phase. The patient was placed on chemotherapy because of disseminated nature of his disease.

The next case was a 39 year old male with skin and lung metastases from a previously excised melanoma. A Technetium-99m Sulphur Colloid scan showed somewhat irregular uptake in the spleen that was slightly enlarged. On the angiogram the intrasplenic vessels were displaced with small areas of tumor vascularity in the late arterial phase. Multiple radiolucent defects were seen in the capillary phase. A defect was also seen in a 2.8 cm accessory spleen.

The next case was a 41 year old female who had a previous excision of a melanoma from the shoulder and was admitted with a left upper abdominal mass. Chest X-ray showed a small nodular density in the left lower lung field. The medial $^{2}/_{3}$ of the left diaphragm was elevated and irregular in contour. A Technetium-99m Sulphur Colloid scan showed the liver to be normal, but multiple defects, measuring up to 8 cm in diameter, were present in the spleen. Splenectomy was performed and at the time of surgery there was no evidence of neoplasm elsewhere in the abdomen. The spleen was markedly enlarged, measuring about 15 $\times$ 30 cm and on cut section showed several well-demarcated large metastatic nodules. Microscopic diagnosis was melanoma of the spleen with many areas of necrosis.

Non-neoplastic masses in the spleen may also be demonstrated by these techniques.

The next patient was a 35 year old cirrhotic who had been assaulted on the day prior to admission and had subsequent abdominal pain and nausea. The abdominal findings of distention and tenderness slowly resolved while in the hospital under observation. A Technetium-99m Sulphur Colloid scan performed 10 days following the trauma showed defects in the posterior border of a grossly enlarged spleen. A selective angiogram revealed several areas of radiolucency in the capillary phase. A splenectomy was performed and a sub serosal hematoma was found on the cephalolateral aspect of the spleen with a rent into the substance of the spleen.

The next patient was a 63 year old male who was admitted with an incarcerated inguinal hernia. A calcified mass was seen in the left upper quadrant on his abdominal film. Following his recovery from the herniorraphy, a selective angiogram showed displacement of the intrasplenic vessels around this mass which was in the inferolateral aspect of the spleen. The area of the mass remained relatively radiolucent during the capillary phase. A Technetium-99m Sulphur Colloid liver scan showed no gross defect in the visualized portion of the spleen and the calcified mass was thought to be on the surface of the spleen. The patient died several months later of a pulmonary infarction, and at autopsy the mass was seen to be a multiloculated calcified fibrous cyst of the spleen.

The last case was a three year old white male who was struck by an automobile and was admitted unconscious, hemiplegic, bleeding from the left ear, with multiple contusions over the chest and abdomen. A diagnostic paracentesis was performed and showed there was gross blood in the abdomen. Angiography was immediately performed. There was demonstration of a subcapsular and pericapsular hematoma of the left kidney. A selective angiogram showed a leak of contrast from a rupture of the spleen. The study was extended to the cerebral vessels demonstrating a complete occlusion of the left internal carotid associated with a fracture of the left temporal bone extending to the petrous ridge. The latter case demonstrated a distinct advantage of angiography over scanning in that multiple organ systems can be studied with great accuracy in a relatively short time during one examination.

In summary, we have demonstrated seven cases of splenic abnormality visualized either by angiography or scanning, and feel that these studies are complementary to each other. The scan is used as a screening procedure while angiography may be necessary to give a definitive diagnosis. Angiography is the preferred method of examination in acute trauma.

Anwendungsmöglichkeiten von Radioisotopen mit kurzer Halbwertzeit in der Milzszintigraphie

G. L. BURAGGI, R. RINGHINI und A. RODARI

Die Anwendung von Radioisotopen kurzer Halbwertszeit ermöglicht es, eine bedeutende Verminderung der Strahlenbelastung des Patienten bei szintigraphischen Untersuchungen zu erreichen. Im Falle der Milz ist die am meisten verbreitete Technik die Markierung der Erythrozyten mit ^{197}Hg BMHP.

Die Verfasser haben Versuche durchgeführt, um die Markierung von menschlichen Erythrocyten mit ^{99m}Tc und ^{113m}In und die darauffolgende Schädigung zu bekommen, um eine schnelle Fixation in der Milz zu ermöglichen.

Was das ^{99m}Tc anbetrifft, wurden Techniken angewendet, die den von anderen Verfassern vorgeschlagenen Techniken ähnlich sind; was das ^{113m}In anbelangt, wurde ein originelles Verfahren angewendet.

Nachstehend werden die durchgeführten Studien dargelegt, um die Stabilität der Markierung zu prüfen und um den Bindungspunkt des verwendeten Radioisotopes an den Erythrocyten festzulegen. Außerdem werden die Ergebnisse der szintigraphischen Untersuchung gegeben, die zuerst am Tier und dann am Menschen durchgeführt wurden.

Diseases of the Pancreas

Combined Angiographic and Scintigraphic Examination of the Pancreas

M. Cen and H.-J. Fernholz

The positive evidence of a pancreas angiography is with about 55% accuracy and 38% wrong negative diagnosis relatively limited.

Even the introduction of the superselective angiography and the pharmaco-angiography have improved minimal the certainty of angiographic diagnosticproce-dure.

Concerning pancreas scintigraphy, 70% accuracy are taken for granted at present, but this percentage seems to need a revision, specially by grouping the different diseases. Most of all the frequency of wrong positive scintigraphic diagnosis has to be considered. The gastro-enteric passage seems a relatively sure method for examining the pancreas as 60% of the diagnosis are correct. This concerns, in first place, the head of the pancreas while the number of diagnostic mistakes of the body and tail of pancreas is by now unknown.

As every examination method in its isolated positive evidence is limited it seemed necessary to check whether the evidence of the morphological condition of pancreas can be improved by the combination of the above-mentioned method. That is the reason why we analysed the test results of 30 persons out of our total patients during the last year. These 30 persons had beside of the routine gastroenteric passage a scintigraphy and an angiography.

16 patients who showed no symptoms of a disease of pancreas the gastro-enteric passage was 13 times without pathological findings, the scintigraphy 6 times and the angiography 10 times.

7 patients with a chronic pancreatitis showed by a scintigram 4 times changes which could be taken for a chronic inflammable pancreas process.

The angiography showed corresponding signs 4 times in comparison to the gastro-enteric passage which made assume twice a chronic pancreatitis.

Out of 6 patients with a pancreas tumor one pancreas insuloma of about 1 cm diameter couldn't be diagnosed, all the other tumors could angiographicly be prooved clearly.

The gastro-enteric passage not only failed the insuloma but also a 4 cm corpus tumor. A pancreas tumor could only be assumed twice by a scintigraphy.

All three examinations combined were once carried out during an acute pancreatitis but only the gastro-entertic passage showed signs for an adequate pancreas process.

The chronic pancreatitis showed scintigraphic twice and angiographic 3 times wrong positive results, while the pancreas tumor showed in the angiography only twice, and in the scintigram and in the gastro-enteric passage, 4 times wrong positive results. The obvious frequency of wrong diagnosis of the gastro-enteric passage is based retrospectively on the ambiguity of an enlarged and displaced duodenal loop.

The following can be stated:

1. the gastro-enteric passage is suitable for diagnosing th head of pancreas tumors. The differential diagnose between a chronic pancreatitis and a neoplasm is improved by an angiography.

2. Valuating diffuse and circumscribed storage defects of scintigraphy you have to be reluctant and try to clear the results by an angiography.

Furthermore, we have tried to find out whether it is possible to improve the evidence about the morphological state of pancreas by a combination of the above mentioned methods.

Diagnosing a chronic pancreatitis an improvement of the accuracy by a combination of all three methods was obtained, even if the total of diagnoses frequency could not reach the number of the final clinical diagnosis.

In case of pancreas-tumors the accuracy of an angiography by combination with the two other methods could not be improved while the combination stomach examination and scintigram reached the positive evidence of angiography.

The reduction of angiographic and scintigraphic wrong positive results from the combination of both methods is remarkable. With the help of angiography three scintigraphic wrong positive pancreatitis diagnosis could be dropped. Even an angiographic wrong positive tumor diagnosis could be corrected by combination with scintigraphy.

Two examples might explain the possibilities and difficulties concerning differential diagnoes.

The first case concerns histologically an inflammable process. The angiographic signs made us assume a tumor in all probability. In the scintigraphy a hot area was seen, there fore what a pancreas tumor was excluded.

Based on principles the statement of a normal storage picture in the scintigram reduces in our opinion the probability of an angiographic tentative diagnoses of an inflammable disease.

The second case showed scintigraphic a cold area. The angiography resulted in no sufficient signs for a pancreas process. In this case the scintigraphic result was not attributed a pathological importance.

Within the clinical pancreas diagnoses, angiography and scintigraphy contribute besides the gastric-enteric passage a part to the final diagnoses.

A combination of these examinations leads to a worth mentioning improvement of accuracy on inflammable and tumerous pancreas disease.

Doppelradionuklid Pankreas–Funktionsszintigraphie mit einem Prozeßrechner

H. Hundeshagen, H. Creutzig und H. Dopslaff

Die Darstellung der Bauchspeicheldrüse ist für die Diagnostik von Pankreasaffektionen, ähnlich wie bei anderen Organen, von großer Bedeutung. Leider existiert bis heute noch kein Verfahren, welches mit der Sicherheit, die für differentialdiagnostische Aussagen gegeben sein muß, eine Beurteilung des Organs durch Strukturanalysen gestattet. Damit ergibt sich aber auch die Schwierigkeit, ein neu eingeführtes Untersuchungsverfahren auf seine klinische Effektivität zu überprüfen, da mangelhafte Vergleichsmöglichkeiten vorhanden sind. Der klinische Verlauf und operative Eingriffe gelten heute immer noch als Vergleichsparameter. Neben diesem erhebt sich noch die Forderung, daß das Untersuchungsverfahren selbst für den Patienten möglichst unbelästigend und leicht durchführbar ist, denn erst dann könnte daraus ein Routineverfahren zur Erfassung einer größeren Zahl von klinisch Verdächtigen werden.

Es ergeben sich also zwei wichtige Forderungen, nämlich:

1. Darstellung der Bauchspeicheldrüse, und zwar so, daß Defekte erkennbar sind und

2. Anwendung eines für den Patienten einfachen und risikoarmen Untersuchungsverfahrens.

Welchen Beitrag kann die Nuklearmedizin hierzu leisten? Blau, Manske und Bender ersetzten das Schwefelatom in der Aminosäure Methionin durch das beim Zerfall Gamma-Strahlen aussendende Radionuklid Selen-75 und versuchten, die Bauchspeicheldrüse mit dem so gewonnenen radioaktiven Indikator darzustellen. Durch die in dem Organ verhältnismäßig große Proteinsyntheserate gelingt eine Anreicherung im Verhältnis 2 bis 5 zu 1 gegenüber der Leber und 2 bis 7 zu 1 gegenüber dem Duodenum, ausgedrückt als Radioaktivität-pro-Gramm-Gewebe.

Unter diesen Bedingungen muß es mit der szintigraphischen Darstellung der Radioaktivitätsablagerung in Organen gelingen, auch die Bauchspeicheldrüse zu erfassen. Doch ergeben sich zwei große Schwierigkeiten. Einmal sind zur Darstellung von außen durch die Szintigraphie die topographischen Beziehungen besonders zur Leber und zum Darm zu beachten und zum anderen handelt es sich um die Erfassung eines Stoffwechselvorganges, der in einer bestimmten Zeit abläuft. Beide Faktoren wirken für das Untersuchungsverfahren erschwerend. Hinzu kommt, daß der applizierte radioaktive Indikator (2–3 μCi/kg Körpergewicht) teuer ist und eine gegenüber anderen nuklearmedizinischen Untersuchungsverfahren hohe Strahlenbelastung von 1–2 rad Ganzkörper bei einer effektiven Ganzkörperhalbwertszeit von 45,5 $\pm$ 10 Tagen erreicht wird.

Aufgrund dieser das Untersuchungsverfahren stark belastenden Faktoren ist besonders die Frage nach der klinischen Wertigkeit zu stellen.

Will man diese beantworten, so muß zunächst das methodische Vorgehen in verschiedenen Entwicklungsstufen aufgeschlüsselt und diese mit bewertet werden. CREUTZIG hat hierzu umfangreiche Untersuchungen durchgeführt.

Wir unterscheiden heute folgende Verfahren:

1. Applikation von ^{75}Se-Methionin und Szintigraphie des Oberbauches mit einem 5''-Kristall-Scanner, dabei Darstellung von Leber, Pankreas und Darm. Untersuchungsdauer 30–60 min.

2. Doppelradionuklid-Szintigraphie nach Applikation von ^{75}Se-Methionin und Verfahren wie unter 1., dann zusätzliche Applikation von ^{198}Au-Kolloid und Darstellung der Leber. Anschließend optische oder elektronische Subtraktion beider Informationen. Untersuchungsdauer 45–90 min.

3. Einsatz einer Szintillations-Kamera oder eines Mehrkristallscanners, Untersuchungsdauer pro Bild 4–12 min und anschließendes Vorgehen wie unter 2.

4. Doppelradionuklid-Szintigraphie, wie bei 2 und 3, mit einer Szintillations-Kamera oder einem 10-Kristall-Scanner, die im "on line"-Betrieb an einen Prozeßrechner angeschlossen sind.

Aufnahme von Selenszintigrammen über 60–90 min in bestimmten Zeitabständen und Verarbeitung der Information im Prozeßrechner durch ein spezielles Rechenprogramm, d. h. nicht einfache Subtraktion und zusätzlich Berücksichtigung der durch den Stoffwechsel gegebenen zeitlich verschiedenen Radioaktivitätsverteilung.

Wir sind aufgrund unserer Erfahrungen und Vergleichsuntersuchungen heute der Ansicht, daß das Verfahren, wie unter 1. beschrieben, im Verhältnis zu seiner klinischen Wertigkeit so ist, daß es für eine gezielte Pankreas-Diagnostik nicht ver-

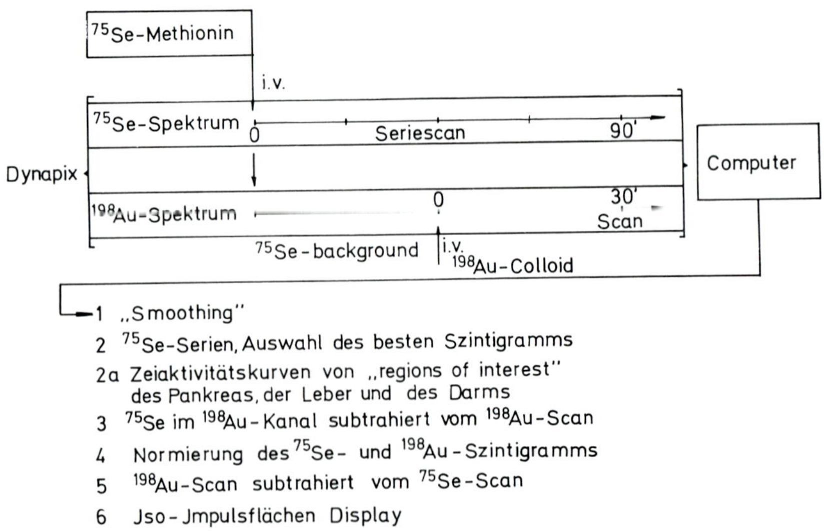

Abb. 1. Schema und Prozeßrechner-Programm zur Doppelradionuklid-Pankreasfunktions-Szintigraphie

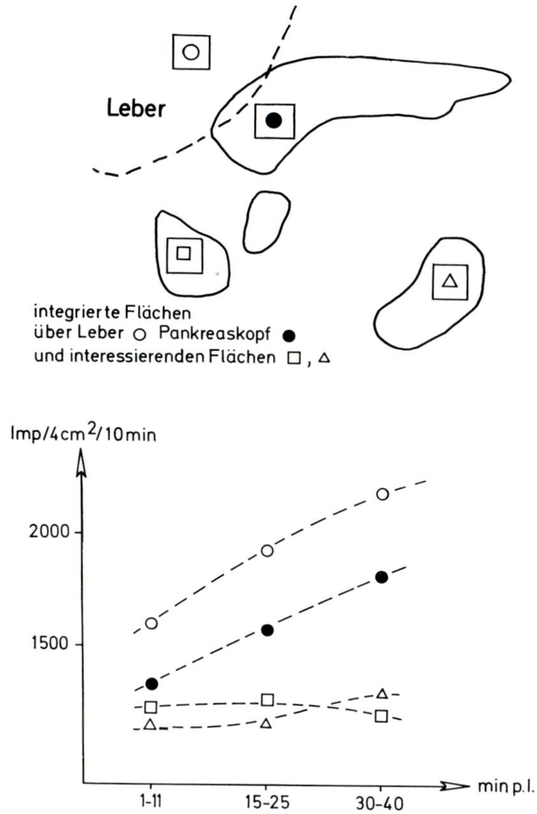

a

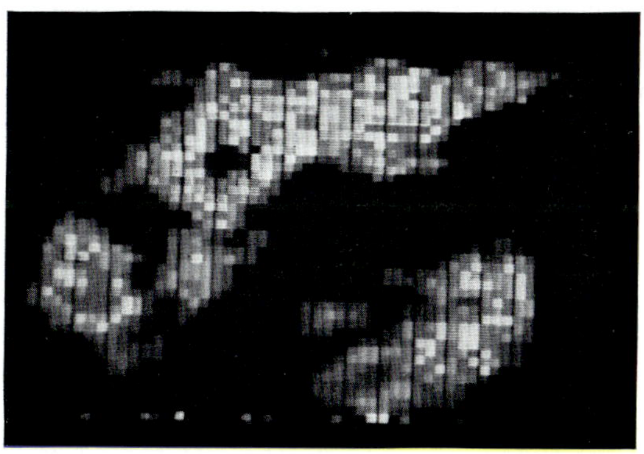

b

Abb. 2. a Szintigramm 30–38 min p. I. von 210 μCi ^{75}Se-Selenmethionin nach Subtraktion der überlagernden Leberradioaktivität. b schematische Darstellung der Abb. 2a mit eingezeichneten „regions of interest“

wendbar ist. Auch mit den unter 2. und 3. angegebenen Methoden ist eine für die klinische Aussagemöglichkeit optimale Lösung nicht gegeben.

Wir sind über die von 1. bis 3. angegebenen Verfahren zu dem 4. gekommen und gehen folgendermaßen vor (Abb. 1).

Methode

Der Patient wird nicht besonders vorbereitet. Er erhält zunächst 3 μCi ^{75}Se-Methionin/kg Körpergewicht i.v. appliziert. Als Untersuchungsgerät dient ein 10-Kristall-Scanner (DYNAPIX), der im "on line"-Betrieb an einen erweiterten LINC-8-Prozeßrechner angeschlossen ist. Der Patient liegt während der Untersuchungszeit mit der linken Seite etwas angehoben und fixiert auf einer Untersuchungsliege. Es werden in 15 min Abstand Szintigramme aufgenommen und die Information gespeichert. Nach 90 min erfolgt die i.v. Applikation von 100–150 μCi ^{198}Au. Vorher wurde jedoch ein ^{75}Se-Szintigramm mit der Einstellung des Szintigraphie-Gerätes auf die ^{198}Au-Energie angefertigt.

Die im Prozeßrechner gespeicherten Informationen werden nach einem speziellen Rechenprogramm verarbeitet. Danach gelingt die isolierte Darstellung der Radioaktivitätsablagerung in der Bauchspeicheldrüse, und zwar so, daß nicht nur das Organ sichtbar wird, sondern auch Speicherungsdefekte mit größerer Sicherheit beurteilbar sind.

In Zweifelsfällen hilft die Auswertung von "regions of interest", von denen aufgrund der Serien-Szintigramme Funktionskurven ausgeschrieben werden. Diese gestatten eine Aussage, ob es sich um Pankreas, Darm oder zu den Nieren zugehöriges radioaktivitätsspeicherndes Gewebe handelt (Abb. 2).

Klinik

Die an uns zur Pankreasuntersuchung überwiesenen Patienten kommen etwa zu $^2/_3$ aus den Kliniken und $^1/_3$ von niedergelassenen Ärzten (Abb. 3).

Die klinischen Symptome und die dem Untersucher zur Verfügung stehenden Unterlagen reichen von unklaren Oberbauchbeschwerden bis zum Verdacht auf einen raumfordernden Prozeß. Die Beurteilung der Szintigramme wurde bei den hier zusammengefaßten Fällen von ein und derselben Person durchgeführt.

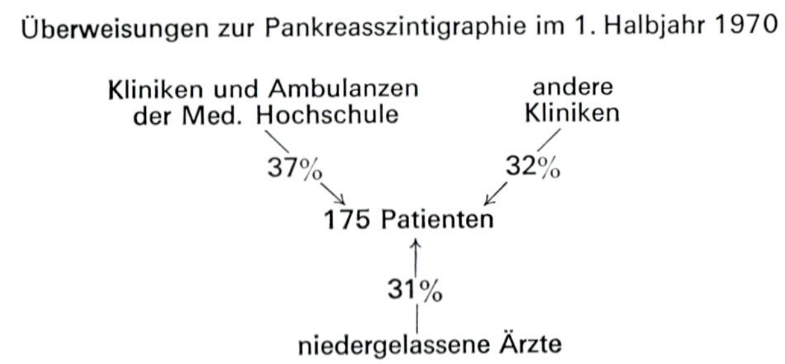

Abb. 3. Aufschlüsselung der Überweisungen zur Pankreas-Szintigraphie an das Institut für Nuklearmedizin und spezielle Biophysik im 1. Halbjahr 1970

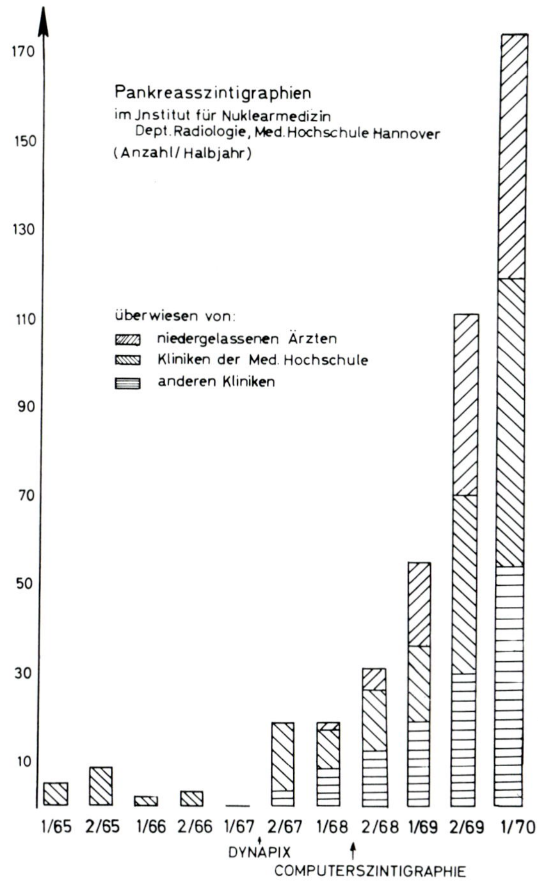

Abb. 4. Übersicht über die Anzahl der Patienten der Pankreas-Szintigraphien im Institut für Nuklearmedizin und spezielle Biophysik pro Jahreshälfte von 1965 bis 1. Halbjahr 1970. Auffällig ist der Anstieg nach Einführung des hier beschriebenen Untersuchungsverfahrens

Die Patientenzahlen stiegen besonders nach Einführung der Doppelradionuklid-Funktionsszintigraphie (Abb. 4), auch dies kann als ein gewisser Wert zur Beurteilung der Effektivität der Methode herangezogen werden. Heute liegen wir aus gerätetechnischen Gründen bei 20–25 Untersuchungen pro Woche.

Die szintigraphischen Bilder von Organen werden im allgemeinen nach Größe, Form, Lage und Speicherungsmuster beurteilt. Die isolierte Darstellung der Bauchspeicheldrüse gestattet dieses Vorgehen nun auch. Man muß sich zunächst über die verschiedenen Formen der Projektion des radioaktivitätsspeichernden normalen Organs auf die Körperoberfläche Klarheit verschaffen. Eine Zusammenstellung von 144 Normalfällen ergibt die in Abb. 5 dargestellten Formen und ihren prozentualen Anteil am Gesamtkollektiv.

Bei diesen normalen Pankreas-Szintigrammen ist die Radioaktivitätsverteilung gleichmäßig vom Rande bis zur Mitte des Organs, und es bestehen keine Bezirke mit verminderter Radioaktivitätseinlagerung (Abb. 6a).

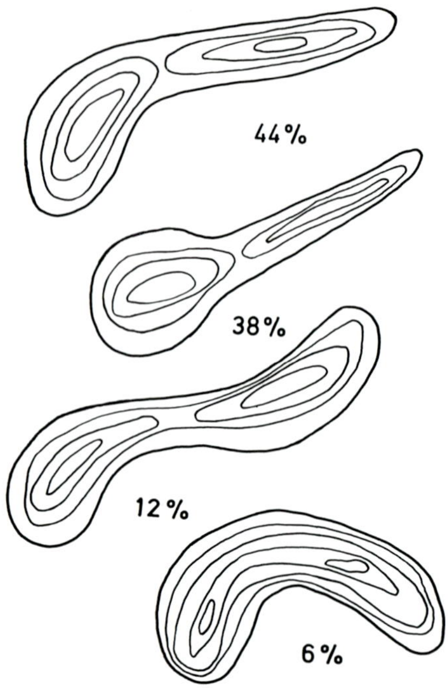

Abb. 5. Formen von normalen Pankreas-Darstellungen im Szintigramm und ihr prozentualer Anteil an der Gesamtzahl von 144 Normal-Fällen

Im Gegensatz hierzu stehen die Befunde, bei denen über ein normal konfiguriertes Szintigramm Stellen mit verminderter Radioaktivität verteilt sichtbar werden (Abb. 6b). Erreichen diese Zonen zusammengenommen mehr als 35% der Organfläche, so geben wir einen Parenchymschaden „Stadium 1“ an.

Tritt zusätzlich zu diesem Befund eine Vergröberung des Organs ein, so geben wir einen Parenchymschaden „Stadium 2“ an (Abb. 7).

Kommt zu diesem Befund eine verstärkte Ablagerung von Radioaktivität im Darmepithel hinzu, so geben wir das „Stadium 3“ an. Diese Ergebnisse sind in Abb. 8 noch einmal zusammengefaßt.

Welche klinische Bedeutung kommt diesen Befunden und dieser Einteilung zu?

Soweit unsere bisherigen Erfahrungen gehen, handelt es sich in diesen Fällen im allgemeinen um eine chronisch rezidivierende Pankreatitis. Hierbei sind die als „Stadium 3“ bezeichneten Befunde repräsentativ für klinisch nachgewiesene und abgesicherte Fälle. Das Stadium 1 und 2 finden wir bei Patienten, die aufgrund ihrer Symptomatik verdächtig sind und aus diesem Grund eingewiesen werden. Ergibt sich bei nicht weiter voruntersuchten Patienten eines dieser Bilder, so schlagen wir in jedem Falle eine größere klinische Durchuntersuchung vor. Erhalten wir bei unklaren Oberbauchbeschwerden ein normales Pankreas-Szintigramm, so können wir aufgrund unserer bisherigen Befunde eine Beteiligung des Organs mit großer Wahrscheinlichkeit als ausgeschlossen betrachten.

Kontrolluntersuchungen sind bei den Stadien 1 und 2 unter Therapie angezeigt und ergeben weitere wichtige Aufschlüsse.

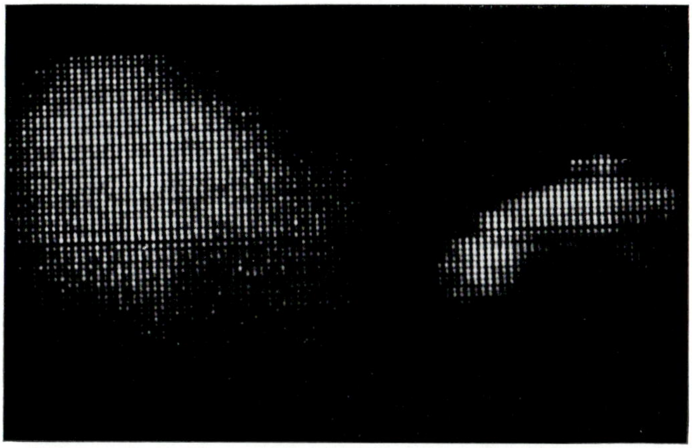

a

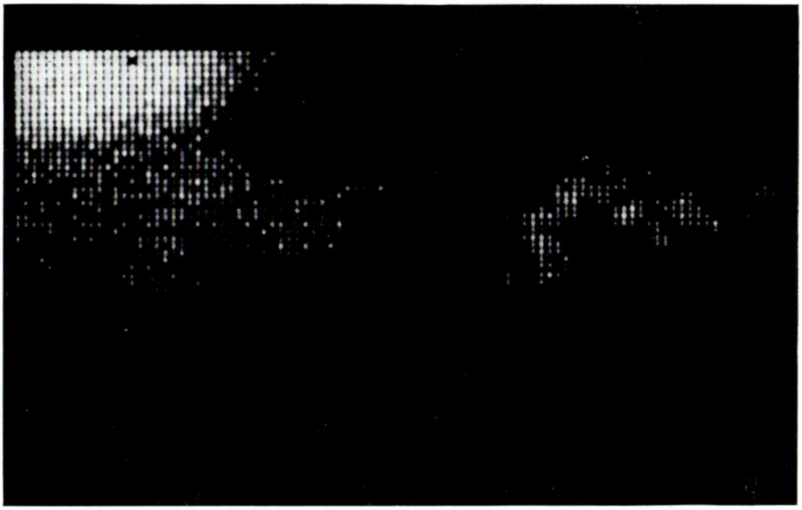

b

Abb. 6a und b. Pankreasszintigraphie. Linke Bildseite: ^{75}Se-Szintigramm Leber und Pankreas; rechte Bildseite: Pankreas nach Auswertungsprogramm. a Normales Pankreasszintigramm. b Szintigramm mit kleinfleckigen Speicherungsdefekten, die mehr als 35 % der Gesamtfläche ausmachen

Raumfordernde Prozesse machen sich im isolierten Pakreas-Szintigramm durch Ausfall eines großen Organ-Areals bemerkbar, wobei das restliche Gewebe sich wie bei einem Pankreasparenchymschaden darstellt. Diese Ausfälle betreffen hauptsächlich den Pankreaskopf, können aber auch den Körper- und Schwanzbereich umfassen (Abb. 9)

Die Pankreas-Szintigraphie mit isolierter Darstellung des Organs ergibt gerade bei den raumfordernden Prozessen einen wichtigen Hinweis. So konnten bei 82 Pa-

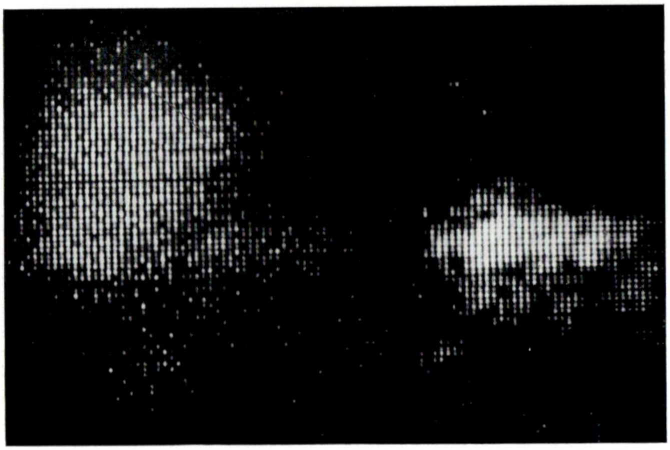

Abb. 7. Pankreas-Szintigraphie: Parenchymschaden „Stadium 2". Links ^{75}Se-Szintigramm Leber und Pankreas; rechts Pankreas nach Rechenprogramm, Vergröberung des Organs und multiple kleine Speicherungsdefekte

	Multiple kleine Speicherungsdefekte (>35% der Organfläche)	Organ-Fläche vergrößert	hohe Radioaktivitäts-Einlagerung im Darm	
Normal	/	/	/	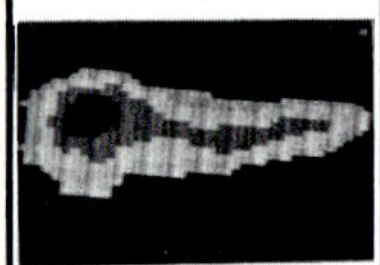
Parenchymschaden Stadium I	+	/	/	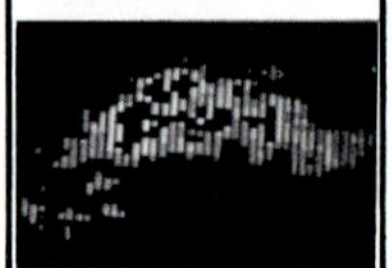
Parenchymschaden Stadium II	+	+	/	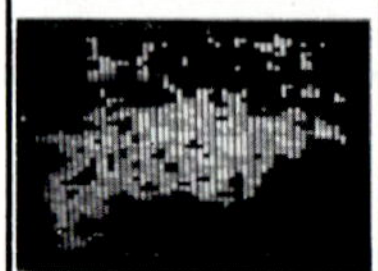
Parenchymschaden Stadium III	+	+	+	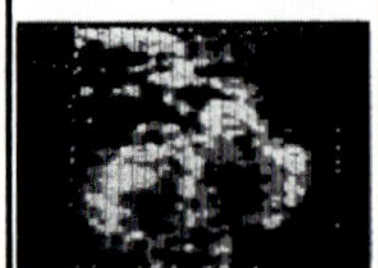

Abb. 8. Schematische Übersicht über die Möglichkeiten von Parenchymschäden des Pankreas, ohne daß ein großer Teil des Organs keine Radioaktivität speichert. Einteilung in 3 Stadien

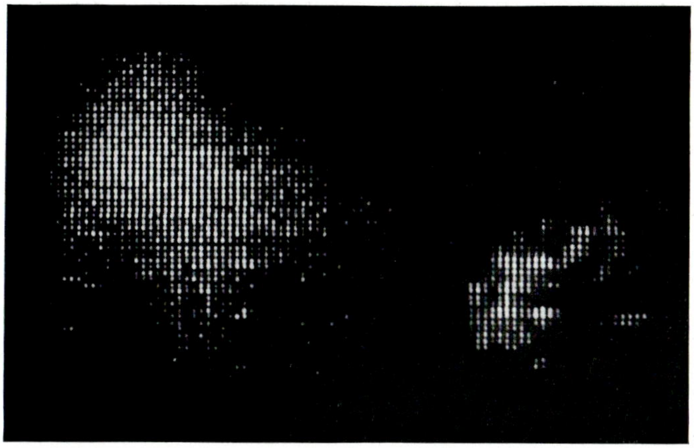

Abb. 9. Pankreas-Szintigraphie: Pankreas-Ca. im Bereich des Körpers und Schwanzes. Keine Radioaktivitätsspeicherung in diesen Teilen des Organs. Pankreaskopf mit multiplen Speicherungsdefekten. Links ^{75}Se-Methionin-Szintigramm Leber-Pankreas, rechts isolierte Darstellung des Pankreas

tienten mittels der hier beschriebenen szintigraphischen Methode 29 Pankreas-Carcinome erkannt werden. 10 Fälle dagegen waren falschpositiv, während kein tatsächlicher Befund übersehen wurde. Wie die Tabelle zeigt, bedeutet dies gegenüber der Subtraktions-Szintigraphie einen Fortschritt.

Tabelle. *Übersicht über 119 Fälle, bei denen nach Doppelradionuklid-Szintigraphie die einfache Subtraktionsmethode [Kernspeicherserie] oder die Auswertung mit dem Prozeßrechnerprogramm [Computerserie] durchgeführt wurde*

	Kernspeicherserie	Computerserie
gesicherte Diagnose	37	82
nicht beurteilbar	2	○
normal ja	20	43
nein	2	○
falsch negativ	9 %	○
übersehene Carcinome	2	○
pathologisch ja	10	29
nein	5	10
falsch positiv	33 %	25 %

Die Doppelradionuklid-Pankreas-Funktionsszintigraphie eignet sich als screening-Methode bei Verdacht auf Pankreasaffektionen. Sehr wichtig erscheint uns dabei die Möglichkeit der Erstellung von Funktionskurven über bestimmte "regions of interest". Hierdurch lassen sich weitere Differenzierungen über das radioaktivitätsspeichernde Gewebe vornehmen.

Eine isolierte Darstellung der Organradioaktivitätsablagerung erlaubt eine sichere Beurteilung. Wenn auch grundsätzlich eine Artdiagnostik durch die Szintigraphie nicht möglich ist, so ergibt die Erfahrung und das Zusammenspiel mit anderen klinischen diagnostischen Verfahren doch einen wichtigen Hinweis. Auch Verlaufskontrollen nach einer eingeleiteten Therapie unterstreichen die klinische Wertigkeit des Untersuchungsverfahrens. Da nunmehr technisch eine Lösung vorhanden ist, die ohne große Belästigung des Patienten eine beurteilbare Darstellung der Bauchspeicheldrüse ergibt, sollte das Hauptaugenmerk auf die Erprobung neuer radioaktiver Indikatoren zur Pankreas-Szintigraphie gelegt werden.

Zusammenfassung

Der metabolische Umsatz des radioaktiven Indikators ^{75}Se-Methionin und die topographischen Verhältnisse der Bauchspeicheldrüse gegenüber Organen wie Leber, Darm und Nieren lassen die normale Pankreas-Szintigraphie im Verhältnis-Aufwand zu klinischer Wertigkeit so nachteilig erscheinen, daß andere Verfahren, wie Einsatz der Doppelradionuklid-Szintigraphie mittels einer Szintillations-Kamera oder eines Mehrkristall-Scanners und der einfachen Subtraktion, eingeführt wurden.

Eine Weiterentwicklung ist die Doppelradionuklid-Funktionsszintigraphie, die hier beschrieben wird. Durch die isolierte Darstellung der Radioaktivitätsablagerung im Pankreas ist eine bessere Beurteilung der Form und des Speicherungsmusters möglich. Funktionskurven von "regions of interest" erlauben eine Aufschlüsselung verschiedener Gewebe. Es wird eine Einteilung von Speicherungsdefekten bei vollständiger Darstellung des Organs in 3 Stadien angegeben. Bei einer Gruppe von Patienten mit Verdacht auf raumfordernden Prozeß wurde kein falsch-negativer Befund erhoben, jedoch lag die Rate der falsch-positiven bei 25%. Für die Klinik ergibt dieses Verfahren wichtige Hinweise, so daß es trotz des erheblichen technischen Aufwandes als Routinemethode vertretbar ist.

Pancreatic Scanning in Clinical Practice and its Comparison with Splanchnic Angiography

A. RODRIGUEZ-ANTUNEZ and R. J. ALFIDI

The pancreatic scintigram presents a challenging problem in interpretation and, in many cases, definite conclusions cannot be reached. The scintigraphic criteria of a normal pancreas are an even distribution of radioactivity and the absence of distortion of the outline of the pancreas.

A fairly common appearance in many normal scintigrams is a narrowing, with diminution of radioactivity, at the neck of the pancreas. In a series of normal pancreatic scintigrams, it is clear that a normal pancreas can be any one of various shapes, a nonuniformity that increases the difficulty of interpretation.

The scintigraphic criteria of an abnormal pancreas are lack of demonstration of the entire pancreas, only partial demonstration of the pancreas, and filling defects within the pancreatic shadow. The lack of demonstration of the pancreas in the scintigram, in my experience, is the most reliable sign of pancreatic disease, as demonstrated on the scintigram. Distortion of the shape of the gland, as well as of some areas of decreased radioactive uptake, has not invariably been a definite sign of abnormality, in my experience.

A fairly common finding in the scintigram is an area of radioactivity on the left side of the abdomen. This finding is considered to be due to the accumulation of radioactive enzymes within the upper jejunum. This finding can be interpreted a proof of the functional integrity of the pancreas. In an effort to correlate the activity of the left side of the abdomen with the status of the pancreas, I reached the following conclusion. Although presence of radioactivity in the upper portion of the jejunum is not always indicative of normality, in doubtful cases in which the pancreas is difficult to identify or its shape is distorted or bizarre, a tentative diagnosis of normality is justified when radioactivity is evident in the upper portion of the jejunum.

For a period of approximately 5 years, over 500 patients have been referred to our department for pancreatic scans. Many of these patients had a clinical diagnosis of pancreatic neoplasm but the majority of them were referred because of vague abdominal symptoms and the clinician could not exclude the possibility of pancreatic tumor. A total of 439 cases has been analyzed for the purpose of this report. I wish to emphasize that, as in previous reports, the scans were not analyzed in a retrospective fashion. The analysis was done by using the original report which was dictated, frequently without clinical information.

The table demonstrates the diagnostic accuracy obtained in all of the cases analyzed.

Table 1. *Analysis of 439 cases*

	Surgical or Clinical Verifications No. of	No.	No.	Correct
Diagnosis	Scintigrams	Right	Wrong	%
Normal	304	281	23	92
Abnormal	135	69	66	51
Total	439			

The material we have reviewed offers a unique opportunity to compare 150 cases where both angiography and pancreatic scanning were performed. The accuracy of both studies is compared in the light of pre-operative diagnoses rather than a retrospective analysis. Methods of catherization, catheter choice, and filming will also be covered extensively. For these reasons we will not discuss the angiographic criteria which were used to determine whether a study was normal or abnormal, except to say that the presence or absence of tumor, pancreatitis, etc., was based upon vessel encasement, displacement, "tumor stain" venous thrombosis and, occasionally, on the presence of arteriovenous shunting.

No attempt was made to differentiate angiographic and scanographic findings as to the presence or absence of tumor, pancreatitis, etc. A correct diagnosis of "normal" or "abnormal" was considered equally important.

Where the scan or angiogram were interpreted as normal in a patient whose follow up or surgery also indicated that the pancreas was normal, the study was listed as correct. Where the scan or angiogram were found to be in disagreement with subsequent findings at surgery, autopsy etc., the study was listed as incorrect.

The first line of the Table 2 deals with instances where both the angiogram and scan were interpreted correctly in the same patient. It can be seen that when both studies were in agreement, accuracy was only slightly better than flipping a coin when all 150 cases were considered. If, however, one compares only those cases where both the scan and the angiogram agreed (97 patients), their combined accuracy was 92%. Therefore, when both studies agree in the same patient, considerable weight must be attached to their significance.

Table 2. *Pancreatic scan vs. angiogram*

150 Cases Stidued By Both Methods		%
Both Correct	89	59
Both Wrong	8	5
Scan Correct Angiogram Wrong	29	19
Angiogram Correct Scan Wrong	24	16

When a comparison of the remainder of the material is made, we have found that either the scan or angiogram was correct in an additional 35% of patients. Angiographic accuracy, taken along, was 75%; the scan was correct in 78%. One of the two studies was correct in 95% of cases. Where there was a difference in interpretation of either test, the question arose as to which of the two was correct. Unfortunately this study does not solve this dilemma as in both instances the scan or the angiogram was incorrect in approximately the same number of cases.

It should be emphasized that better statistics may be available in other studies; however, we feel that this may be tue to patient selection. There are very few patients in this study who had what might be considered advanced signs or symptoms of pancreatic carcinoma. Patients with obstructive jaundice were not studied angiographically but rather with trans-hepatic cholangiography. Despite the fact that our investigations have probably resulted in a number of "early diagnosis". This has not significantly improved survival as regards pancreatic carcinoma. One must unfortunately conclude that by the time the patient begins to experience "early" signs and symptoms, the disease has most often progressed to a presently incurable stage.

As mentioned earlier, it was felt that a correct diagnosis of a normal pancreas was as important as a diagnosis of abnormal pancreas by either method. For those reasons we have not included statistics on which of the correct or incorrect diagnoses were neoplasms, pancreatitis etc. The one area where angiography appeared to have a significant advantage over pancreatic scanning was in the diagnosis of functioning islet cell adenomas. The slide is the pancreatic scan of the patient with well documented hypoglycema. The angiogram shown on the next two slides clearly demosstrates a small vascular neoplasm in the region of the tail of the pancreas supplied by branches of the splenic artery. The scan was interpreted as normal whereas a preoperative diagnosis of an islet cell adenoma in the tail of the pancreas was made by means of angiography. Two additional cases of "insulinoma" and one Zollinger Ellison Syndrome were also correctly diagnosed by means of arteriography. In a fourth case of "insulinoma" the arteriogram was unsuccessful in demonstrating the site of the lesion. The majority of hyperfunctioning adenomas that we have localized angiographically have been quite small but, because of intense straining with contrast media, have been readily identified. It is doubtful that any of these would have been detected by means of pancreatic scanning because of their small mass.

With our present experience, it appears that angiography is the procedure of choice in localizing pancreatic islet cell adenomas. When either the scan or the angiogram is inconclusive the other study should be performed.

Resultats comparés de la scintigraphie et de l'artériographie pancréatique

Ch. Gros, P. Warter, R. Vergnes, M. Truchot, J. Tongio et P. Haehnel

La scintigraphie et l'artériographie pancréatique ont été souvent présentées comme des techniques rivales. En réalité la nature même des informations qu'elles procurent sont dissemblables et complémentaires. Cette constatation explique souvent la difficulté de pratiquer chez un même patient les deux techniques, les cliniciens préférant soit l'une soit l'autre.

D'autre part leur technique complexe et astreignante pour le patient ne permet pas toujour leur mise en oeuvre successive:

1. Scintigraphie

a) jeûne protéique de 48 H.
b) Jeûne total 12 H. avant l'examen.
c) Sevrage tabagique complet.
d) Protocole de Sodee.

2. Pour l'artériographie

a) Mise en place de deux sondes, l'une dans le tronc coelique, l'autre dans l'artère mésentérique supérieure.

b) Modificateur de comportement soit du pancréas par la Sécrétine, soit dans vaisseaux eux-mêmes par l'Adrénaline.

c) Interprétation délicate en raison du faible calibre des arterès.

Sur un total de 16 cas, nombre très réduit en raison de la difficulté à obtenir des cliniciens les deux examens chez le même malade, 9 cas ont été opérés et vérifiés histologiquement.

En gros, les résultats sont comparables sur le plan de l'information dans les pancréatites chroniques (zone froide scintigraphique et vascularisation pauvre avec multiples sténoses artérielles).

Dans les volumineuses tumeurs malignes pancréatiques la concordance entre les 2 techniques est remarquable, d'autant plus que la scintigraphie hépatique simultanée met souvent en évidence des métastases hépatiques visibles également sur les temps tardifs des angiographies coeliaques.

Mais malgré la concordance observée l'artériographie semble cependant apporter plus d'informations. Si l'image élémentaire scintigraphique est la lacune, seule l'exploration vasculaire est le seul examen permettant une cartographie artérielle, toujours intéressante en raison de nombreuses variations anatomiques, ainsi que la mise en évidence du retentissement veineux de la lésion pancréatique (oblitération segmentaire de la veine splénique avec signes angiographiques d'hypertension portale à la splénoportographie de retour).

Enfin l'artériographie permet la mise en évidence de toute autre lésion associée ou d'une étiologie autre à une masse abdominale.

En conclusion, la scintigraphie et l'artériographie ne doivent être considérées comme des techniques rivales, mais bien plutôt complémentaires. Si la scintigraphie pancréatique technique plus facilement réalisable que l'exploration vasculaire permet d'apprécier une zone d'hypofixation et surtout de suivre cette anomalie au cours de l'évolution puisque l'examen peut être pratiqué de façon iterative, l'artériographie seule nous semble apte à apporter des informations précises, non seulement sur la nature même du processus pathologique, mais également sur la distribution artérielle, facilitant ainsi le geste chirurgical.

Angioscintigraphy of the Pancreas

W. Bessler and A. Jucker

In 12 patients transfered to the X-ray department for an angiographic examination of the pancreas, in addition to arteriography, an angioscintigram of the upper abdomen is performed.

The angioscintigrams are made after the injection of 300 μCi macroaggregates of ^{131}I human serum albumin in each of the two catheters placed with their tips in the origin of the celiac and of the superior mesenteric artery. In 7 of the 12 patients previous to arteriography the pancreas is scanned with ^{75}Se-selenmethionine.

The aim of the study is to determine whether angioscintigraphy can give additional information for the interpretation of the arteriogram of the pancreas.

The distribution of radioactivity on the angioscintigram is depending on the course and caliber of the branches of the injected arteries. Due to the individual variations of the arteries, the amount of the uptake of radioactivity in the abdominal organs differs from patient to patient. An accumulation of the tracer substance can be noted in the spleen, pancreas, liver and, to a varying degree, in the stomach and in the small and large bowel. The overprojection of radioactivity in the intestines is often disturbing for the interpretation of the scintigraphic image of the pancreas. However in most cases it is possible to outline at least the head and the body of the pancreas, whereas the pancreatic tail generally disappears within the radioactivity of the spleen and the left colic flexure.

Fig. 1 shows the different studies performed in a 46 year old patient with pain in the upper abdomen, attacks of vomiting, loss of appetite and weight over several months. Selective duodenography demonstrates a filling defect in the region of the inferior flexure of the duodenum (Fig. 1a). A scarcity and irregular caliber of the pancreatico-duodenal arteries can be noted on the arteriogram (Fig. 1b). No tumour stain appears in the later phases of the examination. On the angioscintigram (Fig. 1c) the radioactivity deposited in the pancreas can well be outlined. The radioactivity of the tail merges with the radioactivity accumulated in the spleen and the left flexure of the colon. Irregular storage defects are demonstrated in the marginal portions of the head of the pancreas. Fig. 1d shows the scintigram performed after application of ^{75}Se-selenmethionine. The pancreas is not as well delineated as on the angioscintigram. The head of the pancreas with its pathologic finding is partially superimposed by the radioactivity accumulated in the liver and bowel. With the diagnosis of a pancreatic carcinoma infiltrating the duodenum, the patient ist operated. A duodenal carcinoma is found with infiltration of the head of the pancreas, necessitating the performance of a pancreatico-duodenectomy. The histologic examination

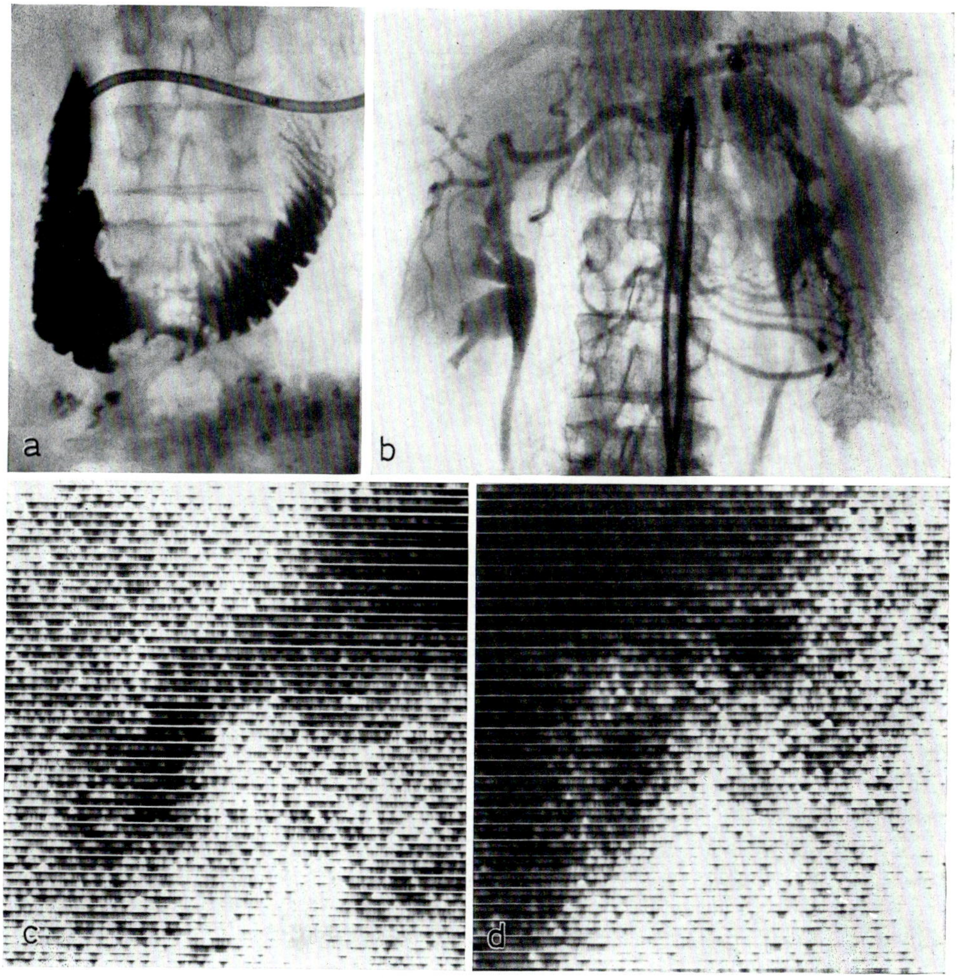

Fig. 1a–d. 58 year old patient with a duodenal carcinoma infiltrating the pancreas. a Selective duodenography: irregular filling defect in the third portion of the duodenum. b Angiography of the celiac artery and of the superior mesenteric artery (simultaneous injection): Scarcity and irregular caliber of the arteries of the pancreatic arcades. c Macroaggregate angioscintigram: clear delineation of the pancreas with filling defects in the pancreatic head. Intensive storage of radioactive material in the spleen. d Selenmethionine scintigram of the pancreas: Radioactive deposits in the head and in the tail of the pancreas due to overprojection of radioactivity present within the increased liver. The pathologic finding in the head cannot be outlined

proves the presence of a carcinoma solidum simplex partim adenomatosum of the third portion of the duodenum.

In the table the arteriographic findings are compared with the angioscintigraphic findings. The final diagnosis made with regard to the clinical course of the disease (2 patients), or to the operative or autopsy finding (10 patients) reveals a normal pancreas in 2 patients, a pancreatitis in 3 patients, a duodenal carcinoma in 2 patients

Table. *Pancreas arteriography and angioscintigraphy. A comparison of the results*

cases	final diagnosis	Arterio-graphy: abnormal vessels	Angioscintigraphy delineation of pancreas	storage of radioactivity reduced	defects	increased
W. F. 62y ♂	no disease	—	—			
B. E. 53y ♂	no disease	—	+	—	—	—
S. J. 60y ♂	pancreatitis	+	+	+	(+)	+
B. S. 41y ♂	pancreatitis	(+)	(+)	+	+	+
K. M. 51y ♀	pancreatitis	—	+	+	(+)	+
	Carcinomas:					
P. J. 74y ♂	duodenum + pancreatitis	++	(+)	++	+	—
H. M. 58y ♀	duodenum	+	++	—	+	—
P. A. 73y ♂	head of pancreas	++	++	—	++	+
G. I. 71y ♀	head of pancreas + pancreatitis	++	(+)	++	++	—
S. H. 65y ♂	head of pancreas + pancreatitis	+++	(+)	++	++	—
G. A. 64y ♀	body of pancreas	+++	++	+	++	—
S. M. 60y ♀	body of pancreas	+++	++	—	++	—

and in 5 patients a pancreatic carcinoma, 3 times carcinomas are combined with pancreatitis. By arteriography in 1 patient with pancreatitis and in 7 patients with carcinomas abnormal vessels are demonstrated.

In 7 of 12 angioscintigraphic examinations the pancreas can be recognized at least partially. In 1 case the pancreas is not visible due to an intensive accumulation of intestinal radioactivity in the upper abdomen. In 4 patients, all affected by pancreatitis, only a small amount of tracer substance is stored within the pancreas which hardly can be outlined on the angioscintigram.

On detailed studies of the angioscintigrams it can be noted that carcinomas lead in all the examined cases to circumscribed filling defects. If a pancreatitis or fibrosis of the pancreas is present, a diffused or a spotty decrease of the storage of radioactivity can be noted in the pancreas. In some cases malignant and inflammatory processes may also cause a circumscribed increase of radioactivity, probably due to reactive hyperemia.

Conclusions

For the radiologic diagnosis of a pancreatic alteration, an arteriography of the celiac and of the superior mesenteric artery is usually necessary. This examination can easily be combined with angioscintigraphy. If an early disease of the pancreas is present, the evaluation of the arteriograms is often difficult and uncertain. In these cases, angioscintigraphy gives additional possibilities for making a diagnosis. It informs of the distribution and the blood supply of the finer pancreatic arteries and capillaries; these vessels are usually not visible on the arteriograms. The angioscintigrams and the ^{75}Se-selenmethionine scintigrams give comparable scintigraphic images of the pancreas. However independant of organ function macroaggregate angioscintigraphy represents a physical means of pancreas delineation based on vascular distribution of radioactive material. On the angioscintigrams more activity is always stored in the spleen than in the liver. On the scintigrams made after ^{75}Se-selenmethionine application the inverse is the case.

The safety of employing macroaggregates of radioiodated human serum albumin has been determined for lung-scanning and, apart from problems associated with arterial puncture, angioscintigraphy of the pancreas does not provide additional hazards. In this series no serious reaction was encountered.

Disturbing for the evaluation of the pancreas are the radioactive deposits in the intestinal tract, which often superimpose the pancreatic region. Therefore, it is advisable to perform a first angioscintigram after injection of the ^{131}I macroaggregate in the celiac artery alone, and to perform a second scan after additional injection of the tracer substance in the superior mesenteric artery. The combined interpretation of the two scintigrams helps to distinguish between radioactive deposits present in the pancreas and an overprojecting radioactivity in intestinal organs. Superselective angioscintigraphy with tracer injection in the gastro-duodenal artery, in the dorsal pancreatic artery and in the splenic artery may be another way to provide a better and clearer demonstration of the pancreas.

Summary

In 2 patients with suspected pancreatic disease, in addition to arteriography, angioscintigrams were performed after injection of ^{131}I macroaggregate human serum albumin in the celiac artery and in the superior mesenteric artery. The angioscintigrams may give additional information about blood circulation within the different portions of the pancreas. It offers an expanded dimension to either pancreatic arteriography or conventional scanning of the pancreas. Arteriography and angioscintigraphy are complementary procedures, the arteriogram showing the macrostructure and the scan displaying the microvascular distribution of macroaggregates within this organ. The demonstration of the scintigraphic image of the pancreas is often impaired by overprojection of radioactive deposits in the intestinal organs. This disturbing factor can eventually be avoided by superselective injection of the tracer substance in the 3 main arteries supplying the pancreas.

Perfusionsangioszintigraphie in der Diagnostik von Erkrankungen der Bauchspeicheldrüse

K. H. van de Weyer, C. Clausen und J. Heckrott

Mit der selektiven Kontrastmittelinjektion in die A. coeliaca und die A. mesenterica superior zur Pankreasangiographie bietet sich die gleichzeitige Injektion radioaktiver Substanzen in dieselben Gefäße zur anschließenden szintigraphischen Darstellung der Bauchspeicheldrüse an.

Im Anschluß an die Gefäßdarstellung haben wir daher bei 37 Patienten radioaktive Substanzen in die genannten Gefäße injiziert und 30–150 min danach Szintigramme des Oberbauches in mehreren Lagerungen angefertigt.

Bei 10 Patienten wurde ^{131}J makroaggregiertes Humanalbumin zur Perfusionsangioszintigraphie verwendet. Wie aus der Tabelle 1 ersichtlich, gelang nur in einem Fall eine mäßige Darstellung der Bauchspeicheldrüse.

Tabelle 1. *Perfusionsangioszintigraphie des Pankreas mit ^{131}J-MAA*

	Applikationsort	Szintigraphisch dargestellte Organe	Diagnose	Erweiterung der radiolog. diagn. Aussage
1	A. coel.	Leber + Milz	Insulinom (Pankreasschwanz)	–
2	A. coel.	Milz	chronisch calcifizierte Pankreatitis	–
3	A. lien.	Milz	Verdacht Pankreasneoplasma: Angio o. B.	–
4	A. coel.	Leber + Milz	chronische Pankreatitis	–
5	A. coel.	Leber + Milz	chronische Pankreatitis	–
6	A. coel.	Milz	Insulinom (Pankreasschwanz)	–
7	A. lien.	Milz	Nierenzyste (Verlagerung von Pankreas + Milz)	–
8	A. coel.	Leber + Milz	Leberechinococcus (Op. inop.)	–
9	A. coel.	Leber	Klin. Verdacht: Pankreasneoplasma (Angio o. B.)	–
10	A. coel.	Pankreas (+) Leber, Milz	Klin. Verdacht: Pankreasschwanzneoplasma (Rö + Angio Tumor im Quercolon)	(+)

Applizierte Aktivitätsmenge pro Patient 200–400 μCi ^{131}J-MAA; Scanning 30–150 min nach Injektion

Tabelle 2. *Perfusionsangioszintigraphie des Pankreas mit* ^{75}*Se-Methionin*

	Applikationsort	Szintigraphisch dargestellte Organe	Diagnose	Erweiterung der radiolog. diagn. Aussage
1	A. coel.	Pankreas, Milz	Klin. Verdacht: Insulinom (Angio + Op. Pankreas o. B.)	+
2	A. coel.	Leber	Pankreaskopfneoplasma	—
3	A. coel.	Leber	Klin. Verdacht: Zollinger-Ellison (Angio + Op. Pankreas o. B.)	—
4	A. hepat. comm.	Pankreas Leber	Pankreaskopfneoplasma (Op. inop.)	+
5	A. coel.	Pankreas Leber	Klin. Verdacht: Pankreasneoplasma (Angio + Szintgr. o. B.)	+
6	A. coel.	Pankreas (+) Leber	Chronische Pankreatitis	—
7	A. coel.	Pankreas (+), Leber, Milz	Lebercirrhose, Milzvenenthrombose	—
8	A. coel.	Pankreas (+) Leber	Labor-Verdacht: Pankreasneoplasma (Angio + Op. Pankreas o. B.)	(+)
9	A. coel.	Pankreas Leber	Echinococcuszyste re. Leberlappen	+
10	A. coel.	Pankreas Leber, Milz	Echinococcus der Leber (Verdrängung des Pankreaskopfes)	+
11	A. coel. + A. mes. sup.	Leber	schwere chronische calcifizierende Pankreatitis	—
12	A. hepat. comm. + A. mes. sup.	Leber	Pankreaskopfzyste	—
13	A. lien.	Milz	chronische Pankreatitis	—
14	A. lien.	Milz + Pankreasschwanz	chronische Pankreatitis	—
15	A. coel.	Pankreas Leber, Milz	Klin. Verdacht: Insulinom (Angio o. B.)	(+)
16	A. coel.	Pankreas Leber	Pankreaskörperzyste	+
17	A. hepat. comm.	Pankreas (+) Leber	Klin. Verdacht: Pankreasneoplasma	(+)
18	A. coel.	Leber, Milz	chronische calcifizierende Pankreatitis	—
19	A. coel.	Pankreas (+) Leber	Klin. Verdacht: Pankreasneoplasma (Angio + Szintigr. o. B.)	(+)
20	A. coel.	Leber, Milz	Klin. Verdacht: Zollinger-Ellison (Angio + Op. Pankreas o. B.)	—
21	A. coel.	Pankreas Leber	Pankreaskopfneoplasma (inop.)	(+)

Tabelle 2 (Fortsetzung)

	Applikationsort	Szintigraphisch dargestellte Organe	Diagnose	Erweiterung der radiolog. diagn. Aussage
22	A. coel.	Milz	ungeklärte Intestinalblutung	—
23	A. coel.	Pankreas	Pankreaskopfneoplasma	+
24	A. coel.	Pankreas (+) Milz	Klin. Verdacht: Verner Morrison (Angio o. B.)	—
25	A. coel.	Pankreas Milz	chronische Pankreatitis	—
26	A. lien.	Pankreas (+) Milz	Pseudozyste Pankreasschwanz	—
27	A. coel.	Milz	Pankreaskopfneoplasma	—

Applizierte Aktivitätsmenge pro Patient 200 μCi ^{75}Se-Methionin; Scanning 30–300 min nach Injektion

Eine Erweiterung der diagnostischen Aussage wurde bei diesen Patienten nicht erreicht, jedoch befand sich unter unseren Erkrankten keiner mit einem Pankreasneoplasma. Wir legen besonderen Wert auf diese Feststellung, da in jüngster Zeit eine japanische Forschergruppe um Kaneko und Sasaki über einen Fall einer positiven Darstellung eines Pankreaskopftumors mit ^{131}J-MAA bei Injektion der radioaktiven Substanz in die A. coeliaca berichtet hat.

Nach Gabe von Selen-75-Methionin in die A. coeliaca oder andere an der Versorgung des Pankreas beteiligte Arterien konnte bei 27 Patienten in 18 Fällen die Bauchspeicheldrüse szintigraphisch zur Darstellung gebracht werden (Tabelle 2).

Um „gute Szintigramme“ handelte es sich dabei in 11 Fällen. Bei diesen Patienten stellte die Perfusionsszintigraphie mit Selen-Methionin in der Regel eine Erweiterung der radiologischen Diagnostik dar. In 6 Fällen bestand diese in einer optimalen szintigraphischen Darstellung der normalen Konturen der Bauchspeicheldrüse; in einem Fall in einer rundlichen Radioaktivitätsaussparung im Körperbereich bedingt durch eine Pseudocyste, in 2 Fällen in einer fast apfelgroßen Radioaktivitätsaussparung im Kopfbereich bei Carcinom. Bei einem weiteren Kopfneoplasma, das sich bei der Operation als inoperabel erwies, war die Radioaktivitätsaussparung im Kopfbereich nicht so eindeutig. Bei einem letzten Patienten fand sich ein Speicherungsausfall im Pankreaskopfbereich, bedingt durch eine Verlagerung desselben durch eine große Echinococcuscyste des rechten Leberlappens.

Beim Insulinom, dem Zollinger-Ellison- und dem Verner-Morrison-Syndrom, bei der chronischen und der calcifizierenden Pankreatitis erbrachte die Perfusionsszintigraphie mit Selen-75-Methionin bei den von uns untersuchten Patienten keine Erweiterung der radiologischen Diagnostik.

Die vergleichende Auswertung der Pankreasangiogramme und Szintigramme zeigte, daß die szintigraphisch oft schwierige Abgrenzung des Pankreaskopfes von der Leber am besten bei Fällen mit einer angiographisch kleinen Leber oder einer hypoplastischen linken Leberarterie gelang.

Zwar liegt die Häufigkeit der „guten“ szintigraphischen Pankreasdarstellungen bei der Perfusion mit Selen-75-Methionin bisher nicht über unserer und der in der Literatur angegebenen Quote von etwa $^2/_3$ der Fälle nach intravenöser Applikation. Die Qualität der Organdarstellung ist jedoch infolge des weitgehend fehlenden Untergrundes besser.

Als vorläufiges Ergebnis möchten wir mitteilen, daß bei unseren Untersuchungen die Perfusionsszintigraphie des Pankreas mit ^{131}J-makroaggregiertem Albumin keine Erweiterung der Diagnostik der Bauchspeicheldrüse erbrachte. Diese radioaktive Substanz strömte bei fast allen Patienten bevorzugt in die Milz ab, so daß wir meist eine optimale szintigraphische Darstellung dieses Organes bekamen. Die Häufigkeit guter szintigraphischer Darstellungen der Bauchspeicheldrüse nach intraarterieller Applikation des Selen-75-Methionin liegt bisher nicht höher als die Quote nach intravenöser Gabe der Radioaktivität, jedoch ist die Qualität der Organdarstellung infolge des weitgehend fehlenden Untergrundes besser.

Kombination von Szintigraphie und Angiographie in der radiologischen Pankreasdiagnostik

H. PRÉVÔT jr.

Erkrankungen der Bauchspeicheldrüse sind verhältnismäßig schwer zu erkennen. Neben klinischen und Labor-Untersuchungsmethoden spielt die radiologische Diagnostik in den letzten Jahren eine zunehmende Rolle. Anhand von Patienten mit operativ gesicherter Erkrankung des Pankreas haben wir geprüft, welche der radiologischen Methoden – konventionelle Magen-Darm-Passage einschließlich hypotoner Duodenographie, Angiographie und Szintigraphie – die besten Ergebnisse liefert. Außerdem stellten wir uns die Frage, ob und wenn ja durch welche Kombination der genannten Untersuchungsverfahren die Diagnostik verbessert werden kann.

Material

Unsere Untersuchungen stützen sich auf das operativ und größtenteils auch histologisch abgesicherte Ergebnis bei 48 Kranken. In allen Fällen wurde eine Bariumkontrastbreiuntersuchung und eine Szintigraphie durchgeführt, bei 25 Patienten zusätzlich eine selektive Darstellung der Arteria coeliaca und mesenterica superior. Bei 29 unserer Patienten fand sich ein Carcinom, bei 15 eine Pankreatitis, 2mal wurde ein Adenom und 2mal wurde eine Cyste gefunden.

Methodik

Für die Bewertung der Röntgenuntersuchung wurden die u. a. von SARLES u. Mitarb. herausgestellten Kriterien wie Impressum am Magen mit oder ohne Abdrängung von der Wirbelsäule, bogenförmige Impression am Bulbus bzw. lacunäre Kontrastmittelaussparung im Stehen, Doppelkonturierung, Stenosen, Nischen oder sog. Spiculae des absteigenden Duodenum, Aufbiegung der duodenalen C-Schlinge mit oder ohne entzündliche Schleimhautveränderung, herangezogen. Die Szintigraphie wurde unter Anwendung von Selen-75-Methionin durchgeführt, auf eine Vorbereitung der Patienten wurde verzichtet. Bei knapp der Hälfte der Patienten wurde zusätzlich Gold-198 injiziert und eine elektronische Unterdrückung der Leber durchgeführt. Szintigraphisch fanden sich teils unspezifische Zeichen, wie herdförmig oder allgemein verminderte Einlagerung der markierten Aminosäure bis zur fast fehlenden Darstellung des Pankreas, teils charakteristische Zeichen, wie ein Abbruch in der Darstellung des untersuchten Organes. Die Angiographie wurde nach der Seldinger-Technik durchgeführt. Die selektive Injektion des Kontrastmittels in die A. coeliaca und mesenterica superior erfolgte teils simultan, teils nacheinander.

Ergebnisse

Das Ergebnis unserer Untersuchungen ist in der Tabelle zusammengefaßt:

Tabelle. *Häufigkeit pathologischer Befunde bei gesicherter Erkrankung der Bauchspeicheldrüse. Die in Klammern angegebenen Ziffern geben die Anzahl der untersuchten Patienten an*

Art der Untersuchung	Raumfordernder Prozeß Kopf	Raumfordernder Prozeß Korpus-Schwanz	Pankreatitis	Gesamt
Magen-Darm-Passage	11 (14)	12 (19)	11 (15)	34 (48)
Szintigraphie	11 (14)	14 (19)	15 (15)	40 (48)
Angiographie	6 (7)	10 (12)	2 (6)	18 (25)

Die konventionelle Magen-Darmdiagnostik in der von uns angewandten Technik ergab bei 11 von 14 Patienten positive Röntgenzeichen, die Nachweisbarkeit gleichartiger Veränderungen im Gebiet von Pankreaskörper und Schwanz ist mit 12 Befunden bei 19 Kranken in der Treffsicherheit schlechter. Die Häufigkeit röntgenologischer Veränderungen bei der Pankreatitis liegt mit 11:15 zwischen diesen beiden Werten. Die Gesamtnachweiswahrscheinlichkeit von Erkrankungen der Bauchspeicheldrüse durch die Magen-Darmpassage ist in unserem Material um 70% anzusetzen.

Bei Gegenüberstellung dieser Ergebnisse mit der Szintigraphie findet sich eine gute Übereinstimmung in der Häufigkeit pathologischer Zeichen bei Pankreaskopfprozessen, hinsichtlich Veränderungen der Korpus-Schwanzregion erscheint die Szintigraphie überlegen. Bei nachgewiesener Pankreatitis war die Einlagerung des markierten Methionin in allen Fällen vermindert, was allerdings nicht heißt, daß aus den entsprechenden Befunden jeweils mit Sicherheit auf eine Pankreatitis geschlossen werden konnte. Die Gesamtnachweiswahrscheinlichkeit liegt um 80% und ist höher als bei der Magen-Darmpassage.

Bei Betrachtung der angiographischen Untersuchungsergebnisse fällt die niedrige Trefferquote bei entzündlichen Veränderungen auf; von 6 untersuchten Kranken war nur 2mal ein sicher von der Norm abweichender Befund erkennbar, wovon einer fälschlich als tumorverdächtig angesprochen wurde. Der geringen Bedeutung der Angiographie zur Erkennung entzündlicher Veränderungen der Bauchspeicheldrüse steht die Häufigkeit positiver Befunde bei raumfordernden Prozessen gegenüber, die in unserem Material unabhängig von der Lokalisation des Tumors war.

Daß die Kombination der beschriebenen Untersuchungsverfahren über das bisher Gesagte hinaus geeignet ist, zu einer richtigen Diagnosetellung zu kommen, möchte ich anhand einiger Beispiele erläutern:

Es handelt sich um die Röntgenaufnahme eines 51jährigen Mannes, der uns zur Primärtumorsuche wegen einer großzelligen Hautmetastase zugewiesen wurde. Es

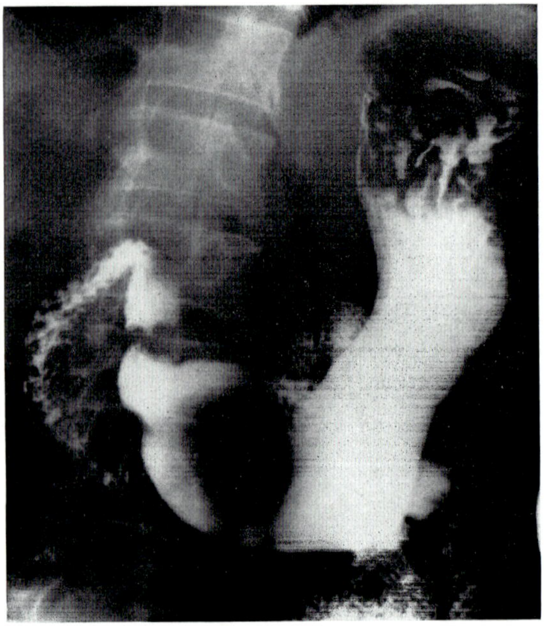

a

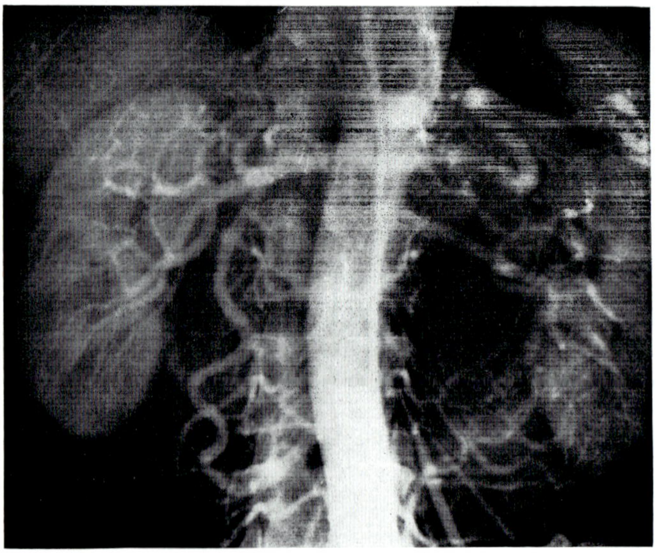

b

Abb. 1. a Übersichtsaufnahme des Magens mit rundlicher Pelottierung im Antrumbereich. b Übersichtsangiographie der Aorta. Keine eindeutige Darstellung des Stammes der A. hepatica. Großes Gefäß das von der A. mesenterica sup. zum Versorgungsbereich der A. gastroduodenalis zieht

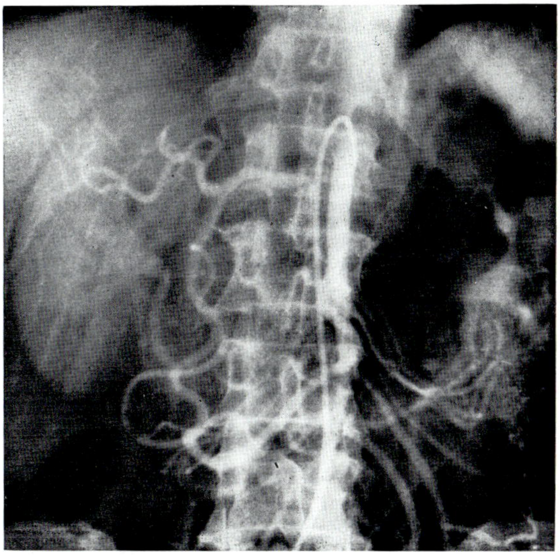

c

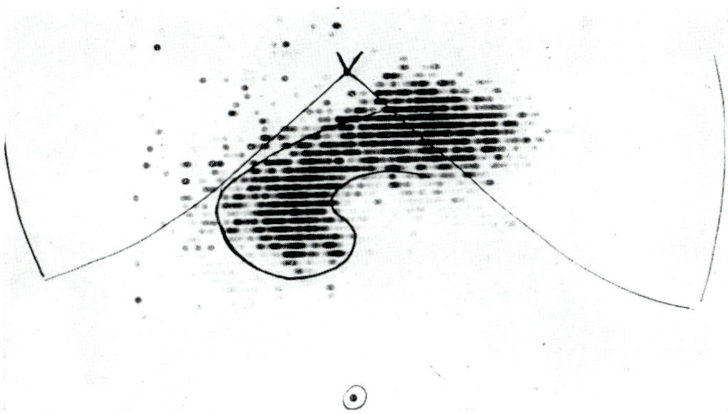

d

Abb. 1. c Selektive Darstellung der A. mesent. sup. Die Versorgung der Leberarterien geschieht über eine Anastomose von der A. mesent. sup. Retrograde Auffüllung der A. hepatica comm. die offenbar dicht hinter ihrem Abgang hochgradig stenosiertist. d Szintigraphische Untersuchung des Patienten von Abbildung 1a–1c. Regelrechte Abbildung der Bauchspeicheldrüse ohne Hinweis für einen Pankreastumor

fand sich eine Pelottierung am Magen, die uns auf die Möglichkeit einer Erkrankung der Bauchspeicheldrüse hinwies (Abb. 1a). Von uns wurde als nächstes die Angiographie durchgeführt.

Die Angiographie schien diesen Verdacht zu bestätigen. Der Versuch einer selektiven Darstellung der A. coeliaca mißlang; die Übersichtsaortographie ließ eine breite Anastomose zwischen A. mesenterica sup. und A. hepatica communis vermuten (Abb. 1b). Abbildung 1c zeigt die Bestätigung und erklärt, warum die Darstellung der A. coeliaca mißlang. Wir konnten durch die retrograde Auffüllung einen Abbruch der A. hepatica communis dicht distal ihres Ursprunges darstellen.

Abbildung 1c zeigt das Pankreasszintigramm des gleichen Patienten; die gute und einwandfreie Darstellung des Organes widersprach allen unseren bisherigen Erfahrungen und veranlaßte uns zur Fortsetzung der Diagnostik. Im Rahmen der

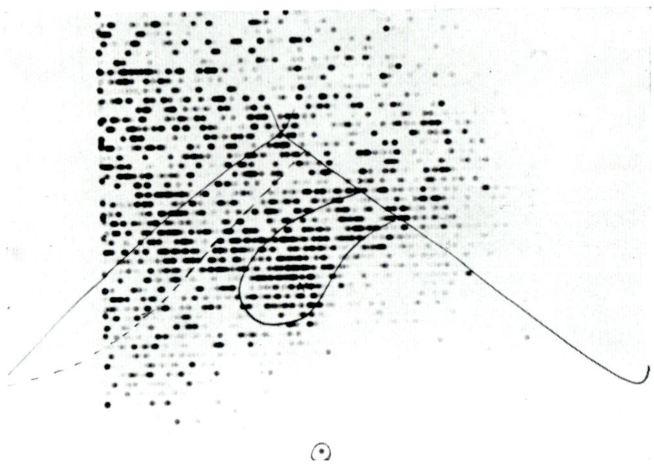

a

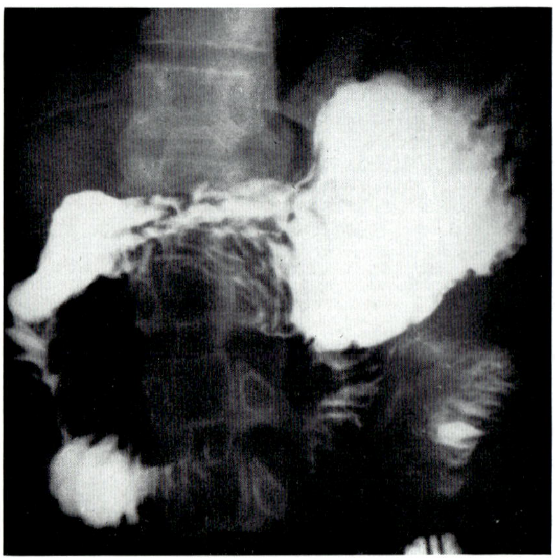

b

Abb. 2. a Pathologisches Pankreasszintigramm. Kaum erkennbare Darstellung der Organkonturen, ungleichmäßige Einlagerung der markierten Aminosäure in das Pankreas. b Übersichtsaufnahme des Magens bei gleichem Patienten wie in Abbildung 2a. Pelottierung der Antrumregion des Magens und stärkergradige funktionell-entzündliche Veränderungen am absteigenden Duodenum weiteren Durchuntersuchung wurde ein später auch histologisch gesichertes Retothelsarkom gefunden. Daß ein pathologisches Szintigramm, auch wenn seine Veränderungen unspezifisch sind, in Kombination mit weiteren Untersuchungen von hohem Nutzen sein kann, zeigen die nächsten Beispiele:

Die Abbildung 2a zeigt eine sehr unvollständige Darstellung des Pankreas im Szintigramm, die auf eine Erkrankung der Bauchspeicheldrüse, welcher Art sie auch sein mag, hinweist. Den zugehörigen Röntgenbefund zeigt Abbildung 2b.

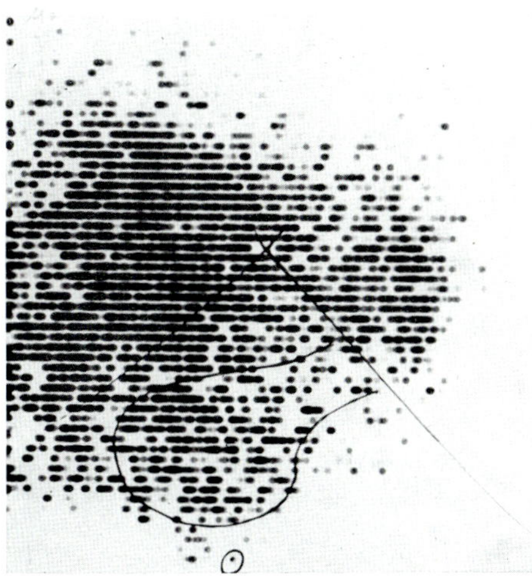

a

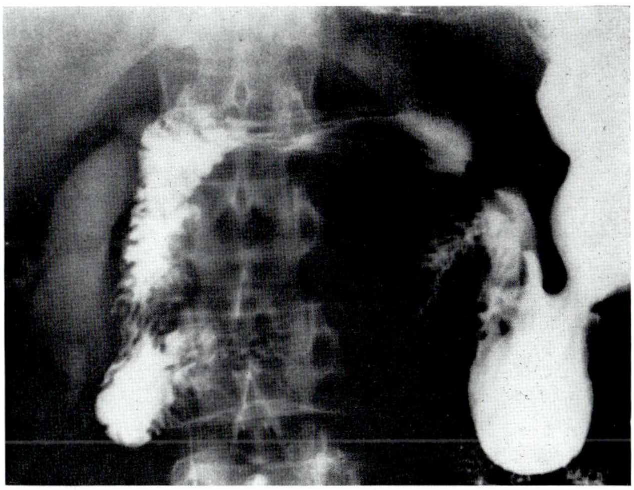

b

Abb. 3. a Pathologisches Pankreasszintigramm. Verdacht auf Auftreibung der Pankreaskopfregion. Ungleichmäßige Einlagerung der Aminosäure wie in Abbildung 2a. b Übersichtsaufnahme der Pankreasregion des Patienten von Abbildung 3a. Pelottierung des Bulbus duodeni ohne entzündliche Begleitreaktion

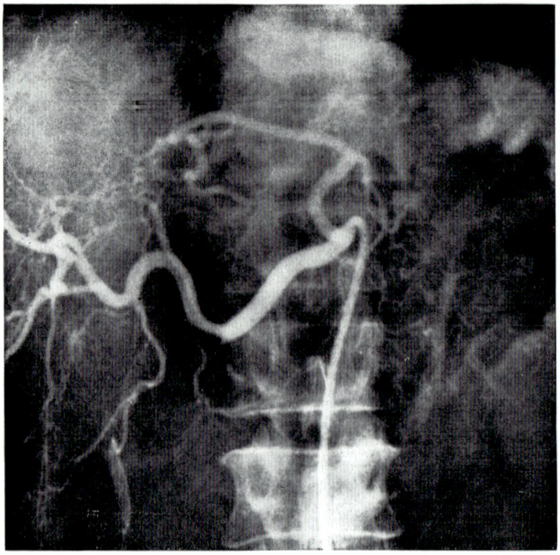

Abb. 3. c Selektive Darstellung der A. coeliaca. Fehlende Auffüllung der A. gastroduodenalis. Stärkergradige Konturunregelmäßigkeit im Abgangsbereich der A. gastroduodenalis. (Bei Op. gesichertes Pankreaskopfcarcinom)

Es bestehen eindeutige entzündliche Veränderungen am Duodenum; als Diagnose bestätigte sich eine Pankreatitis.

Weitgehend gleichartige Veränderungen zeigt das vorstehende Szintigramm.

Die Röntgenuntersuchung von Magen und Duodenum zeigte keine eindeutigen entzündlichen Veränderungen und veranlaßte uns zur Durchführung einer Angiographie:
die zur Diagnose Pankreaskopftumor führte.

Diskussion

Von den vorgestellten Untersuchungsverfahren hat die Szintigraphie mit 40 positiven Befunden bei 48 Patienten die höchste Trefferquote, wenn es um die Frage geht, ob überhaupt eine Erkrankung der Bauchspeicheldrüse vorliegt. Zur Differenzierung der einzelnen Krankheitsbilder ist dieses Untersuchungsverfahren weit weniger geeignet. Mit Ausnahme des Organabbruches, der einem Tumor oder einer Cyste entsprechen kann, haben die übrigen Zeichen für die Zuordnung zu einem bestimmten Krankheitsbild nur eine geringe Wertigkeit. Unsere Befunde stimmen mit den Angaben von Brown u. Mitarb. und den Angaben von Sodee überein, Rotriguez-Antunez u. Mitarb. fanden in ihrem Material in 39% unrichtige Ergebnisse.

Die Nachweiswahrscheinlichkeit von Pankreaserkrankungen durch die Magen-Darm-Passage liegt bei uns um 70% (34 von 48 Fällen). Die Nachweisbarkeit der Carcinome lag in der gleichen Größenordnung. Wir liegen mit diesem Ergebnis zwischen den Angaben von Hodes, der 47% und Salik, der 77% positive Befunde beim Pankreascarcinom angibt. Eine Trefferquote zwischen 50–60% wird von Eyler u. Mitarb., von Gorwitz sowie von Gullik angegeben. Die Wertigkeit von Röntgenzeichen wie Spiculaebildung am Duodenum oder deutliche Verlagerung von Magenabschnitten ist erheblich höher anzusetzen als die üblichen Zeichen der szintigraphischen Untersuchung. Für einen sehr wesentlichen Hinweis halten wir die Tatsache, daß wir bei Patienten mit einem Carcinom der Bauchspeicheldrüse praktisch keine eindeutigen entzündlichen Veränderungen am Duodenum oder Magen gesehen haben. Bis auf einzelne Ausnahmen trifft diese Aussage auch auf ein größeres, von uns jedoch nur mit der Magen-Darm-Passage untersuchtes Krankengut zu.

Die Angiographie liegt mit ihrer Trefferquote von 18:25 in der gleichen Größenordnung wie die Magen-Darm-Passage. Die Wertigkeit ihrer Zeichen ist bei weitem die höchste. So war bei 15 untersuchten Carcinomen 13 mal ein entscheidender Hinweis zu finden. Hierin liegt allerdings auch eine erhebliche Gefahr durch die falsche Bewertung positiver Befunde. Die meisten Versager finden sich in der Gruppe der Pankreatitiden. Unsere Ergebnisse entsprechenden Angaben von LUNDERQUIST. EATON u. Mitarb. und insbesondere NEBESAR und POLLARD geben eine niedrigere Trefferquote für die Angiographie an. Inwieweit an diesem Widerspruch die Größe des Tumors entscheidend beteiligt ist, geht aus den Veröffentlichungen nicht hervor.

Wo liegen nun die besonderen Vorteile der kombinierten Anwendung der genannten Untersuchungsverfahren:

1. Bei klinischen oder röntgenologisch erhobenem Verdacht auf eine Erkrankung der Bauchspeicheldrüse sollte nach Möglichkeit immer ein Szintigramm veranlaßt werden. Dieses Untersuchungsverfahren ist dann in hohem Maße geeignet, zu entscheiden, ob die Bauchspeicheldrüse überhaupt erkrankt ist. Bei sicher unauffälligem Szintigramm darf eine entsprechende Erkrankung mit 80% Wahrscheinlichkeit ausgeschlossen werden.

2. Die Kombination, schlechte Darstellung des Pankreas im Szintigramm ohne entzündliche Zeichen in der Magen-Darm-Passage, halten wir für tumorverdächtig und somit für eine feste Indikation zur Angiographie. Das Gleiche gilt für alle szintigraphischen Organabbrüche.

3. Die Kombination, „schlechte Darstellung" der Bauchspeicheldrüse im Szintigramm mit entzündlichen Veränderungen am Magen oder Duodenum, ist so kennzeichnend für eine Pankreatitis, daß nach unserer Ansicht von einer Angiographie zunächst Abstand genommen werden darf.

Durch konsequenten Einsatz der radiologischen Untersuchungsverfahren in der genannten Form dürfte die Nachweisbarkeit von Erkrankungen der Bauchspeicheldrüse bei 80–90% liegen und somit die frühere diagnostische Unsicherheit bei diesen Krankheitsbildern bald beseitigt haben.

The Endocrine Disorder of the Pancreas and its Comparative Investigations Between Clinical, Angiographical and Operative Findings

H. Scherer, P. Mutzenbach, P. Maurer and H. Scholze

The pancreas shows often some difficulties at diagnosis because of its topographical position. Morphological as well as functional disorders are important. The possibility of angiographic diagnosis is thereby very different.

At the „Klinikum rechts der Isar der Technischen Universität München" 79 angiographies of the celiac and mesenteric artery corresponding to the clinical findings were performed during the last 30 months. In some cases it was necessary to perform additionally the splenoportography in order to get a clear diagnosis and indication for the operation.

We will show you now 4 of our own cases:

1. A tentative diagnosis for a *islet (langerhansian) adenoma* the simultaneous opacification of the celiac and superior mesenteric artery gives best results. If the islets-tumor is located in the tail of the pancreas the superselective angiography of the splenic artery may secure the diagnosis (Fig. 1a, b).

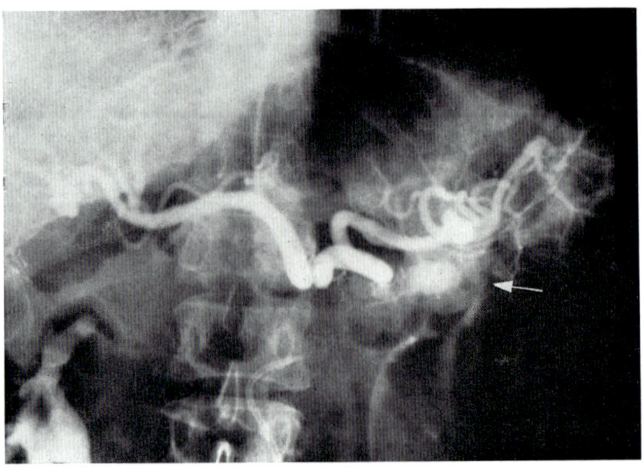

Fig. 1. a Islet-cell-tumor of the pancreas diagnosed by angiography of the celiac artery

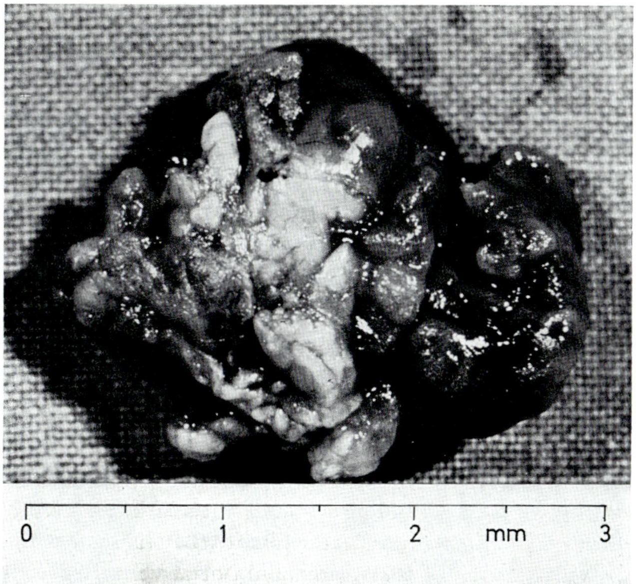

Fig. 1. b The surgical specimen

2. For the diagnosis of the *pancreas-carcinoma* the angiography is indispensablc. A malignant pancreas-tumor early shows displacements, interruptions and pathologic neoformations of vessels (Fig. 2a, b).

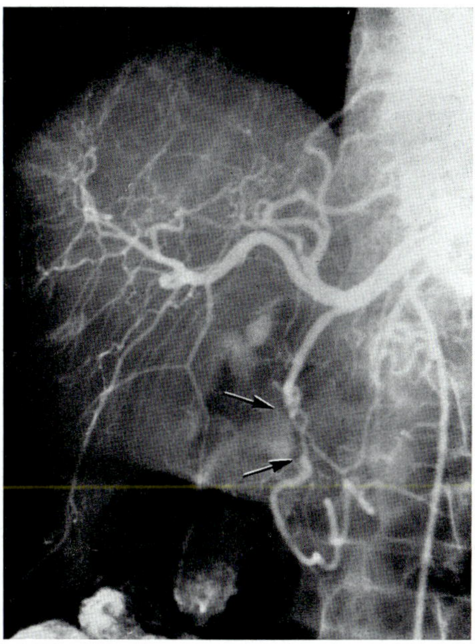

Fig. 2 a and b. Carcinoma of the pancreas. a its angiograph

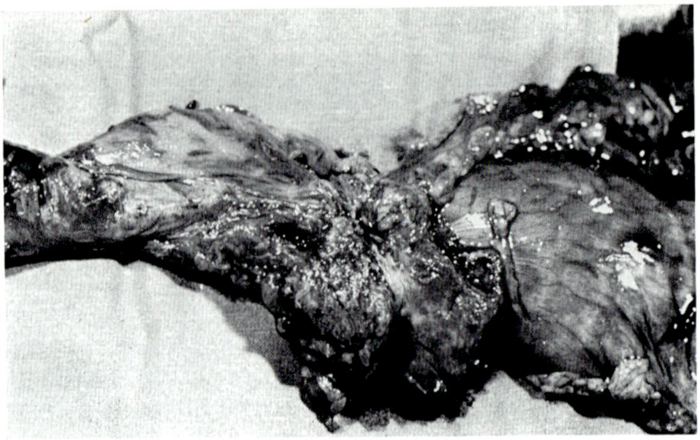

Fig. 2. b its surgical specimen (Whipple's operation)

3. Displacements of vessels and procreated vascularisation at the angiography can be signs of *true or pseudo-cysts*. A clearer picture may be seen at the later phase of arteriography by visualisation of the splenic and portal vein. Especially at these two vessels the changing of the pancreas-outline get very distinct (Fig. 3a, b).

4. The radiologic diagnosis by angiography at the *acute* and *acute recurrent pancreatitis* is most useless. At the progressed *chronically recurrent and chronic pancreatitis* only the superselective arteriography shows some diagnostic importance. There can be seen excentric stenosis of very small vessels. But it is very important to perform the splenoportography, for the chronic pancreatic diseases mostly displace the splenic vein by compressions and clot formations. As consequence there can be seen a slow flowing off and reflux into the collaterals with partial portal hypertension (Fig. 4).

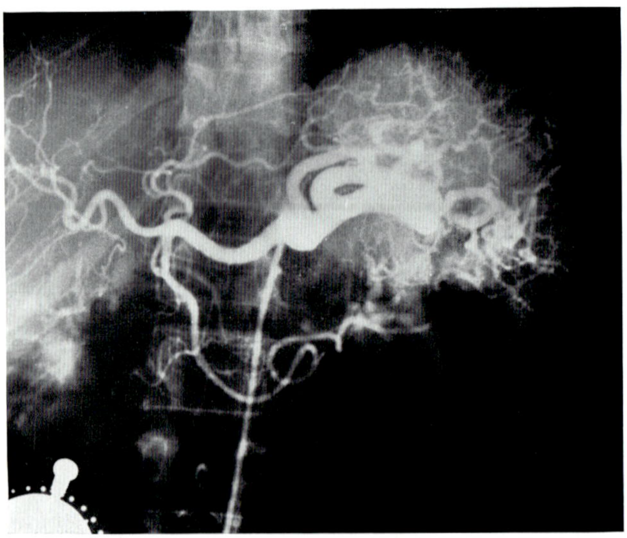

Fig. 3a and b. Cyst of the pancreas, located in its tail. a angiograph

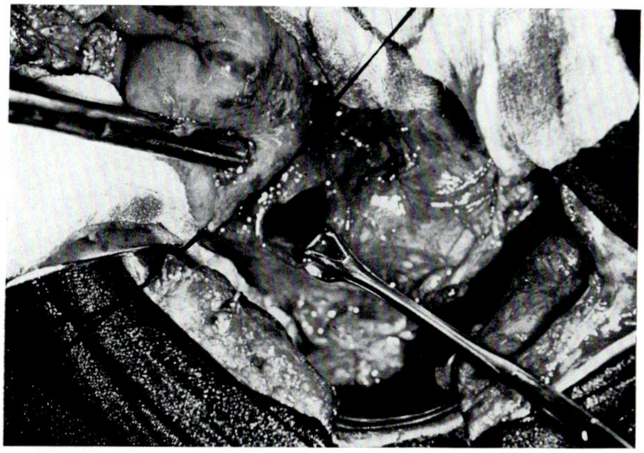

Fig. 3. b intraoperative picture with the opened cyst

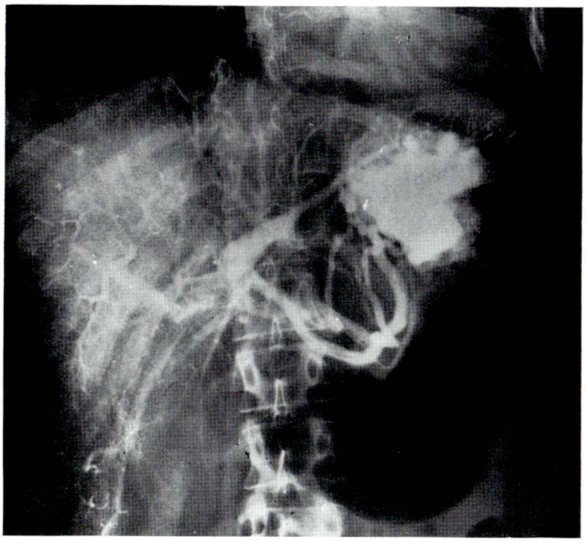

Fig. 4. Splenoportograph showing a case of chronically recurrent pancreatitis

The definite diagnosis clinically can be confirmed with the duodenal probe and its analysis by the "secretin-pancreomycin-test", which mostly shows disfunction of the pancreas.

El tronco celiaco y la mesenterica superior en las pancreatitis Cronica

J. M. Rius Chornet

Dado el creciente auge de las exploraciones angiograficas en las enfermedades del pancreas, hemos querido aportar nuestra experiencia en una serie de enfermos comprobados quirurgicamente y con anatomia-patologica de pancreatitis cronica, y cuyos hallazgos han sido muy variables; tanto que nos hemos replanteado el interes y la rentabilidad de la exploración angiografica en dichos procesos, pues solo el 40% de ellospresentaron las imagenes descritas como típicas de pancreatitis crónica.

Dejando a parte los pacientes en los que ademas existía-pseudo-quiste acompañante, y en los que no habian más imagenes patologicas que las correspondientes a los desplazamintos provocados por el proceso-expansivo, solo en 2 de los 10 casos encontramos angiograficamente imagenes sospechosas de pancreatitis.

Por otro lado las veces en las que el diagnostico diferencialcon una neoplasia de pancreas existia, y en las que no se habían presentado metastasis hepaticas, el difinirse en un sentido u otro nos resultó ser aventurado, ya que la anatomia patologica solo coincidio con el diagnostico radiologico en un 60%.

Quiero aclarar que cuando me refiero a "lesiones descritas como típicas en las pancreatitis" lo hago tanto a las que aparecen sobre la gastroduodenal, pancreatoduodenales, tronco de la mesenterica superior, yeyunales etc. como a las avascularizaciones o hipervascularizaciones radiologicas, y que indistintamente hemos encontrado en las pancreatitis cronicas como en las neoplasias de pancreas.

A continuacion les presentamos una serie de diapositivas en las que el diagnostico angiografico de pancreatitis era obio y que por el contraro la anatomia patologica solo lo confirmó en un 60%.

Queremos pues la atención, a pesar del entusiasmo creciente que la exploración angiografica va despertando sobre la dificultad de interpretar correctamente las imagenes que obtenemos y que con frecuencia nos han llevado a diagnosticos erroneos.

Angiographic Localisation of Insulomas

B. Madsen

The first angiographic demonstration of an insuloma was published by Olle Olsson in 1963. A number of the succesful examinations have been reported since then. Bookstein & Oberman, however, claimed that only tumours with a sinusoidal vascularisation could be demonstrated and estimated that angiography would prove effective in less than 20% of the patients.

Our material includes 10 consecutive cases with surgically verified β-cell tumours All tumours were correctly located preoperatively by angiography.

The examination includes selective catheterisation of the coeliac and superior mesenteric arteries. After distension of the stomach by carbon dioxide, contrast is injected simultaneously into the two catheters.

The principal diagnostic criteria in cases of β-cell adenoma have been: enlarged arterial branches to the tumour, hypervascularisation and accumulation of contrast with a maximum density after 3–8 sec.

A case of β-cell carcinoma presented pathological vessels and only slight accumulation of contrast.

From histological examination of the tumours in our material, it appears that most varieties of vascularisation were represented, – including tumours with and without a sinusoidal structure.

They could *all* be visualized by angiography.

Up to now a total number of 67 verified β-cell tumours in 59 patients have been reported. Approximately 75% of these tumours were demonstrated on the angiograms.

Failure to visualize an insuloma may result from: Technical faults, – obesity of the patient, – superimposition of other structures, – sparse vascularisation of the tumour, – or the tumour being too small to be resolved on the films.

To our experience it is especially important to keep the K. V. lower that 80 either by shortening of the film-focus distance or by using fewer exposures per second. Distension of the stomach by carbon dioxide is also an important aid to better results.

With accuracy in technique and evaluation, angiography offers an extremely valuable method of locating insulomas preoperatively.

The Scintigraphy of the Pancreas

H. K. Deininger and F. Heuck

The possibilities for the early diagnosis of morphological pancreatic diseases became more advantageous by new, angiographic and scintigraphic methods of examination. The 237 scans of the pancreas reported in this paper were performed with ^{75}Se-l-selenomethionine. Only 5–10% of the applicated dose (about 3 μCi per kilogram of body-weight) has been absorbed by the tissues of the pancreas. By means of other radioactive tracers no readable scintigraphic images of the pancreas could be obtained. Better pancreatic scans resulted by using a 3″-scanner than by a 5″-crystal. In these cases more suitable conditions have been existing between the effective counting rate and the background resp. the radioactivity of the adjoining organs and the collimation. The double-tracer-technique, other technical modifications and some modulations of the pancreas scan are able to bring more informative results.

A readable pancreas scan showing a well outlined organ was observed in 73% of the examined patients. The quality of the scans could not be improved by the use of dietetic supplements and injections of drugs. These measures were investigated in a selected number of patients. But it is possible that an empty stomach and a long fasting period could be of importance. In 92 cases the pancreas was inspected at operations or autopsies and the different state of the tissue was confirmed by histological examinations. 77% of them (= 71 patients) correlated with the report of the pancreas scan. Between a great number of specific and relevant biochemical tests and the features of the scans no significant correlations could be noticed. These have been studied in 68 patients. The extent of the scintigraphic alterations was not identical with the endocrine or exocrine loss in function. And vice versa, the biochemical results were not correlating with the degree of the parenchymatous lesions in the pancreas scan. On account of the suspicion of a pancreatic disease angiographic procedures of the celiac and superior mesenteric artery were performed in 186 patients. The analysis of the angiogramms has been completed by the application of photographic and electronic subtraction techniques.

Most frequently, in 84% *healthy persons* showed readable scintigrams; 5 out of 37 scans were alterated pathologically. Therefore, it is likely that tumorous or chronic inflammatory diseases of the pancreas could be excluded if the scan of this organ was normal. The results of the arteriographies were approximately corresponding: None of the healthy persons showed pathological structures of the vessels.

In the cases of an *acute pancreatitis* the scans were least accurate. The informative value of the scan was impaired and the scintigraphic representation of the organ was considerably diminished (only 53% of these scans could be analyzed). Furthermore, scans with lesions suspicous on a tumour, uncharacteristic diffuse alterations and absolutely normal images could be found with the same frequency in this group of acute pancreatitis. The different biochemical tests brought the best results. The great majority of the arteriograms done in the stage of an acute pancreatitis has been normal. Few individual cases and some advanced stages of inflammation showed pathological signs: spasms of the vessels, distortions of the pancreatic arteries and the parenchyma did not dye in later arteriographic phases (but this could be observed in normal pancreas too).

In 84% of the patients with *chronic pancreatitis* and *fibrotic pancreatic disease* the organ could be seen in the pancreas scan. 76 scans out of these 98 (= 78%) has been classified as pathological ones. The various biochemical tests were less reliable. By the angiograms done in this group of patients suspicious results could be found in only 46%. Like the pathological changes in the scan the angiographic alterations were unspecific too. Mostly, the smaller pancreatic arteries were reduced and distorted. In addition, long extending and circular spasms of the vessels could be seen. Sometimes the chronic-cirrhotic processes showed alterations of the splenic and the portal vein. All pancreatic cysts could be diagnosed by the angiographic examinations but only 21 of 27 cysts could be detected by scintigraphic procedures. By means of the scan it was not possible to distinguish between cystic and malignant tumours. But partially, these space-occupying lesions could be differentiated by the angiograms. Some of the cysts showed pathological structures of the small vessels in the border areas and in the cystic walls. However, not in all the cases of malignant diseases of the pancreas typical signs and criterias of malignancy could be proven by the angiograms. Therefore, with a lower degree of diagnostic accuracy it could be concluded to a benigne or cystic, space-occupying lesion if the angiograms showed displacements of the vessels and avascular areas in the parenchyma of the pancreas. And in few cases only, the decreased uptake of the radioactive selenomethionine in the tissue correlated with the real extent of the pancreatic inflammation.

Scintigraphic examinations were also done in 38 *malignant tumours* of the pancreas, and in 14 of them (= 37%) no representation of the organ could be obtained. But no scan was normal and 17 scintigrams were suspected of a tumour because a circumscript decrease of the radioactive accumulation could be seen or the organ was only partially visible. In these cases of malignant diseases of the pancreas the biochemical tests were least accurate. The arteriography was of great importance in the diagnosis of pancreatic tumours. The majority of the angiographic examinations showed alterations of the arteries being suspicious on malignancy, and only in 3 patients with metastatic alterations of the pancreas no vascular lesions could be recognized. Moreover, the abdominal arteriography was superior to the scintigraphy of the pancreas if peripancreatic tumours (e.g. retroperitoneal sarcomas) has been existing.

Summary

The examination of the pancreas by the scintigraphy using ^{75}Se-methionine is not yet an optimal method in nuclear medicine. By this isotope procedure tumours and chronic inflammations can be diagnosed if the scan will be interpreted in connexion with other clinical findings. A severe disease of the pancreas may be excluded if the organ appears normal in the scan. The clinical signs and the biochemical examinations do not correlate with the scintigraphic findings in the diagnosis of pancreatic diseases. The pathological results detected by a pancreas scan has to be completed or proven by other examinations. Selective angiograms of the celiac and mesenteric artery are of a high value to differentiate morphological alterations of the pancreas parenchyma, and tumorous diseases of the organ can be reliably diagnosed by this kind of arteriography. Abnormal scintigraphic or angiographic results require surgical resp. histological exploration of the pancreas.

Tumours of Stomach and Colon

Angiographic Diagnosis and Evaluation of the Extent of Tumors of the Stomach and Colon

J. Wójtowicz

The purpose of this investigation was to evaluate the usefulness of angiography in diagnosing of gastric and colonic tumors which had been already detected with conventional methods.

The material in the present study consisted of 36 patients with gastric tumors and 21 patients with tumors of the colon. In both groups the great majority were carcinomas, while leiomyoma, polyp, accessory, pancreas and inflammatory tumors were also represented (Table 1).

Table 1

Material		
Gastric tumors		36
Carcinoma	31	
Leiomyoma	2	
Polyp	1	
Accessory pancreas	2	
Tumors of the colon		21
Carcinoma	16	
Inflammatory	4	
Polyp	1	

Celiac angiography and superior or inferior mesenteric angiography depending on the localization of the tumor were performed in all patients. Insufflation with gas was made to distend the examined organ and supplemented with pneumoperitoneum in gastric tumors. The diagnosis was confirmed histologically in all the patients except 3, in whom an obvious massive involvement was a contra-indication to surgical exploration.

The diagnostic accuracy of angiography and barium examination was approximately the same in both groups (Table 2).

Among the patients with gastric tumors cases of accessory pancreas and a small antral carcinoma were misdiagnosed by angiography. In the group with tumors of the colon the main cause of failure with both methods was the difficulty to differentiate between neoplasm and inflammatory tumor.

Table 2. *Barium examination versus angiography as compared to surgery*

Organ	Diagnosis		Important supplementary details	
Method	correct	incorrect	correct	incorrect
Stomach				
Barium examination	32	4	—	—
Angiography	33	3	21	4
Colon				
Barium examination	17	4	—	—
Angiography	19	2	14	1

Well known angiographic signs of malignancy and their frequences are given in Table 3.

Table 3. *Angiographic signs*

Carcinoma of the	Arterial invasion	Arterial displacement	Pathological vessels	Contrast accumulation	Early venous filling
Stomach	25	9	21	13	0
Colon	4	5	14	11	7

Invasion of one or more gastric arteries and tumor vessels were found separately or in combination in the great majority of gastric carcinoma. In general, however, carcinomas were poorly vascularized with few pathological vessels and little contrast accumulation within the tumor. Early venous filling was not observed in gastric carcinoma. One of the 2 patients with leiomyoma had no angiographic abnormalities; the other had a poorly vascularized tumor.

Abundant pathological vessels, distinct contrast accumulation and early venous filling were the prevailing findings in tumors of the colon. Avascular carcinomas of the recto-sigmoid were observed as well, while on the other hand, inflammatory tumors presented numerous and irregular arterial vessels.

An essential diagnostic gain was obtained with angiography when local invasion and liver metastases have been revealed (Table 4).

Widespread metastatic foci to the liver or large solitary metastasis were found altogether in 13 patients. There were two false positive and one false negative diagnoses.

Extension of carcinoma through the gastric wall to the diaphragm, spleen, pancreas and to the hilus of the liver were found in 19 instances. Infiltration of the regional lymph nodes and retroperitoneal involvement escaped angiographic detection in all examined cases.

Extension through the wall of the large bowel with involvement of the mesentery were the most frequent findings in carcinoma of the colon.

Table 4. *Important supplementary details*

Neoplasmatic infiltration of the:	Carcinoma of the stomach	Carcinoma of the colon
Diaphragm	4	0
Spleen	6	0
Pancreas	5	2
Liver hilus	4	0
Omentum	3	0
Mesentery	0	8
Stomach	—	1
Kidney	0	1
Liver metastases	10	3

Adrenal Lesions

Adrenal Angiography

H. Reschke

I have been asked to give a brief review of possibilities and limits in angiographic diagnosis of the adrenals. I prefer arteriography to obtain an analysis of the organs as well as of the surrounding tissues. Therefore this method especially shall be described.

Arteriographically the morphology of adrenal structures can be visualized rather compeletly in about 70% of cases. With only few exceptions all organs partially will be demonstrated. In cases of uncertainty in diagnosis phlebography will supplement the findings.

In this short communication the technics of catheterization and the complications can not be discussed. We use seriographic studies employing a focus-film-distance of one meter in sagittal view. In this way, the enlargement factor for the adrenals of adults varies between 16 and 28%. The frontal view may prove important in tumour diagnosis.

The use of arteries to obtain a visualization of the organs as complete as possible does not correspond with the knowledge of descriptive anatomy. In angiographic studies shape, measurements and relations of the adrenals to the kidneys differ remarkably.

A "normal" span of time of blood flow through the organs arteriographically is not to be determined. The main adrenal vein can be seen either $1^1/_2$ sec or 5 sec and later after beginning of injection.

The size of single organs differs from 200/300 mm^2 to 1000/1200 mm^2 (Fig. 1) and the size of pairs of organs from 800 mm^2 to 1500/1800 mm^2.

The measurements in sagittal view are the prerequisite of radiological diagnosis of transformations of the adrenal cortex. Certain shapes, f.i. oval contours do not prove hyperplasia as well as tumour (Fig. 1). Adrenal hyperplasia may only be defined by enlargement of the organ. Sometimes marginal arteries partially may outline their contours (Fig. 2). Hyperplasia can be evident by enlargement of one adrenal. Then the study of only the contralateral organ certainly would cause misinterpretation. An increase of the thickness of the adrenals in hyperplasia must not be expected.

"Nodular" hyperplasia can be visible by punched out defects within stained organs. In some patients the diagnosis of hyperplasia is not possible by any radiological means. This seems to be true more often in Conn-Syndroma, occasionally in Cushing-Syndroma (Fig. 2) and rarely or not at all in AGS.

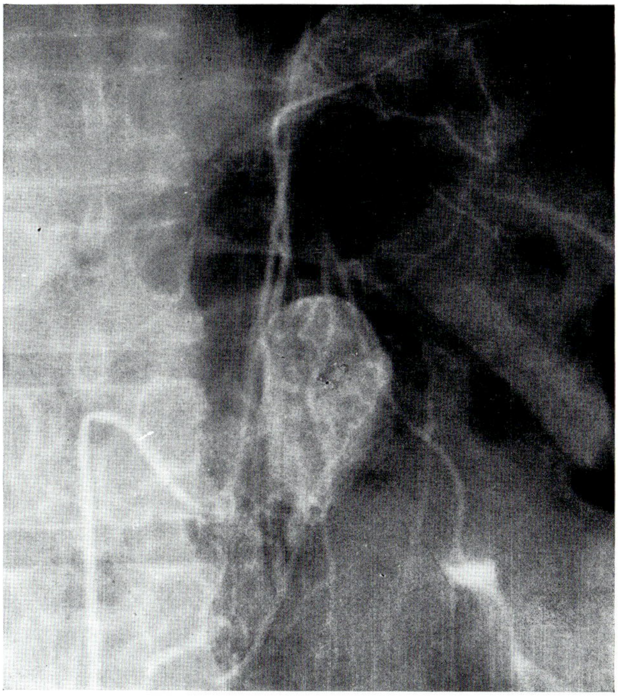

Fig. 1

Regressive transformation can not be demonstrated according to my experiences. Therefore one will not be able to draw any conclusion in respect to a tumour of the contralateral gland or of extraadrenal origin. Opening the discussion of adrenal tumours I shall start with medullary neoplasms in literature often demonstrated by aortograms.

In 80% or 90% neuroblastomas, paragangliomas and pheochromocytomas are developed from the adrenal medulla. The vascularization of the latter often is rather heavy. The diagnosis of chromaffine tumours however, can be impossible by aortography. In case of multiple pheochromocytomas the one or the other only will be seen by selective arteriography because in this way the pararenal space can be better examined.

It is to be mentioned that in-all-seven cases I saw no critical rising of blood preasure during these manipulations.

Tumours of the adrenal cortex may be endocrinologically active or inactive. Rapid tumour growing as well as large dimensions don't prove malignancy.

By demonstration of tumour perfusing suprarenal arteries such neoplasms can not be distinguished from those of the paradrenal space. Beyond this there are no characteristic radiological signs to differentiate adenomas from the one or the other pheochromocytoma (Fig. 3), neuroblastomas or teratomas as well as myomas and several neoplasms of mesenchymal tissues.

An other aortogram only defines a space occupying lesion with attachement to the aorta, the renal artery and to the upper pole of the kidney. In the following selective

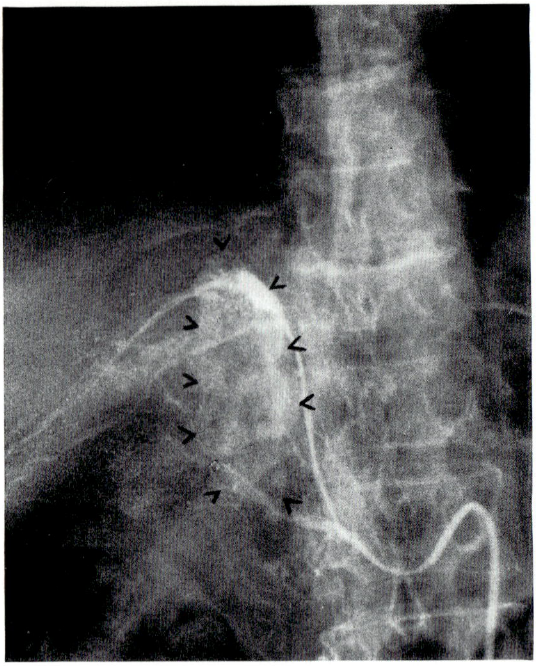

Fig. 2

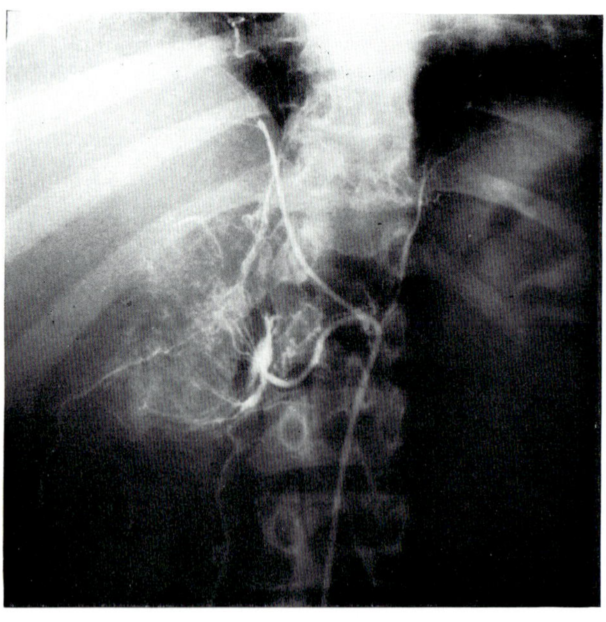

Fig. 3

study of the medial suprarenal artery infiltrative – and irregular – growth up to the renal vessels and hilum can be demonstrated. These findings indicate carcinomas. Metastases should be excluded.

Malignant growth verified histologically by invasion of small adrenal veins and/or of the tumour capsule angiographically may not be discerned. Comparing the vessels of adenomas and pheochromocytomas sometimes an etiological diagnosis may not be possible as mentioned earlier (Fig. 3). Adenomas of a size of 30–40 mm in diameter may destroy the contours of the gland. Similar tumours adjacent to the organ do not differ in their arteriographic signs. In such cases it is not possible to differentiate wether the adenoma originates from the adrenal cortex or extraadrenally.

Smaller adenomas cause irregularities of the contours of the organ and of the density of its contrast. Cortical tumours of a size up to 10 mm will be discerned by ringlike staining or marginal stripes. These tumours are poor in vascularization and give rise to "defects" in opacification.

It is important to know that adenomas "out of function" can be found.

It is to be mentioned also that an early diagnosis of remote metastases of bronchial and/or mammarian carcinomas in about 30–50 % of cases could be gained by adrenal angiography.

Angioszintigraphie der Nebennieren

K. H. VAN DE WEYER

Wie postmortale Gefäßstudien und eigene angiographische Untersuchungen zeigen, bietet die selektive Nebennieren-Angiographie über die obere Arteriengruppe via Arteria phrenica inferior die größten Chancen für die Darstellung des Organes. Weniger Aussichten auf eine Darstellung der Nebennieren bestehen bei der Kontrastmittel-Injektion in die untere Nebennierenarteriengruppe via Arteria renalis. Wie unsere Untersuchungen weiterhin zeigen, hat die selektive Kontrastmittel-Injektion in eine Arterie der mittleren Gruppe die geringsten Aussichten auf eine optimale Darstellung des Organes. Die sich an die Kontrastmittel-Injektion anschließende von uns erstmals durchgeführte Applikation von ^{131}-J makroaggregiertem Human-Albumin in die sondierten Nebennierenarterien mit nachfolgender Szintigraphie stellt eine neue Methode der Nebennierendiagnostik dar.

Wir haben den Versuch einer selektiven angiographischen Darstellung der Nebennieren bisher bei 69 Patienten gemacht, bei 59 gelang er (85%). Bei allen durchgeführten Nebennierenszintigraphien – wir haben bisher 25 Patienten mit dieser Methode untersucht – gelang die szintigraphische Darstellung der Nebennieren, in 6 Fällen jedoch nur einseitig.

Untersuchungstechnik: Anschließend an die abdominelle Übersichtsaortographie erfolgt die selektive Sondierung der A. phrenica inferior oder einer anderen Nebennierenarterie von einer Femoralarterie her mit einem speziell geformten roten Ödman-Ledin-Katheter. 3 Zielaufnahmen werden nach Injektion von 8 bzw. 12 ml Kontrastmittel sowie 2–3 sec nach Beendigung der Injektion belichtet. Daraufhin erfolgt die Injektion von 50 μCi ^{131}J-MAA je Nebenniere in das gleiche Gefäß. Die besten diagnostischen Ergebnisse konnten erbracht werden, wenn die Szintigraphie etwa $^1/_2$–1 Std nach Injektion des Radionukleids erfolgte. Bauchlagerung hat sich der Rückenlagerung bei der Nebennierenszintigraphie als überlegen erwiesen.

Zunächst sollen einige normale selektive angiographische und szintigraphische Darstellungen der Nebennieren gezeigt werden.

Die erste – hier aus Platzmangel nicht wiedergegebene Abbildung – zeigt eine selektive angiographische Darstellung der rechten Nebenniere über die A. phrenica inferior früharterielle und spätarterielle Füllungsphase.

Abbildung 1 zeigt die szintigraphische Darstellung derselben Nebenniere nach Gabe von 50 μCi ^{131}J-MAA, Bauchlage des Patienten. Schwarz-weiß-Wiedergabe eines Buntscanns, die Zonen stärkster Radioaktivitätsanreicherung sind schwarz, die Zonen geringerer grau wiedergegeben.

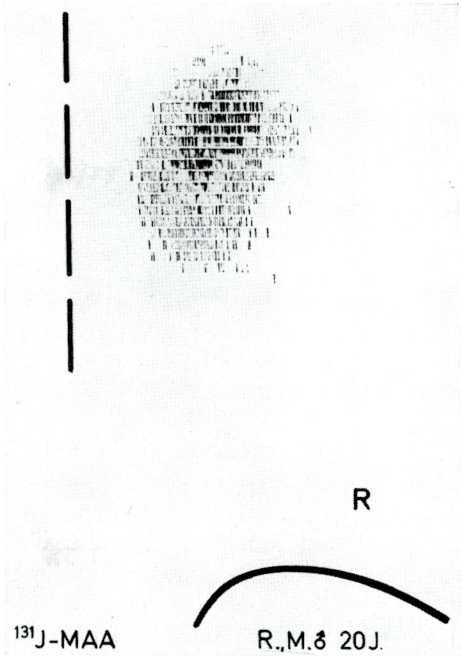

Abb. 1

Abbildung 2a zeigt eine simultane selektive angiographische Darstellung beider Nebennieren über die unteren Zwerchfellarterien, die mit einem gemeinsamen Stamm von der Aorta entspringen, Rückenlage.

Abbildung 2b. Nebennierenszintigramm derselben Patientin wie Abbildung 2a, Bauchlage, 30 min nach Injektion von 100 μCi ^{131}J-MAA. Zum besseren Vergleich

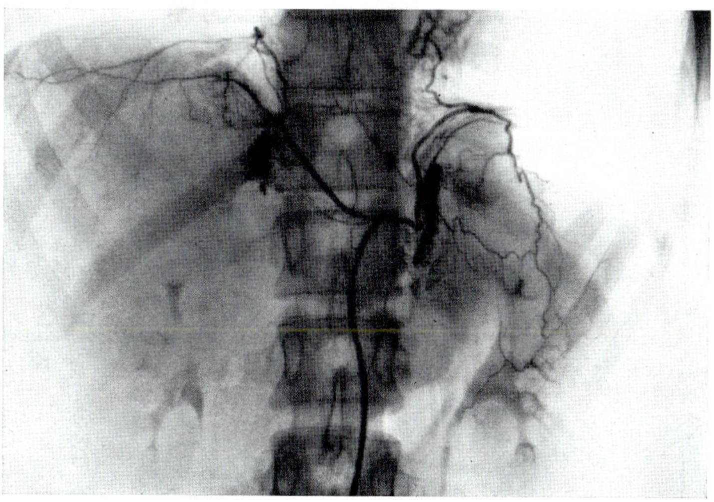

Abb. 2a

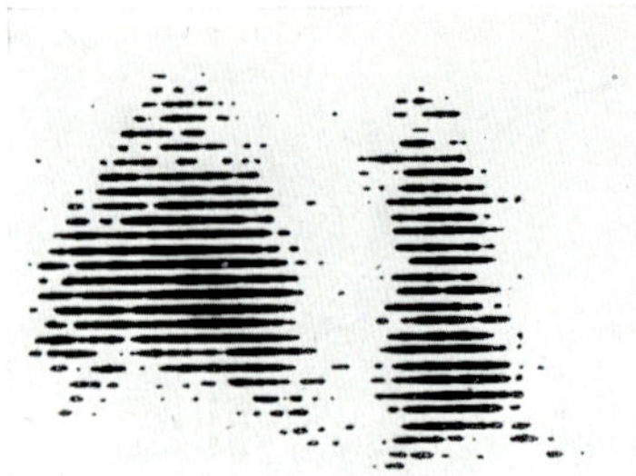

Abb. 2b

mit den Angiographiebildern wird das Szintigramm seitenverkehrt wiedergegeben. Gute Übereinstimmung der angiographischen mit der szintigraphischen Nebennierendarstellung.

Die A. phrenica inferior hat leider nur in 30% der Fälle einen gemeinsamen Stamm von der Aorta. So ist zur selektiven Nebennierenangiographie und Szintigraphie oft eine getrennte Sondierung der Zwerchfellarterien oder anderer Nebennierenarterien notwendig. Diese kleinen Gefäße versorgen oft nicht allein die Nebennieren, sondern darüber hinaus auch andere Gebiete wie Zwerchfell-, Nierenkapsel-, Mediastinal- und Leberanteile. Sowohl bei der Injektion von Kontrastmittel als auch von Radioaktivität kann es also zur Mitdarstellung dieser genannten Bereiche kommen. Ist man über die topographische Beziehung dieser – gegen unseren Wunsch – mit dargestellten Anteile zu den Nebennieren nicht informiert, so kann es leicht zu entscheidenden diagnostischen Irrtümern führen.

Abbildung 3a zeigt die angiographische Darstellung der linken Nebenniere über die untere Zwerchfellarterie. Früharterielle und spätarterielle Phase zeigen auch eine Auffüllung der oberen Nierenkapselarterie. In der spätarteriellen Phase volle Kontrastmittelauffüllung der linken Nebenniere.

Abbildung 3b. Nebennierenszintigramm links bei demselben Patienten wie Abbildung 3a. Nach Injektion von 50 μCi ^{131}J-MAA ist eine sichere Abgrenzung der Radioaktivität im Bereich der linken Nebenniere von derjenigen im Nierenkapselbereich nicht möglich (Rückenlage).

Nach unseren bisherigen Erfahrungen haben wir doch den Eindruck, daß sich die Radioaktivität meist bevorzugt in den Nebennieren anreichert.

Auch durch eine entsprechende Unterdrückung des Untergrundes bei der Szintigraphie kann eine bessere Darstellung der Nebennieren erreicht werden.

Bei der Kombination der selektiven Angiographie mit der Szintigraphie hat uns die größere diagnostische Sicherheit bei der Beurteilung meist die selektive Angiographie erbracht. Die Szintigraphie sehen wir als eine, den Patienten nicht zusätzlich belastende Erweiterung der diagnostischen Aussage an.

Wie Aktivitäts-Messungen in unserem Institut ergeben haben, ist die bei unserer Methode auftretende Strahlenbelastung sowohl für die Nebennieren als auch für die Schilddrüse vertretbar.

Abschließend einige pathologische Befunde.

1. Ein 5 mm großes Conn-Adenom am oberen medialen Pol der rechten Nebenniere. Es konnte durch selektive Nebennierenangiographie über die Aa. phrenicae inferiores dargestellt werden. Am oberen medialen Pol der rechten Nebenniere sah

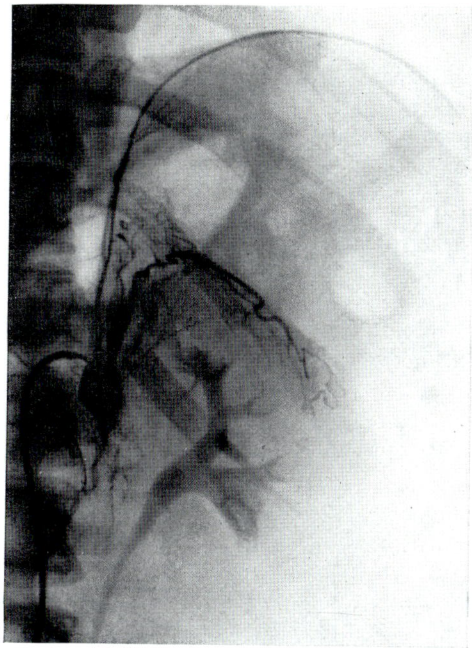

Abb. 3a

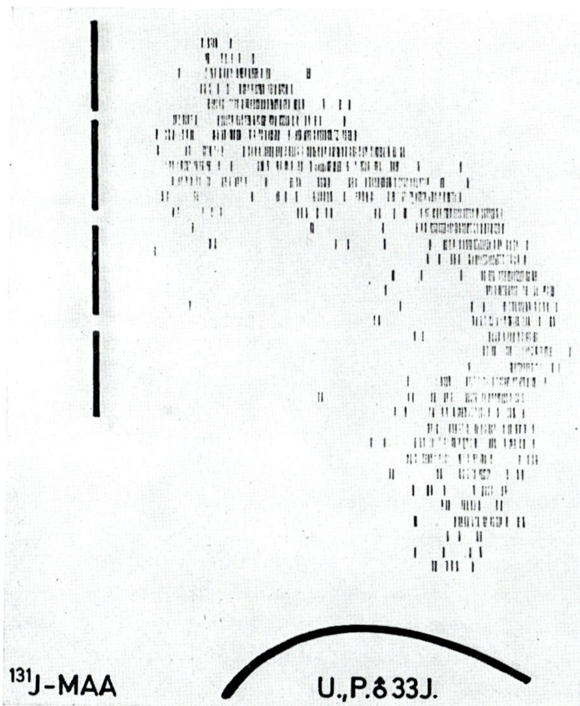

Abb. 3b

man einen rundlichen Bezirk, der nicht vascularisiert war, jedoch in seinen Randpartien vermehrten Gefäßreichtum zeigte.

Die bisher durchgeführten Routine-Röntgenuntersuchungen hatten in Anbetracht der geringen Größe der Conn-Tumoren, die selten größer sind als 1–2 cm im Durchmesser, keine Chance der Erfassung. Das Auffinden des Adenoms ist auch intraoperativ wegen seiner geringen Ausmaße nicht immer leicht. Im selektiven Nebennierenangiogramm ist das Adenom der Nebennierenrinde bei entsprechenden technischen Bedingungen schon ab einer Größe von 5–10 mm diagnostizierbar.

2. Ein weiterer Fall betraf eine beiderseitige Nebennierenhyperplasie bei Cushing-Syndrom. Die Aa. phrenicae inferiores hatten auch hier einen gemeinsamen Stamm aus der Aorta. Die Darstellung der Nebennieren erfolgte über diese unteren Zwerchfellarterien. Die rechte Nebenniere erwies sich als deutlich vergrößert, sie überragte mit ihrem medialen Anteil die Wirbelsäulenkontur und reichte weit nach lateral hin. Die linke Nebenniere war angiographisch nicht sicher beurteilbar.

3. Mit dem letzten Fall möchten wir von einer Beobachtung berichten, bei der die selektive Angiographie, insbesondere aber die Kombination dieser mit der Szintigraphie, eine sichere Aussage über die Beschaffenheit einer chromaffinen Geschwulst erlaubte. Durch die Angioszintigraphie ließ sich bei dieser Patientin ein zentral zerfallenes Phäochromocytom nachweisen. Bei der Übersichtsetagenaortographie nach Hettler sah man, daß die linke Nierenarterie schräg nach caudal-lateral gerichtet war. In der späten Parenchymphase erkannte man eine deutliche Caudalverlagerung der linken Niere. Cranial davon stellte sich ein in den Randpartien vermehrt mit Kontrastmittel angereicherter Tumor dar.

Bei der selektiven Angiographie über die obere Nebennierenarteriengruppe links sah man mit Kontrastmittel angereicherte Nebennierenreste. Nach Injektion von ^{131}J-MAA in das gleiche Gefäß sah man bei der Szintigraphie (Rückenlage, 1 Std nach Injektion) eine Zone vermehrter Radioaktivitätsanreicherung in den medialen cranialen und den lateralen Randpartien. Im Zentrum des Tumors fand sich eine große rundliche Zone verminderter Radioaktivitätsanreicherung. Wir haben aus diesen angiographisch-szintigraphischen Zeichen die Diagnose eines zentral zerfallenden Tumors gestellt. Dieser präoperativ erhobene Befund wurde bei der Operation bestätigt: Es fand sich ein Phäochromocytom mit zentraler Nekrose. Die bei der selektiven Angiographie erfaßten „Nebennierenreste“ wurden histologisch gesichert.

Zusammenfassung

Wir hoffen, daß mit zunehmenden Erfahrungen in der kombinierten Anwendung der selektiven angiographisch-szintigraphischen Darstellung der Nebennieren ein echter Fortschritt in der Nebennieren-Diagnostik erreicht wird. Soweit bisher zu beurteilen, hat sich die Kombination der beiden Verfahren in den meisten Fällen den üblichen radiologischen Untersuchungsmethoden überlegen erwiesen. Dabei ist jedoch zu bemerken, daß die Nebennierenszintigraphie ohne gleichzeitige selektive Angiographie in manchen Fällen eine sichere diagnostische Aussage nicht zuläßt. Die größere Sicherheit bei der Beurteilung hat uns fast immer die selektive Angiographie erbracht.

Retroperitoneal-Tumours

Angiographical Examinations of the Retroperitoneal Space

E. Bücheler

Diseases especially tumours can easily spread in the retroperitoneal space. The clinical symptoms are often interpreted in a false way. Since there is an invasion of a tumour into the neighbouring organs the diagnosis is made per exclusionem. But this fact often already means operative incurability. Nevertheless it is important to get an exact diagnosis, because the surgical indication of removing of the tumour can be made in a wider sense in combination with radiation therapy.

The difficult problem to solve means to apply all the necessary radiological examinations, because improved diagnostics of the retroperitoneal space can only be obtained by combining all methods. In spite of lack of specificity the conventional X-ray examinations are a basic part of the retroperitoneal diagnostics. They determine the application of specific X-ray examinations. First there are the plain X-ray of the abdomen, the urography and the tomography. Above all the nephrotomography seems to be of special value to diagnose the tumours of smaller size for the reason of good contrast and no disturbing superpositions. For excluding intra-abdominal processes, examinations of the gastrointestinal tract and the colon are necessary.

If special angiography is applied at the right time, improved diagnostics of beginning diseases in the retroperitoneal space are possible. The application should be done in the right sequence and the indications and limits should be watched. Usually one special method is insufficient for the preoperative demonstration of the anatomy as well as for the topography and expansion of the tomour.

Since in the diagnostics of the retroperitoneal tumours the pneumoperitoneum has been widely left, the aortography with its modifications is giving definitive informations of the localisation, the expansion and the relation to the neighbouring organs and, with reservation, about the malignancy or benignancy. The poor arterialisation of the retroperitoneal space requires a very good technique. The aortography with fast serial films and sufficient amounts of contrast medium has to consider that the lower intercostal arteries and branches of the arteria iliaca interna besides the lumbar arteries take part in the arterialisation of the spatium retroperitonaeale. Because of the dorsal origin of these arteries, a slow injection of the contrast medium is necessary in order to get a better contrast. The intermediate serial pictures are decisive for the diagnosis, when nearly all the contrast medium has left the other branches of the aorta. The selective angiography of the lumbar, intercostal or iliacal arteries is giving an improved visualisation. In order to get the total expansion of the tumour it is necessary to probe several arteries.

The cavography is able to give informations of the expansion of the tumour and the metastases in the lymph nodes. The proof of a penetration of a tumour into the vena cava inferior and of the fixation to the spine is most important, while for the indirect discovery of metastases and of primary neoplasms of the lymph nodes the lymphography is the method of choice. The expansion of the tumours can be demonstrated better by the combined retroperitoneal venography and lower cavography than by the normal cavography. With the help of this new method the visualisation of the lumbar venous system and the vena cava inferior is possible in one examination. By this, the expansion of the tumour into the paravertebral portion of the spatium retroperitonaeale as well as into the vena cava inferior is provable. This examination has its special value in the case of left-sited neoplasms, for changes of the vena cava inferior do not exist because of the interposed aorta. On the other hand the dorsal expansion of the tumour can be demonstrated by a venogram of the lumbar venous system. Although the venograms are indirect methods of examination and only positive findings are a reliable proof, they are a valuable additional examination to the arteriography regarding the diagnostics of the retroperitoneal space.

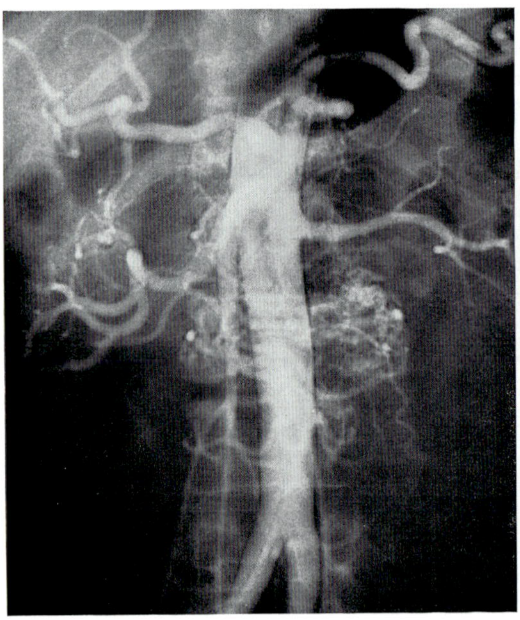

a

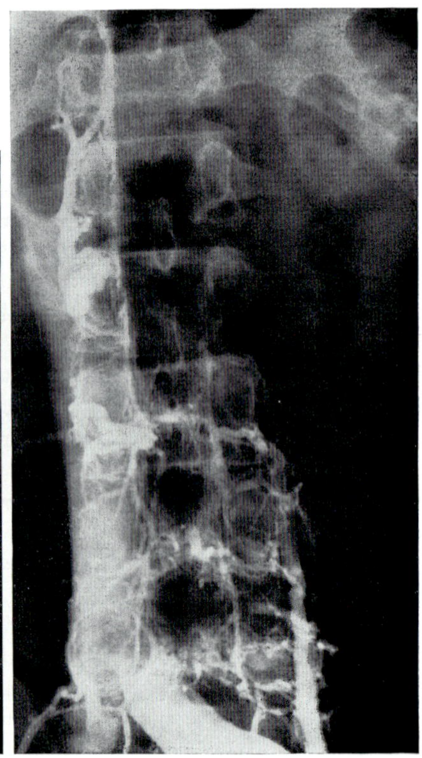

b

Fig. 1a and b. Hemangipericytoma of the retroperitoneal space. a Aortography: Tumour vessels al L 2. b Retroperitoneal veno- and cavography: Occlusion of the vena lumbalis ascendens sinistra at L 3 and of the epidural veins at L 2/3

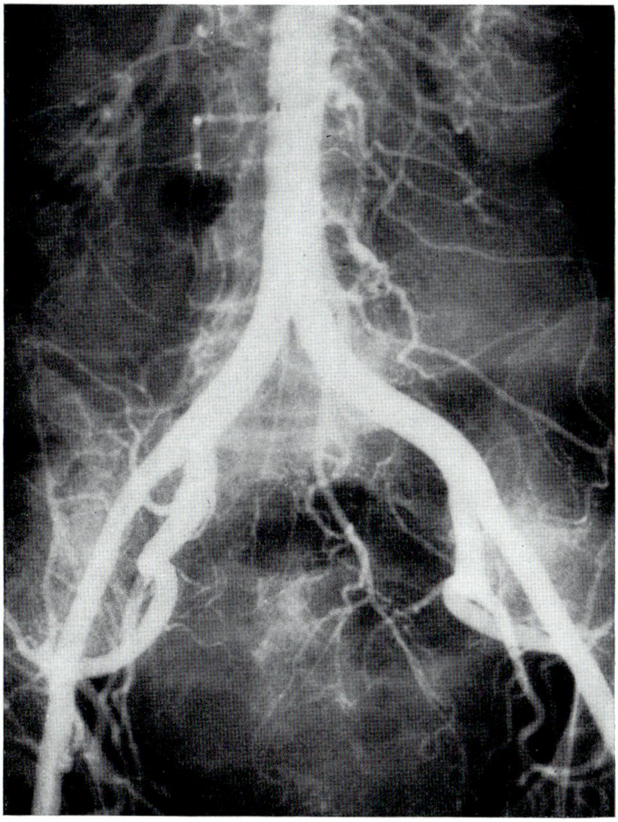

Fig. 2a and b. Hemangiopericytoma of the retroperitoneal space. a Aortography: Sporadic tumour vessels paravertebral on the left side

The arteriographical diagnosis of retroperitoneal neoplasms is absolutely dependent on the grade of vascularisation. The arterial supply of the spatium retroperitoneale is poor. The tumour diagnosis is determined by the quantity of arteries supplying the tumour and by the expansion of the necrosis of the neoplasm. The smaller the quantity and the diameter of the arteries and the larger the area of necrosis, the poorer is the possibility of recognizing the tumour. That is the reason, why the diagnostic and differential diagnosic value of the arteriogram is limited.

The criteria of the common tumour diagnosis are also available for the proof of malignancy of a retroperitoneal space-occupying process. Tumours with a high grade of vascularisation and with pathological formations of the vessels, a.v. fistulas and visualisation of the tumour area are an exception to the rule; here tumour veins are seldom to be found. Arteriographic findings with the same histological result can show the most different pictures. In the case of Fig. 1a of a hemangiopericytoma the aortogram is demonstrating the typical signs of a malignant tumour paravertebral on both sides. In the combined retroperitoneal veno- and cavogram (Fig. 1b) a block of the left paravertebral vein is indicating a dorsal tumour penetrating and an occlusion of the left-sited epidural veins is showing the expansion of the tumour

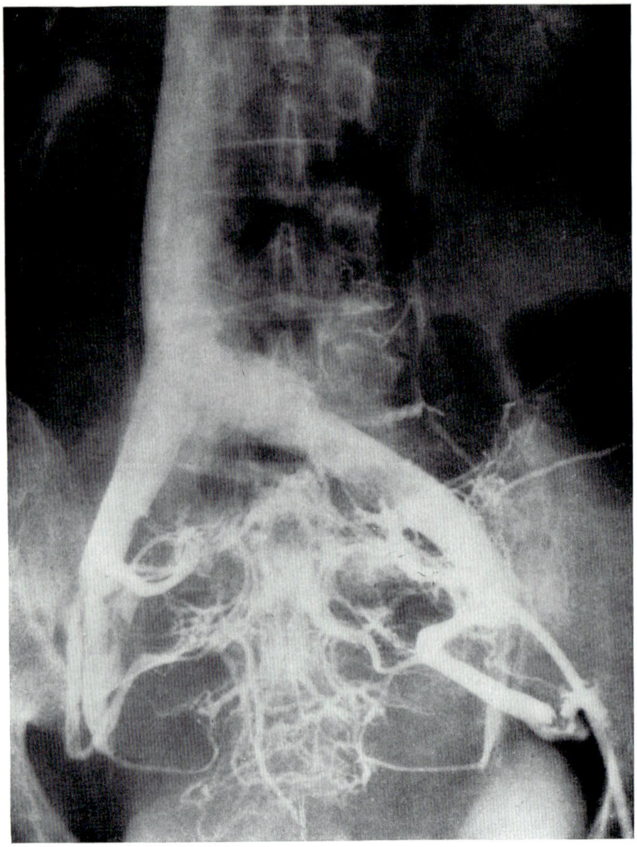

Fig. 2. b Retroperitoneal veno- and cavogram: Occlusion of the vena lumbalis ascendens sinistra at L 4

into the spinal canal. On the contrary the hemangiopericytoma of Fig. 2a has only a few tumour vessels and a low grade of tumour visualisation on the left side. The combined retroperitoneal veno- and cavogram (Fig. 2b) with the occlusion of the left vena lumbalis ascendens is proving the dorsal expansion of the tumour.

In a case of a large tumour necrosis (Fig. 3a) one often finds no signs of a malignoma in the aortogram in spite of numerous nutritive arteries. In this situation the determination of the real size of a tumour by the arteriography seems to be impossible. To solve this problem the lumbar veno- and cavography (Fig. 3b) are the best method because here the displacement of the vena cava inferior and the occlusion of the vena lumbalis ascendens are indications of the expansion of the malignoma.

In the aortogram benign tumours of the retroperitoneal space are characterised by the displacement of the lumbar arteries or of the branches of the arteria iliaca interna (Fig. 4).

These examples of retroperitoneal neoplasms demonstrate, that in many cases the differential diagnosis by arteriography is impossible and the amount of pathological vessels cannot absolutely prove the differentiation of the tumour and the

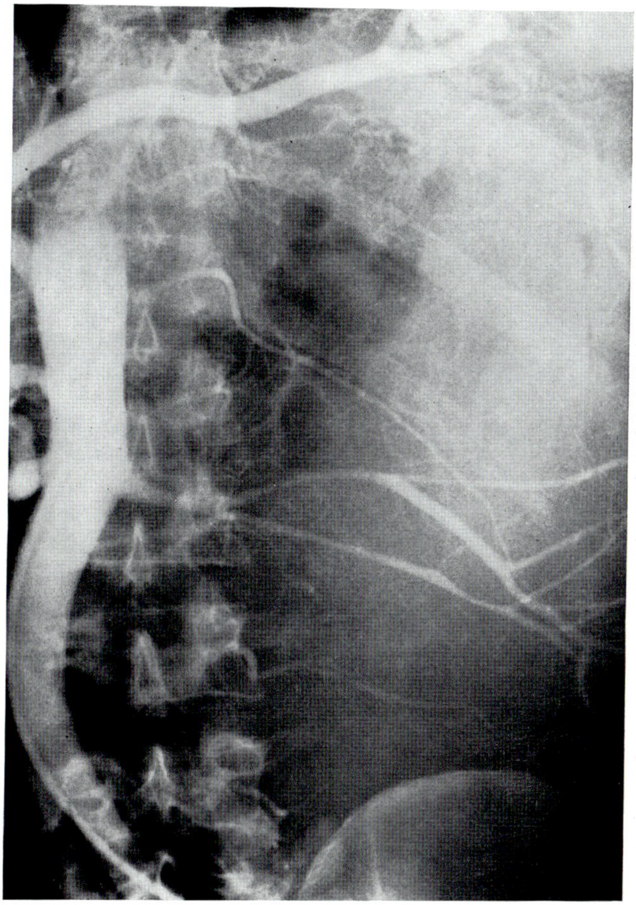

Fig. 3a and b. Retroperitoneal sarcoma. a Aortogram: Extension and contour defects of the lumbar arteries at L 3 and 4 on the left side

grade of malignancy. In some cases only the diagnosis of space-occupying lesions, but no differential diagnosis can be made. Sometimes the malignancy of a tumour, which cannot be classified arteriographically is only recognized by occlusions or vascular defects in the combined retroperitoneal veno- and cavogram. By this the importance of the venous venographie in the tumour diagnostics of the retroperitoneum is emphasized.

In the diagnostics of the recurrence of retroperitoneal tumours after nephrectomies the arteriography is the only method which gives decisive findings by demonstrating tumour vessels and tumour visualisation. These findings should be confirmed by the retroperitoneal venography and cavography. Therefore the angiographical methods should be more often applied in the postoperative control-examinations.

Retropertitoneal metastases or neoplasms of the lymphatic systems usually are not an indication for the arteriography because of their poor vascularisation (Fig. 5a). Here the best method is the cavography especially if combined with the venography

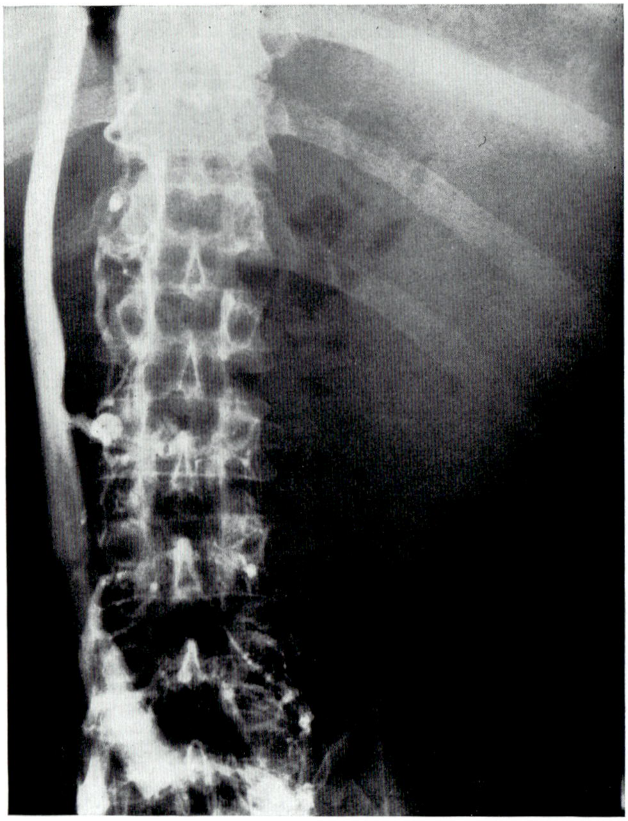

Fig. 3. b Lumbar veno- and cavography: Occlusion of the left vena lumbalis ascendens and displacement of the vena cava inferior

of the vertebral veins (Fig. 5b) because the latter sometimes can show metastases of the spine.

In case of retroperitoneal bleeding the arteriography, if applied during the period of bleeding, is able to localise the origin of the bleeding by demonstrating the contrast medium leaving a lumbar artery.

Summary

While the arteriography can make the diagnosis of a space-occupying lesion, but not always the differential diagnosis, the combined retroperitoneal venography and cavographie is able to give additional hints about the tumour expansion. A reasonable combination of arterio- and venographical examination should bring the best results in the diagnostics of space-occupying processes in the retroperitoneal space if indications and limits of the different methods are watched.

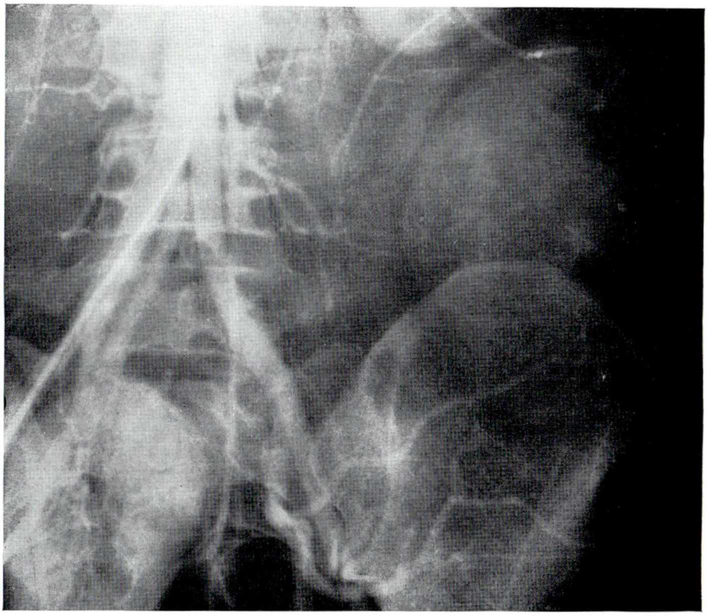

Fig. 4. Partially calcified leiomyoma of the retroperitoneal space. Aortography: Displacement of the lumbar arteries

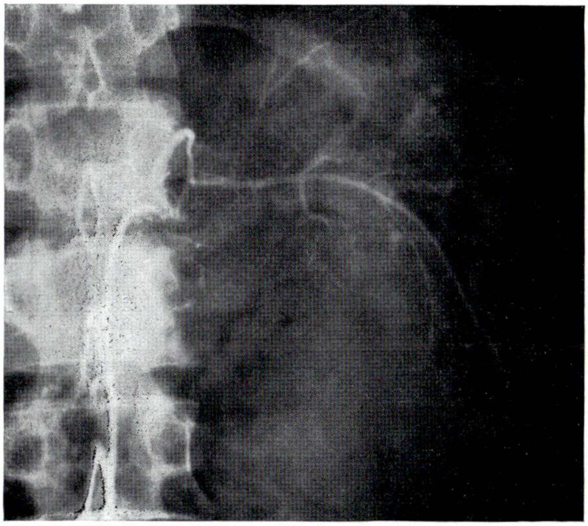

a

Fig. 5a and b. Retroperitoneal metastasis of a seminoma with destruction of the lateral edge of L 2. a Selective lumbar arteriography: A few pathological vessels at L 2

b Retroperitoneal veno- and cavogram: Occlusion of the vena lumbalis ascendens sinistra. Normal visualisation of the vena cava inferior

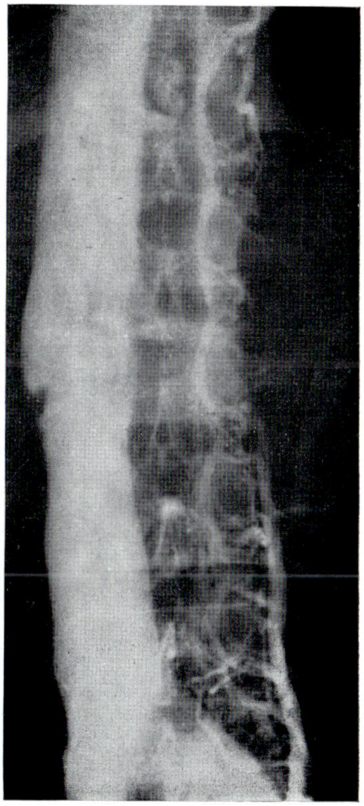

b

Die angiographische Darstellung primärer Retroperitonealtumoren

N. Heger, S. Bayindir, R. Steckenmesser und S. F. Grebe

Die Arteriographie des Spatium retroperitoneale ermöglicht bei raumfordernden Prozessen sicherer als die übrigen sog. indirekten Methoden die Lokalisation und Ausdehnung eines Tumors sowie seine Beziehung zu den Retroperitonealorganen zu bestimmen. Außerdem erlaubt sie in einem hohen Prozentsatz die Differentialdiagnose zwischen gut- und bösartigem Tumor.

Dies setzt eine ausreichende Darstellung des retroperitonealen Arteriensystems voraus, die durch eine abdominale Übersichtsaortographie allein nicht immer gewährleistet ist. Bei der spärlichen arteriellen Versorgung des Retroperitonealraumes über dünnkalibrige Gefäße wie die Aa. phrenicae ascendentes, Aa. supra-

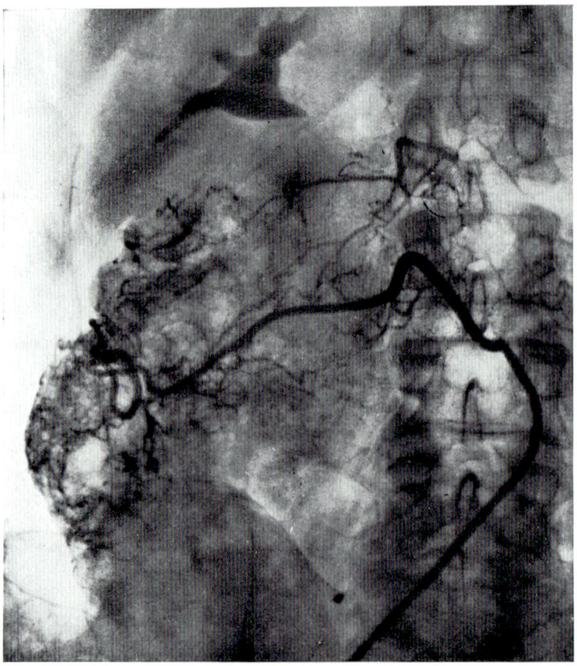

Abb. 1. Selektive Lumbalarteriographie: Maligne erscheinendes Gefäßbild eines ausgedehnten Ganglioneuroblastoms, Cranialverlagerung der rechten Niere

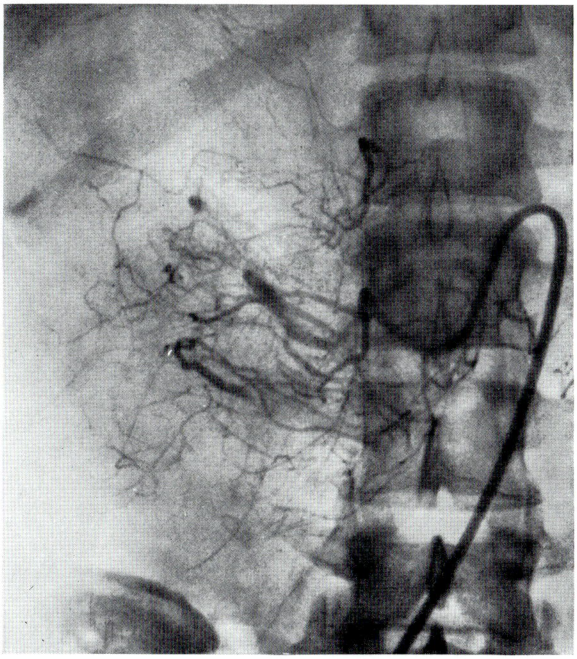

a

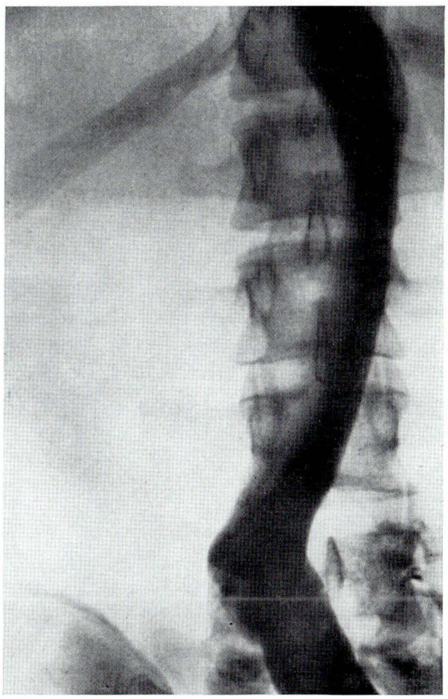

b

Abb. 2. a Selektive Lumbalarteriographie: Pathologische Vaskularisation eines unreifzelligen primären Retroperitonealteratoms. b Cavographie: Verlagerung, Pellottierung und Wandinfiltration der Vena Cava (op. bestätigt) renales, Aa. lumbales und Parietaläste der Aa. iliacae internae ist mit der selektiven Arteriographie (manuelle Injektion von 4–8 ml 60% Conray[1]) eine wesentlich bessere Information zu erzielen.

Für die Retroperitonealgeschwülste gelten die Kriterien der allgemeinen angiographischen Tumordiagnostik.

Die folgenden Beispiele sollen die Aussagekraft der selektiven Lumbalarteriographie demonstrieren.

Abbildung 1 zeigt das Arteriogramm eines 60jährigen Patienten mit einem ausgedehnten rechtsseitigen Retroperitonealtumor. Das im Gefäßbild maligne erscheinende Ganglioneuroblastom wurde pathomorphologisch zunächst prognostisch relativ günstig beurteilt. 3 Jahre nach der operativen Entfernung der Geschwulst besteht jetzt ein massives Tumorrezidiv mit abdominalen Metastasen.

Abbildung 2a zeigt das Angiogramm eines 20jährigen Patienten mit einem unreifzelligen Teratom. Die Cavographie läßt neben der Verlagerung und Pelottierung der unteren Hohlvene die operativ bestätigte Wandinfiltration der Vena cava erkennen (Abb. 2b).

Am letzten Beispiel eines ausgedehnten polymorphzelligen Retroperitonealsarkoms (Abb. 3a) soll die Anwendung des tumoraffinen Radionuklids Ga67 demonstriert werden. 72 Std nach intravenöser Applikation von 1,5 mCi Ga67 fand sich eine selektive Anreicherung der Substanz im Tumor (Abb. 3b).

Wir haben in den letzten 4 Jahren 10 Patienten mit primärem Retroperitonealtumor (Lipom, Lymphcyste, Leiomyom, Neurinom, Ganglioneuroblastom, poly-

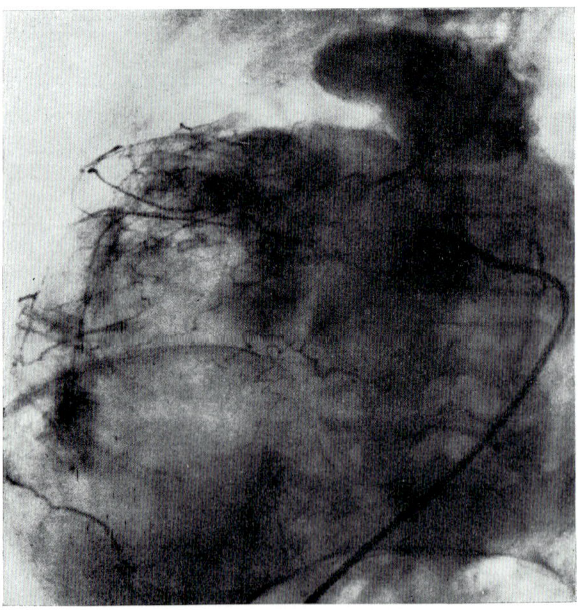

Abb. 3. a Selektive Lumbalarteriographie: Tumorgefäße eines polymorphzelligen Sarkoms, Nierenverlagerung

1 Fa. Byk Gulden, Konstanz

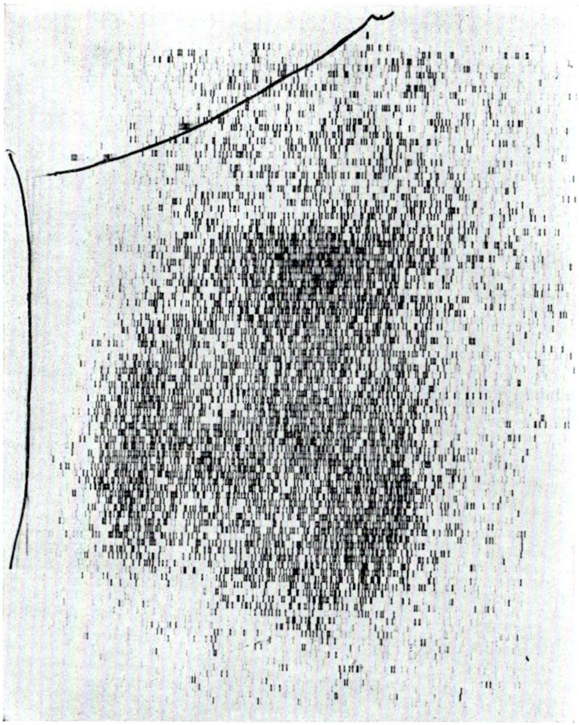

Fig. 3. b Tumorszintigramm (72 Std nach i.v. Applikation von 1,5 mCi Ga 67): Selektive Anreicherung im Tumor

morphzelliges Sarkom, Retikulosarkom, 2 Spindelzellsarkome, undifferenziertes Malignom) angiographisch untersucht. In allen Fällen gelang die exakte Tumorlokalisation, achtmal die Differenzierung zwischen gut- und bösartigem Tumor. Ein Sanduhrneurinom wurde als Malignom, ein cystisch degeneriertes Spindelzellsarkom als gutartige Geschwulst angesehen. In beiden Fällen wurde allerdings noch keine selektive Arteriographie durchgeführt.

In dieser kurzen Übersicht konnte nur auf die Arteriographie des Retroperitonealraumes etwas näher eingegangen werden. Die Bedeutung der retroperitonealen Venendarstellung bzw. der Cavographie für die Operationsplanung konnte nur gestreift werden, die Lymphadenographie mußte unberücksichtigt bleiben.

Angioszintigraphie der retroperitonealen Tumoren

L. Diethelm

Das angiographische Studium von Rezidiven und Metastasen im Retroperitonealraum führt in geeigneten Fällen schon bei der Übersichtsaortographie evtl. unter Verwendung der Angiotomographie zu positiven Tumordarstellungen. Hierbei entdeckte schon Holm eine Kalibervergrößerung der ein Hypernephromrezidiv versorgenden Arteriae lumbales auf das 3–4fache.

Auch bei den primären, nicht von parenchymatösen Organen ausgehenden Tumoren des Retroperitonealraumes lassen sich differenzierte angiographische und szintigraphische Befunde erheben, wenn man die *selektive Angiographie* der Lumbal-

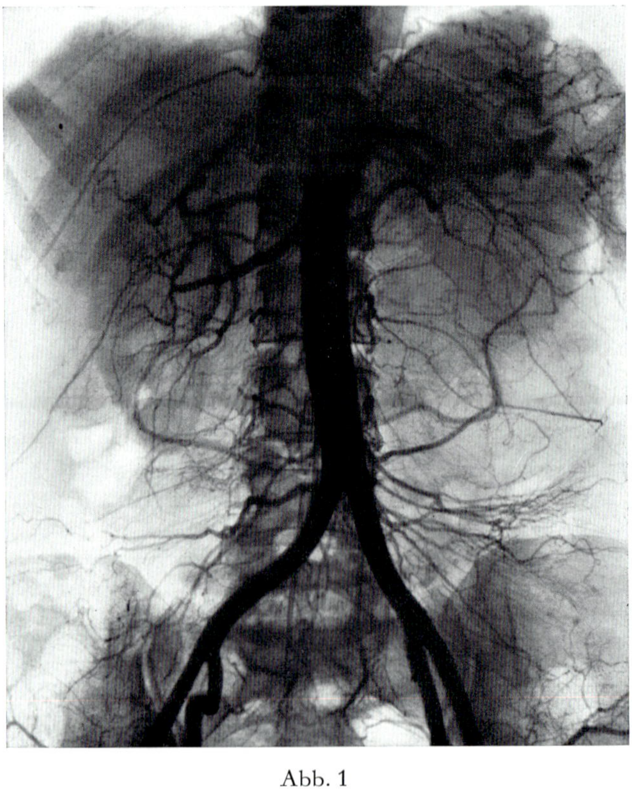

Abb. 1

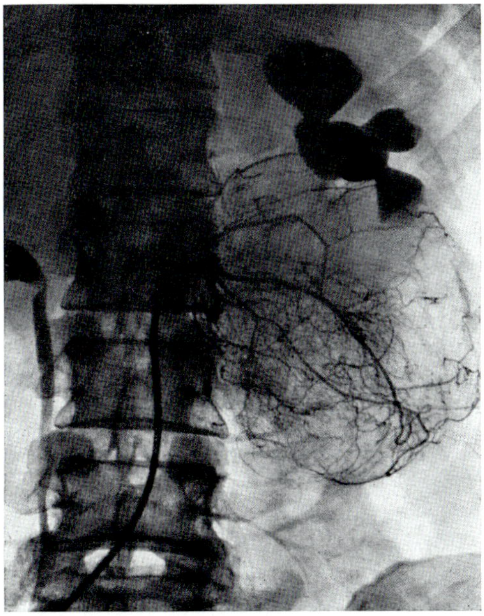
Abb. 2a

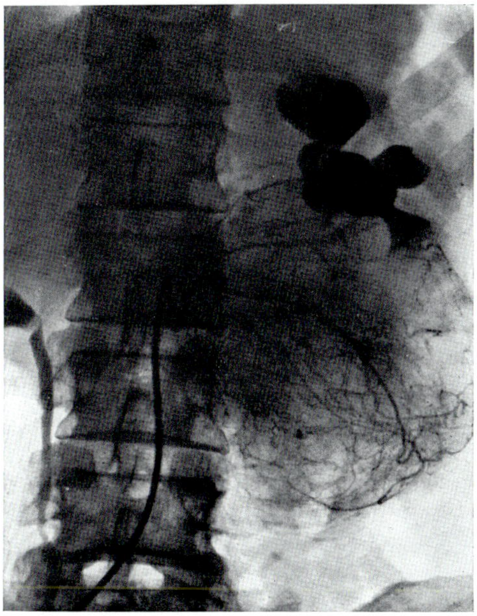
Abb. 2b

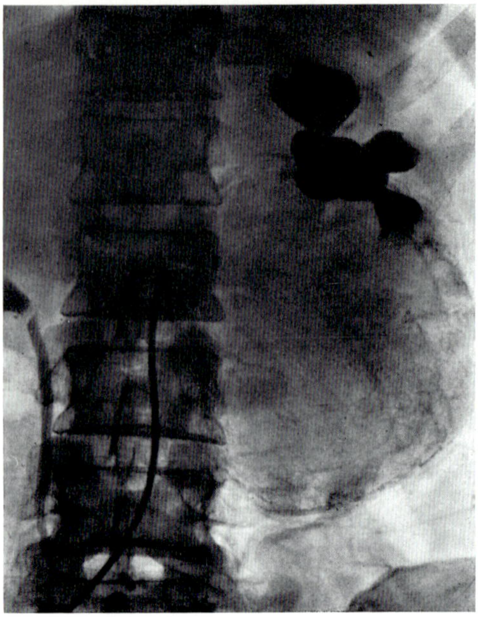

Abb. 2c

arterien heranzieht, die von KAHN und FRATES 1968 schon als eine aussichtsreiche Darstellungsmethode herausgestellt wurde, und wenn man sie zur *Angioszintigraphie* erweitert.

Ein Beispiel: Faustgroßer palpabler Tumor im linken Mittelbauch mit Verdrängung und Abflußbehinderung der linken Niere. Die Übersichtsaortographie zeigt eine Vergrößerung des Gefäßkalibers der 3. linken Lumbalarterie, die über den Weichteilschatten des Tumors ausgespannt ist (Abb. 1).

Die *selektive Angiographie* zeigt keine pathologischen Gefäße, in der Parenchymphase aber eine homogene Kontrastverteilung (Abb. 2a–c).

Das *Angioszintigramm* bestätigt die Durchblutungsstörung in den gleichen Arealen und führt zu guter Darstellung des übrigen Tumors (Abb. 3a und b).

Die radiologische Diagnose „gutartiger Tumor mit Nekrosen" wird durch die Operation bestätigt: es handelte sich um ein von Grenzstrang ausgehendes Neurinom.

Die selektive Angiographie und Angioszintigraphie eröffnet somit eine Verfeinerung der radiologischen Diagnostik auch der nicht von parenchymatösen Organen ausgehenden retroperitonealen Tumoren und vermag die präoperative Differentialdiagnose zu erleichtern.

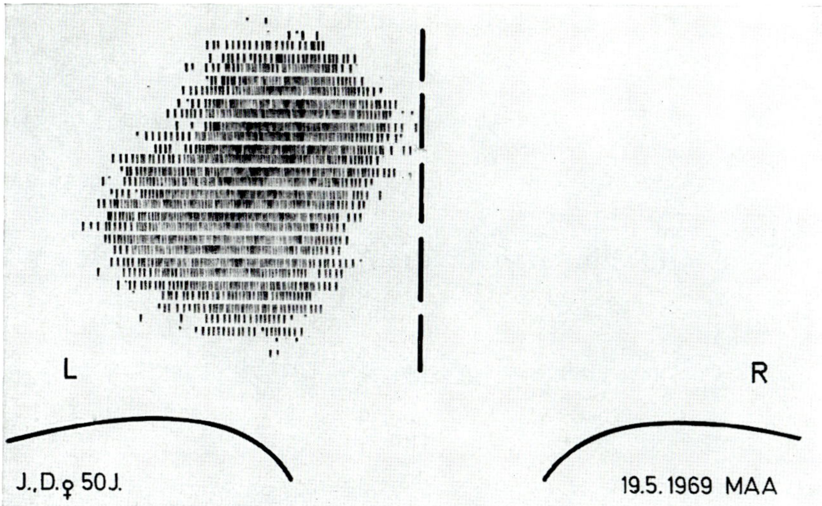

Abb. 3a

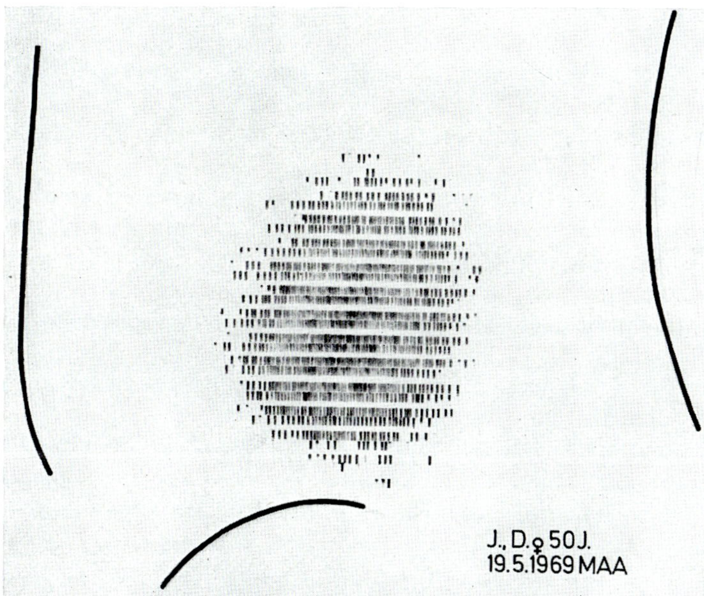

Abb. 3b

Disease of the Kidney

Assessment of Function in the Transplanted Kidney with ^{131}I Hippuran

A. Rodriguez-Antunez

After transplantation of a kidney, several clinical problems or complications may develop. On many occasions, the first step is to determine whether or not the homograft is viable. Complications are acute rejection, ureteral obstruction and leakage of urine into the peritoneal cavity.

Three tests have been found to be valuable and are performed routinely at the Cleveland Clinic in order to evaluate the status of each patient. 339 scans and 160 renograms have been performed in 232 patients who underwent renal transplantation at the Cleveland Clinic in the period through February 1970. The $T^1/_2$ blood clearance was performed only in 34 patients for a total of 61 determinations. The three tests (scintigram, $T^1/_2$ blood clearance and renogram) were performed after the intravenous injection of 30–50 μCi of ^{131}I hippuran. The scintigram covered the area of the transplanted kidney as well as the urinary bladder. The interpretation of the scintigram may provide the following information:

1. The kidney is well visualized and evidence of radioactive material is seen within the urinary bladder. This scanographic presentation appears to be compatible with a functioning kidney. There have been some cases in which the kidney was being rejected and a functioning scan was seen. Therefore, the scintigram is not a reliable test for establishing the presence of rejection.

2. The kidney may be visualized totally and well but radioactivity is not detected within the urinary bladder. This is a typical picture of a vaible kidney with severe oligura (20–50 ml of urine output in 24 h). This picture appeared in many cases immediately in the posttransplant period. This scan we report as viable kidney and the kidney will function sooner or later. Sometimes, we have observed that the output of urine occurs at ten to twenty days after the transplant. Many kidneys have delayed function because of some disturbence that effects the tubular cells. This clinical picture has been called by us. *The bipolar functional dissociation syndrome* (BFD syndrome) of the tubular cells. We feel that the luminal pole of each cell is unable to excrete radioactive hippuran which has been trapped by a properly functioning vascular pole.

3. No visulazion of the kidney on the scintigram is indicative of severe nonreversible renal disease or renal arterial thrombosis. In our experience, those homografts had to be removed.

4. Sometimes, only half of the kidney is visualized on the scan. This is not necessarily a ominous sign. This is indicative of an infarct. In our series, one patient has survived two years after the scintigram demonstrated an infarct effecting the lower half of the homograft.

5. Evidence of radioactive material may be detected outside the urinary tract within the peritoneal cavity, indicating a dehiscence of the surgical anastomosis.

Renography

In addition to the well-known shortcoming of the renogram, we have found that a prolonged functional phase or a constantly rising curve does not necessarily represent renal disease. Usually, the transplanted kidney is so close to the bladder that the accumulation of radioactive substance in the bladder may influence the curve and give a false-positive result. Yet, in all patients who had complications, the renogram was "abnormal" (no false-positive result).

$T^1/_2$ ^{131}I hippuran blood clearance is performed simultaneously with the renogram. The probe is positioned over the inner portion of the right upper quadrant. The data are recorded on the same graph paper as is the renogram. At the same time, a digital print-out gives the actual number of counts. Allowing for mixing, we consider only the portion of the curve between 8 and 20 min. The data are tabulated on semilogarithmetic paper and the $T^1/_2$ is calculated after extrapolation to time zero. In all but 2 patients with good renal status, the $T^1/_2$ was found to be between 15 and 24 min. All patients with poor renal status had a $T^1/_2$ greater than 30 min with only one exception – a $T^1/_2$ of 25 min in a patient who was rejecting the homograft.

The $T^1/_2$ is a reflection of the renal blood flow and it is well known that the early rejection phenomenon is vascular. We have found this to be one of the most sensitive tests in detecting early rejection.

V x 2 Carcinoma as a Tumour Model Induced in the Stomach and Kidney of Rabbits. Pharmacoangiographical Examinations

Gy. Vargha, J. Kelemen, L. Miltényi and L. Szücs

Neither gastric carcinoma, induced or inoculated in animals suitable for X-ray examination, nor malignant renal tumour are includ d in the literature on the subject. In the foregoing experiments malignant lesio s have been produced by cancerogenic substances in the forestomach and glandular stomach of mice and rats; as regards kidney, in 2% of spontaneous renal adenocarcinoma has been observed.

The data of animal experiments being so scanty, we have thought of producing models of gastric and renal carcinoma in a species of animal suitable for X-ray examination. Rabbit seemed to be the best for that purpose, and Vx2 carcinoma has been chosen for producing carcinoma. The pharmaco-angiographical examinations have been carried out on these experimental tumours.

Method and Material

Laparotomy was performed on rabbits in narcosis. After opening the peritoneum, the stomach was mobilized only to such an extent that the pylorus could be visible and the antrum could be fixed in a position suitable for inoculation. In the frontal wall of the antrum 2 ml of Vx2 carcinoma cell suspension was injected praepylorically, submucously and partly intramuscularly. The for one or two minutes the serosa was pressed in order to close the orifice caused by the hypodermic needle.

In another group the serosa of the antrum was opened at a length of 5 mm, the muscular propria was sharply separated, and arriving at the submucous, the tumorous cell suspension was injected towards the mucous membrane. After this the muscular layer and the serosa were closed with "Z"-stitches.

After laparotomy, having found the left kidney and lifted it forward, we induced tumour by injecting 1 ml of Vx2 carcinoma cell homogenizate in the parenchyma on the dividing line between the frontal surface and the convexity in the lower pole; the method in force being transcapsular punction. We penetrated into it by 4–5 mm from the surface of the kidney, consequently the homogenizate got outside the pyelon. The kidney was compressed for one minute then the abdominal wall was closed lege artis.

The aortographical and pharmaco-angiographical examinations were carried out as direct lumbal aortography. Laparotomy was performed in narcosis. The bowels were placed to the right in the abdomen, then the vena cava inf. and the aorta were separated, the peritoneum parietale was peeled off the aorta, and this latter was set free at a length of 3 cm, distal to the art. renalis sin. Two threads were lead under the aorta, it was tied with the more distal one, then a hypodermic needle was placed proximally in the aorta to which an adapter and a teflon tube were connected. In the aorta the needle was fixed by binding the proximal thread to it. The necessary solutions and medicines were administered by syringe and the contrast material by strength of arm. 60% Uromiro was used as contrast material. In the case of gastric Vx2 carcinoma 6 ml, of renal carcinoma 4 ml was injected. Having administered two-thirds of the contrast material, on the basis of an adequate planning we began taking serial roentgenograms by Elema-Schönander rapid film changer. In 95% of the cases the art. mesenterica sup. was tied.

In the pharmaco-angiographical examinations Adrenalin and Isoproterenol were used. 10–20 gamma/kg of Adrenalin, in gastric carcinoma 125 gamma/kg, in renal carcinoma 100 gamma/kg of Isoproterenol, diluted in 5 ml of physiological saline, were given intraaortally immediately before injecting the contrast material.

The rabbits were kept under adequate experimental conditions, they were given standard food and water. They were examined on X-ray before the operation and on the 7th, 14th and 21st day after the operation; in 69 cases aortographical and pharmaco-angiographical examinations were performed. The autopsy was usually done on the 22nd or 23rd day or after the spontaneous death. Histological examinations were carried out in each of the autopsies.

The results of the experiments are summarized in the Table.

In group 1 Vx2 carcinoma, inoculated and growing in the gluteal muscle, was used for transplantation. After adequate preparation and under, as far as possible, steril circumstances cell suspension was obtained by removing 3–4 g of gluteal tumour tissue and homogenizing it with 30 ml of physiological saline, then 30 ml of Penicillin and Streptomycin solution. The homogenizate contains approximately 10^6 cells/ml; the size of detritus is about 40–60 microns. In 41 rabbits 2 ml of it was injected in the frontal wall of the antrum, and in 2 rabbits in that of the corpus.

In group 2, 30 rabbits were studied. In 26 animals marked with (a) of this group the transplant was taken from the carcinomatous lesion in the gastric wall. 4 rabbits were inoculated with 3 ml of this cell suspension and 22 ones with 2 ml. Sub-group (b) of group 2 comprised 4 rabbits. The tumorous cell suspension injected in their gastric wall was obtained from gluteal Vx2 carcinoma, we got, however, this carcinoma by reinoculating the antral carcinoma that had been transplanted repeatedly, in the gluteal muscle.

Group 3 consisted of 17 animals having a carcinoma developed in the antrum and transplanted in the gluteal muscle.

In group 4a gluteal Vx2 carcinoma was transplanted in the renal parenchyma (21 rabbits); in group 4b the homogenizate was taken from antral Vx2 carcinoma (16 rabbits); in group 4c from renal Vx2 carcinoma (5 rabbits).

In group 5th gluteal Vx2 carcinoma was transferred in the gluteal muscle. In the case of 3 rabbits of the 97 ones in the Table renal Vx2 carcinoma was re-injected in the gluteal muscle. This however, there being only a few cases, has not been recorded in the table.

Group 6 consisted of 96 control rabbits, a part of them underwent no operation, another part was inoculated with 1–2 ml of homogenizing material (physiological saline, Penicillin, Streptomycin solution).

Table. *Details of transplantations of Vx 2 carcinoma in the gastric wall and renal parenchyma of rabbits*

Experiment	Number of rabbits		Died in 3 days	Number of appreciable cases	Vx2 carcinoma developed	%	undeveloped
1. Transplantation of *gluteal Vx 2 carcinoma* in the gastric wall							
a) in the frontal wall of the antrum	41						
b) in the frontal wall of the corpus	2	43	2	41	38	92,7	3
2. Transplantation of *antral Vx 2 carcinoma* in the frontal wall of the antrum							
a) from stomach directly in stomach	26						
b) re-injection of antral carcinoma in the gluteal muscle, transplanted again in the antrum	4	30	4	26	24	92,3	2
3. Re-injection of *antral Vx 2 carcinoma* in the gluteal muscle		17	—	17	14	82,4	3
4. *Vx2 carcinoma* transplanted in renal parenchyma							
a) from gluteal Vx 2 carcinoma	21		7	14	13	92,9	1
b) from antral Vx 2 carcinoma	16		1	15	10	66,7	5
c) from renal Vx 2 carcinoma	5	42	—	5	3	60	2
5. Transplantation of *gluteal Vx 2 carcinoma* in the gluteal muscle		97	—	97	92	94,8	5
		229	14	215	194	90,2	21
6. Control group		96	—	96			96
		325	14	311			

In group 1: 6, in group 2: 4, in group 3: 3, in group 4: 10, in group 6: 6 rabbits underwent aortographical examination; in group 1 in 12, in group 2 in 8, in group 3 in 6, in group 4 in 20, in group 6 in 12 cases pharmaco-angiographical examinations were performed.

Results

The results have been summarized in the Table. The cases that died within 3 days, the appreciable cases, the number of the developed Vx 2 carcinomas, the percentage of the transplantational effect and the number of unsuccessful transplantations can be estimated very well from it. In the groups of different transplantation types these data are demonstrated separately; a detailed description would be only a needless repetition. It is only the facts that cannot be inferred from the table and a few instances of gastric and renal Vx 2 carcinoma together with some pharmaco-angiograms that are made account of.

Mention should be made of the fact that, as a rule, both the gastric and the renal as well as the gluteal Vx 2 carcinoma developed in 3 weeks. The animals with tumour perished in the 5th week at the latest if we saw it out without any operation or examination. The rabbits became nothing but skin and bone and lost 30–35% of their weight. In a number of gastric carcinomas there was a histologically proved metastasis in the perigastric lymph nodes and in the liver. In some cases the tumour spread over to perigastric and perirenal tissues.

Spontaneous gastric or renal carcinoma was observed neither in the control animals of group 6 nor in the cases inoculated with Vx 2 carcinoma. In the course of transplantations the stomach and the left kidney were always palpated but in none of the cases could spontaneous tumour be observed. Of course, no Vx 2 carcinoma was found in the animals either in whose stomach and left kidney respectively, only homogenizing solution had been injected.

Figure 1 shows the spot roentgenogram of the stomach of rabbit No. 31 in group 1. The examination was performed on the 21st day. In the praepyloric part of the antrum there is a round filling defect. In the round shadow defect an intensive crater and a faint, pisiform one are discernible in accordance with the exulceration developed in the carcinoma. Radiological statement: exulcerated tumour in the antrum, marked off sharply from the environment and similar to exulcerating human carcinoma. Histology: carcinoma consisting of dedifferentiated anaplastic cells.

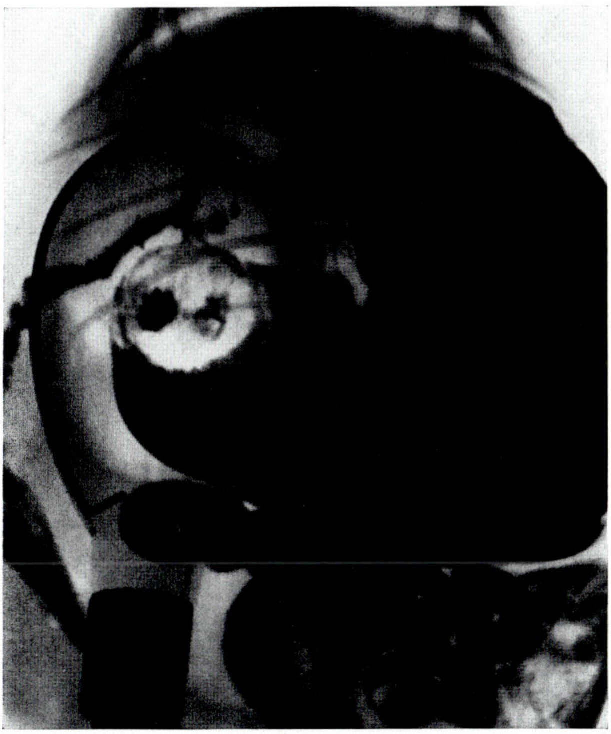

Fig. 1. Spot roentgenogram of the stomach of rabbit No. 31

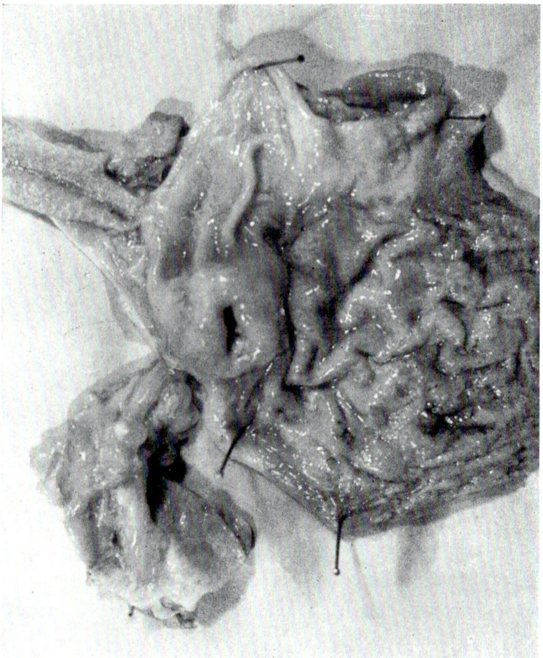

Fig. 2. The macroscopic photo of the stomach of rabbit No. 21. In the antrum there is an exulcerated protuberant Vx 2 carcinoma

The histogram is omitted owing to lack of space. The shape and position of a tumour like this is shown in Fig. 2.

Fig. 3 shows the pharmaco-angiogram of the gastric Vx 2 carcinoma of rabbit No. 09.18.05 in group 2. after having received Adrenalin intraaortally. A wide-spread antral carcinoma was disclosed by autopsy. In the Adrenalin pharmaco-angiogram a wider aorta and the filling of the intercostal arteries are revealed. The art. coeliaca is not filled and the art. renales are narrow, too. The filling of cholecyst is also well demonstrated. The roentgenogram in Figure 4 was taken after the administration of Isoproterenol; here the branches of the art. coeliaca, the art. lienalis and the truncus hepatogastricus, as well as their branches: the art. gastro-duodenalis, the art. gastrica and the art. gastroepiploica dextra are filled well. None of the roentgenograms discloses tumorous capillaries. In Figure 4 no filling of cholecyst can be observed.

Figure 5 shows the normal aortogram of rabbit No. 100 in group 6. The branches of the thoracic and abdominal aorta can be followed well; the art. mesenterica sup. is tied. The pharmaco-angiogram in Figure 6 was taken after the administration of Adrenalin. According to it only the stems of the arteries coming from the aorta are filled, in the farther-off branches there is no evidence of contrast medium. The cholecyst is filled properly. Figure 7 shows an angiogram after injecting Isoproterenol. The peripheric blood-vessels are also filled intensively, and in comparison with Figure 5–6 there is a big difference between them. On the stem of the art. renales

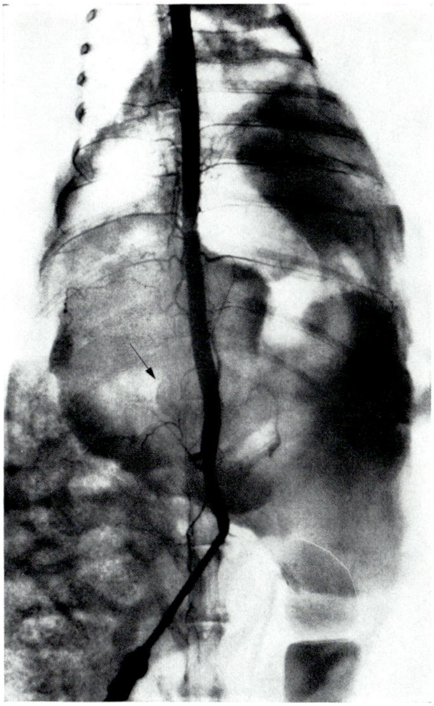

3

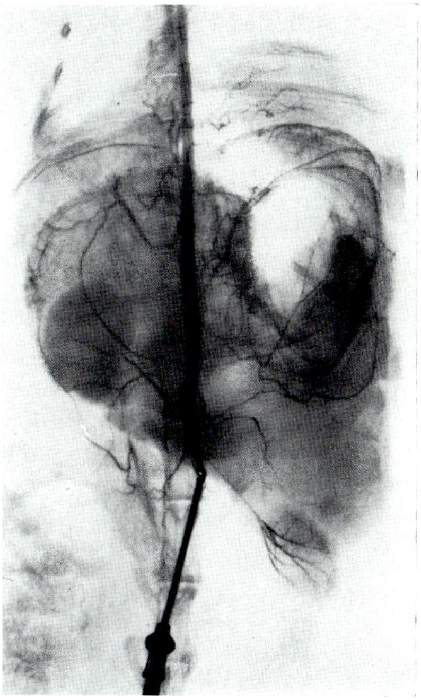

4

Fig. 3. Pharmaco-angiogram of rabbit No. 09.18.05 after injecting 40 gamma of Adrenalin in gastric Vx 2 carcinoma. There is a good filling of the cholecyst (arrow)

Fig. 4. Pharmaco-angiogram of rabbit No. 09.18.05 after injecting 150 gamma of Isoproterenol (0,75 sec) in Vx 2 carcinoma. The bloodvessels described in the text can be seen excellently, there are no tumorous capillaries

there is a circular stenosis (perhaps narcotic effect?) resembling fibro-muscular dysplasia. This rabbit was not operated on, there being no pathological alteration.

Figure 8 shows the macroscopic photo of the left kidney of rabbit No. 09.02.55. In the lower pole of the kidney the transplant of Vx 2 carcinoma can be distinguished very well. The normal aortogram of this rabbit is demonstrated in Figure 9. In the lower pole of the left kidney the renal Vx 2 carcinoma is separated in a semicircular shape; vessels in the tumour cannot be seen. The art. interlobares and the art. interlobulares near the tumour are demaged. This also refers to the fact that renal Vx 2 carcinoma is a tumour that is deficient in blood-vessels. The art. gastroduodenalis and art. gastroepiploica dextra, leading to the stomach turned inside out and thus running in a changed position seem to be hardly discernible, thin branches, whereas in the Isoproterenol pharmaco-angiogram (Fig. 10) these branches are wide and excellently discernible. The peripheral branches of the art. renales, the destruction of the arteries leading to the lower pole of the left kidney, the tumour itself and its area where there are no arteries can be demonstrated in this roentgenogram very

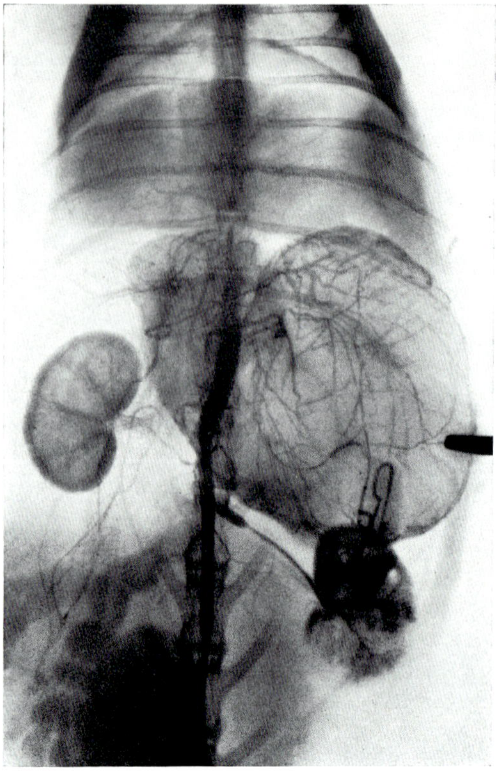

Fig. 5. Normal aortogram of rabbit No. 100 (1,5 sec)

well (Fig. 10). If there were arteries of adequate quality in Vx 2 carcinoma they should be visible in the Isoproterenol pharmaco-angiogram. The pharmaco-angiogram taken in the later phase of the Isoproterenol effect (about after 40 min), after the administration of Adrenalin gave almost the same picture as Figure 10.

Owing to lack of space we are not going to give a histological illustration of the tumours. The reader should consult the publications by VARGHA *et al.* in which the histograms give evidence of dedifferentiated, anaplastic carcinoma of partly solid alveolar, partly trabecular pseudopapillar and pseudotubular structure. The macroscopic description of gastric and renal Vx 2 carcinoma will be omitted here (see VARGHA *et al*).

Discussion

Skin papillomas in hares have been described by SHOPE. These tumours were transplantable and with the help of cell-free filtrate transmissible, in the course of re-inoculation they were transformed malignantly (ROUS and BEARD, ROUS *et al.* SYVERTON and BERRY, SYVERTON *et al.*), and it was at the end of the series that Vx 2 carcinoma developed (KIDD and ROUS). Intracutaneous, subcutaneous, intramuscular and intratesticular injections seem to be the most suitable for inoculation, though

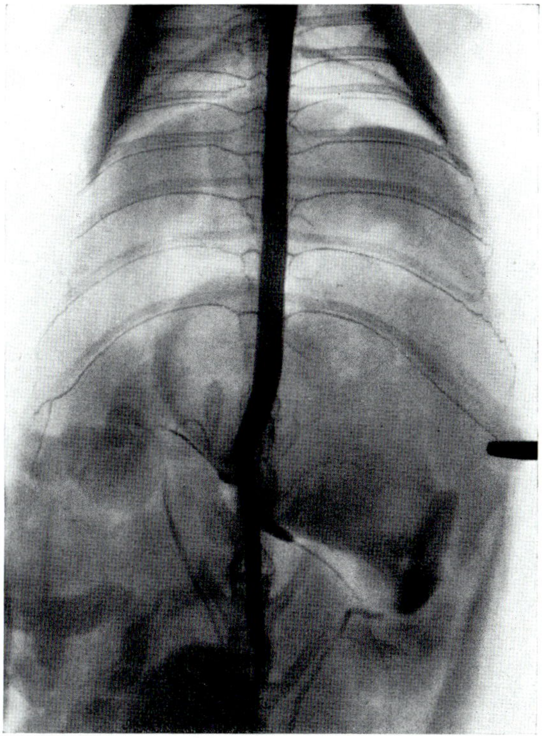

Fig. 6. Pharmaco-angiogram of rabbit No. 100 after injecting 10 gamma of Adrenalin (0,75 sec). Art. intercostales and the main branches of art. renales are filled, the art. coeliaca is not. The cholecyst and the ureters can be seen very well

attempts have been made at intravascular and intracerebral transmission. VARGHA *et al.* have succeeded in performing intraventricular, intrarenal, articular and intra-ossal transplantations.

There have been only scanty results of animal experiment with gastric tumour. In the glandular stomach and forestomach of rats and mice in a certain percentage malignant lesions have been produced by methylcholanthrene. For further references see the works by BONNE, OETTLÉ, SABAD, SEMJAKIN, SZODORAY, WATERMAN.

In connection with renal tumours mention must be made of the writings by LUCKÉ, COMAN *et al.*, DE LONG and COMAN. Transcapsular injection of cell suspension in the renal parenchyma has not been included in the literature on the subject. Our method has the advantage that the amount of cell in the homogenizate is relatively constant, consequently the amount of injected tumour is standard: it does not change in proportion as when transplanting parts of tumours the size of which is given in mm.

The number of publications on human pharmaco-angiographical examinations, introduced in the last ten years, is very little. The papers on animal experiments are even less frequent. The X-ray differences obtained from human material cannot be

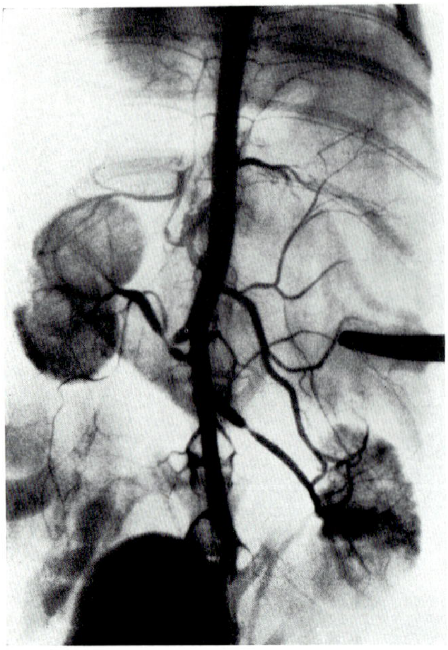

7

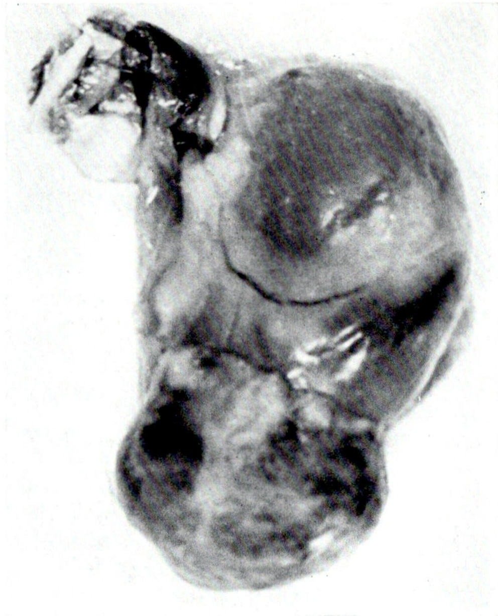

8

Fig. 7. Pharmaco-angiogram of rabbit No. 100 after injecting 100 gamma of Isoproterenol (0,75 sec). Explanation in the text

Fig. 8. Macroscopic photo of the left kidney of rabbit No. 09.02.55. In the lower pole of the kidney the transplanted tumour can be distinguished

estimated uniformly. As regards the localisation of tumours, the possibilities of evaluating X-ray evidences have changed. With animal experiment the situation is relatively easier since the examination is carried out in tumours verified in advance, the X-ray symptoms may change according as whether they are avascular or hypervascularized tumours.

In the evaluation of X-ray symptoms there is no complete agreement, either. Here we refer to the contradictions in the publications by Caplan *et al.*, Olsson and Jönsson, Salmon and Koehler, and the possibilities revealed by Kahn, Abrams.

We have proved by animal experiments that when establishing the diagnosis of gastric Vx2 carcinaoma neither Adrenalin nor Isoproterenol result an appreciable diagnostic difference. Our animal experiments seem to give evidence of the fact that aortography and pharmaco-angiography can be surpassad by routine X-ray examinations of the stomach. In spite of the negative results of the angiograms in every case we have had X-ray evidence of gastric carcinoma.

In the pharmaco-angiographical examinations of renal Vx 2 carcinoma Adrenalin, in contrast to Isoproterenol, seems to be less or not useful for establishing the diagnosis of peripheral renal tumours. In the diagnostics of Vx 2 carcinoma Isoproterenol results appreciable X-ray evidences (avascular regions, blood-vessel destructions, negative nephrographical effect), and in the case of hypervascularized tumours of the

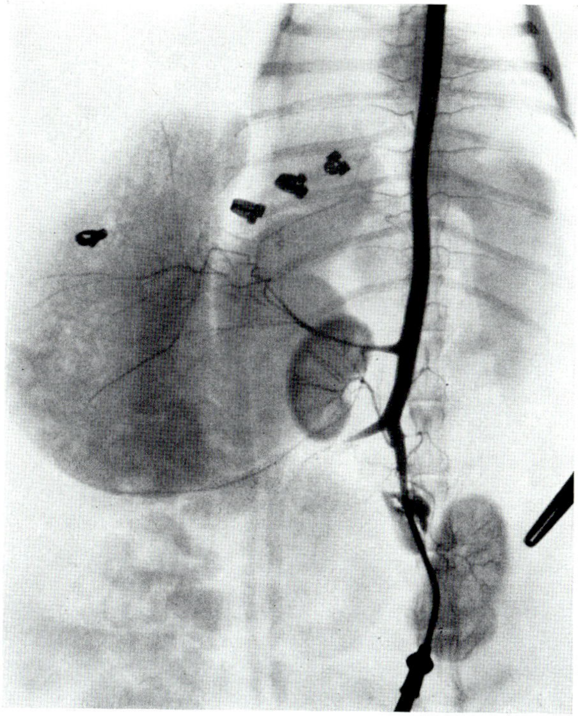

Fig. 9. Aortogram of rabbit No. 09.02.55 (0,6 sec) in renal Vx2 carcinoma. The vessel destructions and the renal tumour described in the text are discernible

kidney it may presumably be used both for those nearby the renal hilums and the peripheral ones. 20 gamma/kg of Adrenalin caused such an arterial spasm that rendered the estimation of peripheral arteries impossible.

It is well-known form the pharmacology of Adrenalin and Isoproterenol that Adrenalin stimulates the alpha and beta receptors of the sympathetic nervous system and Isoproterenol stimulates the beta receptors. Isoproterenol is 3,4 dihydroxy-phenil-ethanol-isopropylamine that is an direct-acting beta adrenerg agent. It may be supposed and our experiment also seem to prove that the arteriolas of the abdominal organs of rabbits have beta receptors that are affected by Isoproterenol directly. From our series of experiment conclusions may be drawn that are applicable to human hypovascularized or avascularized peripheral renal tumours. In such tumours the nephrographic effect and the arterial destructions are suspicious in the pharmaco-angiography with Isoproterenol, whereas Adrenalin does not result appreciable effects.

Our conclusions can be summarized as follows:

1. We have succeeded in transplanting gluteal Vx 2 carcinoma in the gastric wall of rabbits where it stayed affixed and was growing. This carcinoma was transferred in the antral wall of other rabbits, and the gluteal re-transplantations as well as the transmission of this tumour in the renal parenchyma were also successful.

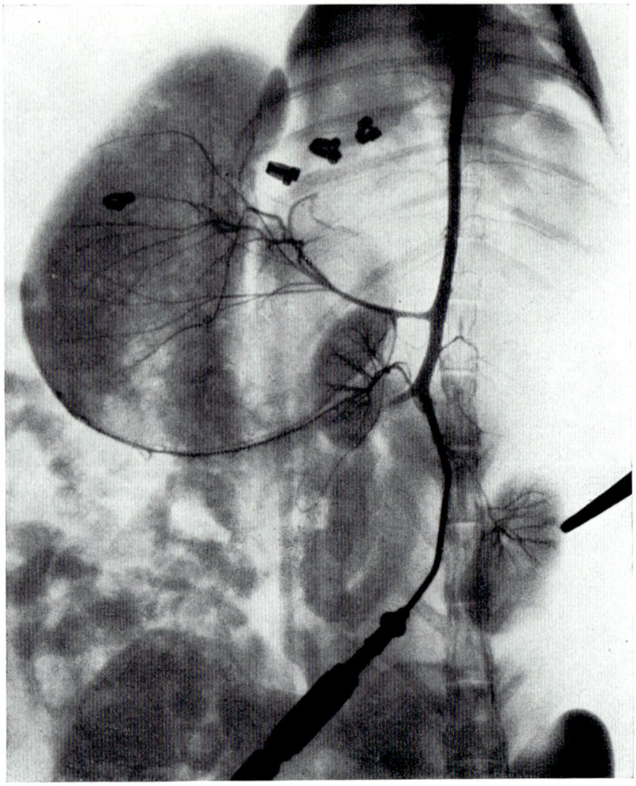

Fig. 10. Pharmaco-angiogram of rabbit No. 09.02.55 after injecting 100 gamma of Isoproterenol (0,3 sec) in renal Vx 2 carcinoma. Explanation in the text

2. The carcinomatous transplantate in the stomach of rabbits is a malignant lesion whose X-ray morphological picture is identical with the roentgenograms of certain human gastric carcinomas.

3. We have succeeded in transplanting gluteal Vx2 carcinoma in the renal parenchyma of rabbits. The carcinoma that had developed there was transferred to the renal parenchyma of other rabbits and we have managed to transplant it into the gluteal muscle.

4. It has been proved by pharmaco-angiographical examinations that in the diagnostics of the peripheral tumours of abdominal organs Adrenalin is less or not employable; Isoproterenol, which stimulates beta-receptors, gives much better results. In the diagnostics of renal Vx 2 carcinoma Isoproterenol, has been made use of effectively, whereas in gastric Vx 2 carcinoma pharmaco-angiography has not revealed a positive deviation.

5. The gastric Vx 2 carcinomas are characterized mainly be expansive growth, but infiltrative one can also be observed. The renal Vx2 carcinomas are more invasive than the gastric ones.

6. The exulceration of the mucosa is mostly not a primary tumorous necrosis but a secondary one, the consequence of compression. In such a case there is no tumour in the mucosa.

7. Histologically these tumours are dedifferentiated, anaplastic carcinomas. The histogram hardly changes during transplantation.

8. The evaluation of the tumorous cell masses in the lymph vessels, as well as the lymph nodes- and liver-metastasis require further observation.

Summary

By submucous and intramuscular injection of Vx 2 carcinoma cell suspension in the gastric wall of rabbits carcinomatous lesions have been produced that revealed X-ray symptoms in 3 weeks and could be discerned by autopsy and histological examinations. In the renal parenchyma, too, carcinoma has been induced by the transplantation of the marked cell homogenizate. The possibility of transplantation from stomach to stomach and from kidney to kidney has been proved, just like the transplantation in the gluteal muscle. The methods of transplantation, the X-ray morphological, angiographical, pharmaco-angiographical and macroscopic photos of the developed Vx 2 carcinoma are described. Attention is called to the fact that this inoculated Vx2 carcinoma is a model that can be used in cancer-researches of the stomach and the kidney, as well as for diagnostic and therapeutical examinations.

Investigations in Connection with the Effect of the Alpha and Beta Stimuli and Blocking Agents of the Sympathetic Nervous System on the Evolution of Renal Angiograms

J. Kelemen, Gy. Vargha, B. Kelentey and M. Kéki

Ever since the observations made by Abrams, Boijsen, and Borgström (1962) in the course of experiments conducted by them on animals and humans, arteriography under the effect of epinephrine has become a generally practised diagnostic system. Experiments on humans show that the bloodvessels of certain types of tumours fail to undergo vasoconstriction under the influence of epinephrine. In fact, under certain conditions they react in a paradox fashion to humoral vasomotor agents. The differences in the reactions of the bloodvessels offer valuable help primarily for determining the extent of tumours and also for diagnosticating various types of tumours, mainly renal malignomes and inflammative changes susceptible to being diagnosed separately (Cen and Rosenbusch, 1968; Kahn, 1965, 1969; Rockoff, Doppman, Block and Ketchxam, 1966; Kahn, Frates, Paul, 1968; Kahn, O'Haloran and Paul, 1969; Doppman, Brown and di Chiro, 1969; Laubenberger, 1969; Hotovy, Losonczy, and Lakos, 1968; and so forth).

Within the framework of the sympathetic nervous system Ahlquist (1948) made a distinction between alpha and beta adrenergic receptors. Both the bloodvessels of striated muscles, and those of the brain are equipped with both types of adrenergic neuroreceptors. The specific cardiac vessels also possess alpha and beta sympathetic innervation; the periferal capillaries, however, are directed only by a beta receptor system. The calices of the kidney and the smooth muscles of the ureters have alpha receptor innervation. However, the role, if any, played by the adrenergic receptor mechanism in regulating renal bloodvessels including urinary outflow, has yet to be clarified.

Notwithstanding the physiological, pharmacological and angiographic experiments conducted up to date, it has still to be settled

a) what kind of effect on the evolution of renal angiograms – beyond that of the hitherto normally studied epinephrine and norepinephrine – is exerted by an equally directly effective beta adrenergic agent synthetic isoproterenol (3,4 dihydroxyphenyl, ethanol-isopropylamine).

b) whether the alpha and beta neuroreceptors presumably existing here too, play any role in intrarenal vasoregulation

c) whether there exist within the kidneys neuroreceptors able to induce adrenergic vasodilatation?

Materials and Methods

We prepared 128 angiograms on 32 dogs under barbiturate-narcosis. In one part of our investigations (20 animals) we made a abdominal aortography, while in the other (12 animals) bilateral selective renal arteriographies were made. The catheter required for photographic presentation of bloodvessels (red Ödman catheter, diameter 2,3/1,3 mm was introduced into the abdominal aorta by way of the duly prepared femoral artery. In the case of 4 animals the catheter was introduced via the external carotid artery in order to find out to what extent the presence of the catheter and the resultant decrease in the bloodflow in the lower extremities exerted their influence on the circulation in the abdominal aorta.

In every instance bilateral selective renal arteriography was made after having introduced a catheter into both femoral arteries; for our studies we used catheters of identical caliber and mould.

As contrast material 60% Uromiro (Bracco, Milano) was used and the doses applied were 2 ml/kg body weight in the case of abdominal aortography, and 2–3 ml/kidney for selective renal arteriography.

When making an aortography the catheter was introduced up to the height of the lockplate Lumbar I.; besids the aperture at the tip of the catheter, three circular lateral apertures were formed by incision of 2 mm each. Infusion pressure amounted to 5 kg/cm^2 (Gidlund injector).

In the case of selective examination no lateral incisions were made, the tip of the catheter entering the renal artery only for a few millimeters in order to carefully avoid plugging renal flow even for a short time. The catheters introduced into the right and left renal arteries were joined to the Gidlund pump in the form of a Y –; pressure used was 3 kg/cm^2. The amount and pressure of the contrast material issuing from the tip of the catheter was not susceptible to change as confirmed by our experiments in vitro.

In the course of our experiments an animals we registered blood-pressure, cardiac frequency and breathing on a kymograph. For our experiments we prepared a control angiogram for each animal, no drugs having been used.

Serial exposures were made by means of an Elema-Schönander- high speed changingfilm apparatus, picture size 35 $\times$ 35 cm: 3 films/sec for 3 sec., 1,5 photos per second for 4 sec. and 1 film/sec. for 22 sec.

Mode of Evaluation

When evaluating the photograms the filling rates of the aorta and its branches were taken into account. The diameter of the aorta directly above the branching off of the more proximal renal artery (mostly the left one in dogs), was then measured; we further measured the diameter of the arteria renalis 1 cm laterally from the contour of the aorta and before the branching off of the arteria renalis. We moreover determined the diameters of the ramus anterior and ramus posterior just after bifurcation, at equal distances from the latter. We furthemore ascertained the duration of the inflow into the arteriae arcuatae and that of the outflow from the aorta and its branches. We then established the time of the appearance of the maximal nephrogram, the point of time of the optimal filling up of the vena renalis and the contours of the latter; we also recorded the change in size of the kidneys and finally, in 5 cases, the intensity of the nephrogram by means of a densitometer.

Results

Effects of Epinephrine

After injecting 5–50 μg epinephrine (Inj. Tonogeni, obtained from the Drug Factory of Köbánya, Hungary) into the aorta or directly into the renal artery, a marked constriction was observable in the renal arteries; this was found to be most pronounced in the interlobar arteries and in the arterioles situated more to the periphery from the former. Constriction was less marked on the main stem of the renal artery, while it was completely absent in the section of the artery at a distance of 10–12 mm. from the aorta. After administering 5 μg of epinephrine intrarenoarterially or 5 μg/kg body weight intraaortally, ringlike local spasms occurred in this transitory section of the renal main stem; ABRAMS *et al.* had previously drawn attention to the significance of these spasms from the point of view of circulatory dynamics. The contrast matter stagnated lengthly in the intrarenal arteries, and the outflow was slowed down. The nephrogram appeared at a later stage, its density being insignificant. An increased flow resistance of the kidneys may be presumed owing to the fact of the reflux, in the case of selective examination, of a comparatively large amount of contrast matter from the renal artery into the aorta, and from the renal artery and the aorta into the smaller arteries branching off near the bifurcation of the renal artery. This reflux causes the pyelar, suprarenal and lumbar arteries to fill up more substantially.

Studies made under the effect of epinephrine revealed an increase in the size of the kidneys in most cases, the transversal and linear diameters decreasing at an average of 1–3 mm, and 3–5 mm, respectively (Fig. 1a and b).

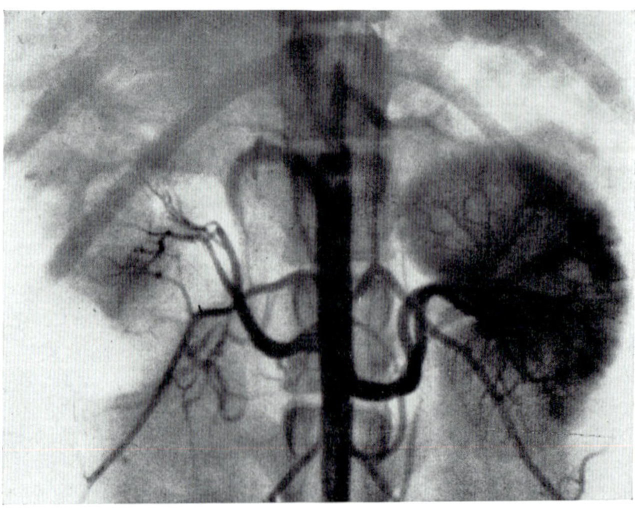

Fig. 1a

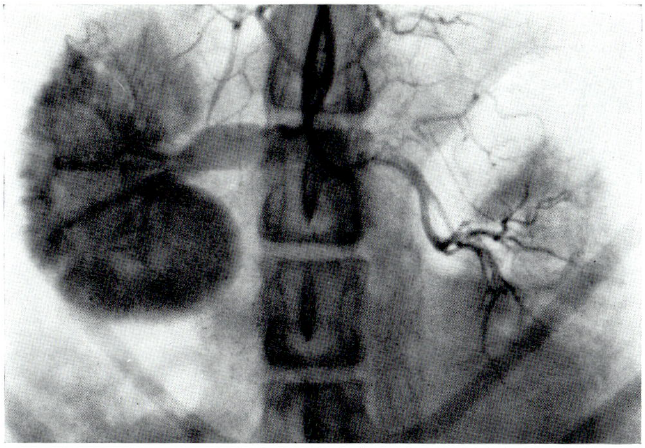

Fig. 1 b

Blood-pressure of the animals was observed to have increased to a marked degree in the course of the tests. Depending on the epinephrine doses applied the increase of systolic and diastolic blood-pressure corresponded to a change in pressure of 40–60 mmHg and 25–35 mmHg, respectively. When larger doses were applied, cummulative extrasystole set in.

After administering a similar dose of norepinephrine intraaortally or intrarenoarterially, the angiogram obtained was identical with that of epinephrine.

Following pretreatment with 5 mg/kg body weight Dibenamine, vasoconstriction as an effect of epinephrine failed to occur; the filling up of interlobar and arcuate arteries was similar to that of the controls. Flow resistance decreased, outflow of the contrast matter was stepped up, attaining, and in some experiments even exceeding the values prevailing in the controls. Similar compensation, though not quite as full, was brought about after pretreatment with 0,30 mg/kg body weight Dihydroergotoxine.

Effects of Isoproterenol and Dichlorisoproterenol

Isoproterenol (obtained from Sigma Chemical Co., St. Louis, USA) in doses of 50–100 μg/kg body weight introduced into the aorta of the animal being tested, produced general vasodilatation accompanied by a fall in blood pressure. Systolic and diastolic pressures decreased, corresponding to a fall of 50–70 and 20–35 mmHg, respectively. A cardiac chronotropic effect asserted itself, the pulse rate almost doubling.

The diameter of the aorta showed no significant changes, aorta-arterial outflow was considerably speeded up. Neither could any changes be observed in the lumen of the main stem of the renal arteries; however, the ramus anterior, posterior and the intrarenal arteries lying more to the perifery of the kidneys, revealed a decisive and characteristic vasodilatation. Filling up of renal arteries of the third and fourth order set in earlier and more intensively.

Renal flow resistance decreased, the nephrogram appeared at an earlier stage, but also diseappeared rapidly owing to a decrease of flow resitance, general circulatory acceleration and the presumable enhancement of excretion.

The filling up of the renal veins could be observed sooner, but was less thorough than in the controls. The kidneys showed a slight, insignificant increase in size (Fig. 2a and b).

Pronounced vasodilatation was shown by the splanchnic arteries too which also revealed a more substantial filling up of their periferal ramifications. The a. coeliaca and mesenterica filled up sooner and more thoroughly; at the same time the contrast tincture of the intestines and chiefly of the stomac lining became more pronounced.

When compared to the controls, contrast density of the pancreas matter proved to by more intensive under the influence of isoproterenol. Vasodilatation of the renal arteries distal from the ramus anterior and ramus posterior, was even more conspicious in the experiments in which, after selective catheterisation renal arteries, 25–50 μg of isoproterenol was introduced into one of the renal arteries, whereupon, immediately after the administration of this drug, 2 ml 60% Uromiro was injected into both renal arteries under identical pressure. The filling up of the interlobular and arcual arteries occured sooner and more intensively. The arterial nephrogram appeared earlier and in contrast to the aortograms recorded under the effect of isoproterenol, outflow was slowed down. The outlines of the nephrogram became more pronounced but this phenomen was of shorter duration. The filling up of the renal veins set in at an earlier stage, while the intensity of the nephrogram decreased. The lumen-diameters of the extrarenal and intrarenal veins failed to reveal any significant changes. After having injected isoproterenol intrarenoarterially, the size

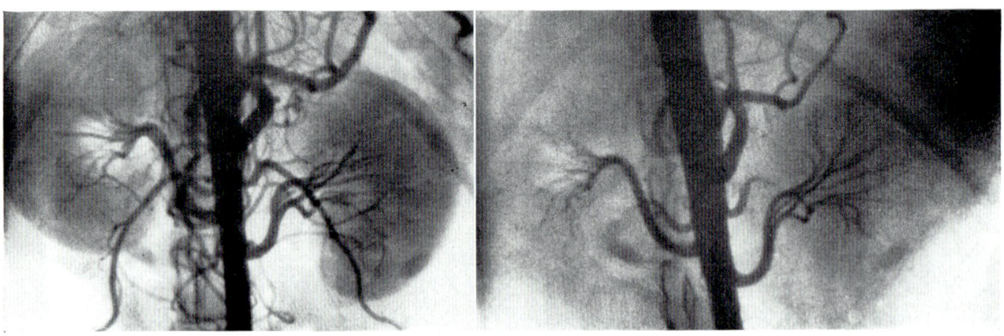

Fig. 2a

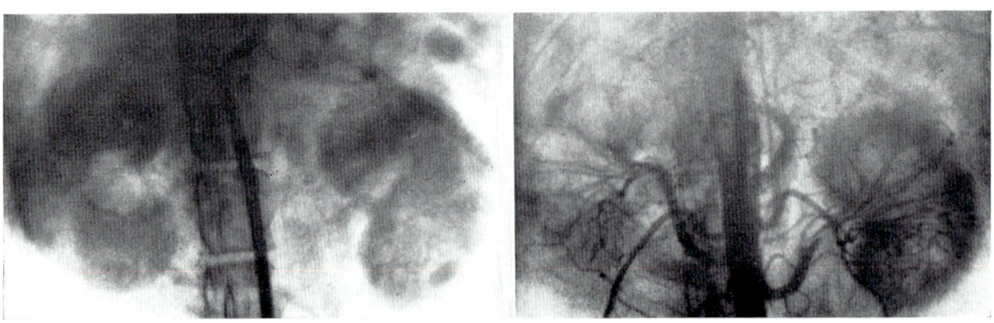

Fig. 2b

of the kidneys increased slightly, but in a continually perceptible manner. After a single injection of 25–50 μg of isoproterenol into the renal artery, average arterial pressure was found to decline by 15–35 mmHg; the enhancement of cardiac frequency amounted to nearly 100%. Tension and pulse rate retourned to normal within 3 min. (Fig. 3).

Following pretreatment with 0,02 g/kg body weight of dichlor-isoproterenol (from a shipment kindly sent by Sigma Chemical Co., St. Louis, USA) and bilateral catheterizing of the renal arteries, vasodilatation due to isoproterenol, as described above, failed to set in after 25–50 μg of isoproterenol had been introduced into one of the renal arteries, followed immediately by injecting 2 ml each of 60% Uromiro, subject to the same pressure, into both renal arteries. The lumen of the main stem of the renal artery failed to show any characteristic changes; the aa. interlobares and interlobulares were subject to a slight vasoconstriction, in contrast to the vaso-

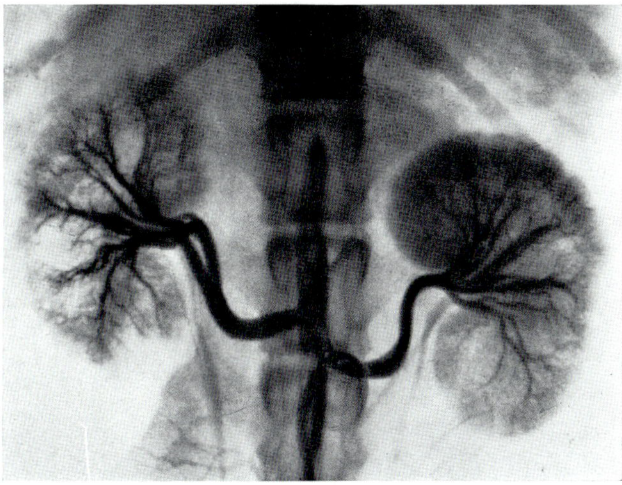

Fig. 3a

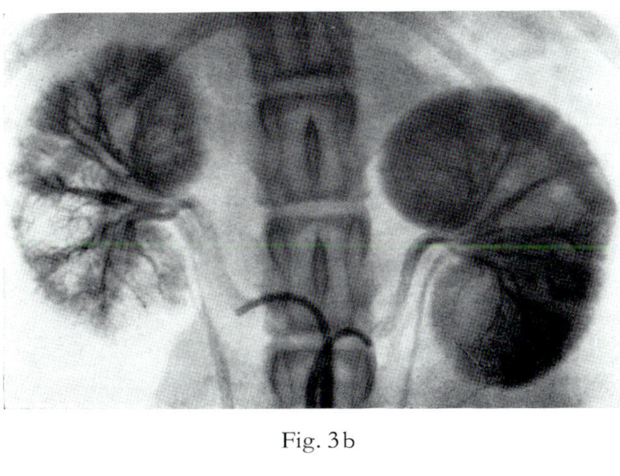

Fig. 3b

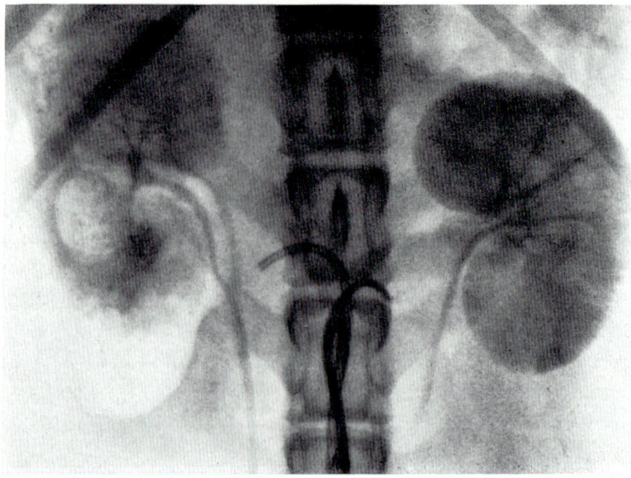

Fig. 3c

dilatation observed in the case of examination made without inhibitory pretreatment; this slight vasoconstrictor action was entirely in accordance with that taking place in the corresponding arteries of the contralateral kidney (Fig. 4). After pretreatment with dichlor-isoproterenol, abdominal aortograms prepared without administering isoproterenol, as well as selective renal arteriograms revealed no characteristic changes as compared to control examinations made without the application of drugs.

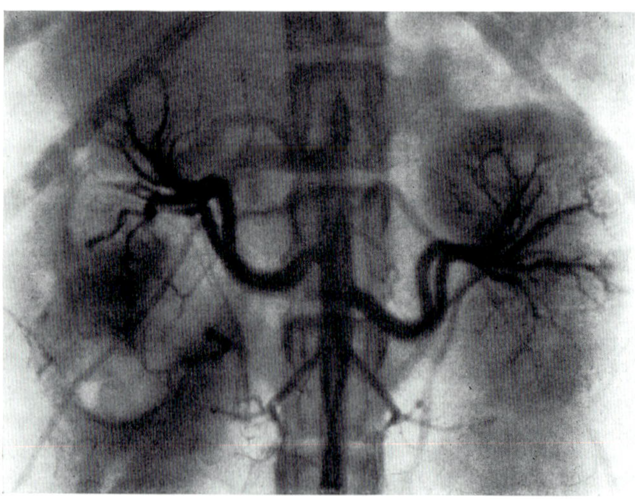

Fig. 4a

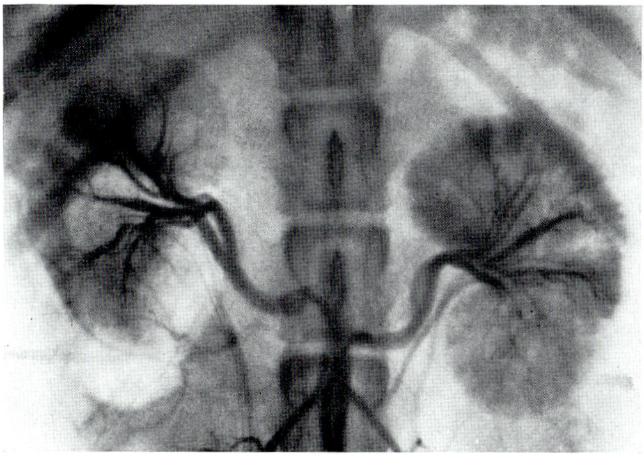

Fig. 4b

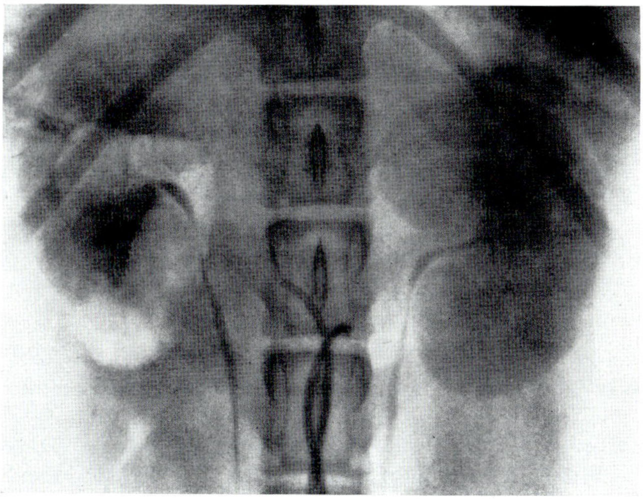

Fig. 4c

Discussion

Alterations appearing in renal angiograms after the intravenal, intraaortal and intrarenoarterial administration of varying doses of epinephrine, were discussed by ABRAMS, BOIJSEN, and BORGSTRÖM, KAHN, ELKIN, and MENG in their papers, on the strength of their findings obtained from experiments on animals and humans. Under the influence of epinephrine and norepinephrine, renal flow resistance was found to increase, thereby diminishing the volume of renal bloodflow. The effect of small doses of epinephrine and norepinephrine was primarily evidenced by the vasoconstriction of the peripheral intrarenal arteries, along with a slight dilatation of the renal main stem and interlobular arteries ("Peripheral type of vasoconstriction"

ELKIN and MENG). The arterial phase was prolonged, the density of the vascular nephrogram decreased, venous filling up was retarded. As a consequence of the reduction of the blood-volume, the kidneys were found to shrink in size. Given larger doses both sympathomimetic amines brought about vasoconstriction already in the section of the renal main stem near its bifurcation. Interlobar arteries became attenuated, renal flow slowed down ("Central type of vasoconstriction" ELKIN and MENG). Contraction of the vessel-lumen distal from the site of the injection was found to markedly decrease, a reflux of part of the contrast matter into the more proximal arteries took place, thus intensifying the filling up to the lateral branches ("Balloon effect"-Kahn). As a consequence of the slowing down of the bloodflow, intravasal sedimentation of the contrast matter became more pronounced ("Layering"-Kahn).

Beyond the observation of the aforesaid phenomena, the experiments we conducted involving the use of our own method evolved for selective catheterisation of the renal artery, proved intrarenal vasoconstriction to be not a result of general changes in circulatory dynamics, but to represent a direct local vasomotor effect, which could be offset by the specific blocking agents of the alpha-receptors of the sympathetic nervous systhem, primarily by the use of Dibenamine. The effects on the evolution of the renal angiogram exerted by the elective action of norepinephrine on alpha receptors, and of the stimulating effect of epinephrine on alpha *and* beta-receptors, do not differ significantly from each other. After elective pretreatment by alpha-receptor-inhibiting Dibenamine, we might theoretically expect not only vasoconstriction induced by epinephrine – alpha-stimulating effect – to fail to appear–which indeed is the case – but instead a slight vasodilatation to occur as an independent action of the henceforth betareceptor stimulating epinephrine. A vasodilatation of this type could, however, not be observed in the course of our experiments.

Isoproterenol electively activates the betareceptors of the sympathetic nervous system, as a result of which bronchial and intestinal relaxation sets in; furthermore, depending on the biological character of the test object, various degrees of relaxation of the myometrium, as well as glykogenolysis assert themselves. Under the influence of isoproterenol a marked vasodilatation of the peripheral vessels took place; pulmonal vessels slightly dilated and coronary flow increased. Positive chronotropic and inotropic effects were elicited in the heart (DI PALMA). As regards the action of isoproterenol on the renal vessels, *Drill's Pharmacology* (DI PALMA) takes the stand that a slight but definite vasoconstriction of the intrarenal vessels is being induced by it. According to this, the renal blood vessels would seem to posses no receptor mechanism apt to produce vasodilatation (AHLQUIST, SPENCER). AVIADO reports that a local vasodilatator response sets in as a result of isopoterenol injected intra-arterially. In the course of our own experiments we found that, beside vasodilatation of the striated muscles and of the splanchnic vessels, *vasodilatation occurs unmistakably in the renal vessels too*, as an effect of isoproterenol. This, however, can be offset by means of the elective inhibitors of the beta-receptors, i.e. of dichlor-isoproterenol. This response of the renal vessels was first recorded by ourselves. Renal flow proved to be more rapid in the case of aortography made under the effect of isoproterenol; conversely, in the case of selective examinations, it was found to be slower. This phenomen may be explained as follows: When making an aortography after injecting isoproterenol intraaortally, this drug stimulated the beta receptors of the heart and, as a consequence, positive chronotropic and inotropic effects set in, and the general change in circulatory dynamics resulting therefrom speeded up the renal flow.

In the case of selective examination and of drugs injected intrarenoarterially, this general change in circulatory dynamics took place at a later stage. The effect of isoproterenol on the renal arteries is consequently primarily a local, direct vasomotor effect, and only secondarily a result of general changes in circulatory dynamics. The succession of our experiments conducted by means of the angiographic method accordingly furnish proof of the existence of a receptor-mechanism apt to induce adrenergic vasodilatation within the renal bloodvessels; the regulating and functional significance of this mechanism is indisputable.

Summary

32 narcotized dogs were used to study the direct effect of certain adrenergic drugs (epinephrine, norepinephrine and isoproterenol) on the evolution of renal angiograms. Furthermore the mechanism of action of the vasomotor effects of these drugs were studied by means of the elective inhibitors of the alpha and beta sympathicus neuroreceptors. The enhancement of vasoconstriction and renal vascular resistance by using epinephrine and norepinephrine may be offset by means of specific alpha-receptor inhibitors; a relative beta-stimulator effect of epinephrine administered after giving Dibenamine could, however, not be shown to supervene.

As an effect of isoproterenol given intrarenoarterially, local vasodilatation and a decrease of renal resistance were found to prevail, which may be offset by the administration of specifically beta-receptor-blocking dichlor-isoproterenol. The experiments furnished proof of the existence of a receptor mechanism apt to induce adrenergic vasodilatation within the renal vessels.

Intraarterial Pressure During Pharmacoangiography

W. Frik and M. Cen

The preinjection of vasoactive substances before the injection of contrast medium has been a well known method in angiography for several years. Our own group with Cen and Rosenbusch is, up to now, mainly occupied with improvement of the angiography of kidneys, pancreas, liver and intestines by preinjection of adrenaline. Increasing practical experience in pharmacoangiography demonstrated, that the theoretical and experimental knowledge, concerning the effect of vasopressive substances in angiography of parenchymatous organs, is not yet sufficient.

Our own experiments deal with measuring intraarterial pressure in the kidneys in the course of pharmacoangiography with adrenaline. We were especially interested to know the dependence of the adrenaline effect on its dosage and to get better information concerning the duration of that effect. We examined moreover, the influence of a preinjection of adrenaline on the increase of intraarterial pressure by the injection of contrast medium.

The following experiments on dogs were made:

1. Measuring of the pressure in the abdominal aorta following intraaortal injection of different doses of adrenaline and following a high pressure injection of 40 ml saline (for simulating an aortography).
2. Measuring of the intraarterial pressure in small peripheric branches of kidney arteries following injection of different doses of adrenaline in the stem of the renal artery and injection of different amounts of saline (for simulating a selective renal angiography).
3. Aortography as non-selective kidney angiography following selective injection of adrenaline in the stem of one renal artery.

The intraarterial pressure was measured by transfemoral catheterization and Statham pressure transducers. Adrenaline was used in a dosage of 0,0006–0,16 μg/kg body weight for intrarenal measurings and up to 2,5 μg/kg body weight for the aorta.

Results

1. The injection of adrenaline in the aorta increases the systolic and diastolic intraaortic pressure only for a short time and on the average not more than 10 mmHg. The pressure in the aorta decreases during a following high pressure injection of fluid.
2. The increase of systolic pressure in peripheric branches of the kidney artery following adrenaline injection in the stem of the renal artery transgresses only in rare cases 25 mmHg. It does exactly depend on the dosage of adrenaline.

3. A high pressure injection of fluid in the stem of the kidney artery increases the systolic and diastolic peripheric pressure in the kidneys by 60–80 mmHg.

4. The increase of pressure in the peripherical branches during fluid injection will be markedly amplified by preinjection of adrenaline. This effect depends on the adrenaline dose up to 0,016 μg/kg body weight. It was not possible to prove the dependence on the dosage for higher doses, because the systolic pressure transgressed in these cases 330 mmHg (Fig. 1).

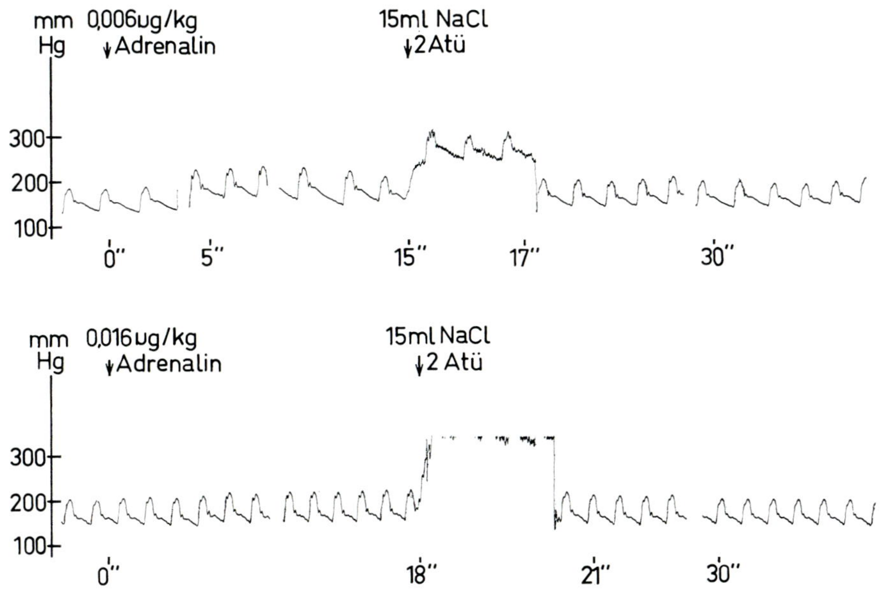

Fig. 1

5. The observation of the typical incisura in the pulse curve, gives an additional hint to the increase of peripheric resistance. The incisura deepens during the adrenaline effect, in consequence of a reflection of the pulse wave in the periphery. The duration of the deepening points to the duration of the adrenaline effect. The increase of peripherical resistance following adrenaline injection in the stem of the renal artery, begins 5 sec after the injection and ends totally 30 sec after injection (Fig. 1).

6. It could be demonstrated that the renal contrast medium excretion after preinjection of adrenaline in one kidney, is also delayed in this kidney for 30 sec. This time corresponds to the time of adrenaline effect demonstrated by pressure measuring, and by observation of the pulse curve.

It could be demonstrated by some additional pressure measurings in the celiac and superior mesenteric artery, that amount and duration of increased pressure following adrenaline injection are in these arteries similar as in the renal artery.

The following practical consequences for the use of adrenaline in pharmacoangiography are derived from our experiments:

1. Due to the early beginning and short duration of the adrenaline effect, it is necessary to inject the contrast medium not later than 20 sec after the adrenaline injection.

2. It is not advisable to replace the preinjection of adrenaline by a mixture of adrenaline and contrast medium. The prolongation of contact with contrast medium and endothelium would be so important by this method, that the local toxic effect of the contrast medium may become dangerous.

3. The marked increase of intraarterial pressure after preinjection of adrenaline in the peripheric arterial branches limits the indication for selective pharmacoangiography to such cases, in which a compensation of the increase takes place by a drainage through anastomoses or tumor vessels. In all other cases, the intraaortic injection of contrast medium is to be preferred.

4. An increase of arterial pressure in the peripheral circulation does not occur after intraarterial preinjection of adrenaline.

Renal Glomerulography in the Diagnosis of Renal Tumor

M. Kaneko

It is the purpose of this paper to investigate the usefulness of glomerulography in the diagnosis of renal tumor.

Method

Selective renal angiography was made by Seldinger's technique using Ödman-Ledin's green catheter. About 10 cc of 76% urografin was used as a contrast medium. In conventional radiography, injection was made by Gidlund automatic injector. However, manual injection was employed in macro-roentgenogryphy. In both techniques, serial angiography was performed for 5–10 sec. In macro-roentgenography, one exposure per second with factors of 125 kVp, 3 mA and 0.2–0.5 sec using a special X-ray tube, with a very fine focal spot less than 0.05 mm in diameter.

Seven cases were subjected to study, including 4 cases of Grawitz's tumor, 2 cases of pelvic tumor and one metastatic renal tumor of uterine cancer.

Result

In a case of clear cell carcinoma, lower part has a normal pattern of renal artery and glomerular opacification by macroroentgenography was observed, whereas the upper portion of the kidney was replaced by a tumor, and tumor vessels with irregular wall proliferated radially from multiple centers in the tumor and no glomerular demonstration was obtained even by macro-roentgenography. These findings were confirmed by micro-angiography and histologically.

In earlier stage of transitional cell carcinoma, when a tumor situated in a pelvis and obstructed the urinal flow, hydro-nephrosis was a main feature and renal arteriography demonstrated hydro-nephrotic pattern. With long standing hydro-nephrosis, renal parenchyma would be destroyed and infiltrated by tumor and in renal arteriography of this stage, only irregular shaped arteries were observed with conventional method. However, in macro-roentgenography fine tumor vessels were radiographed and numerous renal glomeruli among the tumor vessels were also observed. Comparatively intact glomeruli even in a tumor infiltrated portion were found in a histology. Therefore, it is characteristic to have glomerular opacification among the tumor vessels for the diagnosis of transitional cell carcinoma.

In metastatic renal tumor, the vascular pattern depends on the primary tumor and the site of metastasis in the kidney. In case of uterine cancer, infiltration to the renal pelvis demonstrated by hydronephrosis and glomerular opacification among the tumor vessels, but it would be differed from pelvic tumor in the end stage, when the tumor replaced the normal tissue and no further glomerulography was possible.

Conclusion

It is very useful to have glomerulography in a differential diagnosis of renal tumor, for the classification and to know the extension or stage of the disease.

Table 1

No.	Case	Age	Sex	Chief Complaint	Involved Kidney
1.	C. F.	52	♀	General Fatigue and Anemia	left
2.	I. H.	68	♂	Hematuria and Flank Tumor	left
3.	M. H.	63	♂	General Fatigue, Emaciation and Anemia	right
4.	S. T.	73	♂	Flank Pain and Tumor	left
5.	S. H.	62	♂	Hematuria, Flank Pain and Lumbago	right
6.	K. I.	70	♂	Hematuria and Flank Pain	left
7.	F. O.	49	♀	Hematuria and Flank Pain	left

No.	Selective Renal Angiography	Diagnosis
1.	Conventional and Macroradiography (X4)	Clear Cell Carcinoma
2.	Conventional	Clear Cell Carcinoma
3.	Conventional and Macroradiography (X4)	Clear Cell Carcinoma
4.	Conventional	Clear Cell Carcinoma
5.	Conventional and Macroradiography (X4)	Transitional Cell Carcinoma
6.	Conventional	Transitional Cell Carcinoma
7.	Conventional and Macroradiography (X4)	Metastasis of Uterine Cancer

Table 2

	Grawitz's Tumor (Clear Cell Carcinoma)	Pelvic Tumor (Transitional Cell Carcinoma)
Early Stage	Proliferated Tumor Vessels with Surrounding Normal Vessels (Glomerulography +)	Hydronephrotic Pattern
Late Stage	Proliferated Tumor Vessels	Poor Tumor Vessels Scattered in Normal Vessels (Glomerulography +)
	Renal Parenchymal Metastasis	Renal Pelvic Metastasis
Early Stage	Tumor Vessels with Surrounding Normal Vessels (Glomerulography +)	Hydronephrotic Pattern
Late Stage	Tumor Vessels	Tumor Vessels

Außergewöhnliche radiologische Befunde bei Nierentumoren

H. Schmidt

Die Kombination röntgendiagnostischer Methoden mit nuklearmedizinischer Funktions- und Lokalisationsdiagnostik bedeutet für die Nierenuntersuchung einen großen Fortschritt.

Die verschiedenen Methoden gegeneinander abzuwägen und zum richtigen Zeitpunkt einzusetzen ist die Aufgabe des Radiologen. Dabei sind manchmal Radiologen an Häusern mittlerer Größe im Vorteil gegenüber Großkliniken, da sich hier die gesamte Radiologie noch unter einem Dach und unter einer Leitung befindet. Auch unter diesem Gesichtspunkt möchte ich das mir gestellte Thema behandeln.

Das Isotopennephrogramm nützt nicht viel bei der Diagnostik von Nierentumoren. Trotzdem steht es bei uns am Anfang jeder radiologischen Nierenuntersuchung, da ein vorausgegangenes Urogramm oder gar Infusionspyelogramm das Nephrogramm beeinflußt. Danach folgt bei uns das Infusionspyelogramm mit Conray. Das einfache i. v.-Pyelogramm wird bei uns kaum mehr angewandt. Dasselbe gilt vom retrograden Pyelogramm. Schichtuntersuchungen der Nieren werden bei uns relativ selten gemacht. Das mag z. T. daran liegen, daß wir keinen unbeschränkten Filmetat haben, z. T. auch, weil uns das Szintigramm mit wesentlich geringerem Aufwand und weit geringerer Strahlenbelastung etwa vergleichbare Ergebnisse bringt, zum größten Teil aber daran, weil wir wissen, daß bei Tumorverdacht doch am Ende aller Untersuchungen die Angiographie steht.

Bei der oftmals uncharakteristischen Symptomatik der Nierengeschwülste (nicht immer hat man eine Blutung als Wegweiser) zeigt uns die Szintigraphie als Suchmethode den richtigen Weg und rechtfertigt die eingreifende Angiographie. Hier, vor der Angiographie, ist der Platz der Nierenszintigraphie und hier hat sie sich uns bewährt im Gegensatz zur Angioszintigraphie, von der ich bei der Diagnostik von Nierentumoren nicht viel halte.

Anhand von Bilderserien mit außergewöhnlichen Tumorbefunden wird das Gesagte erläutert.

Evaluation of Peripheral Circulation by Angioscintigraphy

H. Shida and I. Ohara

This study was attempted to evaluate the peripheral circulation in those with functional and organic vascular diseases using radioisotope.

96 cases with and without vascular diseases were studied. After intraarterial injection of radioisotope (^{131}I-MAA, ^{19}-Au colloid, ^{133}Xe) into the limbs, 2 channel spectrometers were used to record the movement of radioisotope over the limbs. Profile scanner was used to detect the accumulation of MAA in the lung. The distribution of MAA in the limbs was recorded by scintiscanner or scinticamera.

With regard to ^{131}I-MAA, it was found to be accumulated in the lung after passing from the artery to the vein, which was entirely different from the pattern of MAA seen in lung scintigram. This findings suggested that leakage of MAA through arteriovenous communication existed. Similar observation was made with ^{198}Au colloid particles. High leakage of MAA was noticed in those with organic diseases and distribution of MAA was not uniform on the scintigram. In those with functional diseases, and in control, the leakage was low. However, scintigram showed uniform distribution of MAA. Marked accumulation of MAA in the periphery of feet was observed with prior injection of benzyl imidazolin hydrochloride.

Angiography and Scintigraphy of the Kidney

K. zum Winkel, H.-M. Sonderkamp, H. Jost, F. Marx and H.-J. Hermann

Introduction

The kidneys maintain the water and electrolytes balances of the body and eliminate numerous metabolic products. These tasks are accomplished by the adaption to the volume, the concentration and the composition of the urine. There are 3 different mechanisms serving these purposes

the glomerular filtration,
the tubular reabsorption and
the tubular secretion.

Regarding the renal scintigraphy the introduction of the "tubular piling" as a 4th mechanism seems to be useful. Angiography as well as urography are performed by injecting high doses of triiodinated contrast media, wich are excreted by glomerular filtration, only. In contrary the radiopharmaceuticals applied in order to do renal scintigraphy are excreted in different ways. Thus, labelled Chelates and Inulin are glomerular filtrated exclusively, whereas Ortho-Iodo-Hippuric acid is eliminated by tubular secretion (80%) and glomerular filtration (20%). Mercury compounds as well as Technetium-Iron-Complexes are eliminated by tubular piling within the cells of the proximal tubular convolute or the distal convolute, respectively.

Angiography

The survey aortography and the selective renal arteriography offer a detailed image of the condition, the course and the blood flow of the renal vessels or of any intrarenal or pararenal alteration, respectively. Mostly, the femoral artery ist punctured according to the method of Seldinger, followed by the introduction of an opaque catheter. By means of angiography one can differentiate an arterial from a parenchymatous and a venous phase. The staining of the parenchyma – called the nephrographic effect – is mainly due to the passage of the contrast medium through the capillaries, as the amount of the contrast medium filtrated in the glomerula is only 20%.

Scintigraphy

Renal scintigraphy can be done by a motor driven radiation detector (scanning) or as sequential scintigraphy by using camera systems with stationary detectors.

Using the scanning method the areas of renal tissue are represented, which are able to accumulate radiopharmaceuticals with renal affinity. The scan gives less morphological details compared with the radiograph. Circumscribed lesions of the renal parenchyma can be recognized only, if their diameters are at least 1.5 cm. The scanning ist suitable to detect the position, the size and the configuration of the functioning parenchyma. Furthermore, one can differentiate anomalies- – especially horseshoe kidneys –, irregular renal contours and solitary or multiple parenchymal defects. Solitary defects in the scintigram may represent tumors, solitary cysts, ischemic necrosis or tuberculosis. Among these conditions, no characteristic differences can be seen.

The interpretation of the scintigrams got by using a scanning system is easier because of the higher resolution compared with that of a scintillation camera. The major advantage of the scintillation camera is the performing of sequential scintigrams.

In this way, after the intravenous injection of radiopharmaceuticals eliminated by glomerular filtration or by tubular secretion one can study, except for the site of the functional parenchyma,

the inflow
the intrarenal and
the postrenal transport

of the radioactivity. Using a storage system the slope of the radioactivity within distinct regions of interest can be evaluated. These regions of interest may be determined on the oscilloscope by means of a light pen. In numerous experimental and clinical studies we found in inflammatory diseases of the kidney, that the concentration was mainly reduced within the parenchymal phase (1–3 min after the application of Radiohippuric acid), whereas the intrarenal and the postrenal transport occured delayed (236 patients, FEINE and ZUM WINKEL). Disorders of the evacuation of the upper urinary tract as hydronephrosis or similar diseases (45 patients, FEINE and ZUM WINKEL) cause a prolonged pelvic phase (retention of radioactivity within 15 min and longer in the renal pelvis).

Results

The scintigraphic findings were compared with those of the angiography under different aspects.

In order to control scanning 77 patients were disposable (Table 1). In vascular diseases a diminished size and a reduced accumulation of radioactivity was regarded to be pathological. Usually, the angiography revealed better details for the exact localisation of a pathological process. In many cases angiography allowed the true diagnosis of cysts and malignant tumors. As shown, scanning could not do so. However the results of this method were fairly good in 59 patients with renal tumors either conformed by angiography or operation (Table 2). In 76% parenchymal defect could be proved. It is remarkable too, that in finding of a non-functioning kidney a tumor could not be excluded. In 21 patients (see Table 1) angiography was performed. In 19 patients the angiography findings were positive, one was doubtful and one was negative.

By means of the sequential scintigraphy well vascularized tumors were detectable by the inversion effect. This means, that within 40 sec at the latest an increased radioactivity was seen in a region thereafter missing any uptake.

Table 1. *Results of the renal angiography and the scanning in 77 patients* (zum Winkel *et al.* 1965)

Number of pat.	Diagnosis	Corresponding	Divergent
12	Normal	8	4 (scan 3 parenchym def. and 1 reduced function)
18	Anomalies (dystopia, horseshoe, cysts)	17	1 (ang. polycyst. degener.)
10	Vascular diseases	8	2 (ang. 1 stenosis and 1 arteriosclerosis)
8	Pyelonephritis	6	2 (ang. irregular contours)
4	Hydronephrosis	4	—
1	Pole resection	1	—
24	Tumors (scan parenchymal def. or non-function. kidney)	23	1 (ang. normal)
		67 (87 %)	

Table 2. *Pathological signs in the scanning of 59 patients with renal tumors proved by operation or angiography* (Bachmann, Univ. Strahlenklinik Heidelberg)

Definite defects of the parenchyma	45 (76 %)
Doubtful defects	4
Non-functioning kidney (total destruction)	9
Normal scan	1

74% of 43 patients with renal artery stenosis showed pathological signs (Table 3). These results should to be improved with the aid of a data processing system, because in some of the cases the analysis of equal regions of interest showed the different accumulation of the radioactivity. The most important advantage of the sequential scintigraphy is the discovery of diffuse or circumscribed nephritis in one or both kidneys with the functional or morphological information obtained by this method. In these cases by means of the angiography a rarefaction of the renal vessels, scarredly altered contours and a shrunken parenchyma of the kidney could be revealed, only. We found sequential scintigraphy to be superior in proving inflammatory diseases of the kidney as well as in proving functional disturbances following

Table 3. *Pathological signs in the sequential scintigraphy of 43 patients with renal artery stenosis proved by angiography or operation: 38 unilateral including 4 segmental and 5 bilateral stenoses* (Feine and zum Winkel)

Reduced inflow during the initial phase (15–30 sec)	29 (67 %)
Reduced concentration during the parenchymal phase (1–3 min)	23 (54 %)
Shrunken area of uptake	15 (35 %)
Delayed evacuation out of the pelvis (reduced urine volume)	12 (28 %)
False results (negative 5, false side 6)	11 (26 %)

them (Table 4). However, sequential scintigraphy without data processing system has only limited value in the diagnosis of malignant tumors. For giving sufficient remarks about the accuracy of the sequential scintigraphy together with data processing system as a routine the number of our patients with renal artery stenosis is too small.

Table 4. *Results of the renal angiography and the sequential scintigraphy in 28 patients* (Univ. Strahleninst. Berlin-Westend, May–August 1970)

Number of pat.	Diagnosis	Corresponding	Divergent
9	Parenchymal defects, i.e.	9	
	malignant tumors	1	5 (scint. defects only)
	solitary cysts	3	
1	Polycystic degeneration	1	
1	Horseshoe kidney	1	
2	Renal artery stenosis	2	
11	Pyelonephritis	8	3 (ang. normal)
1	Agenesia left, hypertrophia right	1	
1	Hypertension		1 (scint. unilateral reduced vascular., ang. normal)
1	Nephropexia right, hydronephrosis		1 (scint. bilateral pyelonephritis; ang. stenosis and missed evacuation right, normal left)
1	Normal	1	
		18 (64%)	
Without differentiation of "defects"		23 (82%)	

Some experimental results in 11 untreated dogs with kidney transplantation should be added. After transplantation 26 sequential scintigraphies as well as angiographies on the last examination day, respectively, were performed.

Rejection of a tranplant was marked by a reduced uptake of radioactivity and a delayed evacuation. Due to the edema of the transplant the renal area of accumulated radioactivity was enlarged. The digital evaluation of the transplant revealed a diminished initial concentration. The radioactivity descended within 15 sec and was concentrated contineously afterwards. We explain that sign with the reduced renal extraction rate of Radiohippuric acid due to the rejection. Furthermore, in angiography we found a rarefaction of the vessels and a narrowing of their lumina, whereas the flow rate was slowed down remarkably.

Conclusions

Angiography is the method of choice to examine the morphology of the renal and pararenal vessels. No better method exists, which may informes equally about the quality, width, number and possible pathological new formations of the vessels.

Poorly vacularized tumors, however, can be diagnosed hardly. Especially, the tumors of the renal pelvis show angiographically a quite normal vascular pattern. Thus, in 4 patients with malignant tumors of the renal pelvis we found 3 times normal results in the angiogram and in the sequential scintigram. But, 1 of these 3 patients offered a defect on the conventional scan. 1 patient suffering from a pelvic tumor had pathological findings in the angiogram as well as in the sequential scintigram (Neide).

Scanning is a suitable method for pointing out morphologic anomalies as horseshoe kidneys or dystopia. Also irregular renal contours can be attached. Parenchymal defects caused by tumors, cysts, ischemia or abscesses are easliy detectable. However, the nature of the defect can not be defined. It must be recommanded especially, that the scanning is a very helpful method for proving the polycystic degeneration of the kidney. In these cases angiography should be done only in doubtful results. The *sequential scintigraphy* predominates in diagnosing inflammatory renal diseases. Particularly, subsequent functional disorders can be disclosed. With the analysis of distinct areas, which are to determined on the oscilloscope by means of a lightpen, this method leads to important new results. Flow disturbances of the upper urinary tract can be detected even in patients without accumulation of contrast medium on pyelogram. As a screening test the sequential scintigraphy may be recommanded in patients with hypertension. However, for revealing small differences from the renal vascularization a data processing system should be used. In every case, with the angiography the locality and the extension of a renal artery stenosis are proved exactly.

In future the main importance of the functional scintigraphy seems to be the detection of distinct areas with reduced blood flow. May be, that its results are of prognostic value. When an inversion effect is seen, a well vascularized tumor must be suggested. The sequential scintigraphy is an excellent procedure for the control of kidney transplants. Angiography should be done in these cases only, when strictly indicated.

Angiography and sequential scintigraphy as a single or a combined radiological examination reveal important informations about the renal perfusion, the intensity and the place of the renal excretion and finally, about the intrarenal and the postrenal transports. Regarding the results of these procedures we gain an extensive knowledge of the fundamentals in morphology and pathophysiology of numerous renal diseases.

Summary

After the description of the physiological and pharmacological basics the results of the angiography and the scanning in 77 patients with several renal diseases and 59 patients suffering from tumors of the kidneys are demonstrated. Thereafter, the symptoms of the sequential scintigrsphy in 43 patients with renal artery stenosis proved by angiography are enumerated. Furthermore, the results of the angiography and the sequential scintigraphy in 28 patients are compared. Finally, a report of results in renal transplantation in dogs is given.

Rapid, Sequential Renal Blood Flow Scintiphotography

L. M. FREEMAN

With the use of the Anger Scintillation Camera, the injection of a small bolus containing a large amount of radioactive tracer makes possible visualization of major vascular pathways as well as of the blood supply to certain critical organs, such as the kidney. The technique has been applied to a number of renal problems, which include mass lesions, injury, hypertension, transplantation and infarction. The latter area has been particulary interesting since life saving surgery has been performed after the scintiphotographic study indicated occlusion of major vascular pathways.

An arterio-venous fistula following renal biopsy has also been demonstrated.

As with other studies using isotopic organ visualization, this procedure is meant to complement and not compete with currently available techniques such as intravenous urography and renal angiography. Only further investigative work will determine exactly what diagnositic niche this procedure will occupy in relation to radiographic studies of the kidney.

Selective Angioscintigraphy and Angiography in Kidney Diseases

G. Hör, G. Buttermann, H. G. Heinze, U. Klein, H. Langhammer,
H. Müller-Fassbender and H. W. Pabst

A lot of experimental, metabolic and kinetic studies were performed using (radio-) albumin.

Radioactive particles were also applied for studying renal cortical blood flow, because these are presumably deposited in the peritubular capillaries of cortical parenchyma.

The question of clinical applicability of radioalbumin-aggregated particles (RAMA) for conventional renal angioscintigraphy or-perfusion scanning however remained largely unexplored.

Method

After blocking thyroid we investigated 121 kidneys simultaneously by angiography and by angioscintigraphy.

250 μCi of RAMA were injected selectively into renal artery, ^{113m}In-Fe-Colloid has been abandoned by us, because of additional extrarenal accumulation.

We used a 5 inch cristall rectilinear scanner and a focusing collimator (2111, Fa Picker).

Criteria of Interpretation. For comparative evaluation of angiogram and angioscintigram each kidney area a the scan and angiogram was divided into 6 subareas.

Angiographic Criteria. Alterations in vascular architecture of great and small vessels, quality of nephrographic effect (normal, decreased, lacking).

Angioscintigraphic Criteria. Quality and localization of RAMA in the different kidney areas: normal, reduced, lacking.

Divergence between angioscintigram and angiogram was accepted definitely in those cases, which presented differences in two or more kidney areas according to the criteria outlined above (angiogram normal, angioscintigram abnormal and vice versa).

Partial accordance between radiological and nuclear procedure has been assumed in case, that differences were confined to one kidney area.

Angioscintigram was considered to give additional diagnostic information, when perfusion defects were larger or smaller than it could be expected from angiogram.

Results

1. A case is presented, in which differences were observed between i.v. scintigram and i.a. angioscintigram, in accordance to angiogram.

Table. *Comparison of angiography and angioscintigraphy of the kidneys*

Nephropathy	Number	Accordance Total	Partial	No acc.	No additional information	Additional information Process increased	Process decreased	total	False interpretation
Unspecific inflammatory or arteriosclerotic processes	58	17 (29 %)	21 (36 %)	20 (35 %)	25 (43 %)	26 (45) %	5 (9 %)	31 (54 %)	2 (3 %)
Urogenital tuberculosis	26	2 (8 %)	16 (61 %)	8 (31 %)	8 (31 %)	10 (38) %	6 (23 %)	16 (61 %)	2 (8 %)
Polycystic degeneration and solitary cysts	13	8 (61 %)	5 (39 %)	0 (0 %)	3 (23 %)	0 (0 %)	7 (54 %)	7 (54 %)	3 (23 %)
Hypernephroid carcinoma	6	3 (50 %)	2 (33 %)	1 (17 %)	4 (67 %)	1 (17 %)	1 (17 %)	2 (33 %)	0 (0 %)
Transplanted kidneys	2	2 (100 %)	0 (0 %)	0 (0 %)	1 (50 %)	1 (50 %)	0 (0 %)	1 (50 %)	0 (0 %)
Angiographically normal kidneys	16	12 (75 %)	0 (0 %)	4 (25 %)	9 (56 %)	7 (44 %)	0 (0 %)	7 (44 %)	0 (0 %)
Total	121	44 (40 %)	44 (40 %)	33 (20 %)	50 (41 %)	45 (37 %)	19 (16 %)	64 (53 %)	7 (6 %)

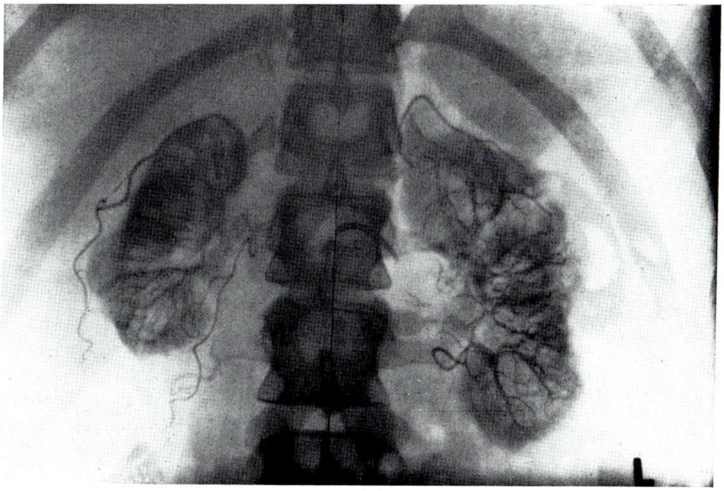

a

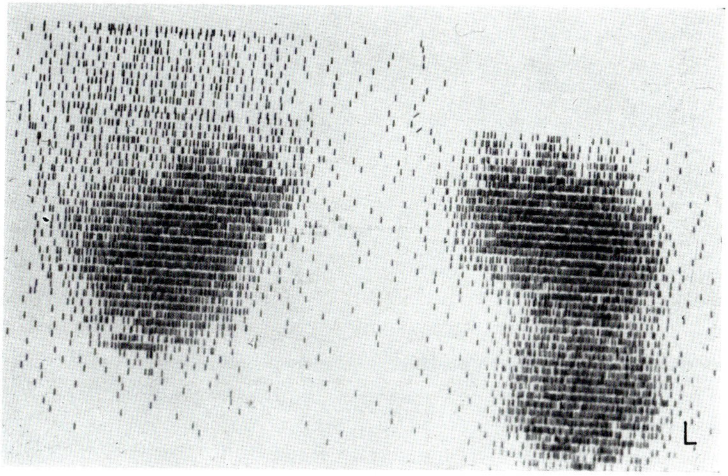

b

Fig. 1. a angiogram, late arterial phase. Marked cortical parenchymal reduction, destructive changes on intrarenal vessels, especially in the middle of the left kidney. b i. v.-scintigram (^{197}Hg-Chlormerodrin) accumulation of radiopharmaceutical is reduced in an area corresponding to the vascular pathology shown by the angiogram

Clinical diagnosis. Cirrhosis of both kidneys consecutive to phenacetin-abusus.

It remains to be explored by further investigations, whether the accumulation of radioalbumin particles as a sign of *redistribution of renal blood flow* within the dilated vessels of inflammatory renal parenchyma is primarily due to a "Trueta-phenomenon" and to a decrease in renovascular resistance.

2. The Table shows, that angioscintigram was of additional diagnostic value in 38–45% of the 121 kidneys, especially in inflammatory diseases, in which angio-

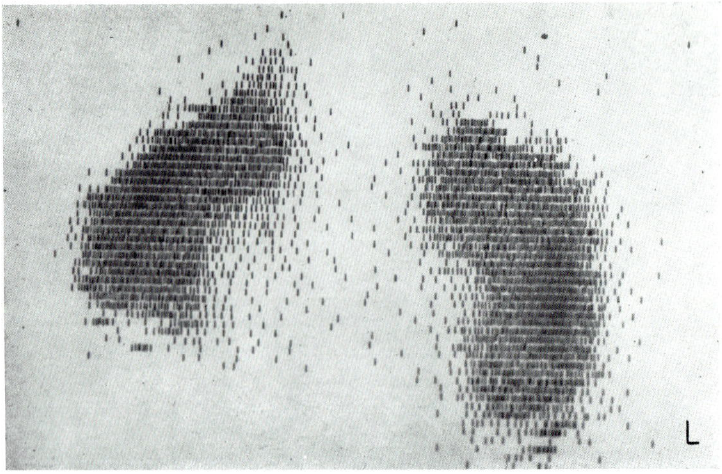

1c

Fig. 1. c i.a.-angioscintigram (RAMA), color scintigrams reproduced in black-and-withe and reserved left to right. There is an increased accumulation of RAMA following the injection of radiopharmaceutical into renal artery: this area corresponds to the angiographic area showing pathological structure of renal vessels

graphy gives minor information concerning pathology of the smallest vessels, which are not discernible by angiography.

Thus angioscintigraphy showed a greater extension of the area of increased or decreased renal perfusion in early and late stages of inflammatory and destructive kidney processes than it was derivable from angiogram.

It seems further remarkable that in 7 out of 16 kidneys (with normal vasculature in the angiogram) the angioscintigram gave strong evidence of renal hypoperfusion.

In summary renal angioscintigraphy is a useful procedure contributory to angiography: it permits the study of renal perfusion and of disturbances of renal blood supply in distinct renal areas.

Angioscintigraphy should not be applied in-cases with severe reduction of renal glomerular filtration because by additional embolization of renal capillaries with albumin or colloid particles in these situations critical decrease of renal blood supply may be induced leading to acute renal failure (data to be published).

Ergebnisse der renalen Angio-Szintigraphie

J. P. HAAS und H. G. CLAUS

Bei 112 aus den verschiedensten Gründen an den Nieren angiographierten Patienten wurden im Anschluß an die selektive Angiographie anfangs 300, später 150–200 μCi ^{131}J-MAA in jedes Organ arteriell injiziert. Etwa 30 min später wurde von jeder Niere in Bauchlage ein Szintigramm geschrieben. Außerdem wurde bei den meisten Patienten 1–2 Tage vor oder nach der Angiographie ein Nierenszintigramm mit ^{99m}Tc-Eisen-Komplex angefertigt.

Für die Auswertung standen 224 Nieren zur Verfügung, deren Krankheitsprozeß aus der Tabelle hervorgeht. Es handelt sich um 26 operativ bestätigte Nierentumoren, 22 Solitärcysten und 17 mal multiple Cystenbildungen oder polycystische Degeneration. Außerdem waren 5 mal eine Nierentuberkulose, 9 Hydronephrosen und 11 Schrumpfnieren verschiedener Ätiologie vertreten. 2 mal lag eine Nierenarterien-

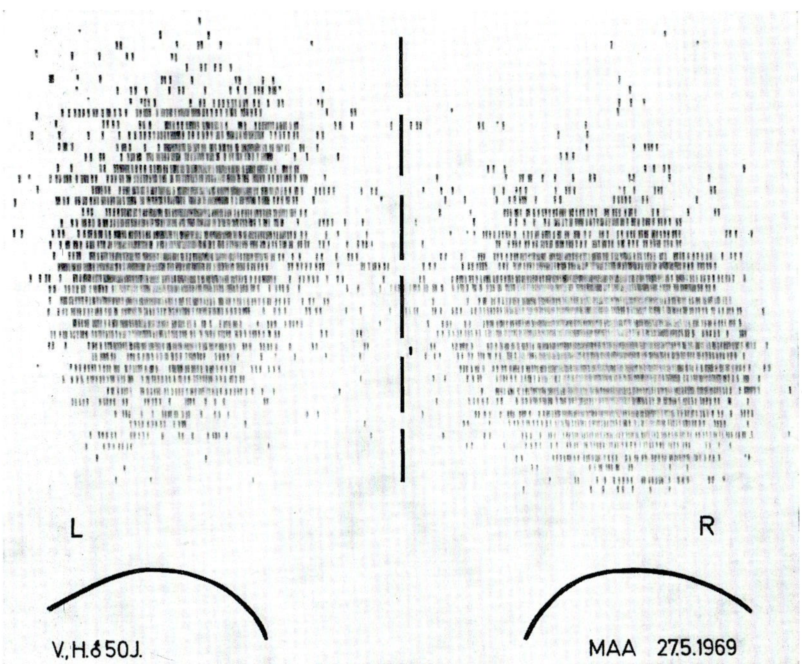

Abb. 1

Tabelle

Nierenerkrankung (Anzahl)	Neue Information		Sehr gute Übereinstimmung		Gute Übereinstimmung		Geringe oder fehlende Übereinstimmung		Path. Szintigramm ohne anatom. Korr.		Nicht geschriebene oder technisch nicht verwertbare Szintigramme	
	^{131}J-MAA	^{99m}Tc-Fe-Komplex	^{131}J-MAA	^{99m}Tc-Fe-Komplex	^{131}J-MAA	^{99m}Tc-Fe-Komplex	^{131}J-MAA	^{99m}Tc-Fe-Komplex	^{131}J-MAA	^{99m}Tc-Fe-Komplex	^{131}J-MAA	^{99m}Tc-Fe-Komplex
Maligne Nierentumoren (26)	**2**		8	4	**14**	**9**	1	6			1	7
Solitärcysten (22)	**2**	**1**	2	2	**16**	**6**	2	7				6
Multiple Cysten u. Cystennieren (17)	**2**	**2**	7	2	8	8						5
Nierentuberkul. (5)	**1**			1	4	2		1				1
Hydronephrose (9)			2		7	6						3
Schrumpfniere (11)			3	2	8	5		2				2
Nierenarterienstenosen (2)					2	1						1
Hufeisenniere u. a. Formatypien (9)			2		5	4		2			2	3
Normalfälle (106)	2	1	2		**84**		1	2	**14**	**12**	3	
Normalfälle m. Gefäßvariationen (17)					**1**	**82**	**16**					26
Gesamtzahl der Nieren: 224	9	4	**26**	**11**	149	123	20	20	14	12	6	54

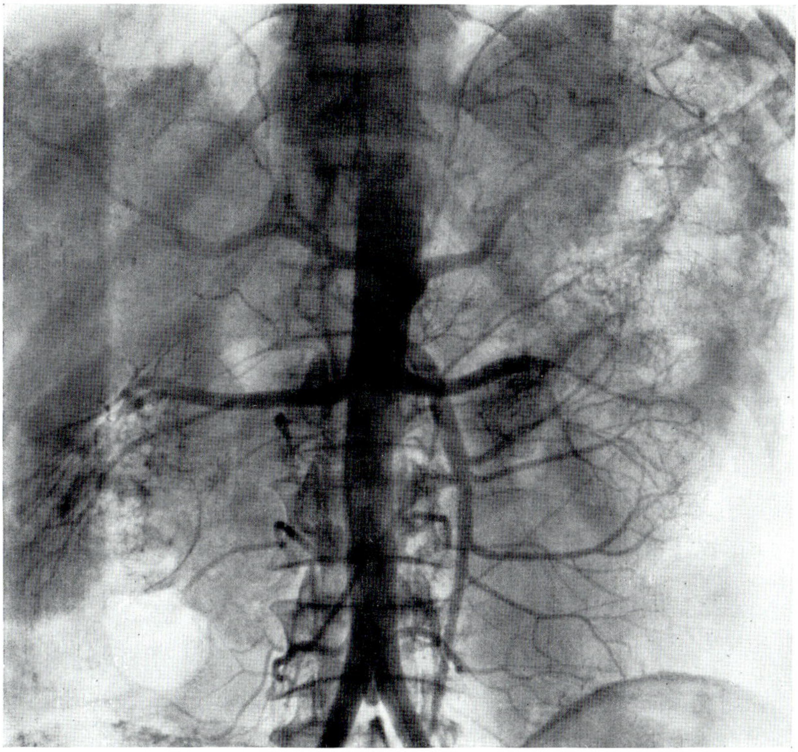

Abb. 2

stenose oder ein Verschluß vor. Die relativ große Anzahl sog. unauffälliger Nieren resultiert aus der routinemäßigen Mituntersuchung des kontralateralen Organes bei einseitig lokalisiertem, angiographiertem Nierenprozeß. Diese sog. Normalfälle stellen die Grundlage für die weitere Auswertung und Deutung der pathologischen Befunde dar, indem vielfache und uneingeschränkte Übereinstimmung ihrer Angiogramme die Brauchbarkeit der Angio-Szintigraphie zunächst einmal dokumentiert. Allerdings war bei kritischer Sichtung und Vergleich der beiden Untersuchungsmethoden eine solche Konkordanz nicht immer gegeben.

Bei 9 Fällen erbrachte die Angio-Szintigraphie zusätzliche über die Aussage der Angiographie hinausgehende Informationen. Hierbei handelte es sich einmal um kleinere Cystenbildungen, die aus dem angiographischen Gefäßbild nicht eindeutig hervorgingen. Die kleineren Raumforderungen wurden erst nachträglich im Angiogramm als solche erkannt. Ein Hypernephrom mit einer walnußgroßen operativ bestätigten Hilusmetastase der kontralateralen Niere stellte sich durch die starke Anreicherung von ^{131}J-MMA (Abb. 1 und 3) im Primärtumor und in der Metastase im Szintigramm wesentlich besser dar, als bei der Renovasographie (Abb. 2). Bei den anderen hier nicht gezeigten Patienten mit frischer Nierentuberkulose kam die Caverne durch ^{131}J-MAA-Anreicherung überzeuggend zum Nachweis. Das Angiogramm zeigte hier einen nur fraglichen Befund. Diese beiden operativ kontrollierten Normalfälle mit neuer Information sind besonders hervorzuheben, da das

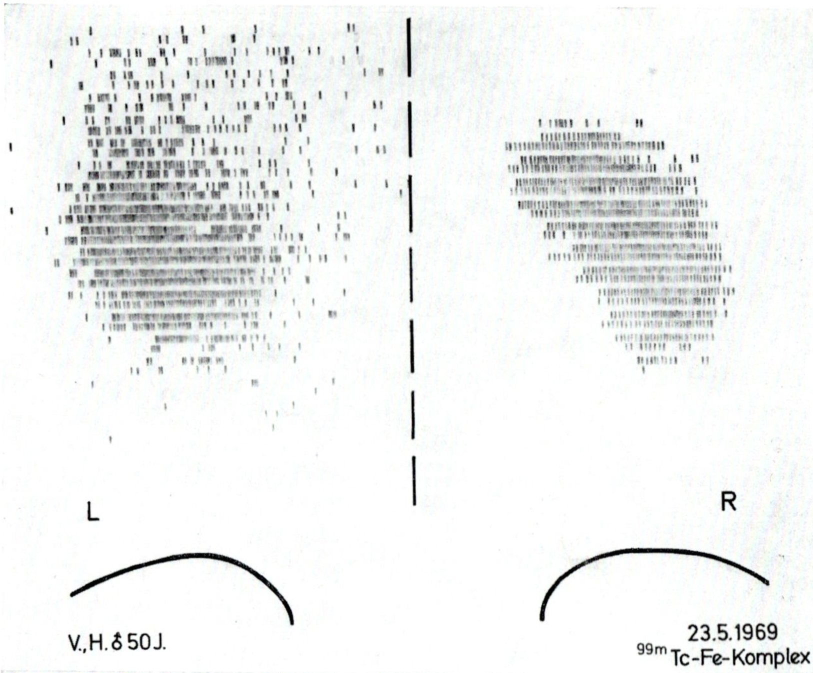

Abb. 3

Angio-Szintigramm den klinisch und angiographisch vermuteten Tumor von vornherein ausschloß.

Unter einer sehr guten Übereinstimmung verstehen wir eine überzeugende angioszintigraphische Darstellung und Bestätigung eines angiographischen Befundes. Dies war bei 26 Nieren der Fall, während das ^{99m}Tc-Eisen-Komplex-Szintigramm eine gleichgute Übereinstimmung nur 11 mal aufwies.

Abgesehen von den in den Spalten 1 und 2 aufgeführten 9 und 26 Nieren bestätigte bei weiteren 149 der untersuchten Nieren das Angio-Szintigramm den angiologischen Befund, und zwar bei 85 Normalnieren und 64 Nieren mit pathologischen Veränderungen. Insgesamt waren somit bei 83% der untersuchten Nieren Informationen aus dem Angio-Szintigramm zu gewinnen. Eine geringe oder gar fehlende angio-szintigraphische Aussage fand sich bei 20 Nieren, das sind 9%. Dies geht fast ausschließlich zu Lasten des Vorhandenseins mehrerer Nierenarterien mit ungleichmäßiger MAA-Injektion.

Unter Fällen mit pathologischem Szintigramm ohne anatomisches Korrelat haben wir solche Nieren eingereiht, die klinisch wie auch angiographisch keine Auffälligkeiten boten, szintigraphisch jedoch sicher nicht als normal anzusehen waren. Als Hauptursache für solche szintigraphischen Befunde möchten wir Störungen in der kapillaren Strombahn zur Diskussion stellen, die mit der derzeitigen angiographischen Technik wahrscheinlich noch nicht erfaßt werden können. Daneben sind, abgesehen von primären Gefäßprozessen, klinisch noch voll kompensierte Parenchymerkrankungen ursächlich zu vermuten.

Was die Aussagefähigkeit des ^{99m}Tc-Eisen-Szintigrammes anbetrifft, so steht diese bei praktisch allen untersuchten Nierenerkrankungen hinter der des ^{131}J-MAA-Szintigrammes. Die Anfertigung beider Szintigramme ist jedoch wegen des dargestellten unterschiedlichen morphologischen Substrates empfehlenswert.

Zusammenfassend möchten wir feststellen, daß die Angio-Szintigraphie der Nieren eine wertvolle Bereicherung der Nierendiagnostik darstellt. Sie bestätigt nicht nur in einem hohen Prozentsatz den angiographischen Befund, sondern gibt in wichtigen Einzelfällen neue über die Angiographie hinausgehende Informationen.

Ergebnisse der radiologischen Untersuchungen bei vaskulären Nierenerkrankungen

E. Vogler

Die Radiologie mit den ihr derzeit zur Verfügung stehenden Untersuchnungsmethoden kann Aufschluß geben über viele, jedoch nicht alle Erkrankungen der Nierengefäße, ferner über die Art derselben, aber auch über die funktionellen Auswirkungen dieser Erkrankungen auf das Nierengewebe.

Folgende radiologische Untersuchungsmethoden haben sich für die Erkennung von Gefäßerkrankungen der Nieren besonders bewährt:

1. Übersichtsaufnahmen des Abdomens,
2. i.v. Urographie,
3. die nuklearmedizinischen Methoden,
4. Angiographie.

Die *Abdomenübersichtsaufnahmen* sollen auch bei Gefäßerkrankungen der Nieren durchgeführt werden, wenngleich damit, außer der etwas zweifelhaften Bestimmung der Nierengröße, nur solche organische Gefäßerkrankungen nachgewiesen werden können, die mit Verkalkungen einhergehen, wie z. B. Arteriosklerose, seltene Fälle von Aneurysmen, Thromben.

Die *i.v. Urographie* mit ihren einzelnen Varianten gibt oft die ersten Hinweise auf das Vorhandensein einer Gefäßerkrankung der Nieren, bzw. läßt im Verein mit den klinischen Daten den Verdacht dafür äußern.

Die *nuklearmedizinischen Methoden* sind für die Erkennung von Gefäßerkrankungen eine Hilfe. Die lokalisatorischen Methoden in Form der Szintigraphie mit rectilinearem Scanner oder mit der Gammakamera, ermöglicht die Bestimmung der Größe, Form und Lage der Nieren und den Grad der Speicherung durch Beachtung des Speichermusters. Die funktionellen Methoden in Form der Renographie geben uns Aufschluß über den globalen Transit des Indikators durch die Nieren und die Möglichkeit des Seitenvergleiches. Mit den nuklearmedizinischen Methoden können wir die aus der intravenösen Urographie gewonnenen Erkenntnisse erhärten und darüber hinaus bessere funktionelle Erkenntnisse gewinnen, wenngleich auch diese Methoden für die exakte morphologische Diagnose nicht geeignet sind.

Die *Angiographie* ist die einzige radiologische Untersuchungsmethode, die das Gefäßsystem der Nieren darstellen kann. Mit dieser Methode ist es möglich, Veränderungen an den Gefäßen der Nieren, aber auch solche, die diese am Nierenparenchym verursachen, morphologisch festzustellen, diese zu lokalisieren und in vielen Fällen zu klassifizieren.

Das Gebiet der Gefäßerkrankungen der Nieren ist zu groß, um hier in seiner Gesamtheit abgehandelt zu werden. Deshalb sollen 3 Erkrankungen als Beispiele herausgegriffen und besprochen werden, und zwar

die arteriellen Aneurysmen,
die arteriellen Angiome,
der arterielle Kollateralkreislauf.

Arterielle Aneurysmen. Diese werden seit der routinemäßigen Anwendung der Angiographie häufiger beobachtet. Vielfach werden sie zufällig im Rahmen einer angiographischen Untersuchung der Nieren gefunden, da die meisten klinisch keine auffallenden Erscheinungen bieten und deshalb nicht gezielt nach ihnen gefahndet wird.

Die Übersichtsaufnahme weist mitunter schon auf das Vorhandensein eines Aneurysmas hin, dann, wenn Wandverkalkungen in typischer Ringform im Nierenbereich nachweisbar sind.

Die intravenöse Urographie läßt bei zentralem Sitz mitunter eine Impression am Nierenbeckenkelchsystem erkennen, ist sonst aber bei unkomplizierten Fällen normal.

Die nuklearmedizinischen Methoden ergeben bei unkomplizierten Fällen keine von der Norm abweichenden Änderungen.

Mit der Angiographie können Aneurysmen exakt nachgewiesen und lokalisiert werden, vorausgesetzt, ihr Lumen ist nicht zur Gänze thrombosiert. Die angiographisch nachweisbare Größe und Form eines Aneurysmas gibt keine sichere Auskunft über die wahre Größe und Form desselben, da mittels Angiographie nur das Lumen eines Aneurysmas dargestellt werden kann.

Die häufigste Komplikation der arteriellen Aneurysmen ist die Ruptur derselben. Die Blutung erfolgt dabei – je nach Sitz des Aneurysmas – in das Nierenparenchym, nach subkapsulär oder auch in den retroperitonelen Raum, seltener nach intraperitoneal. Als weitere Komplikation werden Stenosen der Nierenarterien durch Druck des Aneurysmas selbst oder durch fortgesetzte Thrombosen oder Embolie aus den Aneurysmen mit deren Folgen beobachtet. Nach Ruptur eines arteriellen Aneurysmas besteht auch die Möglichkeit der Ausbildung einer arterio-venösen Fistel. Die genannten Komplikationen können partiellen oder gänzlichen Funktionsausfall der betroffenen Niere hervorrufen, der dann urographisch oder auch mit den nuclearmedizinischen Methoden nachgewiesen werden kann, sie sind aber nicht spezifisch genug, um als Komplikation bei Aneurysmen gewertet zu werden. Die Angiographie gibt bessere Aufschlüsse.

Arterielle Angiome. Als klinisches Leitsymptom steht die Hämaturie im Vordergrund. Der Sitz dieser Hämangiome ist vorwiegend in den Markanteilen der Nieren und da insbesondere in den papillennahen Bezirken derselben. In der Regel sind diese Angiome klein, und können einen wesentlichen arterio-venösen Shunt vermissen lassen, aber auch einen solchen verursachen, wobei dann große Ähnlichkeit mit ausgeprägten arterio-venösen Angiomen, bzw. Fisteln besteht.

Angiome ohne wesentlichen Shunt beeinflussen die Nierenfunktion meist nur indirekt, und dann, wenn bei Blutungen in das Nierenbeckenkelchsystem und Abgang von Koagula über die Ureteren eine temporäre Harnrückstauung hervorgerufen wird. Die Abdomenübersicht gibt keine Hinweise. Die Urographie läßt mitunter bei papillennahem Sitz kleine Defekte am entsprechenden Kelch erkennen und bei Koagulaabgang Funktionsbehinderung, bzw. temporären Funktionsausfall.

Die nuclearmedizinischen Methoden ergeben keine wesentlichen Hinweise. Angiographisch sind die Angiome als kleine, zentral gelegene Gefäßkonvolute zu erkennen.

Angiome mit vorhandenem Shunt verursachen durch den Shunt außerdem eine Ernährungsstörung der regionären Parenchymbezirke mit ihren morphologischen Folgen und damit auch eine Behinderung der Funktion der Niere, die um so größer ist, je größer die Shuntrate ist. Die Übersichtsaufnahme des Abdomens ergibt keine Hinweise. Die Urographie zeigt verzögerte und verminderte Ausscheidung in die dazugehörigen Kelche, bzw. Kelchgruppe, meist mit Verkleinerung derselben oder auch retrograde Füllung dieser. Die nuclearmedizinischen Methoden ergeben im Szintigramm eine Verkleinerung der Nieren, sowie eine verminderte Speicherung. Im Renogramm findet man eine Abflachung des 2. Segmentes und eine Verzögerung des Abtransportes (3. Segment). Diese Veränderungen entsprechen der verminderten Durchblutung des Parenchyms, eingeschränkte tubulo-sektetorischer Sekretion, sowie verminderten Harnfluß.

Mit der Angiographie kann die Ausdehnung und Lokalisation des Angioms, die Größe des Shunts, die erweiterten zuführenden arteriellen, als auch abführenden venösen Anteile nachgewiesen werden und darüber hinaus auch oft morphologische Veränderungen des Nierenparenchyms.

Arterieller Kollateralkreislauf. Ganz allgemein bildet sich ein arterieller Kollateralkreislauf dann aus, wenn die das Erfolgsorgan versorgende Arterie hochgradig eingeengt oder verschlossen ist, so daß die für das Erfolgsorgan notwendige Mindestblutmenge über andere präformierte Bahnen, unter Umgehung des Hindernisses, herangeführt werden muß. Auch im Bereiche der Nieren ist die Möglichkeit der Ausbildung eines arteriellen Kollateralkreislaufes im Prinzip gegeben und ist abhängig von der Lokalisation des Hindernisses und davon, welche präformierten Gefäße für den Kollateralkreislauf zur Verfügung stehen. Man kann vorwiegend 3 Hauptsysteme des arteriellen Kollateralkreislaufes unterscheiden, über die das Blut letzten Endes zu den intrarenalen Gefäßen auf retrogradem Wege gelangt:

Kollateralsystem über die Aa. capsulares.
Kollateralsystem über die Aa. pelvicae und dem pelvinen Plexus.
Kollateralsystem über die Aa. uretericae.

Die Abdomenübersicht ergibt in der Regel eine kleinere Niere der betroffenen Seite, mitunter auch Verkalkung der Gefäße, vorwiegend dann, wenn das Hindernis arteriosklerotischer Natur ist. Die Ergebnisse der intravenösen Urographie und der nuklearmedizinischen Methoden hängen weitgehend von der Ausbildung des Kollateralkreislaufes ab. Bei schlecht ausgebildetem Kollateralkreislauf und Funktionsausfall im intravenösen Urogramm erfolgt im Szintigramm keine Darstellung des Organes und im Renogramm kein Nachweis renaler Funktion.

Bei gut ausgebildetem Kollateralkreislauf kann die Ausscheidung normal sein, ja die Dichte des Kontrastharnes kann sogar erhöht sein. Am Nierenbeckenkelchsystem und an den Ureteren sind Impressionen durch die erweiterten Kollateralgefäße nachzuweisen (scalloping und notching); im Szintigramm stellt sich gewöhnlich ein kleineres Organ mit verminderter Speicherung dar. Im Renogramm ist ein abgeflachtes 2. Segment und eine verlängerte intrarenale Transitzeit und verlangsamter Harntransport zu beobachten.

Die Angiographie, zur Darstellung des Kollateralkreislaufes am besten geeignet als Aortographie, mit pulssynchron gesteuerter Kontrastmittelinjektion durchgeführt, ergibt in allen Fällen und in allen Einzelheiten Aufschlüsse bezüglich des Hindernisses und des ausgebildeten Kollateralkreislaufes.

Zusammenfassend darf gesagt werden, daß derzeit für die exakte radiologische Diagnostik von Gefäßerkrankungen der Nieren, die Angiographie als die Methode der Wahl anzusehen ist. Alle anderen Methoden sind nicht spezifisch genug, um damit gleichwertige diagnostische Ergebnisse zu erreichen, es kommt ihnen die Rolle von Suchmethoden zu.

Die klinische Bedeutung der Weite und Konfiguration der Nierenarterien

H. LUDIN

Bei der Beurteilung von renalen Angiogrammen fällt auf, daß die Hauptstämme der Nierenarterien sich von Fall zu Fall hinsichtlich ihres Kalibers und ihrer Form beträchtlich voneinander unterscheiden. Da die Vermutung bestand, daß diese Verschiedenheiten nicht nur zufällig, sondern Ausdruck einer nierenphysiologischen Größe seien, wurde eine Untersuchung angestellt mit dem Ziel, einen Zusammenhang zwischen Nierenarterienkaliber und -form und gewissen Krankheitsgruppen zu finden. Die Serie, über welche nächstens in einer Publikation berichtet werden wird, umfaßt 458 Erwachsene und 127 Kinder. Gemessen wurden erstens der Durchmesser der Arterien, zweitens das Verhältnis des Quadrates des Arteriendurchmessers zum Nierengewicht, welches nomographisch aufgrund der Länge und Breite des radiologischen Nierenschattens geschätzt wurde, und schließlich noch die prozentuale Kaliberabnahme zwischen zwei Querschnitten, 1 und 3 cm vom aortalen Arterienabgang entfernt gemessen.

Sowohl frühere Untersuchungen unserer Gruppe in Form einer Korrelation zwischen Arterienweite und der PAH-Clearance, wie auch eine quantitative Behandlung von Rodbards Theorie ergaben, daß innerhalb nicht zu weiter Grenzen, die Nierendurchblutung eine quadratische Funktion des Nierenarterienkalibers ist. Für normale Nieren von Säuglingen, Kindern und Erwachsenen nimmt der Wert B eine annähernd konstante Größe, nämlich etwa $0{,}42 \pm 0{,}09$ mm^2 per Gramm geschätzten Nierengewichtes, an. Daraus und aus den erhältlichen tierexperimentellen und humanphysiologischen Daten wurde eine Korrelation zwischen Arterienweite und Nierendurchblutung errechnet. Die Untersuchungsreihe ergab auch Normalwerte für die Weite von Nierenarterien beim Kind in Abhängigkeit vom Alter und der Körperlänge sowie, im Zusammenhang mit zwei anderen Untersuchungsreihen, für das normale Nierengewicht beim Kind.

Die innerhalb gewisser Grenzen konstante Beziehung zwischen Arterienweite und geschätztem Nierengewicht spricht dafür, daß einerseits die Arterienweite eine Funktion der Nierendurchblutung, und daß andererseits die Nierendurchblutung von der Menge des vorhandenen funktionstüchtigen Nierenparenchyms abhängig ist. Tierexperimentelle Untersuchungen schwedischer Autoren sowie eigene und von anderen Untersuchern stammende klinisch-radiologische Beobachtungen sprechen dafür, daß sich die Arterienweite nur relativ langsam, d. h. innerhalb Wochen und Monaten an Veränderungen der durchschnittlichen Durchblutung anpaßt. Erfolgt eine solche Anpassung an eine Durchblutungsveränderung im späteren Kindesalter oder im Erwachsenenalter, so findet dieser Prozeß meistens seinen Ausdruck in einer Kaliberabnahme der Nierenarterien nach distal hin; ist die Durchblutungsverminderung extrem, so nimmt der Übergang des Ursprungs von der Aorta in die enge Renalis die Form eines abgerundeten Trichters an. Hat das Wachstum einer Niere durch eine frühkindliche Pyelonephritis aufgehört, d. h. bevor das Arteriensystem die Dimensionen des Erwachsenen angenommen hat, so wird die enge Nierenarterie einen konstanten Durchmesser aufweisen; dasselbe wird auch bei der sehr seltenen Nierenhypoplasie beobachtet, gleich wie eine kompensatorische Hypertrophie der gegenseitigen Niere.

Eine Abnahme des Nierenarterienkalibers ist also ein Zeichen für die Abnahme des Volumens von funktionstüchtigem Nierenparenchym, sei diese nun durch Druckatrophie bedingt wie z. B. bei der Hydronephrose oder bei Cystennieren oder aber durch entzündlich bedingten Parenchymuntergang wie hauptsächlich bei der Pyelonephritis, der interstitiellen Nephritis, aber auch bei der Glomerulonephritis, Tuberkulose, Nephrokalcinose usw. Entsprechende Veränderungen zeigen sich dann auch beim Parameter B wie oben definiert.

Wenn auch die Aortographie nicht die Prozedur der ersten Wahl bei der Abklärung parenchymatöser Nierenerkrankungen ist, so scheint sie doch eine wichtige Information zu liefern: nämlich die Menge des noch vorhandenen funktionstüchtigen Parenchyms bei chronischen Nierenerkrankungen.

Comparison of Angiographic and Scintigraphic Findings in Localized and Generalized Alterations of the Renal Arteries

G. Stephan and R. Zimmer

Localized alterations of renal vessels, such as arterial stenosis or infarcts, can easlily be demonstrated by renovasography. Difficulties arise, however, in the angiographic diagnosis of generalized changes of the renal vessels in arteriosclerosis or pyelonephritis.

We compared the angiographic and scintigraphic findings in order to define the possible value of renal scintigraphy as an additional method.

Patients with hypertension, in whom localized or generalized alterations of renal vessels could be demonstrated by angiography, were selected. Renal angio-

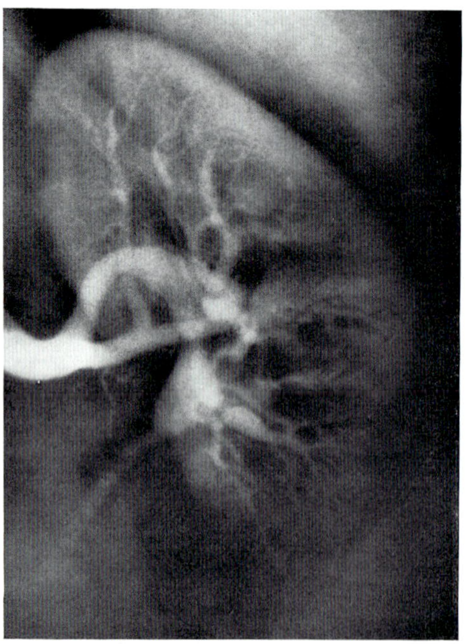

a

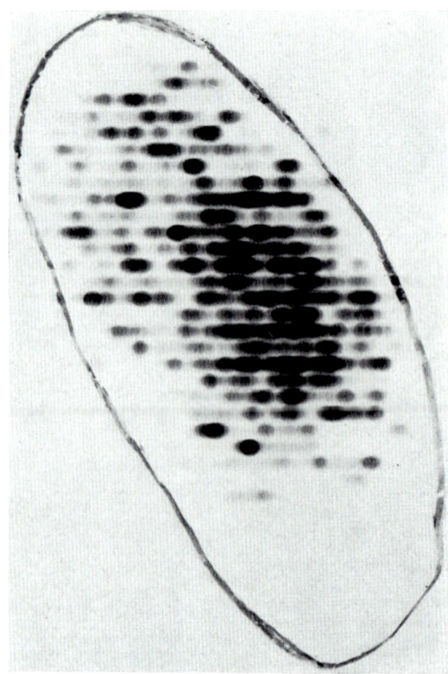

b

Fig. 1. a Selective angiography of the left kidney: Intrarenal stenosis of a segmental artery in the lower part. b Scintigram: Patches of diminished activity in the whole kidney, particularly distinct in the area of hypoxaemia as shown by angiography

graphy was performed in all cases using the Seldinger-Technique. In most cases also selective angiography was carried out. Renal scintigraphy followed after the application of 150–200 μCi ^{197}Hg-Chlormerodrin.

The results of our comparison are demonstrated by the following examples:

Localized Alterations of the Renal Arteries

Where infarcts had recently occured we found in the scintigram a localized decreased activity in the affected area. Other cases in later stages showed scarred deformations of the kidney. Intrarenal stenosis of segmental arteries appeared likewise in the scintigram as localized areas of reduced radioactivity where the hypoxaemia occured and occasionally patches of diminished activity in the remaining parts of the kidney (Fig. 1).

These patches of diminished activity with or without reduction in kidney size, where stenosis of the renal artery was present, were scintigraphically particularly impressive.

We found in accordance with the examples above that in localized processes of the renal arteries, the scintigraphic and angiographic findings corresponded. Such scintigraphic results, however, can not be considered specific, as emphasised by ZUM WINKEL. The existence of a vascular process is demonstrated first of all by renovasography.

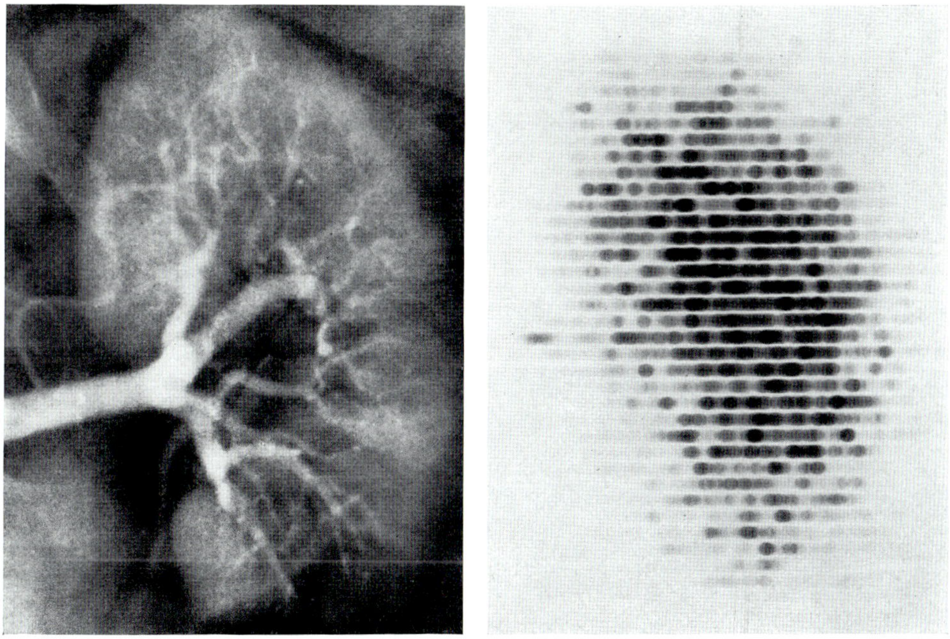

a b

Fig. 2. a Selective angiography of the left kidney: Barely indicated rarefaction, coiling and changing calibre of the intrarenal arteries. b Scintigram: Reduced density of activity, irregular shape of the whole organ

Generalized Alterations of Renal Arteries

Our angiographic diagnosis of a generalized renal vascular process is based on the following criteria:

1. Elongation and narrowing of the renal trunk artery.
2. Rarefaction, coiling and changing calibre of the intrarenal arteries.
3. Thinning of the renal cortex.
4. Irregular shape and shrinking of the kidneys.

We dispensed with the differentiation between arteriosclerosis and pyelonephritis by angiography because of the problems described by PYTEL and WILLMANN *et al.* In cases where rarefaction, coiling and changing calibre of the intrarenal arteries are barely hinted at by angiography, areas of reduced density of activity were to be found in the scintigram (Fig. 2). Irregular outlining, without shrinking of the kidneys, could often be seen. In advanced stages, with bilateral elongation and multiple stenosis, a diminution of the kidneys could be seen in the scintigram. The pathological pattern of distribution of activity was distinctly shown in these cases.

We established that also in generalized renal processes the angiographic and scintigraphic findings correspond. Renovasography often only hints at intrarenal vascular changes. In these cases renal scintigraphy is able to confirm or refuse the angiographic findings.

Angiography and Scintigraphy of Inflammatory Renal Diseases

TH. LAUBENBERGER and G. OBERHAUSEN

This statement is basing on 70 cases of inflammatory renal diseases and 62 cases of renal tuberculosis.

Angiography and scintigraphy are of no value for the diagnosis of acute pyelonephritis. Reduced blood flow of the parenchyma and decreased activity as results of the oedema of renal tissue will give no characteristic findings.

Advanced chronic pyelonephritis shows a diffuse or patchy distribution in the organ. Atherosclerotic changes of intrarenal vessels will be early found in scarred tissue. The concerned arteries are shortened towards the periphery and often tourtuous. Renal vessels of scarred tissue appearing like "cutted trees". Irregular accummulations of contrast medium are found because of shrinking and contraction. There is an unsharp border between medulla and cortex. Infarct – like defects and scar tissue of the parenchyma may be best shown by angiotomography.

Scintigraphy is less successful, approximately a half of our cases of chronic pyelonephritis will be detected by this method.

There will be a delayed renal medulla phase, inhomogenous activity, irregular surface of the kidney caused by scarring changes.

32 patients with advanced renal shrinkage had no activity enrichment in scintigraphy. Angiography is of great value to detect secondary renal shrinkage. With angiography it is possible to distinguish secondary renal shrinkage from renal hypoplasia.

The normal pattern of intrarenal vessels and their uninjured appearence gives the chance to decide for the diagnosis renal hypoplasia. We could demonstrate this in 6 cases. Scintigraphy will have a distinct activity in hypoplasia, activity will be missed in advanced renal shrinkage. Pyonephrosis and renal carbuncle can be diagnosed by angiography. Scintigrams of this diseases are not typical.

Perinephritis and paranephritis cannot be recognized by scintigraphy or angiography. Internal atrophy of the kidney, the lipomatosis renalis can be demonstrated by scintigraphy and angiography.

Selective angiography is indispensible in renal tuberculosis. It shows not only the vascular pattern and changes in the region of the tuberculosis focus but also the state of remaining parenchyma. The investigator will be informed about the kind of progress of the disease, shrinkage or necrosis. With scintigraphy normal parenchyma will show activity. Activity in tuberculous focus will be diminished or vanished.

The important aspect is that angiography shows simultaneously pathological vessels and normal vascular structure.

Advanced tuberculosis without excretion of contrast medium in urogram will have no renal isotope activity by scintigraphy.

In this cases angiography will reveal the whole destructions of tuberculous changes of the kidney.

Table. *Comparison of the diagnostic value of angiography and scintigraphy*

	Angiography	Scintigraphy
Acute pyelonephritis	—	—
Chronic pyelonephritis	+	+
Pyonephrosis and carbuncle	—	—
Paranephritis and perinephritis	+	—
Tuberculosis tuberculous focus	+	+
Advanced renal tuberculosis (without excretion of contrast medium in urography)	+	—

Comparison of Angiographic and Scintigraphic Findings in Unilateral Renal Lesions Accompanied by Hypertension

H. WIENERS and D. NOVAK

Urography, renovasography and split clearence examination are methods of choice in the preoperative evaluation of patients with unilateral renal lesions as a cause of hypertension. Opinions are contradictory regarding the validity of renal scanning in the assesment of renal ischemia (HAYNIE *et al.*, 1961; WESTPHAL *et al.* 1962; COHEN *et al.*, 1963; ZUM WINKEL, 1964). Therefore the value of renal scanning in patients with angiographically demonstrated destruction of renal parenchyma was studied in order to localise and to evaluate the degree of renal demage. The correlation of findings of renovasography and renal scanning in assesment of unilateral loss of renal parenchyma accompanied by increased prerenal or intrarenal renal blood flow resistance as a cause of hypertension is demonstrated in typical cases.

Methods

Renovasography was performed by Seldinger technique. After placement of catheter in the abdominal aorta the contrast medium (60–70 ml Angiographin[1]) was injected by means of Gidlund automatic injector with a pressure of 6–7 kg/cm^2. Serial roentgenogramms (2–3 per sec) were taken using automatic film changer. For better evaluation of intrarenal vasculature as a rule a selective catheterisation of renal artery and manual injection of contrast medium was performed additionally.

Renal scanning was performed after injection of 150–200 μCi ^{197}Hg-labeled chlormerodrin. Renal scanning was followed by registration of count rates over cranial, middle and caudal regions of each kidney. The radioactivity of the given region was compared with the highest count rate registered over contralateral kidney (R_{max} = 100%). The difference calculated was expressed in percentage of maximal accumulation of ^{197}Hg-Chlormerodrin. A deviation from 20–35% was considered as slight reduction of the accumulation of Chlormerodrin as a measure of destruction of functioning renal parenchyma. Differences from 35–60% were concerned as medium and differences over 60% as severe reduction of functioning renal parenchyma.

The correlation of angiographic and scintigraphic findings as well as the results of radioactivity measurements over three defined regions of the kidney were performed in the following cases of renal diseases:

1 (® Schering A.G.)

1. congenital hypoplastic kidney with pyelonephritis
2. hypoplastic renal artery accompanied with parenchymal lesions
3. multiple renal arteries with lokalised pyelonephritis
4. fibromuscular hyperplasia of renal artery
5. renal artery aneurysm
6. unilateral chronic pyelonephritis
7. unilateral or localised atherosclerotic plaques with renal arterial thrombosis
8. unilateral thromboangitis obliterans of renal arteries
9. ischemia due to renal artery embolism and infarction.

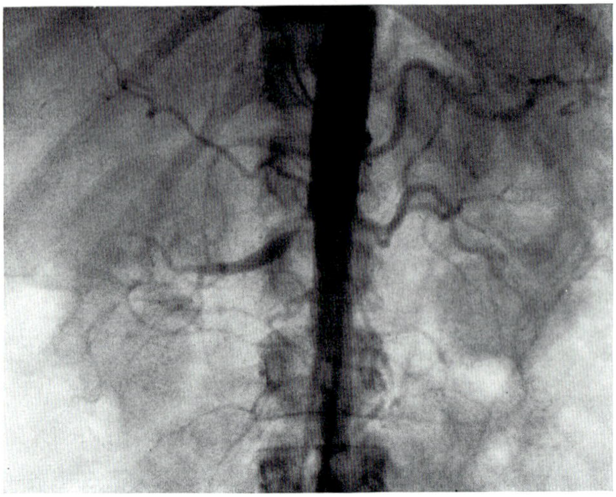

a

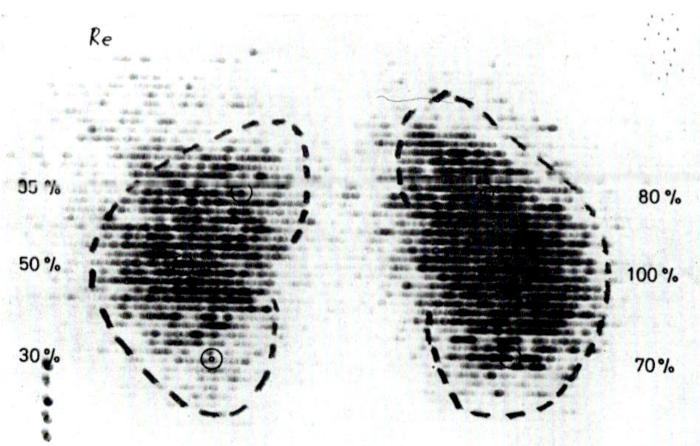

b

Fig. 1a and b. Angiogram (a) demonstrates stenosis of right renal artery and atrophic right kidney with the signs of pyelonephritis. Renal scan (b) shows an irregular radioactivity pattern and an overall reduction of radioactivity for about 50 %

Case Reports

Case 1: 32 year female with histologically proven unilateral pyelonephritis and destruction of renal parenchyma as sequelae of right renal artery stenosis. Angiogram (A) demonstrates stenosis of right renal artery and atrophic right kidney with the signs of pyelonephritis. Renal scan (B) shows an irregular radioactivity pattern and an overall decreased chlormerodrin uptake. In comparison with contralateral kidney reduction of radioactivity for nearly 50 % over the total kidney. Operation showed an atrophic right kidney with complicating pyelonephritis. Nephrektomie was performed.

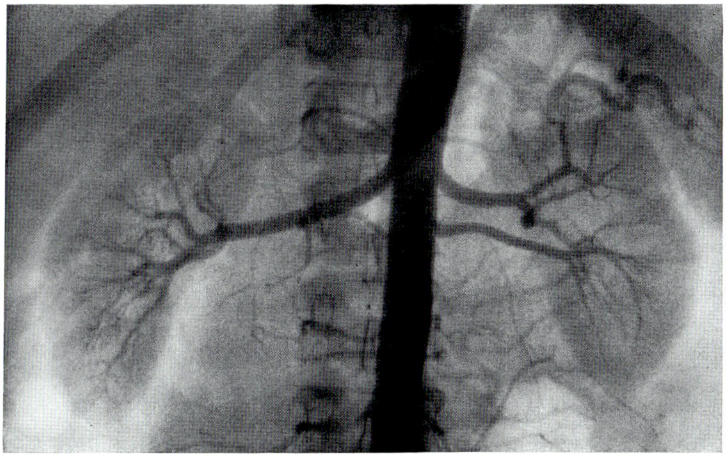

a

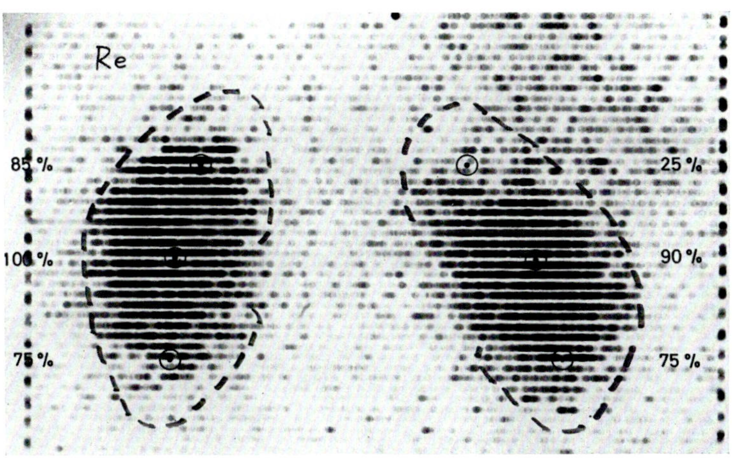

b

Fig. 2a and b. Angiogram (a) shows multiple renal arteries left and signs of renal parenchymal demage of the upper pol. Renal scan (b) demonstrates reduction of radioactivity over the cranial pol of the left kidney for 60 % in comparison with the cranial pol of the contralateral kidney

Case 2 : 29 year male with hypertension and operatively proven localised pyelonephritis in cranial pol of the left kidney. Angiogram (A) demonstrates multiple renal arteries and signs of renal parenchymal damage. Renal scan (B) shows reduction of radioactivity over the cranial part of the left kidney. Measurement of radioactivity in comparison with contralateral kidney shows a reduction of 60 %. Cranial pol resection of left kidney was performed. Hypertension was significantly decreased.

Discussion and Conclusions

Correlation of findings of renovasography and renal scanning demonstrates that evaluation of pathological changes of renal vasculature and damage of renal parenchyma is a topic of renovasography. The quantification of destruction of renal parenchyma based on visual evaluation of angiographic as well as scintigraphic findings could not be performed with sufficient accuracy. Since accumulation of Radiochlormerodrin is highly specific for functioning renal parenchyma, the simple method of quantification and comparison with the accumulation of Chlormerodrin in the contralateral kidney is proposed for preoperative assesment of patient with unilateral or localised renal diseases accompanied by hypertension.

According to our studies the final diagnosis of unilateral renal disease should be based on a combination of renovasography and renal scanning. A very reliable criterion of comparing the function of one kidney with the other is the ratio of the rate of radiochlormerodrin accumulation measured over three defined regions of each kidney. Renovasography and renal scanning are complementary examination methods in evaluation of the etiology of renovascular hypertension. The correlation of findings of both methods facilitates a decision, whether nephrectomy or more conservative operations (heminephrectomy, segmental resection or plastic surgery of renal artery) should be performed. Both methods allow to predict the effect of corrective surgery in the treatment of renal hypertension due to unilateral renal diseases.

Comparative Angiographic and Scintigraphic Studies in Chronic Renal Disease

L. V. Habighorst and K. J. Schmidt

About 100 patients were studied with reference to the yield of angiographic and scintigraphic methods in chronic renal disease. For kidney scanning we have used since 1966 ^{99m}Tc-Iron (II)-Ascorbic-Acid Complex, a tracer which is primarily returned and excreted in the renal tubules. It can be accumulated only by a functioning renal parenchyma. Angiography was performed according to Hettler's technique as abdominal aortography, followed in most cases by selective renal arteriography.

Unilateral decrease in scanning activity may be prerenal in origin. Restricted perfusion in patients with renal artery stenosis can lead unilaterally to a spuriously small

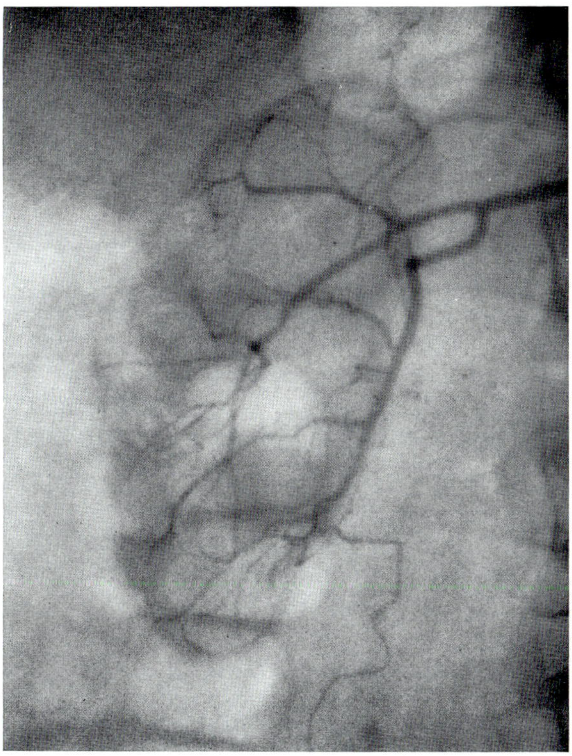

Fig. 1a and b. Shrunken kidney (hydronephrosis). a Selective arteriogram

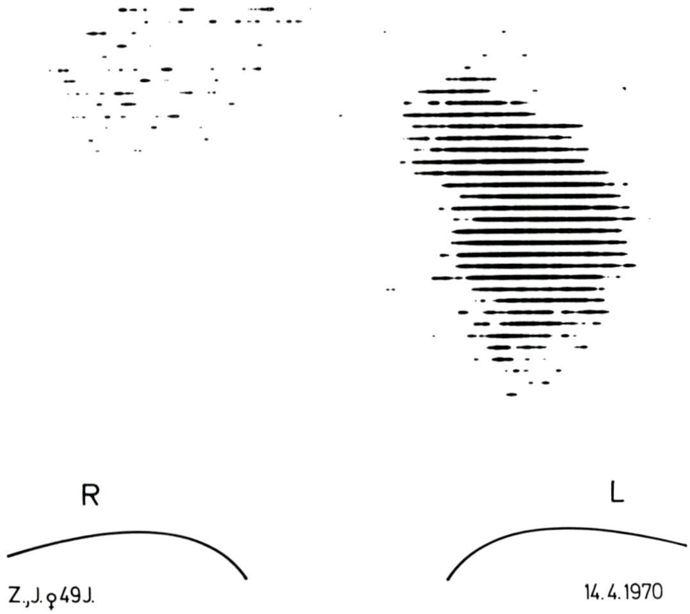

Fig. 1. b Scintigram, completely absent tracer activity

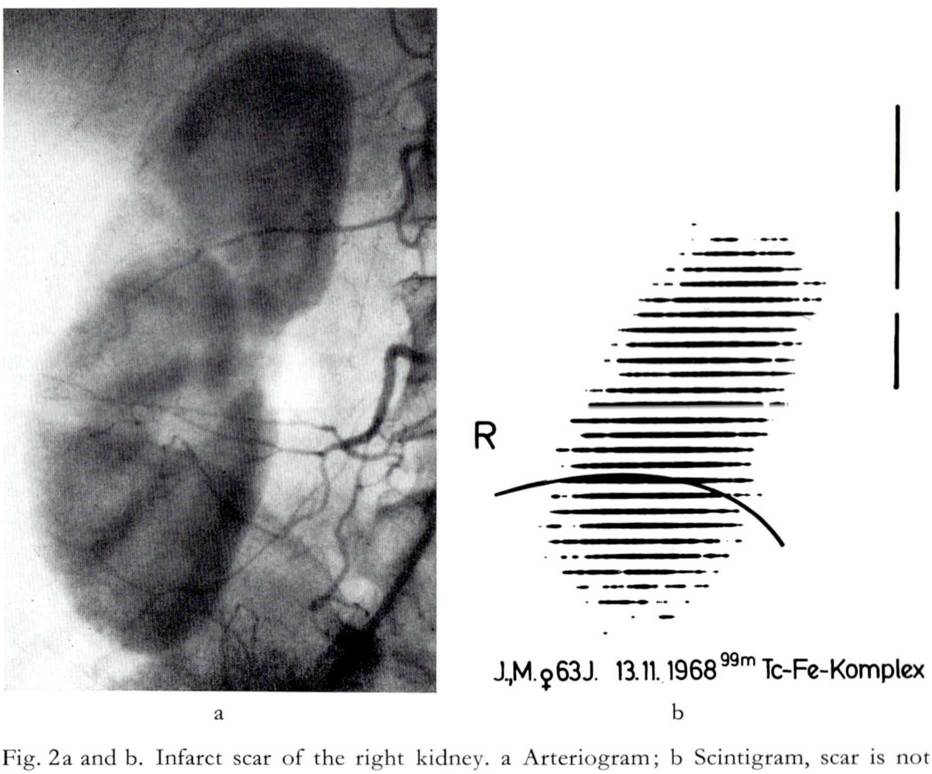

a b

Fig. 2a and b. Infarct scar of the right kidney. a Arteriogram; b Scintigram, scar is not recognizable appearing kidney. Differences in activity can be determined by calculation of impulse-rate quotients.

Whereas angiography in uni- or bilaterally decreased kidney size is productive of considerable morphologic detail, the scan usually shows only reduced, nonhomogenous, or completely absent tracer activity. Scanning is not helpful in the elucidation of unilateral renal insufficiency. The diagnosis can often be made angiographically. This patient (Fig. 1) demonstrates a shrunken kidney as a result of hydronephrosis.

The recognition of discrete parenchymal lesions with scanning is limited by its relatively minimal resolution. An infarct scar on the lateral aspect of the kidney is just barely discernible in the scan (Fig. 2). Smaller scars in the cortex are not definitely recognizable.

The scan in renal tuberculosis shows defective accumulation, deformities, differential activity from one side to the other, and, in cases with compromised ureteral flow, tracer activity in the renal pelvis. Diminished or absent tracer activity in advanced renal tuberculosis reflects the marginal collecting capacity of the renal parenchyma. Scans are nonspecific, yet yield in many cases a good impression of the extent of parenchymal destruction. In contrast, angiography can delineate essential morphologic details, especially important with regard to intended operative measures.

The renal scan alone is not sufficiently informative in the majority of patients with chronic renal disease. Entirely different pathologic processes can produce similar, thus nonspecific, scans. Advantages of renal scanning include simplicity of performance without special preparation and minimal risk even for the severly ill patient, as well as repeatability as a control study throughout the course of the illness. The scan affords an impression of renal size, form and position even in the presence of azotemia. In renal disease with reduced parenchyma, angiography in the arterial and nephrographic phase offers differential diagnostic information in addition to the individual findings obtained.

Comparing Scintigraphic and Angiographic Tests with Peripheral Renal Processes

M. Nuic and H. H. Wagner

Morphological and functional changes of the parenchyma in its cortex zone can only be determined by means of specific radiological and nuclear medical methods of examination.

By means of the scintigraphy and angiography which are different in their contents of information, the character, the localisation and the stage of spreading of such processes can extensively be analysed.

The storage picture of the kidney represents the distribution of function within individual sections of the parenchyma. This is based on the maintained storage function of the renal tubule. With that a finer differentiation is possible between diffuse nephropathies with unilateral and bilateral involvement of the parenchyma and circumscribed processes. Focal, tumoral and nontumoral processes, difficult to be determined by means of other methods, can scintigraphically be visualised also in peripheral localisation. This applies also to the circumscribed lesions of inflammatory geneses (Heptinstall, 1965) which remain compensated for a long time defying any functional diagnosis. The said lesions provide most frequently characteristic findings in the scintigram by a typical image form and localisation (Hodson) whereas the differentiation of other focal processes by means of the scintigram is limited. In this respect scintigraphy requires further diagnostic criteria.

In comparison with it, the angiogram demonstrates changes of the intrarenal vascular structures in respect of a deficiency, a rarefaction or a vascular neogenesis. In the phase of the nephrographic effect diverse densities of the parenchyma are demonstrated. Furthermore changes of the larger vessels can be determined definitely. Whilst intrarenal processes richly vascularized in the angiogram mostly intimate malignant changes, the differential diagnosis with poorly vascularized processes is often very difficult. The complementary possibilites of both methods were investigated in 280 cases. In the following some cases will be demonstrated:

The considerable shrinkage of the parenchyma shown in the scintigram and in the infusion pyelogram with the missing representation of the upper calyx formation and the amputation of the upper renal pole intimated a tumoral process (Figs. 1 and 2).

The layer aortogram as well as the selective presentation of the left kidney show an excessive shrinkage in the area of the upper renal pole with a hypoplastic upper pole artery and missing parenchyma presentation. The criteria present in the vascular and parenchyma phase of the angiogram intimate a shrinking process in the area

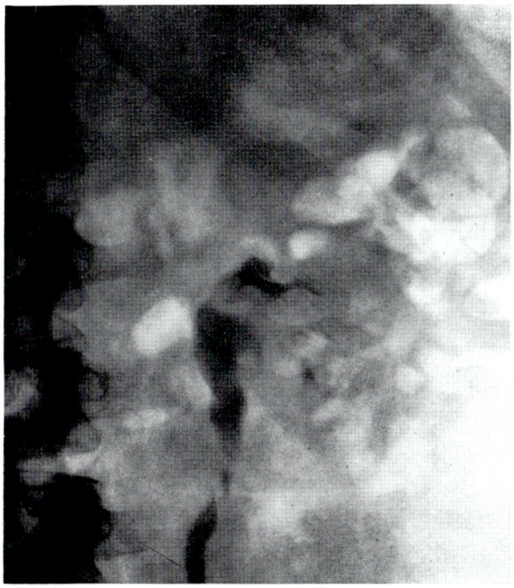

Fig. 1a

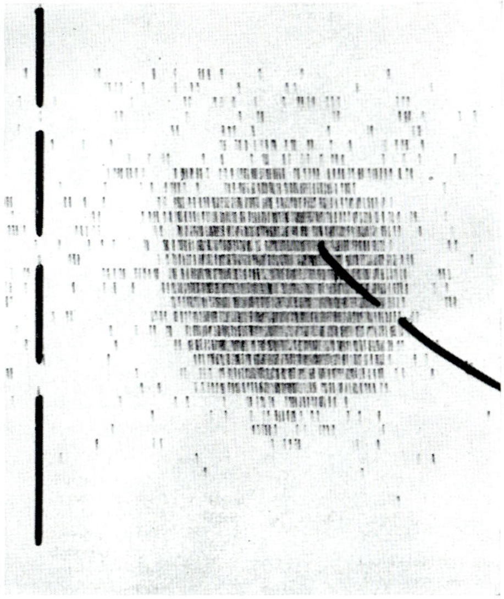

Fig. 1b

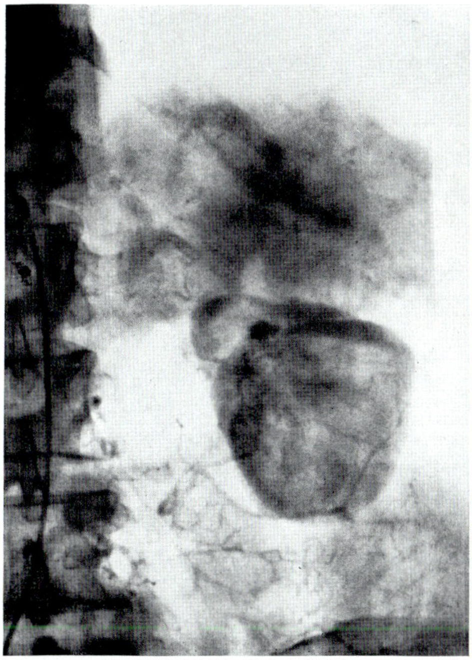

Fig. 2a

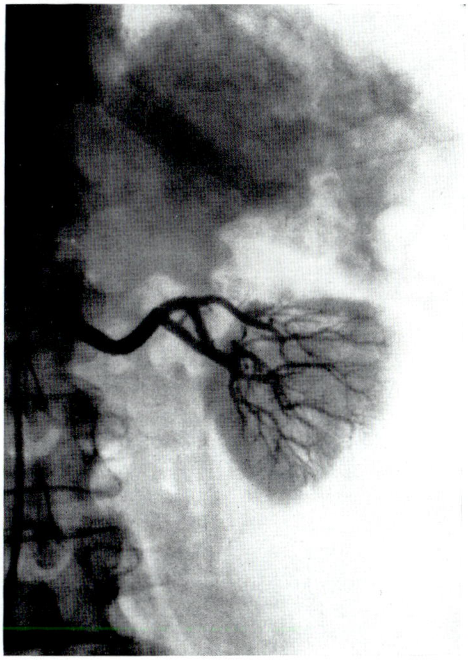

Fig. 2b

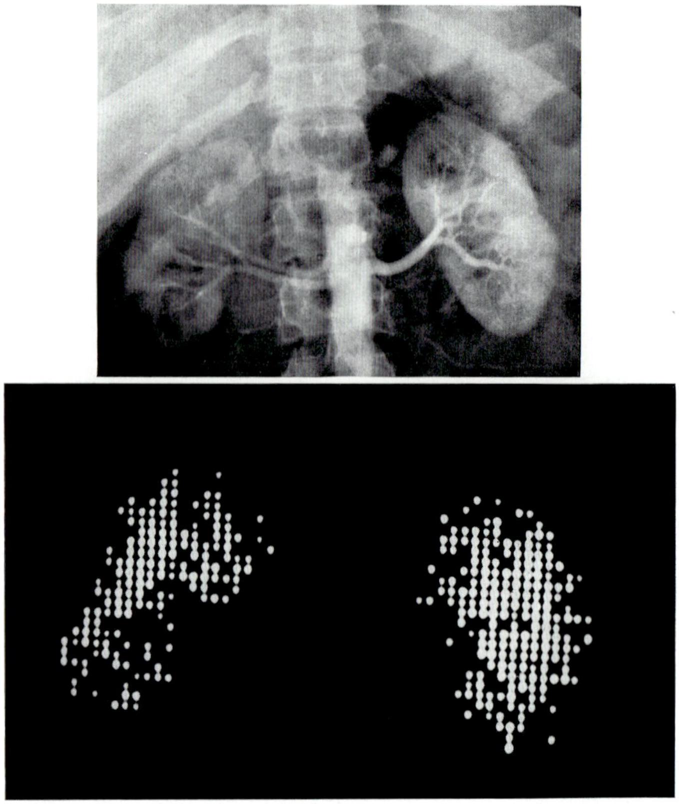

Fig. 3

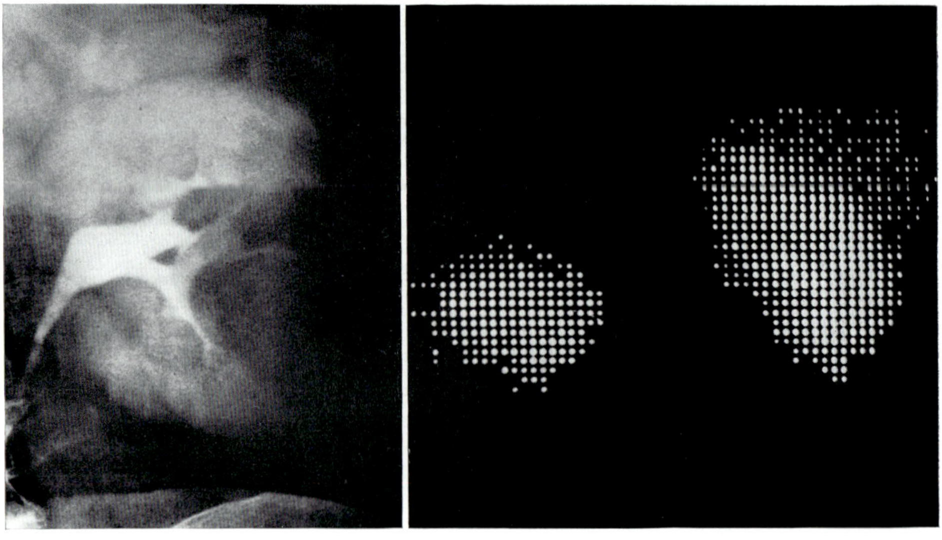

Fig. 4

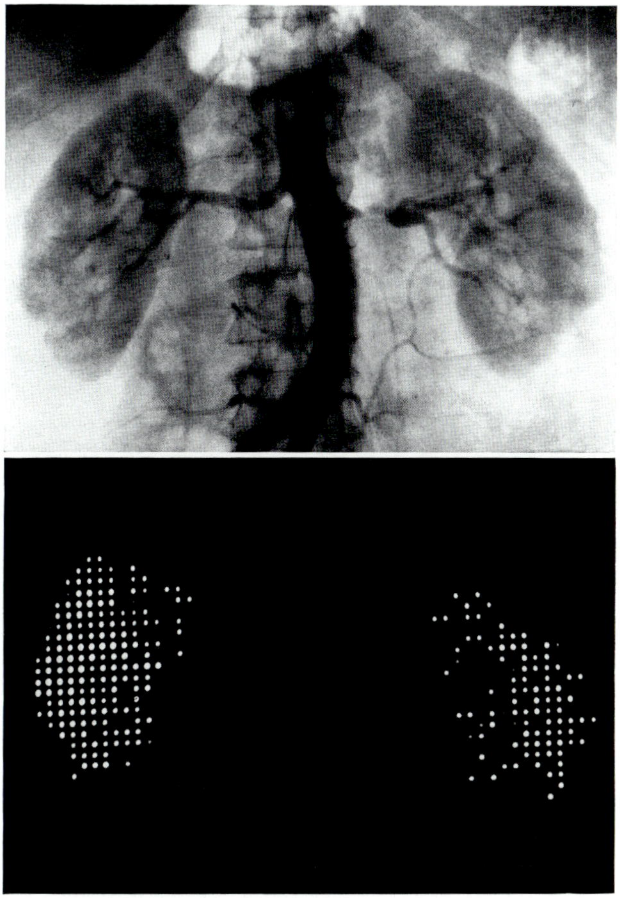

Fig. 5

of the upper renal pole. The operation report confirmed this assumption. There were no criteria intimating the existence of a tumoral process.

Figure 3 demonstrates the form of a clinically evidenced chronic pyelonephritis with rarefaction of the peripheral vessels in the aortogram and circumscribed recesses in the scintigram.

Renal cyste of the size of a small apple – evidenced by operation – in the infusion pyelogram and the renal scintigram (Fig. 4).

With a unilateral arteriostenosis in the angiogram, a strongly reduced concentration on the stenosed side is shown in the nuclear storage scintigram as a result of a reduced blood circulation. Slight deficiency of function in the upper pole of the contralateral kidney (Fig. 5).

With a circumscribed storage deficiency in the medium part of the right kidney with reduced global storage capacity (as a result of compensatorily increased liver concentration) (the patient had been referred to the hospital because of haematuria and decrease in weight) no unequivocal vascular or parenchyma changes could

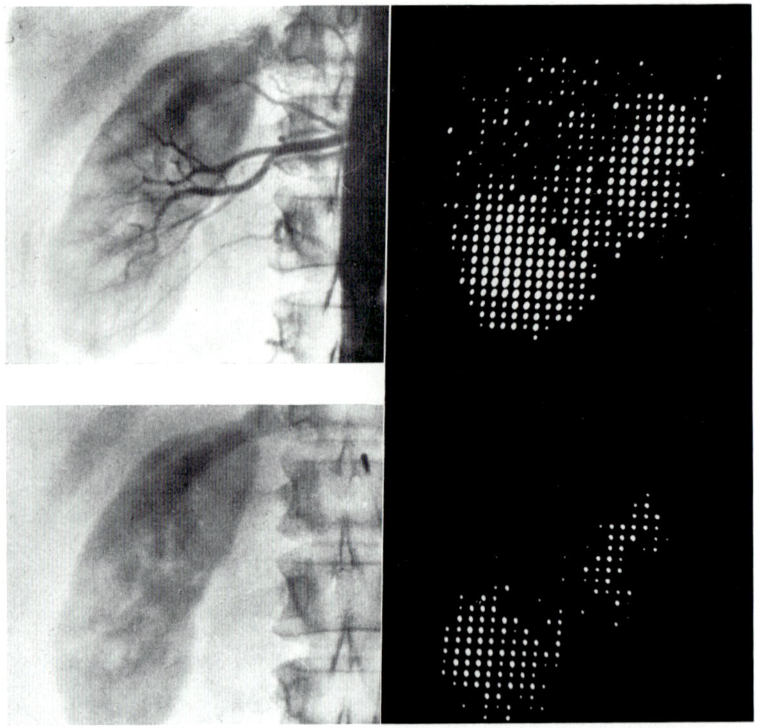

Fig. 6

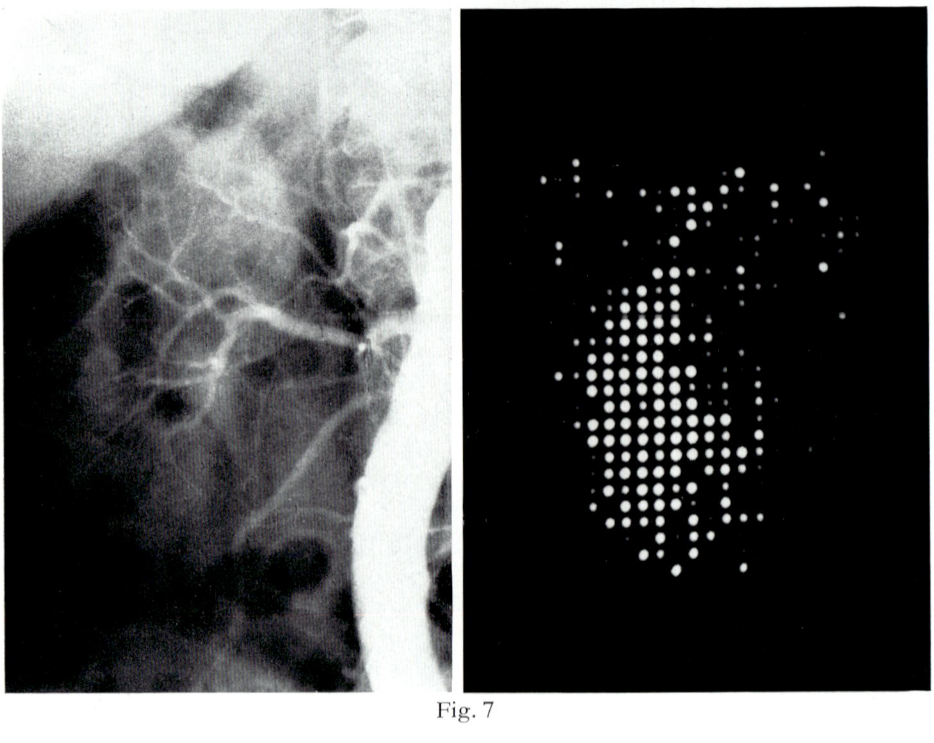

Fig. 7

angiographically be evidenced. This case represents a renal tumor evidenced by operation (Fig. 6).

Contrary to this, the case on Figure 7 shows a rarefaction – evident in the angiogram – of the vascular structure in the area of an enlarged upper renal pole. The scintigram showed in the same zone circumscribed recesses with convex renal contour. Both methods correspond in indicating the functional and morphological changes in the sense of a chronic inflammation.

Summary

In 280 cases the representability of peripheral parenchyma processes by means of scintigraphy and angiography is analysed. Whereas the scintigraphy demonstrates also discreet focal lesions of the parenchyma, differential diagnostic evidence – especially with respect to vascular and tumoral processes – is only possible by means of angiography. The two methods complement each other well in their efficiency of evidence and are superior to any other methods in the diagnosis of circumscribed renal processes. The indicated examples of some cases demonstrate evidence value and limits of the method.

Comparative Angiographic and Isotope Studies of the Kidneys

F. S. Fuchs, E. Ogris and F. Olbert

Patients presenting with a clinical symptomatology suggestive of renal processes, whose urograms are equivocal, are generally subjected to topographic angiography and selective angiographic studies of either one or both kidneys. These may be supplemented by the applikation of adrenalin. Causes underlying regional differences in intrarenal ^{131}I Hippuran transport can be clarified by Scintillation Camera isotope nephrography. By converting the analogue tracing into digital patterns with the help of a 4096 channel analyser, functional deficits can be traced with a high measure of accuracy.

Finally isotopes, which yield data of the regional blood flow of an organ (serial scintigrams using ^{99m}Tc or ^{131}I-MAA) intra-arterial, serve to establish whether areas with loss of function which manifest themselves as deficits on the chlormerodrin scan are vascularized or not, thus permitting, to a large extent, a differentiation of tumors and cysts (Fig. 1).

From January to July 1970 90 patients with urologic conditions, including 45 with suspected space occupying renal processes, underwent differentiated isotope stubies. 31 patients with suspected renal tumors were, in addition, subjected to angiography.

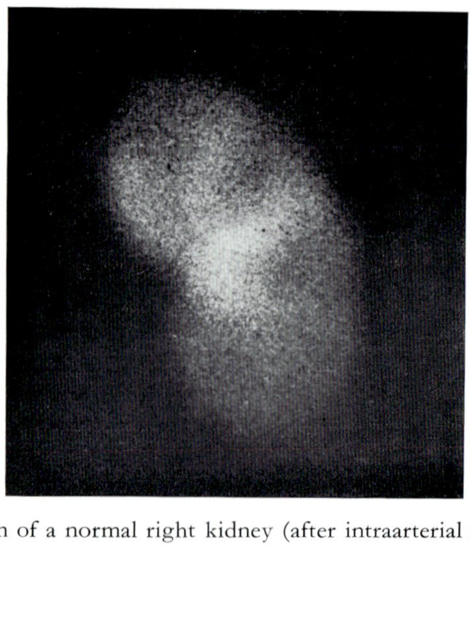

Fig. 1. Angioscintigram of a normal right kidney (after intraarterial injection of ^{131}I-MAA)

Table. *Isotope studies for urologic conditions*

90
patients

suspected renal tumor
45 patients

angiography and scintigraphy
31
patients

20
surgery omitted

15
both tests
negative

5
Ang. neg.
Isot. pos.
but not
grave

11
surgery performed

7
preop.
diagn.
corrob.

4
Ang. false
incl. 2 false
Isot. results

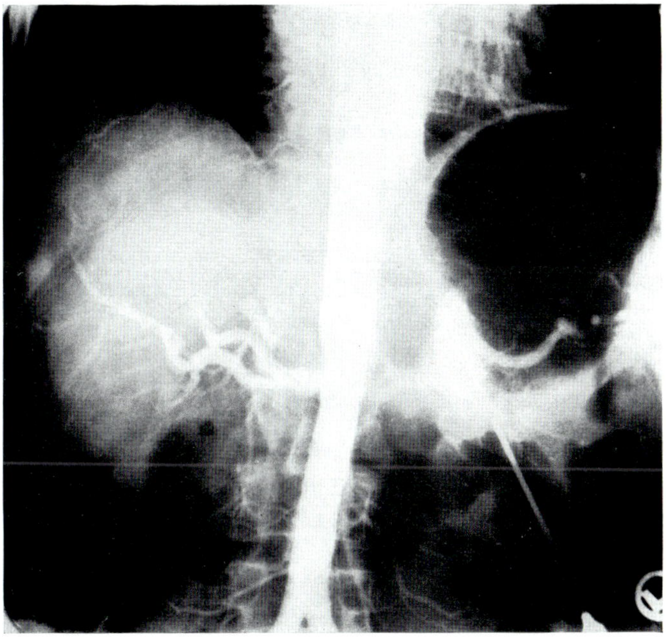

Fig. 2a. Topographic angiogram

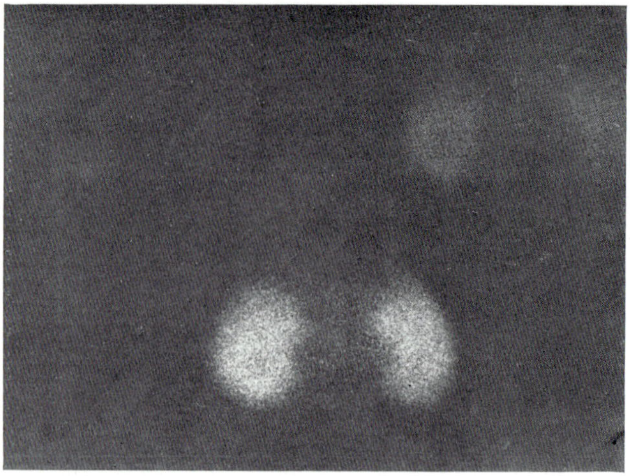

Fig. 2b. ^{197}HG-Chlormerodrin scintigram showing reduced activity in lower part of the left kidney

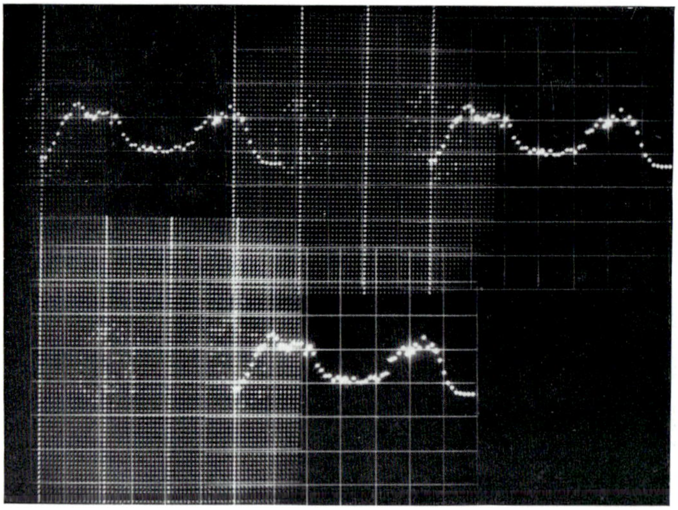

Fig. 2c. Digital display of the picture 2b showing activity profile through lower part of both kidneys

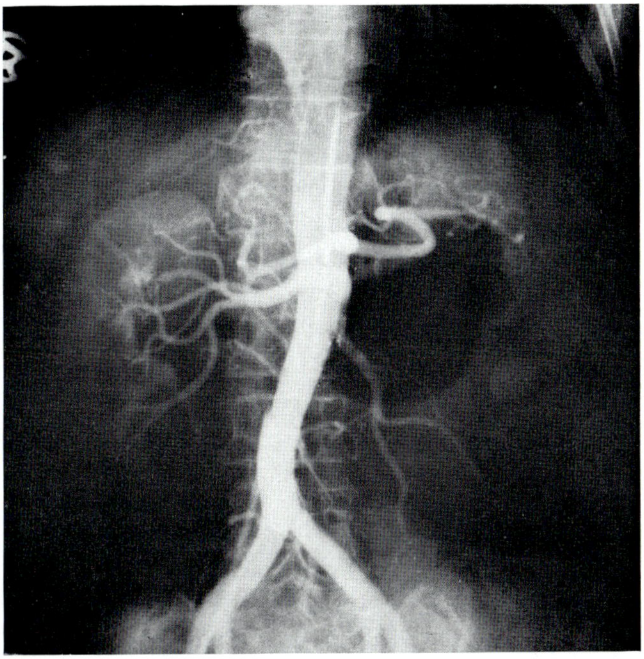

Fig. 3a. Topographic angiogram

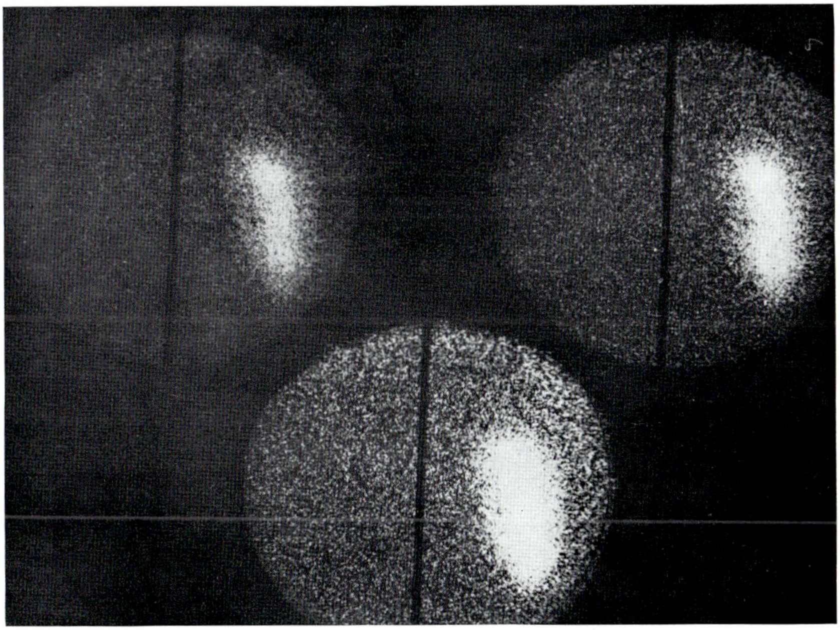

Fig. 3b. ^{131}I-Hippuran scintigram

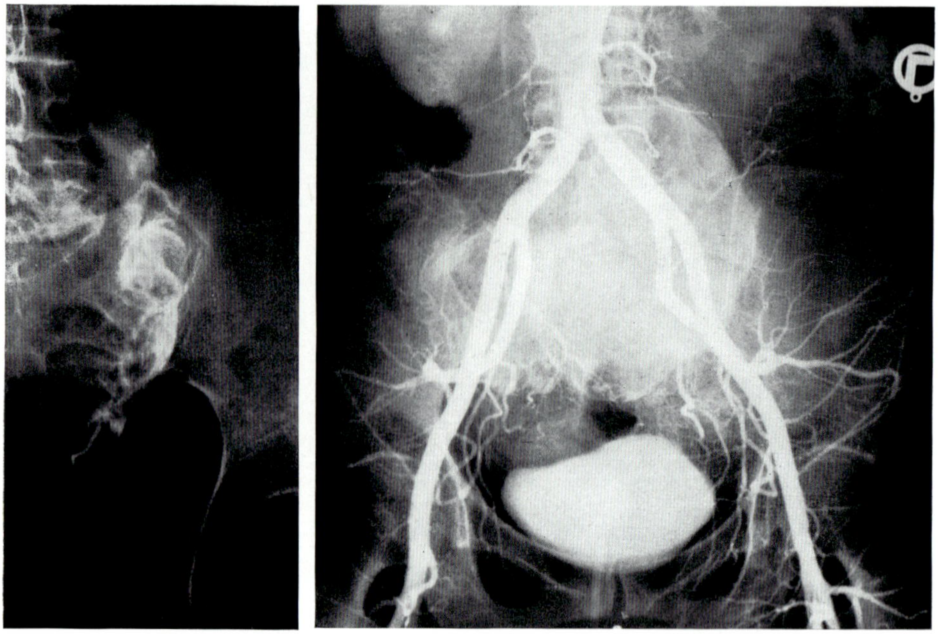

c d

Fig. 3c. Retrograde Pyelography. d Pelvic Angiography

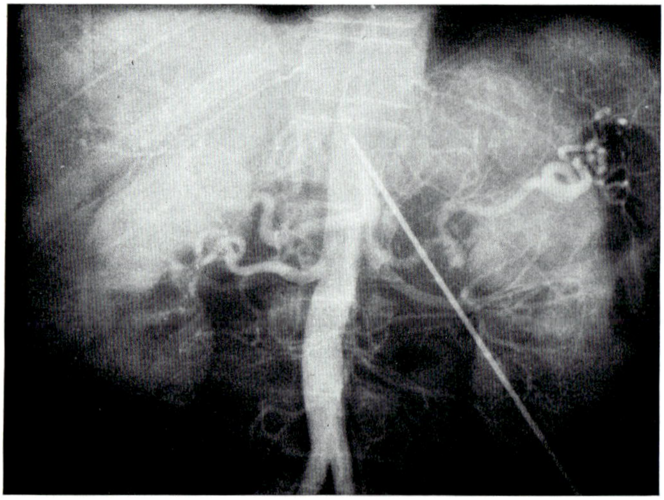

Fig. 4a. Topographic angiography

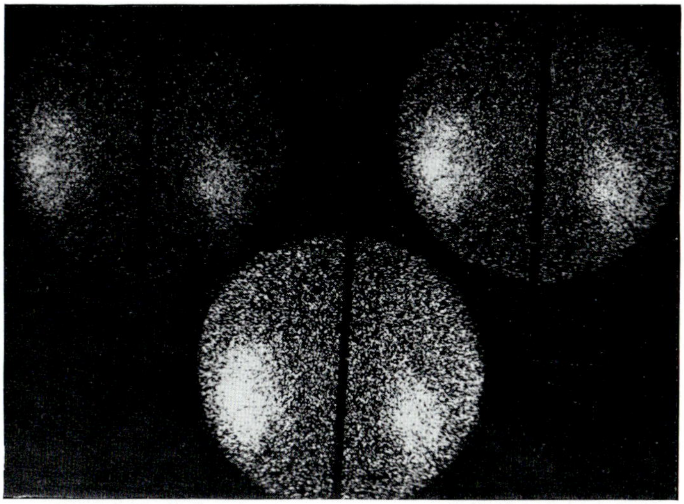

Fig. 4b. ^{131}I-Hippuran scintigram

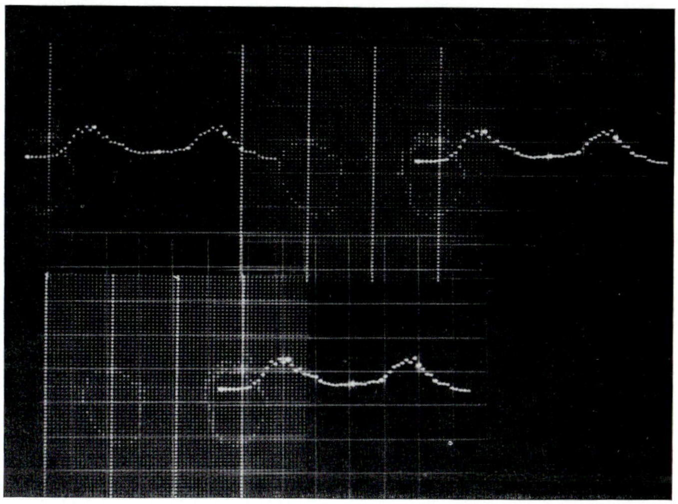

Fig. 4c. Digital display of ^{197}Hg scintigram showing normal activity profiles through upper part of both kidneys

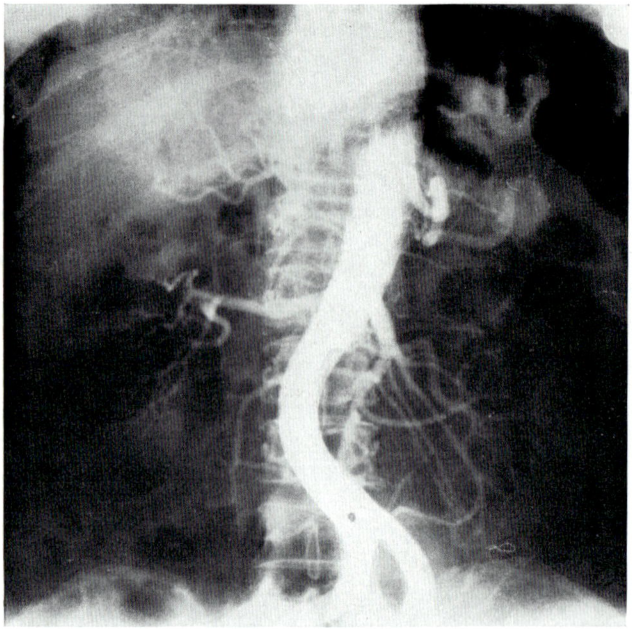

Fig. 5a. Topographic angiography

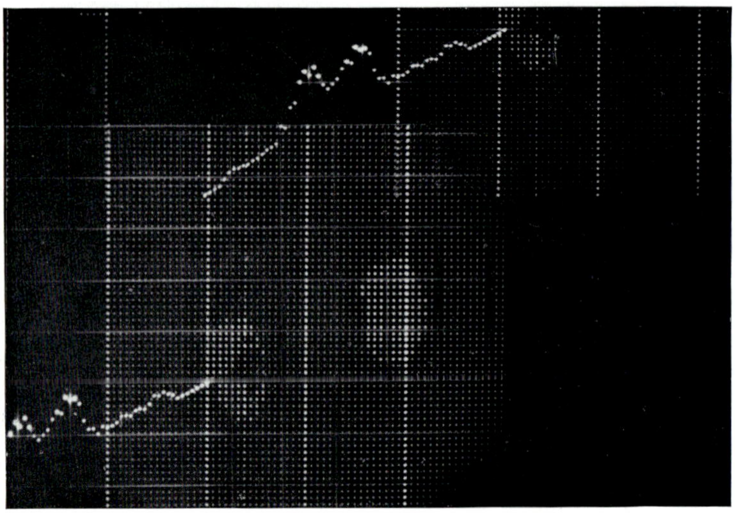

Fig. 5b. Digital display of ^{197}Hg-Chlormerodrin scintigram with activity profile showing large defect in left kidney

In 20 of these patients surgical exposure of the kidney proved to be unnecessary. Both procedures yielded negativ results in 15 cases. In the remaining 5 cases angiologic data were noncontributory, while the results of the isotope studies were not grave enough to warrant exposure of the organ. These 5 patients were scheduled for follow-up examinations.

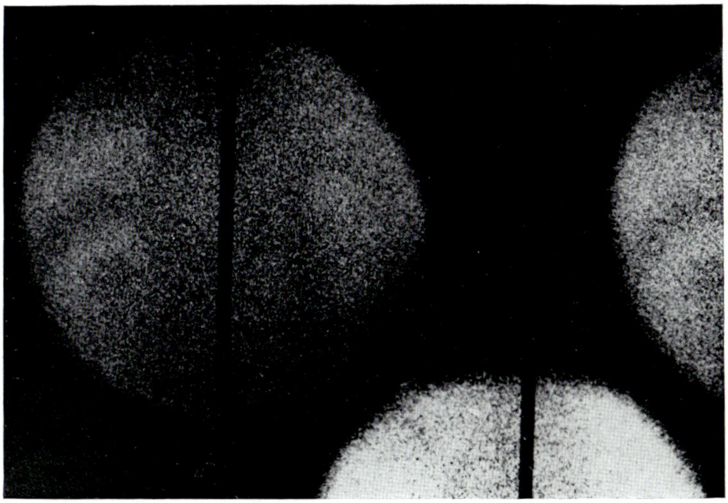

Fig. 5c. Perfusion scintigram (^{99m}Tc i. v.) showing activity defect in corresponding area

Surgery was performed in 11 patients, and the preoperative diagnosis established both by angiologic and isotope procedures was upheld in 7. Angiography furnished false data in 4 patients, 2 of which were also misdiagnosed in isotope studies.

In one case exposure of the left kidney was required to rule out a tumor. Angiography in this case was suggestive of an adenoma. As suspicion of a tumor could not be dispelled on account of the reduced activity observable on the chlormerodrin scan, surgery was performed and revealed an extensive pyelonephritic scar (Fig. 2a, b, c).

In a female both topographic angiography and the scintigram failed to visualize the left kidney (Fig. 3a, b).

It took retrograde pyelography and pelvic angiography to obtain evidence of a tumor of a pelvic kidney, which was subsequently confirmed by surgery (Fig. 3c, d).

In another case an adrenal metastasis of a N. bronchi simulated a tumor of the left kidney in angiography. The tumor of the kidney was, however, ruled out by isotope studies (Fig. 4a, b, c).

Once angiography failed to visualize a walnut-sized cyst of the left kidney, which was clearly visible on differentiated isotope studies (^{197}Hg Chlormerodrin and ^{99m}Tc), (Fig. 5a–c).

Summary

The joint evaluation of angiograms, particularly those obtained in selective angiography, and the results of differentiated isotope studies further adds to the subtilety of renal diagnostics. Many a patient can thus be spared a surgical intervention. Patients whose angiographic and isotope data fail to be congruent should be given special attention. In these cases immediate surgery to rule out any tumor or a strict follow-up schedule are imperative.

Vergleichende szintigraphische und angiographische Untersuchungen der Nieren

H. Kempe, P. Pfannenstiel, G. Hoffmann und H. Weissleder

Die Lesbarkeit szintigraphischer Darstellungen von Organen und von Bereichen unterschiedlicher Aktivität innerhalb eines mit radioaktivem Nuclid angereicherten Organs ist im wesentlichen abhängig von der applizierten Dosis, vom Funktionszustand des Organs, von den verwendeten Collimatoren, der Abtastgeschwindigkeit und dem Untersuchungszeitpunkt.

Während das i.v. und retrograde Pyelogramm Veränderungen des Kelchsystems durch entzündliche oder raumfordernde Prozesse bzw. die Angiographie Gefäßanomalien erkennen lassen, ist der renale Scan von Destruktionen funktionstüchtigen Nierenparenchyms abhängig, das dann eine verminderte oder aufgehobene Anreicherung in dem betroffenen Bezirk erkennen läßt. Eine Art-Diagnose läßt das Nierenszintigramm nicht zu, lediglich mit weiteren klinischen und röntgenologischen Untersuchungen lassen sich bisweilen für eine bestimmte Erkrankung typische szintigraphische Veränderungen finden.

Bei unseren 100 vergleichenden Nierenszintigrammen, die mit einem Picker-Magna-Scanner durchgeführt wurden, und den röntgenologischen Untersuchungen, handelte es sich um Patienten, bei denen der Verdacht auf einen raumfordernden Prozeß im Bereich der Nieren bestand.

Der szintigraphische Befund wurde in nicht vorhandene, verminderte oder vermehrte Anreicherung der Aktivität auf einer Seite, inhomogene Anreicherung und in „kalte Zonen“ unterschieden. Dabei wurden in 70% der Fälle szintigraphisch Veränderungen bei pathologischen angiographischen Befunden gesehen. 18% der Szintigramme ließen keine Veränderungen erkennen, die angiographisch zu erheben waren. 12 Fälle stimmten bei beiden Untersuchungsmethoden als Normalbefunde überein.

Die Nierenszintigramme, die eine verminderte oder inhomogene Anreicherung oder verkleinerte Nieren zeigten, wiesen vorwiegend entzündliche oder vaskulär bedingte Erkrankungen auf, sie werden aber auch bei infiltrativ wachsenden Nierencarcinomen gesehen.

Bei 44 Patienten, die angiographisch Nierentumoren hatten, wobei es sich in 21 Fällen um Nierencysten und in 23 Fällen um Carcinome handelte, zeigte das Nierenszintigramm in 18 bzw. 22 Fällen pathologische Befunde.

Wie weit Parenchymdefekte erfaßt werden, hängt von der Größe und Tiefenlage ab, dabei können selbst größere Defekte durch Überstrahlung von darunter oder darüber gelegenem intakten Gewebe verborgen bleiben. Unsere Vergleichsuntersuchungen reichen noch nicht aus, um über fraktionierte Kamera-Szintigramme eine Aussage machen zu können.

Zusammenfassend können wir sagen, daß die Nierenszintigraphie röntgenologischen Untersuchungen, insbesondere der Angiographie nicht gleich kommt, daß aber das Szintigramm in Verbindung mit dem hier nicht aufgeführten nephrographischen Befund als positiver Screening-Test wichtige Hinweise liefert, die Anlaß zu weiteren diagnostischen Maßnahmen sein sollten.

Es scheint denkbar, daß Untersuchungen mit einer Anger-Kamera trotz des schlechteren Auflösungsvermögens durch die Möglichkeit unterschiedlicher Zeiten im Bild verfolgen zu können eine Verbesserung der Nierendiagnostik bringt, so daß im Vergleich zu röntgenologischen Untersuchungen die Aussagekraft noch zu erhöhen ist.

Comparison of the Diagnostic Value of Renal Scan and Angiography (together with I.V.P. and Isotope Nephrogram)

K. J. Pfeifer, K. W. Frey, H. G. Heinze, U. Klein, H. Müller-Fassbender and H. Langhammer

202 kidneys of 104 patients were compared. Diagnosis of renal diseases was based on the results of intravenous pyelography (I.V.P.), angiography and clinical investigation.

Of 141 pathological renal arteriographs 107 showed also abnormal scans, that is 74%, and 93 (68%) pathological isotope nephrograms (RIN).

In *renal vascular diseases* $^1/_3$ of the investigated cases, especially bilateral processes, yielded no abnormal scans. In contrast to this, cases of uni-lateral renal vascular diseases showed more often differences in activity of each side indicating pathological lesions.

In $^3/_4$ of the cases of *kidney tumors* and *solitary cystes* we found corresponding results. The scans were negativ for smaller space-occupying processes up to 3.5 cm in diameter, or also for larger tumors located either at the lower or upper pol of the kidney or primarily with extrarenal extension. Exact diagnosis is possible only by angiography.

In all cases of *progressive polycystic degeneration* we found abnormal scans. Renal scan is also of high diagnostic value in *congenital malformation* of the kidney such as horseshoe kidney, hypoplasia, aplasia and pelvic kidney.

Isotope nephrograms and I.V.P. proved to be most efficient methods in diagnosing initial stages of *hydronephrosis*, whereas the scans were less yielding. The scans are mor often abnormal as urinary stasis increases and thus they gain importance together with angiography in diagnosis of parenchym reduction. They are also very suitabel for follow-up studies.

Slight *unspecific kidney* inflammations revelaed in $^2/_3$ of our cases negativ results in conventional scintigraphy, whereby only 2 of 14 angiograms were also inconspicuous. Quite on the contrary, good corresponding results were achieved in all cases of inflammatory contracted kidneys.

Stage I of renal tuberculosis were not diagnosed by scans. In stage II $^1/_3$ of our cases yielded abnormal scans. In stage III the scans were all pathological. In all stages angiography was superior in exact localisation and diagnosis of the extent of the lesions.

Summarizing, the comparison demonstrated the following:

1. The scans are inconspicuous in cases of discrete lesions of renal vessels.

2. The diagnostic value of scintigraphy is larger for space-occupying and destructive processes than for diffuse vascular and inflamatory processes.

3. In contrast to angiography an exact diagnosis can not be achieved by scintigraphy, but it is an adequate and simple methode for follow-up studies.

4. The additional functional information of renal scan is of diagnostic and prognostic value, especially in hydronephrosis.

5. Conventional scintigraphy is thus primarily a screening test supplementary to I.V.P. in diagnosing uni-lateral and progressive kidney diseases. The capacity of angiography can not be achieved.

Results

N	Diagnosis	RIN		Scan			Angio	
		norm.	path.	norm.	susp.	path.	norm.	path.
25	vascular diseases	8	15	9	—	16	—	25
30	space-occupying processes	9	18	2	5	23	—	30
13	polycystic degenerations	7	5	—	—	13	—	13
7	congenital malformations	—	7	—	—	7	—	7
29	unspecific inflammations	9	20	11	—	18	2	27
13	hydronephrosis	1	12	4	—	9	2	11
28	tuberculosis	9	16	7	—	21	—	28
145	total	45	*93*	33	5	*107*	4	*141*

Selective Nephrophlebography

J. Anatkov and Chr. Kumanov

In recent years, the interest in the venous side of renal circulation increases, chiefly on account of the opportunity of obtaining morphologic information substantial to the diagnose. Difficulties in visualizing the venous renal system led to the development of various techniques and methods, some of them rather cumbersome for clinical use. In spite of certain sceptic judgements of the potentialities of nephrophlebography, its indications go on widening and comprise already a wide range of renal diseases and retroperitoneal processes.

In 25 patients, we made use of the technique of retrograde selective nephrophlebography by overcoming the venous blood outflow after Kahn as well as by the method of reducing the renal blood-flow previously by intra-arterial injection of adrenaline after Olin and Reuter. To prevent the direction of the contrast medium jet straight against the wall of the vein, we give the catheter tip a slight terminal reversed bend of about 10–15 degrees (Fig. 1).

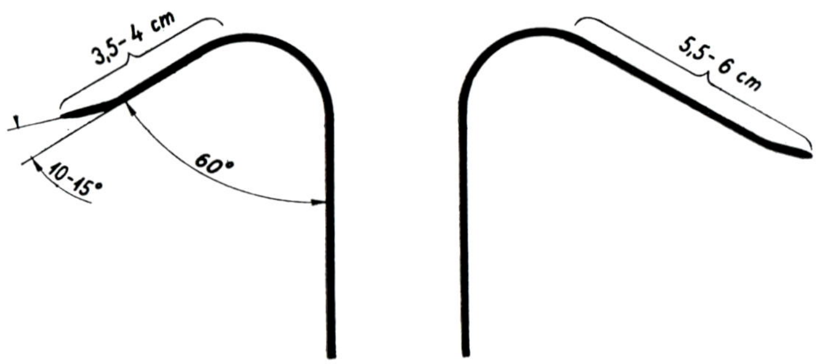

Fig. 1

The renal veins and their intrarenal tributaries are larger than the respective arteries; their walls are softer. That's why, in many a renal disease and retroperitoneal, process respectively, earlier and more strongly pronounced alterations are inflicted on renal veins rather than on renal arteries. In one female patients of ours, for instance, V.P.A., 42 years of age (case history no. 15236/24.9.1969), with myxoblastic retroperitoneal carcinoma (Fig. 2), selective nephrophlebography (Fig. 3) furnished a better visualization of the tumour infiltration into the renal pelvis and the parenchyma of the left kidney than selective arteriography did (Fig. 4).

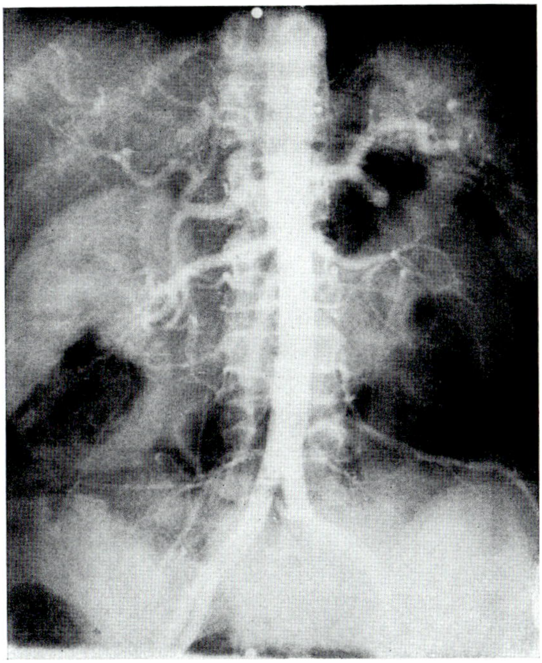

Fig. 2

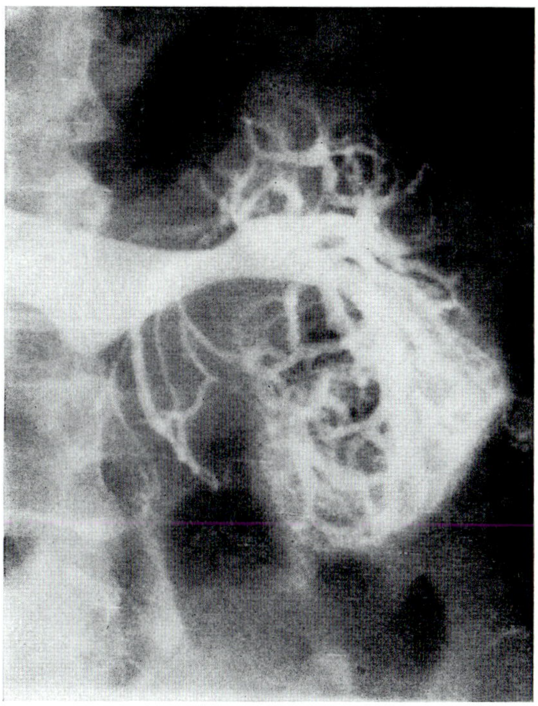

Fig. 3

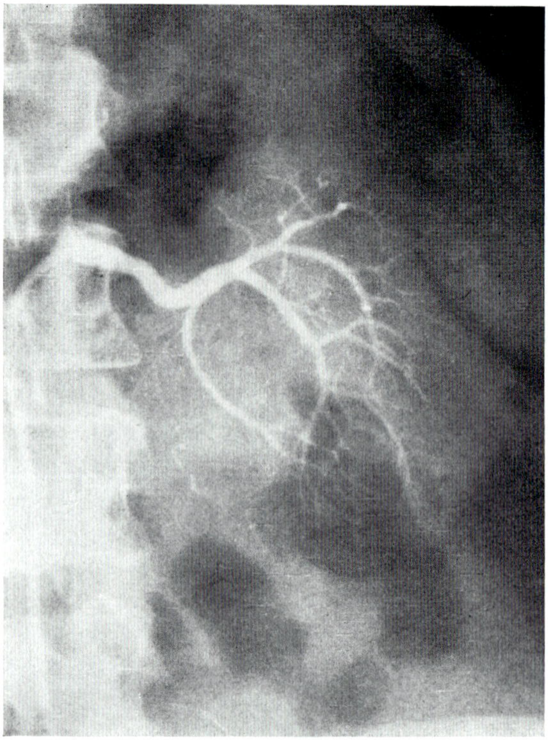

Fig. 4

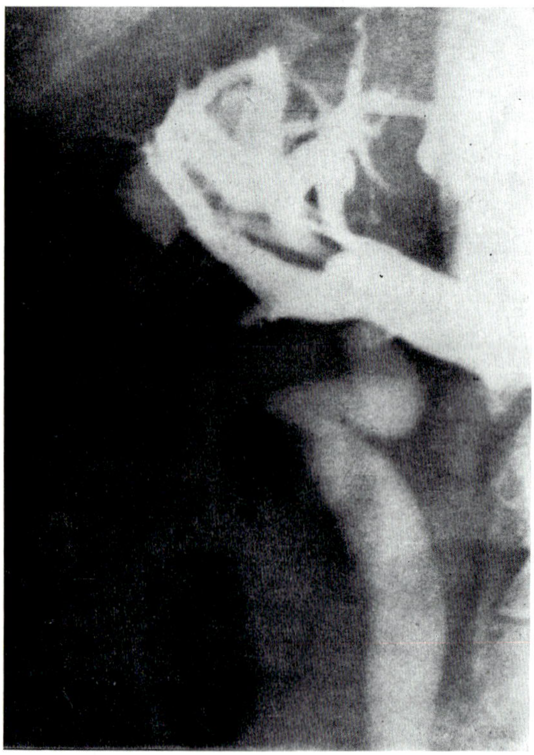

Fig. 5

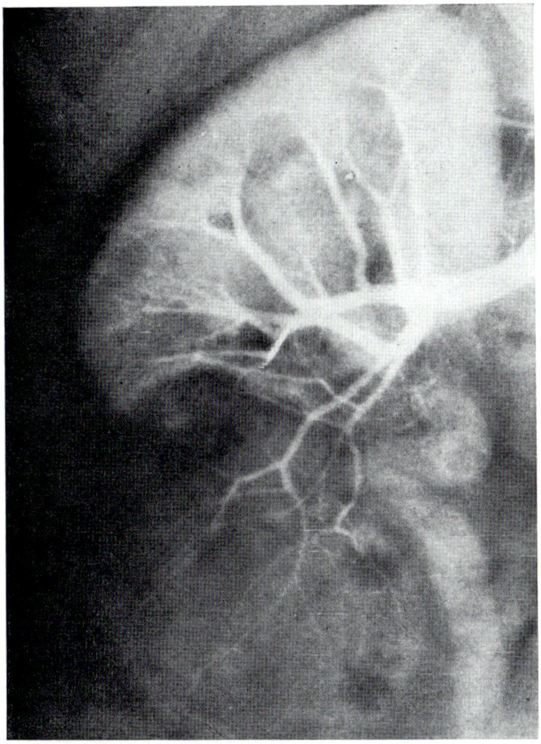

Fig. 6

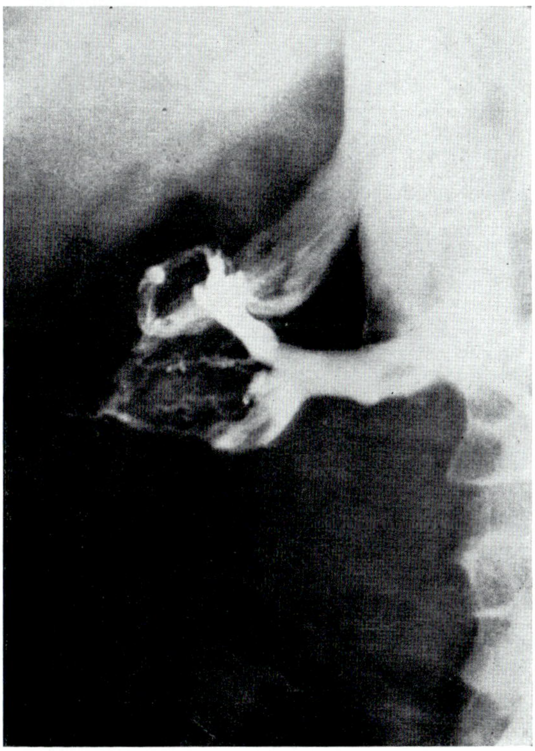

Fig. 7

In another female patient, E.D.M., 42 years of age (case history no. 16187/ 10.10.1969), superselective nephrophlebography (Fig. 5) revealed a clear-cut deformation and rarefaction of intra-renal veins in the upper half of the right kidney affected by productive tuberculosis, whereas selective arteriography (Fig. 6) established slithter alterations only. Thus, the uselessness of segment resection was demonstrated and nephrectomy indicated.

As a shortcoming of the method, we would like to point out the fact that sometimes no satisfactory retrograde filling of all intrarenal veins can be obtained. This occurs rather frequently in the right kidney (Fig. 7), whenever two renal veins exist. On account of the wide communications between both the venous areas, the contrast medium, when injected through one of the veins, flows out through the other rendering opaque only the segment veins and some of the interlobar ones to a satisfactory degree.

Moreover we can not help insisting on the necessity of a very cautious manoeuvring of the catheter, in order to avoid any injury or even perforation of the venous wall. The inappropriate orientation of the catheter tip straight against the renal vein wall may entail its perforation, either by the very contrast medium jet, or by back-blow of the catheter at the moment of injection. Such a case, the only rather serious incident we had (Fig. 8) occurred at an injecting rate of 21 ml/sec. Flooding of about 20 ml of Urografin 60% round the renal pelvis and the upper third of the

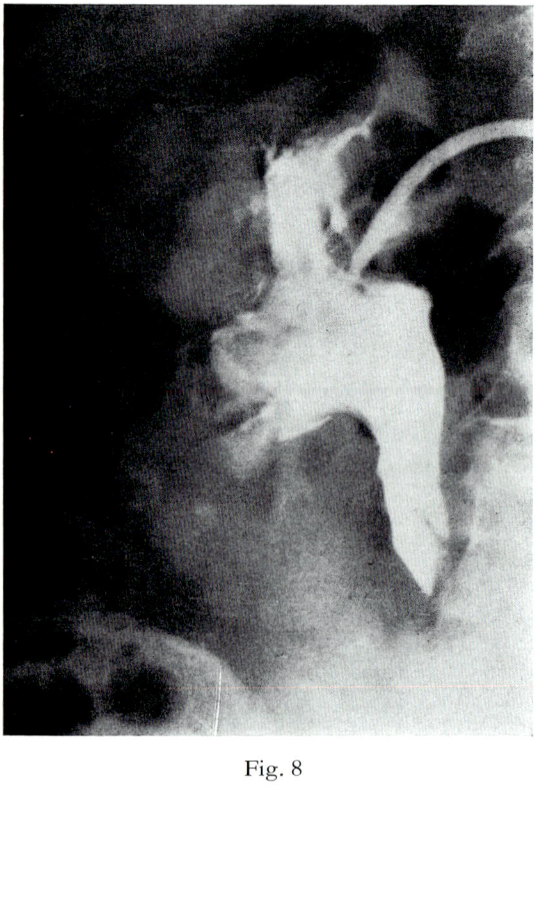

Fig. 8

right ureter called forth intense pains in the right renal area for about 10 min without entailing further complications, however.

Our own restricted experience shows that selective nephrophlebography is a valueable additional angiographic method which may be helpful in resolving certain diagnostical problems. For the result of such explorations, a good visualization of all intrarenal veins, cortical ones included, is a decisive criterion. With the techniques applied by us, it does not always work to an equally satisfactory degree and depends on factors varying individually, inappreciable beforehand. In this respect, occlusive techniques, as developped recently by TAKARO and his associates for clinical purposes, excel. It is likely, however, that they entail greater risks too.

Obviously, the technique of nephrophlebogtaphy needs further improvement, in order to obtain pictures of higher quality with reduced risks.

Further clinical and pathomorphologic studies are necessary to establish to what extent the alterations found are really sequelae of the morbid process and to what extent the significance of evaluation may be influenced by mere technical factors.

The more precise definition of "venous symptomatology" in various renal diseases will undoubtedly increase the potentialities of the angiographic differential diagnostics.

The Role of Angiography in the Detection of Polycystic Renal Disease and Associated Aneurysm of the Splenic Artery

D. CATALANO

The adult type of polycystic renal is a congenital hereditary disease in which both kidneys show advanced cystic pathology. In the majority of cases a radiological diagnosis can be made by urographic methods. Utilizing this technique one can demonstrate enlarged kidneys with the distortional changes in the pelvi-calyceal systems due cystic pressure effects. In some patients the characteristic urographic features are absent or equivocal. This is usually the case in the early stages when the cysts are small and renal enlargement is not particularly significant, or in the advanced stages when there are signs of renal insufficiency.

In these patients selective renal arteriography makes possible a very dependable method for the recognition of renal pathology not reliably possible by any other radiological method.

Since the development of polycystic renal disease may be asymmetrical, renal arteriography has its values in the radiological differentiation from the multicystic kidney disease.

Angiography is necessary in the demonstration of a possible concomitant carcinoma in the polycystic kidney; this has been reported in at least 17 instances (HOWARD and YOUNG).

The typical angiographic pattern of polycystic kidney has been reported by other Authors (BILLING, MEANEY, and CORVALAN; KLEMENCIC and KRAUS; ETTINGER, KAHN, and WISE, CORNELL etc.). During the arterial phase, the main stem of renal artery is reduced in size, while the intrarenal vessels are narrowed, elongated and displaced, producing a "dead tree" appearance. In the nephrographic phase there is a characteristic lack of homogeneity due to the presence of small, well-defined areas of cystic trabslucency ("swiss cheese appearance") (HALPERN, DARYMPLE, and YOUNG).

In patients with this pattern, it is necessary to extend the angiographic investigation to other major abdominal vessels, such as the celiac and superior mesenteric arteries, in order to demonstrate possible associated cystic disease of the liver and of the pancreas. This has been our experience in two patients in our service (we made intravenous urography, aortography and selective celiac arteriography in the arterial and venous phase).

Previously unreported finding shown in 70% of our patients has been the association of polycystic renal disease with splenic artery aneurysmal changes.

The radiological aspects of these aneuryms are not substantially at variance from those of splenic arterial changes due to other causes. In this instance there was no radiological evidence of splenic artery aneurysm on the scout film. The aneurysm may be single or multiple.

The association of polycystic renal disease with intracranial aneurysm has been reported on a number of occasions (Poutasse, Gardner, and McCormack), but the association with splenic artery aneurysm has not previously described. We have on record a 42 years old patient in whom a small aneurysm of anterior left cerebral artery and multiples plenic arterial aneurysmal changes, associated with polycystic kidney, was found.

In conclusion it may be said that the value of angiography in the establishment the diagnosis of polycystic kidney disease can not be overemphasized. At the same time it makes possible to investigate for the co-existence of cystic disease of liver and pancreas. The not infrequent association of intracranial or splenic artery aneurysm must be kept in mind during the investigation.

We stress that angiographic study of splenic artery or intracranial vessels is indicated in every case of polycystic kidney disease – conversely a renal study would be useful in all cases of splenic or intracranial aneurysms.